Mosby's
Critical Care Nursing Reference

Fourth Edition

Mosby's
Critical Care Nursing Reference

Fourth Edition

Susan B. Stillwell, MSN, RN, CNE
Clinical Associate Professor
Arizona State University
College of Nursing
Tempe, Arizona

Illustrated

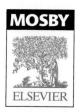

MOSBY

ELSEVIER

MOSBY
ELSEVIER
11830 Westline Industrial Drive
St. Louis, Missouri 63146

Mosby's Critical Care Nursing Reference   ISBN-13: 978-0-323-03214-8
                                                 ISBN-10: 0-323-03214-1

Notice

Knowledge and best practice in this field are constantly changing. As new research and experience broaden our knowledge, changes in practice, treatment and drug therapy may become necessary or appropriate. Readers are advised to check the most current information provided (i) on procedures featured or (ii) by the manufacturer of each product to be administered, to verify the recommended dose or formula, the method and duration of administration, and contraindications. It is the responsibility of the practitioner, relying on their own experience and knowledge of the patient, to make diagnoses, to determine dosages and the best treatment for each individual patient, and to take all appropriate safety precautions. To the fullest extent of the law, neither the Publisher nor the Author assumes any liability for any injury and/or damage to persons or property arising out of or related to any use of the material contained in this book.

The Publisher

ISBN-13: 978-0-323-03214-8
ISBN-10: 0-323-03214-1

Executive Publisher: Barbara Nelson Cullen
Senior Developmental Editor: Victoria Bruno
Editorial Assistant: Blair Biscardi
Publishing Services Manager: Deborah L. Vogel
Senior Project Manager: Ann E. Rogers
Book Design Manager: Paula Ruckenbrod

Printed in United States of America

Last digit is the print number: 9 8 7 6 5 4 3 2 1

Contributors

Cindy L. Boyer, PhD, RN
Teaching Specialist
University of Minnesota
Minneapolis, Minnesota
Principal Clinical Research Scientist
Guidant Corporation
St. Paul, Minnesota
Chapter 6, Monitoring the Critically Ill Patient

Claudia E. Campbell, BSN, ADN, RN
Manager, Anesthesia Pain Management Services
Intermountain Healthcare, LDS Hospital
Salt Lake City, Utah
Chapter 2, Acute Pain in the Critically Ill Patient

Margaret L. Campbell, PhD, RN, FAAN
Nurse Practitioner
Detroit Receiving Hospital
Detroit, Michigan
Chapter 8, Palliative Care in the Critical Care Unit

Kerry H. Cheever, PhD, RN
Associate Professor and Chairperson
Department of Nursing and Health
DeSales University
Center Valley, Pennsylvania
Chapter 5, The Critically Ill Patient
Chapter 7, Therapeutic Modalities

Ellen Dooling, MSN, RN, CNP
Certified Nurse Practitioner
The Cleveland Clinic Foundation
Cleveland, Ohio
Chapter 5, The Critically Ill Patient
Chapter 7, Therapeutic Modalities

Debra Hagler, PhD, APRN, BC, CCRN, CNE
Clinical Associate Professor
Arizona State University
Tempe, Arizona
Chapter 5, The Critically Ill Patient
Chapter 7, Therapeutic Modalities

Mary Hodges, MS, BSN, RN
Faculty Associate
Arizona State University
Tempe, Arizona
Chapter 7, Therapeutic Modalities

Jacqueline Keuth, MS, BSN, RN, CCNS, CCRN
Cardiothoracic Clinical Nurse Specialist
Banner Good Samaritan Medical Center
Phoenix, Arizona
Chapter 5, The Critically Ill Patient
Chapter 7, Therapeutic Modalities

Pamela J. Manning, BA
RN Lead Case Manager
University of Colorado Hospital
Denver, Colorado
Chapter 3, Concepts Common in the Care of the Critically Ill Patient

Claudia M. McCormick, MSN, BSN, RN
Duke Trauma Program Director
Duke University Hospital
Durham, North Carolina
Chapter 9, Nursing Care of the Child in the Adult Intensive Care Unit (ICU)

Doris Milton, PhD, RN
Director, Nursing Research and Education
Scottsdale Healthcare
Scottsdale, Arizona
Chapter 11, Complementary Therapies

Chris Pasero, RN-C, MS, FAAN
Pain Management Educator and Clinical Consultant
El Dorado Hills, California
Chapter 2, Acute Pain in the Critically Ill Patient

Deborah Pool, MS, RN, CCRN
Instructor, Department of Nursing
Glendale Community College
Glendale, Arizona
Chapter 5, The Critically Ill Patient
Chapter 7, Therapeutic Modalities

Sharon Roberts, PhD, RN, FAAN
California State University Long Beach
Long Beach, California
Chapter 4, Psychosocial Concerns of the Critically Ill Patient

Nicolle L. Schraeder, BSN, RN
Charge RN
University of Colorado Hospital
Denver, Colorado
Chapter 3, Concepts Common in the Care of the Critically Ill Patient

Susan B. Stillwell, MSN, RN, CNE
Clinical Associate Professor
Arizona State University
College of Nursing
Tempe, Arizona
Chapter 1, Critical Care Patient Assessment Guides
Chapter 3, Concepts Common in the Care of the Critically Ill Patient
Chapter 5, The Critically Ill Patient
Chapter 7, Therapeutic Modalities
Chapter 10, Pharmacology in the Critically Ill Patient

Chris Winkleman, PhD, RN, CNP, CCRN
Assistant Professor
Case Western Reserve University
Cleveland, Ohio
Chapter 5, The Critically Ill Patient
Chapter 7, Therapeutic Modalities

Reviewers

Jennifer Kane, RN, BSN
Massachusetts General Hospital
Boston, Massachusetts

Sharon M. Lee, RN, BS, CCRN
Kettering Medical Center
Miamisburg, Ohio

Tracy Pasek, RN, MSN, CCRN
Children's Hospital of Pittsburgh
Pittsburgh, Pennsylvania

Susan C. Vaughn, RN, BSN
Carolinas Medical Center-Mercy
Charlotte, North Carolina

Preface

The fourth edition of *Mosby's Critical Care Nursing Reference*
expands and updates the acute care management of the patient hospitalized in the adult critical care unit and has revised the separate
chapter on Nursing Care of the Child in the Adult Intensive Care
Unit (ICU). In addition, a new section on Case Management in the
Critical Care Unit is included in Chapter 3, Concepts Common in the
Care of the Critically Ill Patient. Also new to this edition is Chapter
8, Palliative Care in the Critical Care Unit. Appendixes have been
expanded to include the Confusion Assessment Method for the
Intensive Care Unit (CAM-ICU).

Mosby's Critical Care Nursing Reference remains a reference book
that provides easy access to information. Tools that have continued
to make this reference useful include organ donation guidelines, cardiopulmonary formulas, and drug dosage charts and conversion factors. This reference is not intended to be a critical care textbook or a
procedure manual and assumes that the clinician is familiar with critical care technology and the pathophysiology associated with life-
threatening illness.

Novice critical care nurses and student nurses, as well as seasoned
nurses who "float" to various critical care units, will find the fourth
edition of *Mosby's Critical Care Nursing Reference* a valuable
resource. I welcome your comments and suggestions on this edition.
Please contact me at sstillwell@asu.edu.

Susan B. Stillwell

Contents

1

Critical Care Patient Assessment Guides

CULTURAL ASSESSMENT

Although the critically ill patient may come to the critical care unit with physiologic needs that take priority for survival, consideration should be given to planning and implementing care that is culturally sensitive. The following guide can provide the nurse with an initial assessment of a patient's cultural influence on health and health practices. This guide is not intended to be a comprehensive cultural assessment tool. The information can be used to begin a plan of care that is sensitive to needs of patients and families from diverse cultural populations. The nurse can consider the questions in Box 1-1 to plan culturally competent care for the critically ill patient and family.

Box 1-1 Culture Assessment

How would you like us to address you?
Is there a key person who makes or shares in making health care decisions?
What do you want us to know about:
    Your traditions and beliefs about your health and health care practices?
    The cultural sanctions or restrictions you want to observe?
    Preferences or restrictions to touching, to making eye contact, or to other behaviors
        when communicating?
    Specific objects you would like to wear or have nearby?
    Any healing practices you would like to carry out?
    How you express pain or discomfort?
    How respect or disrespect is shown in your culture?

FAMILY ASSESSMENT

Understanding families of the critically ill patients and meeting their needs are essential to holistic care of the patient. Although family needs can change throughout the critical care experience, the nurse can consider the following assessment questions to understand the patient's illness, coping mechanisms, and support systems:

How many members are in your family?

Who is the decision maker in your family?

Who is the designated spokesperson in your family?

Have you ever had a family member hospitalized in a critical care unit?

What is your understanding of your relative's illness?

How have you coped with stressful situations?

Do you need any assistance with lodging or transportation or have any financial concerns?

See Interventions for Interrupted Family Processes, p. 45.

ANALYZING A SYMPTOM

A positive finding can be analyzed using the following guide. It is equally important to obtain pertinent negative information about the patient's health status.

Location: site, including any radiation of the symptom

Timing: onset, progression, and duration of the symptom

Setting: place the symptom began

Quality: characteristics or properties of the symptom

Quantity: degree of symptom—amount, extent, and size

Alleviating factors: factors that improve or relieve the symptom

Aggravating factors: factors that make the symptom worse

Associated factors: concomitant symptoms

SELF-REPORT SCALES

A visual analog scale and a modified Borg scale are self-report instruments that can be used to assess subjective sensations such as pain and dyspnea (Figure 1-1 and Box 1-2). However, 1-to-10 numerical scales (10 being the worst) may be more beneficial to use with individuals who have visual problems.

HEAD-TO-TOE SURVEY

When a critically ill patient is admitted to the unit, a routine assessment should be performed and repeated at least every 4 hours thereafter. A more frequent and more selective or detailed assessment may be necessary, depending on the patient's clinical disorder or a change

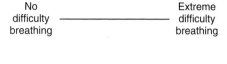

Figure 1-1 Sample visual analog scales. Patient places an X on the line to indicate the severity of the symptom.

in his or her condition, or both. Keep in mind the physiologic changes that normally occur with aging (Figure 1-2).

NEUROLOGIC ASSESSMENT

Level of Consciousness (LOC)

Note the patient's state of wakefulness and awareness. First, observe the patient for spontaneous activity; if none is noted, verbally stimulate the patient. If the patient is unresponsive to verbal stimuli, use noxious stimuli such as applying pressure to the nail bed, pinching the trapezius muscle, or pinching the inner aspect of the arm or

Box 1-2 **Modified Borg Scale**	
0	None/nothing at all
0.5	Very, very _____ (just noticeable)*
1	Very _____
2	_____
3	Moderate
4	Somewhat severe
5	Severe
6	_____
7	Very severe
8	_____
9	Very, very severe (almost maximal)
10	Maximal

Modified from Borg GAV: Psychophysical bases of perceived exertion, *Med Sci Sports Exerc* 14:377-381, 1982.
*Descriptors such as mild, weak, or slight can be inserted to assess symptoms such as pain, exertion, or breathlessness. Patients rate the symptom on a scale of 0 to 10 according to the descriptor that best indicates the severity of the symptom.

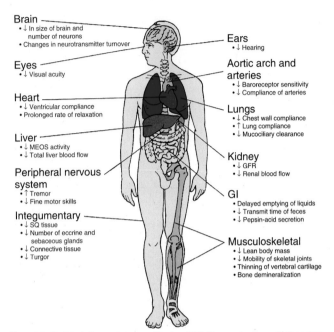

Figure 1-2 Physiologic changes that occur with aging. *MEOS,* Microsomal enzyme oxidative system. (From Urden LD, Stacy KM, Lough ME: *Thelan's critical care nursing: diagnosis and management,* ed 4, St Louis, 2002, Mosby.)

thigh. Avoid rubbing the sternum with knuckles, applying pressure to the supraorbital area, and pinching the nipples or testicles.

Stuporous: eye opening to painful stimuli; verbal responses are inappropriate

Semicomatose: nonpurposeful or reflexive movement of eyes to verbal or noxious stimuli; no response to verbal commands

Comatose: no response to stimuli

The Glasgow Coma Scale is a tool for assessing consciousness (Table 1-1). The best or highest response is recorded for the purpose of assessing the degree of altered consciousness. If a patient's abilities cannot be evaluated, a notation of the condition should be documented and the subscore should be labeled untestable.

Pupillary Reaction and Reflexes

Check position, size, shape, and response of the pupils. Photophobia may be associated with increased intracranial pressure or meningeal irritation. No direct pupillary response occurs in a blind eye;

Table 1-1 GLASGOW COMA SCALE

Ability	Response	Score*
Best eye response	Spontaneously (as nurse approaches)	4
	To verbal stimulus (nurse speaks/shouts)	3
	To painful stimulus (pressure on nail bed)	2
	No response to painful stimulus	1
Best motor response	Obeys simple command	6
	Localizes pain (locates and attempts to remove pain source)	5
	Withdrawal (attempts to withdraw from pain source)	4
	Abnormal flexion (Figure 1-3)	3
	Abnormal extension (see Figure 1-3)	2
	No response to painful stimulus	1
Best verbal response	Oriented to time, person, place	5
	Confused, but able to converse	4
	Inappropriate words—makes little or no sense; words are recognizable	3
	Incomprehensible sounds—groans or moans; words are not recognizable	2
	No verbal response	1

*Possible score ranges between 3 and 15 (15 = alert and oriented; <8 = coma).

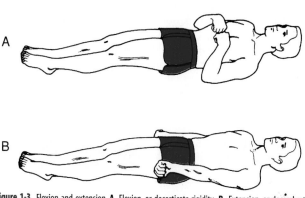

Figure 1-3 Flexion and extension. **A,** Flexion, or decorticate rigidity. **B,** Extension, or decerebrate rigidity. (From Sheehy SB: *Mosby's manual of emergency care*, ed 5, St Louis, 1999, Mosby.)

however, a consensual response can occur in the blind eye when the light is shined in the normal eye. Pinpoint pupils can result from miotic drugs, opiate drugs, or a pontine hemorrhage. Dilated pupils may result from use of cycloplegic drugs (atropine) or pressure on cranial nerve III (e.g., from a tumor or clot). Fixed pupils may be the result of barbiturate coma or hypothermia. Irregularly shaped pupils may occur as a result of cataract surgery.

Position: pupils should be midposition.

Size: note size in millimeters (Figure 1-4).

Shape: pupils are normally round.

Direct light reflex: the tested pupil should constrict briskly.

Consensual light reflex: nontested pupil constricts as light is shined in other eye.

Accommodation: pupils constrict and eyes converge as the patient focuses on an object moved toward the nose.

Corneal reflex: an absent reflex (lack of blinking or eyelid closure) indicates trigeminal or facial nerve damage, necessitating eye protection with artificial tears and eye shields.

Cranial Nerve Assessment

Cranial nerves V, IX, and X control protective reflexes (corneal, cough, gag, and swallow). Table 1-2 lists the cranial nerves and components to test.

Motor Function

Observe the patient's resting posture and note any spontaneous or involuntary movement; also note any rigidity, spasticity, and flaccidity. Test gross muscle strength by assessing hand grasp and testing dorsiflexion and plantar flexion of the lower extremities. Compare both sides of the body. Observe for arm drift by having patient hold both arms (palms up) out while the eyes are closed. Pronator drift is present if one arm drifts with palm turning down.

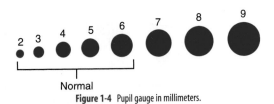

Figure 1-4 Pupil gauge in millimeters.

Table 1-2 Cranial Nerves

Nerve	Evaluate
Olfactory (I)	Sense of smell
Optic (II)	Vision: visual fields and acuity
Oculomotor (III), trochlear (IV), and abducens (VI)	Pupil reactions, extraocular movements: III—evaluate eye movement up and outward, down and outward, and up and inward; IV—evaluate eye movement down and inward; VI—evaluate eye movement outward
Trigeminal (V)	Sensation on both sides of face, opening and closing of jaw, corneal reflex
Facial (VII)	Facial muscle movement: eyebrows, smile, frown, eyelid closing; taste sensation
Acoustic (VIII)	Hearing
Glossopharyngeal (IX), vagus (X)	Gag reflex, swallowing, soft palate elevation
Spinal accessory (XI)	Shoulder shrug and head movement
Hypoglossal (XII)	Tongue position, movement, and strength

Sensory Function

A gross evaluation of sensory function includes light touch to the forehead, cheeks, hands, lower arms, abdomen, lower legs, and feet. Other types of sensations can be used (e.g., pain, heat and cold, vibration, position changes, and deep pressure pain). Use a dermatome chart to determine level at which the change in sensation has occurred. Compare both sides of the body.

Spinal Cord Assessment

The motor strength of each muscle group should be evaluated in patients with spinal cord dysfunction (Table 1-3). A 5-point system can be used to assess overall muscle strength of the extremities (Table 1-4). A less complex system such as 0 = absent, 1 = weak, and 2 = strong may be used.

Specific dermatomal areas (Figure 1-5) should be evaluated in the patient with a spinal cord dysfunction. Terms used to describe sensory dysfunction can be found below.

Analgesia: loss of pain
Anesthesia: complete loss of sensation
Dysesthesia: impaired sensation

Hyperesthesia: increased sensation
Hypesthesia: decreased sensation
Paresthesia: burning, tingling sensation

Peripheral Neurovascular Assessment

Peripheral nerves and circulation should be evaluated in patients with injury (e.g., fractures, burns) to upper or lower extremities.

Table 1-3 SPINAL CORD ASSESSMENT

Level of Innervation	Function	Reflex
C4	Neck movement, diaphragmatic breathing	
C5	Abduction of the shoulder	Biceps (C5)
C5-6	Elbow flexion	Brachioradialis (C6)
C7-8	Elbow extension	Triceps (C7)
C6-8	Wrist dorsiflexion	
C8	Hand grip	
C6-8, T1	Finger extension and flexion	
L2-4	Hip flexion	
L4-5, S1	Hip extension	
L2-4	Knee extension	
L4-5, S1	Knee flexion	Patellar (L4)
L5	Dorsiflexion of the foot	
S1	Plantar flexion of the foot	

Table 1-4 MUSCLE STRENGTH SCALE

Description	Score
Normal power or muscle strength in extremities	5
Weak extremities, but patient can overcome resistance applied by examiner	4
Patient can overcome gravity (can lift extremities) but cannot overcome resistance applied by examiner	3
Weak muscle contraction, but not enough to overcome gravity (movement, but cannot lift extremities)	2
Palpable or visible muscle flicker or twitch, but no movement	1
No response to stimulus, complete paralysis	0

Both sensory and motor function of the ulnar, radial, median, and peroneal nerves should be assessed.

5 Ps: pain, paresthesia, paralysis, pulse, and pallor.

Circulation: check presence and amplitude of pulses, capillary refill, and skin temperature.

Movement: upper extremities—have patient hyperextend the thumb or wrist (radial), oppose the thumb and little finger (median), and abduct all fingers (ulnar). Lower extremities: have patient dorsiflex the foot (peroneal) and plantarflex the foot (tibial).

Sensation: upper extremities—use a pin to prick the webbed space between the thumb and index finger (radial), distal fat pad of

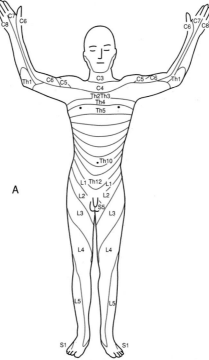

A

Figure 1-5 A, Dermatomes from anterior view. Landmarks are clavicle—C4; deltoid—C5; nipples—T4; navel—T10; knee—L3-4; great toe—L5; little toe—S1; sole of foot—L5-S1.

Continued

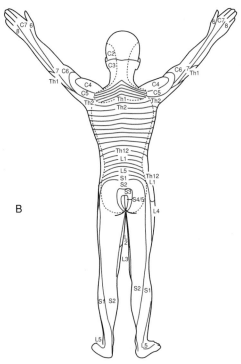

Figure 1-5, cont'd B, Dermatomes from posterior view. Landmarks are clavicle—C4; deltoid—C5; knee—L3-4; great toe—L5; little toe—S1; sole of foot—L5-S1.

small finger (ulnar), and distal fat pad of index and middle finger (median). Lower extremities: use a pin to prick the dorsal surface of the foot near the webbed space between the great and second toes.

Reflexes

Abnormal reflexes may be early signs of upper motor neuron disease, lower motor neuron disease, or disease of the afferent sensory component of muscles.

Deep tendon reflexes: jaw, biceps, brachioradialis, triceps, patellar, and Achilles reflexes can be assessed on a scale from 0 to 4+ (Table 1-5).

Pathologic reflexes: positive Babinski sign—great toe pointing upward (extension) and fanning of the other toes. Grasp reflex—patient

Table 1-5 SCALE FOR DEEP TENDON REFLEXES

Score	Description
0	Absent
1+	Diminished
2+	Normal
3+	Increased, more brisk than average
4+	Hyperactive, clonus

does not release an object that has been placed in the patient's hand. Snout reflex—pursing of lips when the mouth is tapped above or below the midline.

Brainstem Function

An alteration in brainstem function can affect the state of consciousness; respiratory, circulatory, and vasomotor activities; and a number of reflexes.

DERM mnemonic: the mnemonic device DERM can be used to assess brainstem functioning; D = depth of coma; E = eye assessment; R = respiration assessment; M = motor function (Table 1-6).

Oculocephalic reflex—doll's-eye maneuver: tested in the comatose patient to assess brainstem function. Presence of doll's eyes (both eyes move in the direction opposite to the head rotation) is normal and indicates an intact brainstem. If this response is absent, the patient's airway may not be protected by gag and cough reflexes.

Oculovestibular reflex—caloric testing: usually tested in the comatose patient to assess brainstem function. With an intact brainstem, eyes deviate, with nystagmus toward the ear that is irrigated with cold water. An absent reflex (both eyes remain fixed in midline position) may indicate impending brain death. Neuromuscular blocking agents, barbiturates, and antibiotic agents can inhibit this reflex.

Determining Brain Death

Reversible conditions such as sedation, neuromuscular blockade, shock, hypothermia, and metabolic imbalances must be excluded. The clinical examination is most important; however, transcranial Doppler and somatosensory-evoked potentials and electroencephalogram tests may be used in conjunction with the clinical examination to confirm brain death. Cerebral blood flow studies are

Table 1-6 Assessing Brainstem Function Using the DERM Mnemonic

Brainstem	Herniation Levels	D = Depth of Coma	E = Eyes	R = Respirations	M = Motor Function	Posturing
	None	Aware, alert, oriented	Equal and reactive	Eupnea	Normal	None
	Thalamus	Painful stimulus causes nonpurposeful response	Small; react to light	Cheyne-Stokes respirations	Hyperactive deep tendon reflexes	Abnormal flexion (decorticate)
	Midbrain	Painful stimulus causes nonpurposeful response	Midpoint to dilated; fixed; no reaction to light	Central neurogenic breathing	Decreased deep tendon reflexes	Abnormal extension (decerebrate)
	Pons and cerebellum	Painful stimulus causes no response	Pinpoint; fixed; no reaction to light	Biot's respirations	Flaccid	No tone
	Medulla	Painful stimulus causes no response	Midpoint to dilated; fixed; no reaction to light	Ataxia; apneusis	Flaccid	No tone

From Budassi SA, Barber J: *Mosby's manual of emergency care,* ed 3, St Louis, 1989, Mosby.

confirmatory tests. The absence of cerebral circulation is diagnostic of brain death regardless of cause.

Clinical examination: The following findings must be present:

Patient must be comatose.

Pupils must be nonreactive.

Corneal reflex must be absent.

Gag reflex must be absent.

Cough reflex must be absent.

Oculocephalic reflex must be absent.

Oculovestibular reflex must be absent.

Spontaneous respirations must be absent. (See "Apnea Testing," following.)

After atropine administration, heart rate should not increase.

Apnea testing: To test for the presence of apnea, 100% oxygen is administered to the patient to a PaO_2 exceeding 200 mm Hg. The patient continues to receive passive flow of 100% oxygen, and the ventilator is disconnected. Spontaneous breathing must be absent during this time. Lack of spontaneous respirations in the presence of adequate carbon dioxide stimulus ($PaCO_2$ >60 mm Hg or >20 mm Hg from baseline and respiratory acidosis) indicates that the brainstem is not functioning. The test should be stopped if cardiac arrhythmias, hypotension, or arterial desaturation ensues, and a confirmatory test should be performed.

Incisions, Drainage, and Equipment

Assess the condition of incisional sites, including ventriculostomy site, from neurosurgical surgeries and procedures. Assess for cerebral spinal fluid leaks (e.g., rhinorrhea or otorrhea) by testing suspicious clear drainage for glucose or observing the presence of a "halo" or "ring" sign on a dressing or on bedclothes from a serosanguineous blood stain. Assess equipment and devices for proper functioning.

Intracranial Monitoring

Obtain intracranial pressure (ICP) and calculate cerebral perfusion pressure (CPP). (See ICP monitoring on p. 462 and formula on p. 786.)

PULMONARY ASSESSMENT

Respirations

Determine respiratory rate and rhythm (Figure 1-6). Assess the chest for depth of respirations, paradoxic movement, and symmetry of

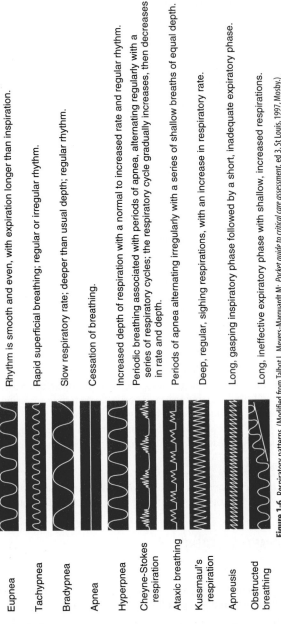

Eupnea	Rhythm is smooth and even, with expiration longer than inspiration.
Tachypnea	Rapid superficial breathing; regular or irregular rhythm.
Bradypnea	Slow respiratory rate; deeper than usual depth; regular rhythm.
Apnea	Cessation of breathing.
Hyperpnea	Increased depth of respiration with a normal to increased rate and regular rhythm.
Cheyne-Stokes respiration	Periodic breathing associated with periods of apnea, alternating regularly with a series of respiratory cycles; the respiratory cycle gradually increases, then decreases in rate and depth.
Ataxic breathing	Periods of apnea alternating irregularly with a series of shallow breaths of equal depth.
Kussmaul's respiration	Deep, regular, sighing respirations, with an increase in respiratory rate.
Apneusis	Long, gasping inspiratory phase followed by a short, inadequate expiratory phase.
Obstructed breathing	Long, ineffective expiratory phase with shallow, increased respirations.

Figure 1-6 Respiratory patterns. (Modified from Talbot L, Meyers-Marquardt M: *Pocket guide to critical care assessment*, ed 3, St Louis, 1997, Mosby.)

respirations. Note any tracheal deviation and any chest deformities that may interfere with respirations. Note use of accessory muscles, retractions, nasal flaring, and cough. Note sputum—purulent (pus), fetid (foul smelling), hemoptysis (blood, blood streaked), or mucoid (clear and thick). Palpate the chest for crepitus or pain. Tactile fremitus is increased with lung consolidation and decreased when the bronchus is obstructed or in the presence of pleural effusion or pneumothorax. Check for tracheal alignment by palpating the trachea at the suprasternal notch. The trachea should be midline in the suprasternal notch.

Breath Sounds

Auscultate all lung fields. (Figures 1-7 and 1-8 illustrate the location of lobes and normal breath sounds.)

Bronchial sounds: high-pitched and normally heard over the trachea. Timing includes an inspiration phase less than the expiration phase. If heard in lung fields, this usually indicates consolidation

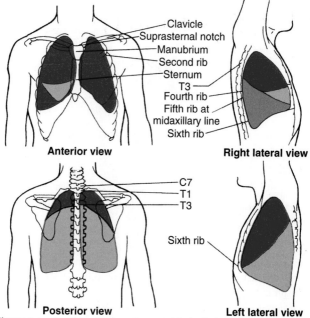

Figure 1-7 Location of lobes of the lung using anatomic landmarks. (From Talbot L, Meyers-Marquardt M: *Pocket guide to critical care assessment*, ed 3, St Louis, 1997, Mosby.)

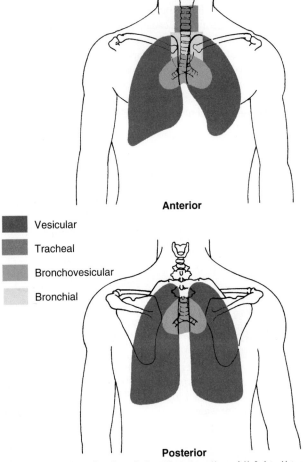

Figure 1-8 Location of normal breath sounds. (From Talbot L, Meyers-Marquardt M: *Pocket guide to critical care assessment*, ed 3, St Louis, 1997, Mosby.)

Vesicular sounds: low pitched and normally heard in the periphery of the lungs. Timing includes an inspiration phase greater than the expiration phase

Bronchovesicular sounds: medium pitched, with a muffled quality. Timing includes an inspiration phase equal to the expiration phase

Adventitious Sounds

Assess breath and voice sounds.

Crackles: discontinuous sounds heard during inspiration that can be classified as fine (similar to rubbing strands of hair together next to the ear) or coarse (bubbling quality similar to carbonated soda). Crackles associated with fluid in the airways often clear when patient coughs.

Rhonchi: low-pitched continuous sounds represent air flow through narrowed airways.

Wheezes: high- or low-pitched continuous sounds that may be heard during inspiration or expiration.

Pleural friction rub: grating, harsh sound, located in an area of intense chest wall pain.

Bronchophony: spoken words (have patient say "ninety-nine") that are heard clearly and distinctly upon auscultation are indicative of lung consolidation.

Whispered pectoriloquy: extreme bronchophony, such that a voice sound (have patient whisper "ninety-nine") is heard clearly and distinctly through the stethoscope upon auscultating the lungs.

Egophony: upon auscultation, the spoken word assumes a nasal quality (have patient say "E"; it is heard as "A" through the stethoscope) indicative of consolidation or pleural effusion.

Artificial Airway

Check placement and patency of an artificial airway (e.g., oral or nasal airway, endotracheal tube, tracheostomy). Determine cuff pressure of endotracheal tube or tracheostomy.

Oxygenation/Ventilation

Check the oxygen delivery system, ventilator settings, and alarms. Obtain oxygen saturation and carbon dioxide readings.

Chest Drainage

Assess the system for proper functioning and note the amount, color, and character of chest drainage.

Oxygenation Calculations

Monitor relevant parameters. (See Cardiopulmonary Parameters, p. 779.)

Chest Radiograph

A chest radiograph is used to provide information about gross anatomic proportions and the location of cardiac structures, including the great vessels; to evaluate lung fields; and to confirm placement of airways, central venous catheters, pulmonary artery catheters, chest tubes, and transvenous pacemaker leads. The least dense (air-filled) structures (e.g., lungs) absorb fewer x-rays and appear black on the radiographic film. Structures that are as dense as water (e.g., heart and blood vessels) appear gray. Bone and contrast materials are most dense and appear white on the radiograph. Figure 1-9 depicts a normal chest radiograph, with underlying structures outlined; Figures 1-10, 1-11, and 1-12 identify conditions commonly evaluated in intensive care unit (ICU) patients. Normal findings are identified in Table 1-7. Serial assessments of endotracheal tube, central lines, and chest tube placement should be done. An endotracheal tube should be 2 to 3 cm above the carina. Table 1-8 lists abnormal radiographic findings common to ICU patients.

CARDIOVASCULAR ASSESSMENT

Heart Rate and Rhythm

Note monitor lead placement and obtain a rhythm strip to determine rate and rhythm. (See Rhythm Strip Analysis, p. 441.)

Integument

Note color, temperature, and moisture. Check the anterior chest wall for capillary refill (>3 seconds reflects poor tissue perfusion). Evaluate the severity of edema (Table 1-9) by applying pressure for 10 seconds and noting the depth of the finger imprint. Approximately 5 L of fluid accumulation is required for the appearance of peripheral edema.

Central Venous Pressure (CVP)

Check neck veins to estimate CVP (Figure 1-13). Note presence of Kussmaul's sign (a pathologic increase in jugular venous pressure on inspiration). If right ventricular failure is suspected, the hepatojugular reflex (HJR) is tested by applying firm pressure with the palm of the hand to the upper quadrant of the patient's abdomen for 30 to 60 seconds. An increase in venous level >3 cm during the application of pressure is a positive HJR.

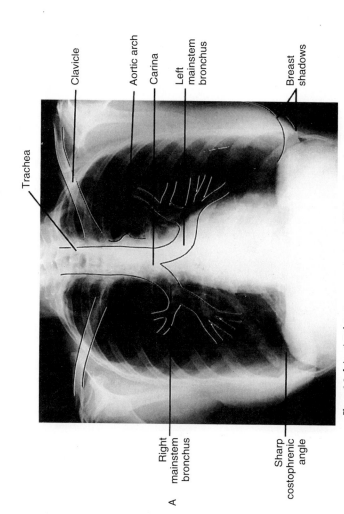

Trachea

Clavicle

Aortic arch

Carina

Left mainstem bronchus

Breast shadows

Right mainstem bronchus

Sharp costophrenic angle

A

Figure 1-9 A, Location of structures on a posteroanterior (PA) chest radiograph.

Continued

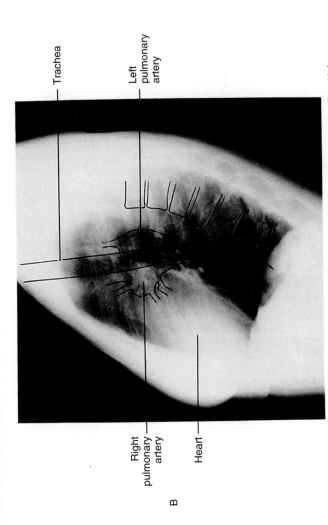

Figure 1-9, cont'd B, Location of structures on a lateral view chest radiograph. (From Talbot L, Meyers-Marquardt M: *Pocket guide to critical care assessment,* ed 3, St Louis, 1997, Mosby.)

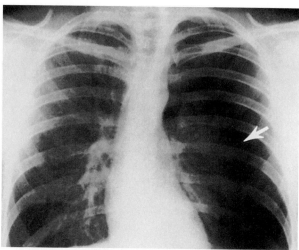

Figure 1-10 Radiograph of a spontaneous pneumothorax. (From Sahn SA: Pneumothorax and pneumomediastinum. In Mitchell RS, Petty TL, Schwarz MI, eds: *Synopsis of clinical pulmonary disease,* ed 4, St Louis, 1989, Mosby.)

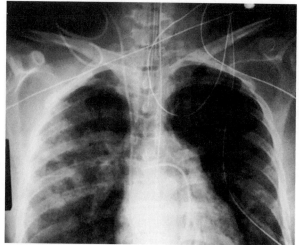

Figure 1-11 Radiograph of patient admitted with acute respiratory distress syndrome. (From Petty TL: Adult respiratory distress syndrome. In Mitchell RS, Petty TL, Schwarz MI, eds: *Synopsis of clinical pulmonary disease,* ed 4, St Louis, 1989, Mosby.)

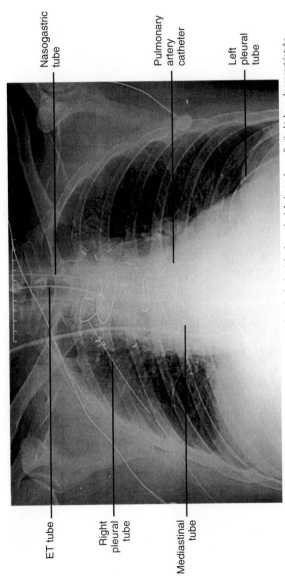

Nasogastric tube

Pulmonary artery catheter

Left pleural tube

ET tube

Right pleural tube

Mediastinal tube

Figure 1-12 Chest radiograph with pulmonary artery catheter, endotracheal tube, right chest tube, left chest tube, mediastinal tube, and nasogastric tube.

Table 1-7 NORMAL FINDINGS ON CHEST RADIOGRAPH

Assessed Area	Usual Adult Findings
Trachea	Midline, translucent, tubelike structure found in the anterior mediastinal cavity
Clavicles	Equally distant from the sternum
Ribs	Thoracic cavity encasement
Mediastinum	Shadowy-appearing space between the lungs that widens at the hilum
Heart	Solid-appearing structure with clear edges visible in the left anterior mediastinal cavity; cardiothoracic ratio should be less than half the width of the chest wall on a posteroanterior film
Carina	Lowest tracheal cartilage at the bifurcation
Mainstem bronchus	Translucent, tubelike structure visible approximately 2.5 cm from the hilum
Hilum	Small, white, bilateral densities present where the bronchi join the lungs; left should be 2 to 3 cm higher than the right
Bronchi	Not usually visible
Lung fields	Usually not completely visible except for "lung markings" at periphery
Diaphragm	Rounded structures visible at the bottom of the lung fields; right side is 1 to 2 cm higher than the left; costophrenic angles should be clear and sharp

Modified from Talbot L, Meyers-Marquardt M: *Pocket guide to critical care assessment*, ed 3, St Louis, 1997, Mosby.

Table 1-8 ABNORMAL RADIOGRAPHIC FINDINGS

Finding	Possible Diagnosis
Nondistinct or widened aortic knob	Aortic dissection
Silhouette sign (loss of border visibility)	Infiltrates or consolidation of RML or lingula
Enlarged cardiac silhouette	HF, pericardial effusion, pulmonary edema
Blackened area without tissue markings	Pneumothorax
Patchy infiltrates or streaky densities	Pneumonia, atelectasis
Fluffy infiltrates (Kerley B lines)	Pulmonary edema
Loss of costophrenic angle sharpness	Pleural effusion

HF, Heart failure; *RML,* right middle lobe.

Table 1-9 GRADING SCALE FOR EDEMA

Depth of Pitting Edema	Score
<¼ inch	+1
¼ to ½ inch	+2
½ to 1 inch	+3
>1 inch	+4

Pulses

Check pulses simultaneously bilaterally except for carotids. Note rate, rhythm, equality, and amplitude. Figure 1-14 shows variations in arterial pulses. The following scale can be used to describe pulses: 0 = absent, +1 = weak, +2 = normal, +3 = bounding.

Heart Sounds

Systematically auscultate each area of the precordium (Figure 1-15), concentrating on one component of the cardiac cycle at a time. The bell of the stethoscope accentuates lower-frequency sounds (e.g., S_3, S_4). The diaphragm of the stethoscope accentuates high-pitched sounds (e.g., S_1, S_2). Figure 1-16 illustrates heart sounds in relation to electrocardiogram (ECG). Table 1-10 lists the various heart sounds and differentiating components.

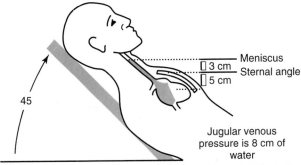

Figure 1-13 Estimation of central venous pressure. Identify the highest level of pulsations in the internal jugular vein (meniscus). Determine the vertical distance between the sternal angle and meniscus. Add that distance to the constant 5 cm (sternal angle is 5 cm above mid-right atrial level). Normal is 5 to 12 cm H_2O.

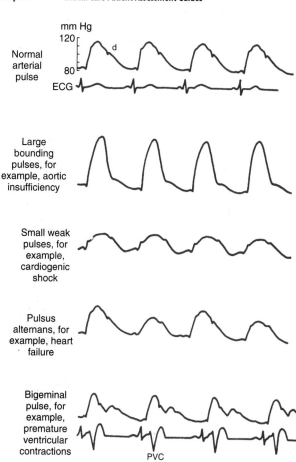

Normal arterial pulse

Large bounding pulses, for example, aortic insufficiency

Small weak pulses, for example, cardiogenic shock

Pulsus alternans, for example, heart failure

Bigeminal pulse, for example, premature ventricular contractions

Pulsus paradoxus, for example, pericardial effusion, cardiac tamponade

Figure 1-14 Variations in arterial pulse. (From Kinney MR et al: *Comprehensive cardiac care*, ed 8, St Louis, 1995, Mosby.)

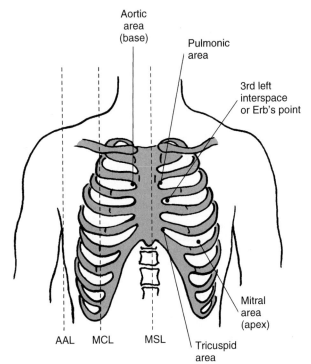

Figure 1-15 Cardiac auscultatory sites. S_1 is heard loudest at mitral and tricuspid areas. S_2 is heard loudest at aortic and pulmonic areas. S_3 and S_4 are heard best at the mitral area. *AAL,* Anterior axillary line; *MCL,* midclavicular line; *MSL,* midsternal line.

Heart Murmurs

Describe murmurs according to location (e.g., distance from midsternal, midclavicular, or axillary lines); radiation—where the sound is transmitted; loudness—grades I to VI (Table 1-11); pitch—high or low; shape—crescendo, decrescendo, crescendo-decrescendo, plateau; and quality—harsh, rumbling, musical, blowing.

Blood Pressure (BP)

Use a BP cuff (length of cuff bladder) 20% wider than the diameter of the limb to avoid false high or low pressures. Assess BP on both arms. A pressure difference of <10 mm Hg is not significant unless the radial pulses are not of equal intensity or quality. If there is a

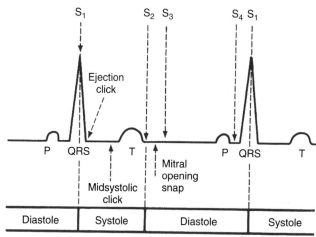

Figure 1-16 Heart sounds in relation to the ECG.

pressure difference, use the arm with the higher BP. Suspect subclavian artery stenosis when there is a 20 mm Hg or greater difference in systolic values and a palpable difference in radial artery pulses.

Ankle brachial index (ABI) is the ratio of dorsalis pedis systolic blood pressure (SBP) to brachial SBP. ABI identifies obstruction

Table 1-10 DIFFERENTIATING HEART SOUNDS

Heart Sound	Best Area to Auscultate	Timing
S_1	Apex	Systole
S_2	Base	Diastole
S_3	Apex, LSB	Early diastole, after S_2
S_4	Apex, LSB	Late diastole, before S_1
Split S_1	4ICS, LSB	Systole
Split S_2	2ICS, LSB	End of systole
Aortic ejection sound	2ICS, RSB; apex	Early systole
Pulmonic ejection sound	2ICS, LSB	Early systole
Midsystolic click	Apex	Mid to late systole
Opening snap	Lower LSB, 4ICS	Early diastole
Pericardial friction rub	Loudest among LSB	Systole and diastole

ICS, Intercostal space; *LSB,* left sternal border; *RSB,* right sternal border.

Table 1-11 MURMUR GRADING SCALE

Grade	Description
I/VI	Faint, barely audible
II/VI	Quiet, heard immediately on auscultation
III/VI	Moderately loud, no thrill
IV/VI	Loud, thrill
V/VI	Very loud, requires a stethoscope; thrill present
VI/VI	Same as V/VI, but can be heard with stethoscope off the chest

between proximal aorta and the large vessels and lower extremities. ABI <0.5 may occur with atherosclerosis of the aorta or femoral or popliteal vessels; coarctation of the aorta; or the presence of a dissecting aneurysm.

Auscultatory Gap

Determine the presence of an auscultatory gap (Figure 1-17), a common finding in patients with hypertension or aortic stenosis.

Pulsus Paradoxus

Determine the presence of pulsus paradoxus. Slowly deflate the BP cuff (1 mm Hg per respiratory cycle) and note when the first sound is heard. Sounds heard intermittently correspond with expiration. Note when sounds begin again and are heard continuously (during inspiration and expiration). If the difference between the first sound and the continuous sound is >10 mm Hg, pulsus paradoxus is present. Pulsus paradoxus may be present in pericardial effusion, cardiac tamponade, pulmonary embolus, and severe obstructive airway disease.

Hemodynamic Monitoring

Obtain readings and calculate cardiopulmonary parameters. (See Hemodynamic Monitoring on pp. 426, 435, and 471, and Cardiopulmonary Formulas on p. 779.)

Pacemaker

Validate settings. Assess for failure to capture and failure to sense. Assess what percentage of the patient's rhythm is paced.

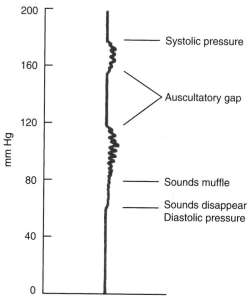

Figure 1-17 Auscultatory gap. Systolic sounds are first heard at 180 mm Hg. They disappear at 160 mm Hg and reappear at 120 mm Hg; the silent interval is known as the *auscultatory gap*. Korotkoff sounds muffle at 80 mm Hg and disappear at 60 mm Hg. Blood pressure is recorded at 180/80/60 with auscultatory gap. If the cuff was inflated to 150 mm Hg, the reading may have been interpreted as normotensive. (From Kinney MR et al: *Comprehensive cardiac care,* ed 8, St Louis, 1995, Mosby.)

GASTROINTESTINAL ASSESSMENT

Bowel Sounds

Auscultate all quadrants (Figure 1-18). Bowel sounds normally are 5 to 35 per minute.

Absent sounds may be associated with intestinal obstruction, paralytic ileus, or peritonitis. Listen for at least 2 to 5 minutes in each quadrant. Temporarily turn off any nasogastric (NG) suction if not contraindicated.

Intensified or gurgling sounds may be associated with early intestinal obstruction, increased peristalsis, or diarrhea.

Abdomen

Note size, shape, and symmetry. Measure abdominal girth at the level of the umbilicus. Palpate for tenderness or masses.

Right upper quadrant

Right lobe of liver
Gallbladder
Pylorus
Duodenum
Head of pancreas
Upper right kidney

Right lower quadrant

Lower right kidney
Cecum
Appendix
Ascending colon
Right fallopian tube (female)
Right ovary (female)
Right ureter
Bladder (distended)

Left upper quadrant

Left lobe of liver
Spleen
Stomach
Left kidney
Body of pancreas
Splenic flexure of colon

Left lower quadrant

Descending colon
Sigmoid colon
Left fallopian tube (female)
Left ovary (female)
Left ureter
Bladder (distended)

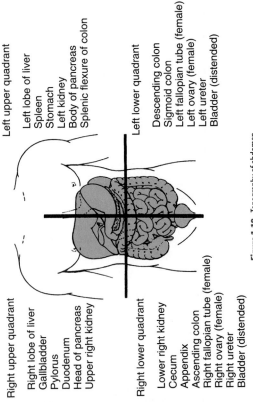

Figure 1-18 Topography of abdomen.

Bowel Elimination

Note characteristics of stool.

Nasogastric Tube

Check placement, patency, drainage, and amount of suction. Check the pH of gastric secretions and test secretions for occult blood. If the NG tube is used for enteral feeding, check placement and residual. Note skin condition at tube insertion site.

Drains

Note type and location of drain. Check for proper functioning of the drainage system and the characteristics and amount of drainage. Assess skin condition.

Incisions and Stomas

Assess color, approximation, and presence of any swelling or drainage of incisions. Assess color and moisture of stoma and note if the stoma is flush, retracted, or prolapsed. Assess condition of peristomal skin.

GENITOURINARY ASSESSMENT

Genitalia

Check external genitalia for any drainage, inflammation, or lesions.

Fluid Status

Check weight daily. An increase of 0.5 kg/day suggests fluid retention. Measure intake and output (I&O); 1 L of fluid is approximately equal to 1 kg of body weight. Table 1-12 lists findings associated with volume excess or deficit. An accumulation of approximately 5 kg of excess fluid is associated with pitting edema.

Bladder

Percuss the abdomen for bladder distention.

Urine

Identify type of urinary drainage tube and assess proper functioning. Measure urinary output. Note color and consistency.
Anuria: <100 mL/24 hr
Oliguria: 100 to 400 mL/24 hr

Table 1-12 Signs and Symptoms Associated with Volume Disturbances

	Hypovolemia	Hypervolemia
Weight	Acute loss	Acute gain
Pulse	Decreased pulse pressure	Bounding
	Tachycardia	
Blood pressure	Postural hypotension	Hypertension
Mucous membranes	Dry	Moist
Turgor	Decreased skin elasticity	Pitting edema
Peripheral veins	JVP flat when supine	JVP elevated
	Slow-filling hand veins	
Hemodynamics	CVP <2 mm Hg	CVP >6 mm Hg
	Decreased PAWP	Increased PAWP
Other	Thirst	Cough
	Urine output <30 mL/hr	Dyspnea
		Crackles
		S_3
Laboratory data	Increased hemoglobin	Decreased hemoglobin
	Increased hematocrit	Decreased hematocrit
	Increased serum osmolality	
	Increased specific gravity	Decreased serum osmolality
	Increased BUN/ creatinine ratio	Decreased specific gravity

BUN, Blood urea nitrogen; *CVP,* central venous pressure; *JVP,* jugular venous pressure; *PAWP,* pulmonary artery wedge pressure.

SCORING SYSTEMS FOR THE INTENSIVE CARE UNIT (ICU) PATIENT

Acute Physiology and Chronic Health Evaluation (APACHE III)

APACHE III[1] is a prognostic scoring system (see p. 769). The score, which can range from 0 to 299, is determined from physiologic values, age, and the presence of chronic illness. The APACHE III risk equation can be used to calculate a predicted risk of hospital mortality and takes into account the patient's APACHE III score, major disease category, and treatment location before the ICU admission.

Trauma Score

The trauma score (see p. 765) is a system for estimating the severity of patient injury.[2,3] The patient's level of consciousness (LOC) and cardiopulmonary function are assessed. A numeric value is assigned to each of the assessment parameters. The total score reflects the severity of the injury, and a survival estimate for the patient can be projected from the score.

Therapeutic Intervention Scoring System (TISS)

TISS has been used to determine severity of illness, establish nurse-patient ratios, and assess current bed use and need.[4] Patient classification of severity of illness is based on points: class I is less than 10 points, class II is 10 to 19 points, class III is 20 to 39 points, and class IV is 40 or more points (see p. 766).

It has been proposed that class IV patients receive a 1:1 nurse-patient ratio and that an accomplished critical care nurse should be capable of managing 40 to 50 patient TISS points. TISS has been used to differentiate intensive care and high-dependency patients.[5]

REFERENCES

1. Knaus WA et al: APACHE III prognostic system, *Chest* 100:1619-1636, 1991.
2. Champion HR et al: Trauma score, *Crit Care Med* 9:672-676, 1981.
3. Champion HR, Gainer PS, Yackee E: A progress report on the trauma score in predicting a fatal outcome, *J Trauma* 26:927-931, 1986.
4. Keene R, Cullen D: Therapeutic intervention scoring system: update 1983, *Crit Care Med* 11:1-3, 1083.
5. Pirret AM: Utilizing TISS to differentiate between intensive care and high dependency patients and to identify nurses' skill requirements, *Int Crit Care Nurs* 18:19-26, 2002.

BIBLIOGRAPHY

Alspach, JG: *Core curriculum for critical care nursing,* ed 5, Philadelphia, 1998, WB Saunders.

Borg G: Psychophysical bases of perceived exertion, *Med Sci Sports Exerc* 14:377-381, 1982.

Budassi SA, Barber J: *Mosby's manual of emergency care,* ed 3, St Louis, 1989, Mosby.

Darovic GO: *Hemodynamic monitoring: invasive and noninvasive clinical application,* ed 3, Philadelphia, 2002, WB Saunders.

Fink MP: *Textbook of critical care,* Philadelphia, 2005, WB Saunders.

Guidelines for the determination of death: report of the medical consultants in the diagnosis of death to the President's Commission for the Study of Ethical Problems in Medicine and Biomedical and Behavioral Research, *JAMA* 246:2184-2186, 1981.

Kinney MR et al: *Comprehensive cardiac care,* ed 8, St Louis, 1995, Mosby.

Kinney MR et al: *AACN clinical reference for critical care nursing,* ed 4, St Louis, 1998, Mosby.

Leith BA: Transfer anxiety in critical care patients and their family members, *Crit Care Nurse* 18:24-32, 1998.

Parrillo JE, Dillinger RP: *Critical care medicine: principles of diagnosis and management,* ed 2, St Louis, 2002, Mosby.

Petty TL: Adult respiratory distress syndrome. In Mitchell RS, Petty TL, Schwarz MI, eds: *Synopsis of clinical pulmonary disease,* ed 4, St Louis, 1989, Mosby.

Purnell LD, Paulanka BJ: *Transcultural health care: a culturally competent approach,* Philadelphia, 2002, FA Davis.

Sahn SA: Pneumothorax and pneumomediastinum. In Mitchell RS, Petty TL, Schwarz MI, eds: *Synopsis of clinical pulmonary disease,* ed 4, St Louis, 1989, Mosby.

Seidel HM, Ball JW, Dains JE, Benedict GW: *Mosby's guide to physical examination,* ed 5, St Louis, 2003, Mosby.

Sheehy SB: *Mosby's manual of emergency care,* ed 5, St Louis, 1999, Mosby.

Smith TL, Bleck TP: Determination of death by neurologic criteria. In Fink MP, *Textbook of critical care,* ed 5, Philadelphia, 2005, WB Saunders.

Talbot L, Meyers-Marquardt M: *Pocket guide to critical care assessment,* ed 3, St Louis, 1997, Mosby.

Teasdale G, Jennett B: Glasgow Coma Scale, *Lancet* 2:81-83, 1974.

Urden LD, Stacy KM, Lough ME: *Thelan's critical care nursing: diagnosis and management,* ed 4, St Louis, 2002, Mosby.

2

Acute Pain in the Critically Ill Patient

CLINICAL BRIEF

Most critically ill patients experience significant pain as a result of their underlying condition or disease or the aftermath of their care. The sources of pain for these patients include surgical incisions, turning, chest tubes, endotracheal intubation and suctioning, and mechanical ventilation.[1] In fact, turning is the most painful and distressing procedure for adults ages 18 and older,[2] and pain intensity scores taken at rest nearly doubled immediately after trauma patients were turned.[3]

HARMFUL EFFECTS OF UNRELIEVED PAIN

Unrelieved pain stimulates a number of physiologic stress responses in the human body. These physiologic stressors can have a significant negative impact on the stability, healing, and outcome of critically ill patients (Table 2-1).[4]

PAIN ASSESSMENT

Pain is always a subjective and personal experience. The patient's self-report of pain is the most sensitive and reliable indicator of its presence and intensity.[5] Pain assessment in the critically ill patient is often complicated by endotracheal intubation, administration of sedatives and neuromuscular blocking agents, and physiologic instability. *Critically ill patients who are unable to communicate are at risk of undertreatment of their pain.* Efforts should be made to obtain the patient's self-report whenever possible. Use the following strategies to improve pain assessment of the critically ill patient.[6]

- Assess pain in alert and oriented patients using a valid and reliable pain rating tool (e.g. 0 to 10 numeric rating scale).
- If a patient is unable to verbalize a self-report, determine if the patient can point to a number on the pain rating scale or blink

Table 2-1 HARMFUL EFFECTS OF UNRELIEVED PAIN

Systems	Stressors	Outcomes
Endocrine	Increased release of stress hormones (e.g., epinephrine, catecholamines, aldosterone) Decreased insulin	Lipolysis, catabolism, and increased blood glucose, insulin resistance
Cardiovascular	Activation of the sympathetic nervous system	Increased cardiac workload: tachycardia, hypertension, vasoconstriction, hypercoagulation, and increased myocardial oxygen consumption
Respiratory	Limited thoracic and abdominal muscle movement ("splinting")	Atelectasis, shunting, hypoxemia, sputum retention, infection
Genitourinary	Urinary retention	Fluid overload and hypokalemia
Gastrointestinal	Decreased gastric and bowel motility	Constipation and ileus
Musculoskeletal	Increased muscle spasm	Impaired muscle function, fatigue, and immobility
Cognitive	Hypoxemia, sleep disturbances	Mental confusion
Future pain	Repeated stimulation of nociceptive pathways (nerve fibers carrying pain message)	Increased potential for chronic pain syndromes

    or nod in response to questions about pain as an acceptable option to document yes or no per the patient's report.

- When self-report is not possible, assume that pain is present for patients who have undergone surgery, have injuries or illness, or require procedures that are known to be painful. Document APP (assume pain is present).

- Assessment of behaviors (e.g., restlessness, grimacing) and physiologic signs (e.g., elevated heart rate and blood pressure) should be used cautiously and only when other assessment efforts are not successful because these indicators do not consistently correlate with the absence or presence of pain.

The intensity, quality, and even the location of pain can be variable depending on when the pain assessment is completed. Pain should be assessed while the patient is at rest to determine their persistent or baseline pain. In addition, breakthrough pain and pain caused by common activities (e.g., turning, endotracheal [ET] suctioning) and procedures (e.g., placement of invasive lines) also should be assessed. The Joint Commission on Accreditation of Healthcare Organizations (JCAHO) recognizes the importance of pain assessment in reducing the undertreatment of pain. Its pain management standards require systematic initial assessment and ongoing reassessment of pain for *all* patients.[7]

PAIN MANAGEMENT

Pharmacologic interventions are the cornerstone of managing moderate to severe acute pain in all patients including the critically ill.[8] Drugs from each of three analgesic groups—(1) nonopioid analgesics (acetaminophen and nonsteroidal antiinflammatory drugs), (2) opioid analgesics, and (3) adjuvant analgesics (local anesthetics, benzodiazepines, corticosteroids, and others)—may be used in a combination approach called *multimodal, balanced analgesia.*[1] Multimodal, balanced analgesia uses lower doses of each analgesic, thereby producing fewer side effects and achieving comparable or better pain relief than is possible with any single analgesic. For example, a patient may receive low-dose fentanyl and bupivacaine by continuous epidural infusion along with intravenous (IV) ketorolac every 6 hours following major surgery.

Characteristics of the patient's pain are used when determining appropriate analgesic treatments and timing of administration. For example, most patients in the intensive care unit (ICU) can be expected to have continuous pain, which is treated with around-the-clock (ATC) analgesics. Additional analgesic doses should be available as needed (PRN) to treat episodes of breakthrough pain. If an activity or procedure is known to cause pain, a local anesthetic or the breakthrough analgesic should be administered before the onset of pain, allowing sufficient time for the medication to reach its peak effectiveness; 5 minutes for IV fentanyl, 10 to 15 minutes for IV hydromorphone and morphine.[1]

Consider the following:
- Anesthetic agents (e.g., enflurane, halothane, isoflurane) are short acting and provide little if any analgesia postoperatively.

- Naloxone may have been administered at the end of surgery, reversing the analgesic effects of opioids administered during surgery.
- Sedatives, such as propofol, or neuromuscular blocking agents such as vecuronium, do not provide analgesia.
- Subanesthetic doses of the *N*-methyl-D-aspartate (NMDA) antagonist ketamine (0.15 to 1.5 mg/kg/hr IV) may be helpful to optimize opioid therapy when pain is difficult to control or during extremely painful procedures such as burn debridement.[1,9] Administer benzodiazepines, such as midazolam, to reduce unpleasant experiences of dissociation associated with ketamine should they occur.

KEY CONCEPTS

Concerns often arise when opioids must be administered over a long time or in significant doses to relieve severe pain. Because opioid analgesics are the mainstay drug treatment, these concerns are a potential barrier to adequate pain management for the critically ill. It is important that the patient, the patient's family, and the health care team have an adequate understanding of the key concepts of tolerance, physical dependence, and addiction.

Tolerance to opioids is a physiologic response that should be expected when an individual takes an opioid drug regularly for several days or longer. As tolerance develops, a higher dose of drug is needed to maintain the original effect. After the opioid is titrated to an acceptable dose when opioid therapy is initiated, the dose stabilizes unless there is a change in the pain.[1] The need for further dose increases in patients with stable pain is unusual. However, if analgesia declines either because of tolerance or worsening disease, the treatment is to increase the opioid dose, usually by 50% until adequate pain relief is achieved. Tolerance should not be confused with addiction, and it is not a predictor of abuse.

- Opioid-tolerant patients (those who have been taking regular daily doses of opioid for a week or more) may require higher starting doses than are required by opioid-naive patients.

After 1 to 4 weeks of regular opioid administration, physical dependence, a physiologic phenomenon, should be expected. It is manifested by the development of withdrawal syndrome after abrupt discontinuation of the opioid, substantial dose reduction, or administration of an antagonist drug such as naloxone (Narcan). Signs of withdrawal include restlessness, agitation, runny nose, abdominal cramping, and diarrhea. Physical dependence does not lead to addiction and requires no treatment unless withdrawal symptoms occur or are anticipated. Withdrawal can be avoided or suppressed with gradual reduction in the opioid dose over several days.[1]

- Do not abruptly discontinue opioids in patients who have been receiving opioids for a week or more; taper doses by 25% or less every other day.
- Avoid abrupt discontinuation of opioids before ventilator weaning and extubation; suggest instead a slight decrease (25%) in opioid dose and the addition of nonopioids to provide additional analgesia during weaning.

Fear of addiction continues to pose a significant barrier to effective pain management in the critically ill. *The American Pain Society defines addiction as "a primary, chronic, neurobiological disease, with genetic, psychosocial, and environmental factors influencing its development and manifestations"* (p. 38).[8] Characteristics of addiction include compulsive use of opioids and continued use despite harm. The medical use of opioids for pain relief is not the major factor in the development of addiction. Opioids should never be withheld from critically ill patients with pain because of concerns about causing addiction.[1]

Nursing Diagnosis: ACUTE PAIN

OUTCOME CRITERIA

Patient states or demonstrates decreased pain as evidenced by one or all of the following indicators:

Patient's reported pain score at rest, with activity and during procedures

Improved function and tolerance of recovery activities

INTERVENTIONS

1. Perform systematic initial and ongoing pain assessment (intensity, location, quality, and aggravating and relieving factors) at rest, with activity, and during painful procedures.
2. Use a self-report pain rating scale, such as 0-to-10 numeric rating scale (NRS), to assess pain intensity in patients who are awake and oriented.
3. Assume pain is present and document painful pathologic condition or procedures to support the need for analgesics in patients who are unable to use a self-report pain rating scale.
4. Document behaviors such as grimacing, groaning, grunting, sobbing, crying, irritability, withdrawing, or hostility because they may be signs of pain. However, the absence of these behaviors does not necessarily mean the absence of pain.

5. Document physiologic indicators that may be signs of pain, such as increased respiratory rate, heart rate, and blood pressure; dilated or constricted pupils; and pallor. However, the absence of these physiologic indicators does not necessarily mean the absence of pain. *Note that some of these symptoms can also indicate other conditions such as hypoxia.*

6. Collaborate with physician regarding the use of a balanced analgesic approach to manage pain with ATC dosing for persistent pain and PRN dosing for breakthrough pain (see preceding section on pain management).

7. Suggest intraspinal analgesia for patients with major thoracic, abdominal, or orthopedic injuries or surgery (see Intraspinal Analgesia, p. 590)

8. Suggest patient-controlled analgesia (PCA) for patients who are alert and able to understand the relationships between pain, pressing a button, and pain relief.

9. Suggest continuous opioid infusions with nurse-administered bolus doses via the PCA pump (nurse-activated dosing) for patients who are too ill to manage their pain using PCA.

10. In patients who are unresponsive, initiate opioid therapy at the recommended starting dose for moderate to severe pain (e.g., 1.25 to 2.5 mg of IV morphine equivalent per hour). Observe for changes in behaviors that might indicate response to treatment (e.g., more or less restlessness or facial grimacing). If a pain indicator is present or changes, adjust the treatment plan accordingly (e.g., increase analgesic dose or add analgesics if behavior increases). In the absence of response, continue the starting analgesic dose.

11. Avoid meperidine (Demerol); it is no longer recommended as a first-line opioid for pain management primarily because it produces the active metabolite normeperidine, which is a central nervous system (CNS) stimulant and can cause irritability, tremors, muscle twitching, jerking, agitation, and seizures. Appropriate candidates for meperidine are those with acute pain *who are otherwise healthy and are allergic to other opioids such as morphine, fentanyl, and hydromorphone.* Meperidine should not be used at doses greater than 600 mg/24 hr or for longer than 48 hours.

12. Suggest nonopioids with reduced adverse gastrointestinal (GI) effects or those with minimal inhibition of platelet function, such as celecoxib or choline magnesium trisalicylate.

13. Identify patients at higher risk than others for respiratory depression, such as patients with sleep apnea syndrome, myasthenia gravis, or chronic obstructive pulmonary disease (COPD). Suggest a pain management plan that includes nonopioids and local anesthetics in addition to low-dose opioid analgesics to manage pain in these patients.

14. Monitor level of sedation and respiratory status to identify sedation and prevent opioid-induced respiratory depression; decrease opioid dose if increased sedation is detected (Table 2-2).

15. Determine if the patient has impaired renal or liver function and provide analgesics such as hydromorphone or fentanyl, which have no clinically relevant metabolites.

16. Prevent nausea by routinely administering nonsedating antiemetics, such as ondansetron, prophylactically in patients at high risk for nausea (e.g., after abdominal surgery).

17. Treat adverse effects, such as nausea, itching, hypotension, urinary retention, and increased sedation (see Table 2-2), with prescribed medications and consider decreasing analgesic dose by 25% to eliminate the adverse effect rather than repeatedly treating with medications; add or increase dose of nonopioids for additional analgesia.

Table 2-2   SCALE FOR ASSESSING OPIOID-INDUCED SEDATION

Level of Sedation	Intervention
S = Sleep, easy to arouse	None
1 = Awake, alert	None; may increase opioid dose
2 = Slightly drowsy, easily arousable	None; may increase opioid dose
3 = Frequently drowsy, arousable, drifts off to sleep during conversation	Reduce opioid dose by 25% to 50%, add or increase the dose of an opioid-sparing nonopioid, such as acetaminophen and ketorolac or celecoxib
4 = Somnolent, minimal or no response to physical stimulation	Stop opioid and consider administering naloxone (Narcan); add or increase the dose of an opioid-sparing nonopioid, such as acetaminophen and ketorolac or celecoxib

18. Observe patient outcomes affected by pain (see Table 2-1) and increase and decrease analgesic doses based on patient response. Collaborate with the physician to revise the pain management plan if pain is not adequately controlled. Request a referral to a pain management specialist for complex pain problems.

19. Explain to patient and family that preventing pain is easier than trying to reduce it once it becomes severe.

20. Assure patient and family that addiction is rare when opioids are taken for pain relief and explain that pain control is beneficial and necessary for healing.

21. Expect that terminally ill patients may experience an increase in pain at the end of life (restlessness, grimacing, or moaning may be signs); increase doses of analgesics appropriately.

22. Do not discontinue opioids in comatose patients; the point at which pain is no longer felt is not known.

REFERENCES

1. Pasero C, McCaffery M: Multimodal balanced analgesia in the critically ill, *Nurs Clin North Am* 13:195-206, 2001.

2. Puntillo KA et al: Patient's perceptions and responses to procedural pain: results from Thunder Project II, *Am J Crit Care* 10(4):238-251, 2001.

3. Stanik-Hutt JA et al: Pain experiences of traumatically injured patients in a critical care setting, *Am J Crit Care* 10(4):252-259, 2001.

4. Pasero C, Paice JA, McCaffery M: Basic mechanisms underlying the causes and effects of pain. In McCaffery M, Pasero C. *Pain: clinical manual,* ed 2, St Louis, 1999, Mosby.

5. Agency for Healthcare Policy and Research (AHCPR): *Acute pain management: operations or medical procedures and trauma: clinical practice guidelines,* AHCPR pub no 92-0032, Rockville, Md, February 1992, US Public Health Service, AHCPR.

6. Pasero C, McCaffery M: Pain in the critically ill: new information reveals that one of the simplest procedures—turning—can be the most painful one, *Am J Nurs* 102(1):59-60, 2002.

7. Joint Commission on Accreditation of Healthcare Organizations (JCAHO): *Hospital accreditation standards,* Oakbrook Terrace, Ill, 2000, JCAHO.

8. American Pain Society (APS): *Principles of analgesic use in the treatment of acute and cancer pain,* ed 5, Glenview, Ill, 2003, APS.

9. Berger JM et al: Ketamine-fentanyl-midazolam infusion for the control of symptoms in terminal life care, *Am J Hosp Palliat Care,* 17:127-134, 2000.

BIBLIOGRAPHY

Pasero C, Portenoy RK, McCaffery M: Opioid analgesics. In McCaffery M, Pasero C. *Pain: clinical manual,* ed 2, St Louis, 1999, Mosby.

Radnay PA et al: The effect of equianalgesic doses of fentanyl, morphine, meperidine, and pentazocine on common bile duct pressure, *Anaesthetist* 29:26-29, 1980.

3

Concepts Common in the Care of the Critically Ill Patient

FAMILY

The hospitalization of a family member can be very stressful and can create specific needs for the family. These include need for information, comfort, support, assurance and anxiety reduction, and proximity and accessibility. If these needs go unmet, tension may mount, leading to major disorganization and ineffective coping. Although the critical care nurse intervenes to resolve life-threatening problems, a holistic approach to the patient, which includes the family, is essential to the well-being of the patient.

Nursing Diagnosis: RISK FOR INTERRUPTED FAMILY PROCESSES

Outcome Criteria

Family will state that their needs are met.
Family will demonstrate adequate coping behaviors.

Interventions

1. Introduce yourself to the family and prepare the family for the intensive care unit (ICU) environment. Anticipate the need for supportive services for the patient and family during this crisis. Provide continuity of caregivers and identify a primary nursing contact for the family whenever possible.
2. Display competence in caring for the patient. Families want to be assured that the best possible care is being provided for their relative.
3. Demonstrate personal knowledge of the patient. Be respectful of cultural and religious beliefs and integrate them into nursing care.
4. Approach the family with a relaxed and humanistic attitude and volunteer information frequently without waiting to be

asked. Listen to their expressions of fear, anger, or anxiety. Avoid defensive retorts. Provide the family a time away from the bedside to vent their concerns. Answer questions honestly and provide facts frequently regarding their relative's condition. Anticipate repeating information and allowing time for them to digest the information during this crisis period. Assign a family advocate, if available, to meet psychosocial needs.

5. Assess critical junctures or risk points that may affect family expectations and satisfaction (e.g., family expressing anger, patient awaiting surgery or near discharge).

6. Provide the family with written information about the unit policies and services available. Information should include the phone number of the unit and location of the waiting room.

7. Obtain the family contact phone number and contact the family spokesperson at least daily with information about the patient's condition and any changes in medical or nursing care.

8. Clarify the family's perception of their relative's illness and validate their understanding of the situation. Let them know the staff cares for their relative and that the best care is being given.

9. Individualize visiting hours, explain the equipment being used and why things are being done, assess family members' need to participate in their relative's care, and allow as much participation as is reasonably possible. Be sensitive to the family's need to be left alone with their relative. Arrange equipment so that family members can touch the patient.

10. Reassure the family that they will be contacted if the relative's condition worsens.

11. Offer the family an opportunity to meet with the hospital chaplain, social worker, financial officer, and other supportive services as needed.

12. Encourage the family to meet their own physical and personal needs such as eating and sleeping. Suggest complementary and alternative therapies such as journaling and relaxed breathing.

13. Provide palliative care and support for terminally ill patients.

14. Allow family members to be present during cardiopulmonary resuscitation (CPR) to assist them through the grieving process.

INFECTION CONTROL

Critically ill patients are exposed to many factors in addition to their underlying illness that depress the immune system and lower the body's defenses. The patient's own organisms, as well as environmental sources of organisms, or cross-contamination, can cause infection. The first, second, and third lines of defense can be adversely affected by therapeutic interventions, thus placing the patient at risk for infection.

The patient's first line of defense includes epithelial surfaces and secretions that provide a barrier between the internal and external environments. Table 3-1 outlines the patient's first line of defense and examples of things that interrupt the system.

Table 3-1   FIRST LINE OF DEFENSE

Body System	Protective Barrier	Conditions Disrupting Protective Barriers
Integument	Skin	Pressure ulcers
		Surgical incisions
		Invasive lines
		Invasive procedures
		Burns
		Steroids
Pulmonary	Mucociliary escalator	Intubation
	Reflexes: sneeze, cough, gag	Endoscopic procedures
	Normal flora	Sedation (decreased LOC)
		Cranial nerve impairment
		Antibiotics
Gastrointestinal	Gastric pH	NG intubation
	Motility	H_2 antagonists
	Intact mucosal epithelium	Antacids
	Normal flora	Endoscopic procedures
		Antibiotics
		Electrolyte imbalance
Genitourinary	Micturition	Urinary catheterization
	Urine pH	Incontinence
	Bladder mucosa	Glycosuria
	Vaginal pH	Antibiotics
	Normal flora	

LOC, Level of consciousness; *NG,* nasogastric.

The patient's second line of defense involves the inflammatory response, which occurs when the first line of defense fails or as a result of the patient's condition (e.g., cancer, myocardial infarction). The response can be localized (red, edematous, warm, painful) or systemic (fever, malaise, leukocytosis, neutrophilia). The inflammatory response always accompanies infection; however, the inflammatory response also can occur without an infection (e.g., trauma, burns). Factors that impair the inflammatory response include stress, hyperglycemia, and pharmacologic agents such as corticosteroids, immunosuppressants, and aspirin. Patients who are human immunodeficiency virus (HIV) positive, neutropenic, organ transplant recipients, asplenic, diabetic, or on corticosteroids are more susceptible to specific pathogens.

The patient's third line of defense involves acquired immunity. Malnutrition, age, anesthesia, radiation, and chemotherapy can adversely affect the third line of defense.

Antibiotic-resistant organisms are increasing. Of concern are methicillin-resistant *Staphylococcus aureus* (MRSA), penicillin-resistant *Streptococcus pneumoniae* (PRSP), and vancomycin-resistant enterococci (VRE), among others.

Nursing Diagnoses: RISK FOR INFECTION; INEFFECTIVE PROTECTION; IMPAIRED TISSUE INTEGRITY; IMPAIRED SKIN INTEGRITY; IMPAIRED ORAL MUCOUS MEMBRANE

Outcome Criteria

Temperature 36.5° C to 38° C (97.7° F to 100.4° F)
Absence of chills, diaphoresis
Skin without redness and exudate
Mucous membranes intact
Clear breath sounds
Absence of dysuria
Urine clear yellow
Serum glucose 80 to 120 mg/dL
White blood cells (WBCs) 5 to 10×10^3/mL

Interventions

1. Avoid cross-contamination: wash hands, avoid sharing equipment, use sterile equipment, and avoid "dirty" to "clean" activities. Note: MRSA and VRE remain viable on environmental surfaces and clothing for days.
2. Obtain temperature every 4 hours and assess for diaphoresis and chills. Monitor serial serum glucose and WBC counts.
3. Maintain ICU environmental temperature at approximately 75° F (23.8° C).

Integument

1. Provide meticulous skin care.
   a. Assess pressure points (Figure 3-1). Nonblanchable erythema of intact skin is a sign of a pressure ulcer. Hardness, discoloration, or warmth of the skin may also indicate skin ulceration.
   b. Turn and reposition the patient frequently because continued pressure can result in ischemia; provide range of motion (ROM) exercises every 2 to 4 hours to increase circulation.
   c. Use pressure-relieving or pressure-reducing devices such as an air mattress or specialty bed. Avoid "doughnuts" because these devices may increase pressure.
   d. Moisturize skin sparingly because too much moisture can macerate skin. Avoid vigorous massaging because further damage to underlying tissue can occur.
   e. Clean skin of feces or urine immediately. Apply petrolatum ointment or a spray that protects against moisture to perianal area.
   f. Avoid skin stripping by using gauze or a stockinette to secure dressings if at all possible or Montgomery straps to avoid multiple tape applications.
2. Consult with nutritionist regarding the dietary needs of the patient. Patient should be hydrated and in positive nitrogen balance.

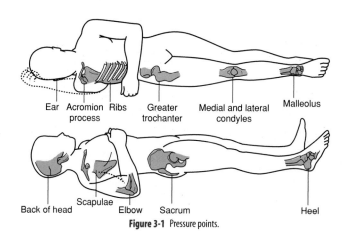

| Ear | Acromion process | Ribs | Greater trochanter | Medial and lateral condyles | Malleolus |

| Back of head | Scapulae | Elbow | Sacrum | Heel |

Figure 3-1 Pressure points.

3. Avoid shearing forces by limiting head of bed (HOB) to no greater than 30 degrees. Use sheepskin elbow and heel protectors to prevent friction. Keep topsheets loose and lift patients to reposition them. Turning sheets can decrease shear and friction.

4. Assess nares for pressure areas associated with nasogastric (NG) or endotracheal (ET) tubes; assess peristomal skin for chemical irritation; assess mouth and lips for dryness associated with nothing by mouth (NPO) status.

5. Closely monitor patient receiving vasopressors for tissue ischemia.

6. Use sterile technique with invasive lines, incisions, tubings, drains, and so on. Keep stopcocks covered with sterile caps. Change wet or soiled dressings immediately.

7. Follow infection control protocol for changing intravenous (IV) sites, dressings, tubing, and solutions.

Pulmonary

1. Assess cough and gag reflexes to evaluate presence of protective reflexes.

2. Assess lungs for adventitious sounds.

3. Provide pulmonary hygiene: cough and deep breathing (C&DB), chest physiotherapy, incentive spirometry.

4. Position the patient to facilitate chest excursion. Mobilize patient as soon as possible.

5. Keep HOB elevated or place the patient in side-lying position if level of consciousness (LOC) is decreased or the patient is receiving tube feedings. Turn tube feedings off 30 to 60 minutes before and during chest physiotherapy and other activities, such as weighing patient on a bed scale, to prevent aspiration.

6. If the patient is intubated, check cuff pressure to prevent mucosal injury; drain respiratory circuit of water accumulation.

7. Use sterile technique when suctioning.

8. Ensure that respiratory equipment is replaced periodically.

Gastrointestinal (GI)

1. Assess the patient's abdomen for distention or change in bowel sounds.

2. Prevent GI contamination by changing tube feeding container every 24 hours. Rinse container before adding new feeding to the bag. Fill container with enough tube feeding for

8 hours (see manufacturer's recommendations). Refrigerate unused feeding.

3. Assess for tube feeding residual every 4 hours.

Genitourinary

1. Inspect urinary meatus for any drainage.
2. Assess urine for cloudiness, presence of glucose, or foul odor.
3. If the patient is incontinent of stool, clean the patient and the catheter tubing; avoid a back-and-forth motion on tubing, which could lead to fecal contamination of the urinary meatus.
4. Check indwelling urinary catheter tubing for any kinks that may obstruct urine flow. Do not irrigate the catheter unless an obstruction is suspected. Keep the drainage bag lower than the patient's bladder. Secure the catheter to the patient's leg and avoid excessive manipulation of the catheter. Provide individual patient-labeled containers for emptying the drainage bags.
5. Remove the urinary catheter as soon as possible. When the urinary catheter is removed, assess the patient for dysuria, frequency, urgency, and flank or labial pain.

Education

1. Instruct patients and visitors on handwashing.
2. Explain the importance of antibiotic therapy to reduce the risk for antibiotic-resistant pathogens.

OXYGENATION IN THE CRITICALLY ILL

The critically ill patient is at risk for tissue hypoxia, the underlying event that results in cellular dysfunction, organ failure, and death. Thus it is important to understand the concepts of oxygenation and the relevant parameters that can be monitored in the critically ill. Concepts of oxygenation include (1) oxygen transport or delivery ($\dot{D}o_2$), (2) oxygen consumption ($\dot{V}o_2$), (3) oxygen extraction, (4) cardiac output/cardiac index (CO/CI), (5) hemoglobin (Hgb), (6) hemoglobin saturation (So_2), and (7) partial pressure of oxygen (Po_2).

Tissue oxygen consumption is independent of oxygen delivery during steady states. The amount of oxygen used by the cells (oxygen consumption) determines the amount of oxygen delivered to the cells. If tissue oxygen demand increases, more oxygen is extracted from the blood without requiring additional blood flow (i.e., CO/CI). As the demand increases, however, an increase in blood flow will be necessary to provide adequate supply. The more blood flow, the more oxygen is extracted, up to a point. The point at which oxygen consumption becomes dependent on oxygen delivery is referred to as "critical oxygen delivery." If there is a further increase in metabolic demand, these compensatory mechanisms may not be adequate, and an oxygen debt results.

In addition to cardiac function, the lungs also play a role in tissue oxygenation. Conditions such as atelectasis, pneumonia, and pulmonary edema may cause arterial hypoxemia (decreased PaO_2 and SaO_2). To assess the extent to which the pulmonary system contributes to inadequate tissue oxygenation, intrapulmonary shunting can be evaluated. Efficiency of gas exchange can be estimated with a number of equations (e.g., Qs/Qt, $P(A - a)O_2$, $P(a/A)O_2$ ratio, or the PaO_2/FIO_2 ratio).

Oxygen extraction ratio (ERO_2) is a fractional comparison of oxygen consumption with oxygen delivery. It is an index of the efficiency of total tissue extraction of oxygen from the extracellular environment. Normally 22% to 28% of all oxygen that is transported to the cells is removed from the hemoglobin by the cells. An increased extraction ratio ≥ 0.60 reflects either an inadequate cardiac output or inadequate arterial oxygen content (SaO_2, PaO_2, Hb) to meet oxygen demands and is thought to be associated with anaerobic metabolism. Oxygen extraction can be estimated with SvO_2 monitoring and analysis (see p. 482). Some conditions (e.g., septic shock, cyanide poisoning, and adult respiratory distress syndrome [ARDS]) interfere with oxygen extraction. Adequate levels of $\dot{D}O_2$ may exist, yet tissue ischemia may occur. These conditions may benefit from supranormal levels of $\dot{D}O_2$ to optimize $\dot{V}O_2$.

When oxygen content, delivery, and extraction are inadequate the cells depend on anaerobic metabolism. This results in lactic acidosis. A serum lactate level can provide information about cellular oxygenation; however, a single value does not necessarily reflect immediate changes and is not always reliable. There is a lag time between the generation of lactate in the cells and the accumulation of lactate in the serum. Thus the absence of lactate does not reflect the absence of anaerobic metabolism. Serial lactate levels may provide more helpful information.

When the patient's cellular oxygenation is being threatened, efforts to increase oxygen content and oxygen transport or to decrease oxygen consumption should be made. Table 3-2 lists factors interfering with oxygen delivery and oxygen consumption.

Table 3-2 SOME FACTORS AFFECTING OXYGEN DELIVERY AND CONSUMPTION

Factors that impede $\dot{D}o_2$	HR: dysrhythmias
	SV: MI, HF, hypovolemia, elevated SVR
	O_2 content: hypoxic anemia, intrapulmonary shunt, histotoxic anemia
Factors that increase $\dot{V}o_2$	Anxiety
	Shivering
	Fever
	Increased WOB
	Pain
	Hypermetabolism
Conditions that impair ERo_2	Septic shock
	ARDS
	Cyanide poisoning
	Edema

ARDS, Acute respiratory distress syndrome; *HF,* heart failure; *HR,* heart rate; *MI,* myocardial infarction; *O_2,* oxygen; *SV,* stroke volume; *SVR,* systemic vascular resistance; *WOB,* work of breathing.

Nursing Diagnosis: RISK FOR INEFFECTIVE TISSUE PERFUSION

Outcome Criteria

CI 2.5 to 4 L/min/m^2
$\dot{D}o_2$I 500 to 650 mL/min/m^2
$\dot{V}o_2$I 115 to 165 mL/min/m^2
Svo_2 60% to 80%
Pao_2 80 to 100 mm Hg
O_2 sat ≥95%
ERo_2 22% to 28%
Qs/Qt 0% to 8%
Pao_2/Fio_2 >250
$P(a/A)o_2$ ≥0.75
Hematocrit (Hct) 37% to 47% (females); 40% to 54% (males)

Interventions

1. Correct hypoxemia and increase oxygen saturation. Administer supplemental oxygen as ordered; intubation and mechanical ventilation may be needed.
2. Increase cardiac output by manipulating heart rate or stroke volume: optimize preload, contractility, and afterload.

Administer antidysrhythmic agents as ordered. Administer fluids or diuretics as ordered to maintain effective blood volume, generally not to exceed a pulmonary artery wedge pressure (PAWP) of 15 mm Hg. Fluid volume overload can potentially impair oxygen diffusion. Administer electrolytes as ordered to correct imbalances, administer inotropes (dobutamine) and titrate vasopressors (dopamine or norepinephrine) as ordered. Vasodilators (nitroprusside) may be needed in some cases to decrease systemic vascular resistance (SVR).

3. Administer blood products or blood substitutes as ordered to improve oxygen carrying capacity.

4. Decrease metabolic demands: relieve pain, keep patient warm and dry, relieve or reduce anxiety, maintain bed rest, and allow for periods of uninterrupted rest; suction if patient is unable to handle secretions; prevent infection. Anticipate sedation and possible neuromuscular blockade.

5. Monitor intramucosal pH (if available) to assess tissue oxygenation of the gut.

6. Anticipate supranormal levels of $\dot{D}o_2$ to optimize $\dot{V}o_2$ in some patients.

7. Monitor CI, Spo_2, and Svo_2. Note trends and patient response to therapy and activities and nursing interventions.

8. Calculate $\dot{D}o_2I$, $\dot{V}o_2I$, ERo_2 and estimate intrapulmonary shunt. Note trends and patient response to therapy.

9. Monitor arterial blood gases (ABGs), Hb, and Hct levels.

10. Monitor patient's mentation, urine output, skin temperature, and capillary refill in addition to blood pressure (BP) and trends in arterial lactate levels.

11. See Svo_2 Monitoring, p. 482.

NUTRITION

Adequate nutrition is essential in critically ill patients to decrease the risks of malnutrition-associated complications. Patients with fevers, burns, or trauma may require as much as 8000 to 10,000 kcal/day to meet their metabolic needs. Inability to ingest food orally because of unconsciousness, weakness, dysphagia, intubation, vomiting, or trauma rapidly results in muscle catabolism. Not only can fluid and electrolyte imbalance cause severe cardiopulmonary problems, but also protein and mineral loss can delay healing and recovery and lead to shock.

To supply the calories needed for seriously ill patients to regain their strength, most patients in the ICU receive nutritional support either by enteral or parenteral routes. Enteral nutrition is considered superior to parenteral nutrition because it is physiologic and maintains the integrity of the GI tract. (Disruption of intestinal mucosa may lead to hypermetabolism, translocation of bacteria, and multiple organ failure.) Parenteral nutrition is instituted when the GI tract is not functioning properly. Ongoing nutritional assessments are required and adjustments are made based on the patient's response and changing caloric needs. Excess energy intake with enteral or parenteral nutrition influences the risk of sepsis. Euglycemia results in improved outcomes, e.g., decreased morbidity and mortality.

Nursing Diagnosis: IMBALANCED NUTRITION: LESS THAN BODY REQUIREMENTS

Outcome Criteria

Stabilized target weight
Serum glucose 80 to 120 mg/dL
Prealbumin 15 to 32 mg/dL
Serum albumin 3.5 to 5 g/dL
Serum transferrin >200 mg/dL
Lymphocytes >1500 cells/mm^3
Positive nitrogen balance

Interventions

1. Assess energy needs using the Harris-Benedict equation (see Appendix D) or assist with indirect calorimetry. Daily caloric needs for the critically ill patient are based on actual body weight and estimated at 20 to 30 kcal/kg.
2. Estimate ideal body weight with the following formula: 50 kg (males) or 45 kg (females) + 2.3 (for each inch above 5 feet) ±10%.
3. Compare serial weights; rapid (0.5 to 1 kg/day) changes indicate fluid imbalance and not an imbalance between nutritional needs and intake.
4. Assess GI status: vomiting, diarrhea, or abdominal pain may interfere with nutritional absorption.
5. Review nutritional profile to evaluate patient response to therapy. Prealbumin is the most sensitive indicator of nutrition; however, glucose, electrolytes, magnesium, blood urea nitrogen (BUN), and triglycerides are also monitored.
6. Consult with the nutritionist for formal nutritional evaluation.

7. Provide mouth care to prevent stomatitis, which can adversely affect the patient's ability to eat.
8. Create a pleasing environment to improve patient's appetite; avoid offensive sights at the bedside; prepare the patient by making certain that hands and face have been washed.
9. Assist the patient as necessary because fatigue and weakness or the presence of invasive equipment may discourage the patient from self-feeding.
10. Administer enteral nutrition as prescribed (see p. 561).
11. Administer parenteral nutrition as prescribed (see p. 565).

TRANSPORT OF THE CRITICALLY ILL

Moving the critically ill patient for diagnostic tests or procedures or to another facility for treatment can involve some risks to the patient. Risks should be weighed against the benefits before a decision to transport the patient is made. Hospitals should have policies and protocols for interhospital and intrahospital patient transfers. Critical elements for transporting the patient include pretransport coordination and communication, competent personnel to accompany the patient, appropriate level of monitoring for the patient's condition that includes appropriate equipment, and patient and family preparation.

Nursing Diagnosis: RISK FOR INJURY

Outcome Criterion

Patient's condition will not deteriorate.

Interventions

1. Stabilize the patient before transport.
2. Consider intubating before the transport, inserting NG tube to prevent aspiration, and stopping enteral feedings.
3. Secure all tubes, catheters, and monitoring lines, and so on.
4. Anticipate potential emergencies (e.g., chest tube removal, accidental extubation) and include necessary replacement equipment with transport.
5. Communicate the patient's condition to the receiving end; confirm that the receiving end is ready.
6. Contact ancillary services to assist in transport and notify the responsible physician of the transfer.
7. For interhospital transport, select the mode of transportation and send a copy of the current medical record.

8. One critical care nurse plus one additional health care member, generally a respiratory therapist if the patient is mechanically ventilated, should accompany the patient. If the patient is physiologically unstable and may require interventions beyond the scope of standing orders or nursing practice, a physician should accompany the transport.

9. For interhospital transport, select personnel with the appropriate competencies and qualifications (e.g., able to intubate) to accompany the patient.

10. Continually monitor the cardiac rate and rhythm and the oxygenation status with pulse oximetry.

11. When appropriate, monitor hemodynamic measurements including pulmonary artery (PA) pressures; PAWP; central venous pressure (CVP); cardiac output; and other measurements such as intracranial pressure (ICP), capnography, and airway pressures in patients who are intubated and receiving mechanical ventilation.

12. Standard resuscitation drugs, defibrillator, oxygen source and airway management equipment, and blood pressure cuff should accompany the patient. Battery-operated infusion pumps should be used for IV fluids and medications during the transport.

13. Scheduled medications should be administered during the transport.

14. A plan to access a resuscitation cart and suction equipment (within 4 minutes) should be made.

15. Meet the needs of the patient and family; explain the reason for moving the patient and answer any questions they may have.

16. For interhospital transport, explain the reason for transfer and give the location of the receiving facility to family.

TEACHING-LEARNING

The critically ill patient requires constant intensive nursing care of life-threatening physiologic problems. However, critical care nursing also focuses on supporting psychologic and social integrity and restoring health. Teaching is an independent nursing activity that can assist the patient and family in understanding the disease process and prescribed therapies so that the patient and family are provided the necessary information and resources to maintain optimal health.

Questions should be answered honestly and procedures explained; however, teaching should not be initiated when the patient and family are feeling the impact of the illness and expressing feelings about dying, loss of control, and hopelessness. Once the patient and family express the need for explanations or discuss the events that led to the ICU hospitalization, the patient and family may be ready to learn. Learning everything one must know will not occur during the ICU hospitalization; however, the process can be initiated in the ICU.

Nursing Diagnosis: DEFICIENT KNOWLEDGE

Outcome Criteria

Patient and family will verbalize accurate understanding of illness and treatment plan.

Patient will demonstrate self-management skills.

Interventions

1. Anticipate the need for supportive services for patient and family during this crisis because ineffective coping may be a barrier to education.
2. Assess the patient's and family's perception of the illness. Be sensitive to questions asked about the illness or a demonstrated interest in the treatments and care rendered. Validate the learning need.
3. Provide an environment that is as private as possible, comfortable, and free of interruptions (e.g., reduce volume of alarms of bedside monitors while providing information to patient and family); have comfortable chair available and pull curtain or close door to patient's room.
4. Provide information by answering questions immediately, or, if possible, schedule a time to include the family and to discuss the disease process, medications, dietary restrictions, activity level, or signs and symptoms to report to a health care professional, or any procedure or therapeutic measure in which the patient is interested. Include other health care team members as needed to meet the learning needs of the patient and family. Provide interpreters to help provide important information.
5. Tailor the teaching to the patient's strengths. Take into account that fever, pain, fatigue, lack of sleep, fear, and some medications may interfere with the patient's learning. "Teaching sessions" may be incidental, but an overall plan should be developed based on the assessed needs. The plan

should include outcomes, content to be learned, and strategies to facilitate learning.

6. Recognize that signs of restlessness and inattention are barriers to learning. Teaching should be postponed and the patient's immediate needs should be addressed.

7. Provide printed materials and written information to increase patient and family recall of information. Allow opportunities for answering questions and clarifying misconceptions.

8. Discuss available support services and resources including credible health-related websites; offer to contact the service if the patient or family requests it (e.g., social worker, dietitian).

9. Forward a copy of the teaching-learning plan to the nursing staff when the patient is transferred from the ICU. Communicate the degree of learning (outcome achievement) to the staff and document the information in the chart.

10. If the patient is undergoing surgery, provide information about the surgical experience: preoperative expectations including NPO status, breathing exercises, surgical preparation, and preoperative medications. Include specifics regarding the surgical procedure. Discuss the postoperative experience: nurse availability, pain control, ET tube and communication, IV lines, tubes and equipment, C&DB, and early mobilization, and any specifics on the surgical procedure.

CASE MANAGEMENT IN THE CRITICAL CARE UNIT

Case management in the critical care unit is a collaborative team approach to providing care for critically ill patients. The team involves multidisciplinary members such as a social worker and utilization management/diagnosis-related group (DRG) specialist, among others. However, two key team members are the critical care case manager and the critical care nurse. The critical care nurse "case manages" the needs and services of the patient on a daily basis, and can identify the patient's acuity level, required treatments and services needed, and physiologic stability, whereas the critical care case manager "case manages" global activities such as insurance issues, financial needs, and discharge planning to ensure the patient receives the needed care and services delivered in an efficient cost-effective manner.[1] The case manager, in most institutions, is a registered professional nurse who assumes an advanced practice role and is viewed as the "gatekeeper" or "conductor" of the care team who coordinates, facilitates, and evaluates patient needs across the continuum of care.

Patients can be referred to the case manager from a variety of sources (Box 3-1) and for a variety of reasons, e.g., severity of illness, financial need, lodging assistance, insurance coverage, and coordinating outpatient care. Critical care nurses are in a key position to identify high-risk patients and make referrals to the case manager as well as contribute to an in-depth high-risk assessment that is instrumental in developing the plan of care. See sample tool (Figure 3-2).

The plan is monitored and evaluated to ensure the patient's needs are being met in a timely manner and that resources are being used to promote cost-effective outcomes.

Preestablished criteria and guidelines, such as those of Milliman and Robertson or InterQual, are used to ensure that acceptable utilization management practices are being met. The criteria are divided into three main categories: intensity of service (IS), severity of illness (SI), and discharge screen (DS) (Table 3-3). The patient's clinical condition and needed diagnostic and therapeutic interventions are matched to the appropriate level of care and appropriate care setting. Thus, the following questions can be asked by the critical care nurse on a daily basis:

- How sick is the patient?
- What treatments/services is the patient receiving?
- What resources does the patient require?
- Is the patient in the appropriate setting/level of care (ICU, step-down, wards, or discharge)?

PROGRESSION OF CARE ACROSS THE CONTINUUM

As the critically ill patient improves, the case manager coordinates the transfer to the next level of care. Examples of the various levels of care can be found in Table 3-4. Placement options dependent on patient needs and financial resources, location of facility, and patient/family choice. The placement referral process may take a few

---

Box 3-1 Sources of Patient Referrals

- Unit census lists
- Critical care RN
- Physicians
- Diagnosis/diagnosis-related groups (e.g., respiratory failure, subarachnoid head bleed, burn)
- Self-referrals from patients/families
- Other disciplines (e.g., dietitian, pharmacist, physical therapists)

days; thus, to optimize patient care and alleviate discharge delays, it is important that the discharge process begin when the patient is admitted to the health care setting.

Transferring to another level of care can be frightening for both the patient and family. The critical care nurse plays an important role in supporting the patient/family during this time as the patient may be physically stable, yet psychologically insecure about the move (see Intensive Care Unit Discharge on page 62).

University of Colorado Hospital
4200 E. Ninth Avenue
Denver, CO 80262

**Case Management Care Team
Initial High Risk Assessment**

Addressograph

Date of Assessment: _____

Source of info: ☐ Patient ☐ Family/Caregiver ☐ Medical Record ☐ Physician ☐ Nurse ☐ OTHER: _____
Readmission: ☐ No ☐ Yes <15 days, <30 days, <60 days
Diagnosis and Chief Complaint: _____

(Check box for each potential discharge need)

Demographics
Potential ability for returning to prior living situation
Excellent   Good   Poor   Unable to assess
☐ Home/family/friends
☐ Home/primary caretaker or other
☐ Home alone/self care
☐ Home/unable to care for self
☐ Home/home care (agency_____)
☐ Homeless/shelter
☐ Extended care facility
☐ Any person admitted who does not reside in area usually served by hospital and may need follow-up care
☐ Transfer from other hospital
☐ Financial resource issues
☐ OTHER: _____

Behavioral Factors
☐ History of non-compliance with health care plan
☐ Prior or active substance abuse
☐ Suicide attempt/Suicide ideations
☐ Active psychiatric issues
☐ Manipulative/aggressive/behavioral issues
☐ OTHER: _____

Special Care Regimen
☐ Wound care
☐ Diabetes education/coordination
☐ Renal Failure – dialysis
☐ Tube/drain/access line care
☐ Tracheotomy/Stoma care
☐ Ostomy care
☐ Nutrition needs – i.e. TPN/enteral/parental feeds
☐ SC/IM/IV therapy at home
☐ Oxygen
☐ Multiple/complex medicine regimen
☐ OTHER: _____

Age
☐ >70, living alone or with a non-capable caregiver
☐ under age of 18
☐ OTHER: _____

Social/Familial
☐ Legal: Conservator/guardianship
☐ Durable POA issues
☐ Adoption/Parenting issues/Foster care
☐ No identification of patient – John/Jane Doe
☐ No next of kin known
☐ Inter-family dilemma
☐ No known social support system
☐ Emotional/Spiritual distress/Adjustment to illness
☐ Language Barriers
☐ Transportation issues
☐ Domestic violence – suspected/actual
☐ Neglect/abuse – physical/psychological/FTT
☐ OTHER: _____

Neurological Status
☐ Chronic cognitive deficits
☐ Acute cognitive deficits
☐ OTHER: _____

Medical/Functional/Emotional Status
☐ Sensory deficits
☐ Problems with Mobility/ADL's/Swallow
☐ Chronic health conditions
☐ Trauma/Burn/CVA
☐ Joint replacement/fractures
☐ Terminal illness
☐ Head/Spinal Cord Injury
☐ New life altering diagnosis
☐ Neuromuscular degenerative disease
☐ OTHER: _____

CSM 46020 E/– (03/03) DOD   Page 1 of 2

Figure 3-2 Case management care team initial high-risk assessment. (University of Colorado Hospital, Denver. Used with permission.)

Continued

University of Colorado Hospital
4200 E. Ninth Avenue
Denver, CO 80262

Case Management Care Team
Initial High Risk Assessment

Addressograph

Anticipated Care Plan: _____
_____
_____

Anticipated Length of Stay: _____

Consultations/Referrals: (include Name, Pager, Date, Time and Reason)
☐ Clinical Social Worker: _____
☐ Financial Counselor: _____
☐ Pastoral Care: _____
☐ Interpreter: _____
☐ Rehabilitation: _____
☐ Pain Service: _____
☐ Respiratory Therapy: _____
☐ OTHER: _____

Anticipated Discharge Needs: (Check all that may apply)
☐ Home, No Identified Needs   ☐ Acute Rehabilitation
☐ Medication coordination   ☐ Sub-acute Rehabilitation
☐ Establishing PCP/Follow-up care   ☐ Long-term Care Facility Placement
☐ Home Care   ☐ Shelter/Respite Bed
☐ Long-term Care Facility Placement ☐ Hospice Care
☐ Short-term Care Facility Placement ☐ OTHER SPECIAL SERVICES: _____

Primary Care Physician: _____
                   Phone# _____

Payer Source: Primary: _____
                   Phone#: _____

                   Secondary: _____
                   Phone#: _____

                   OTHER: _____

Additional Contacts: (e.g. Community Case Manager): _____
_____

Signature _____ Title _____ Pager _____

Continuum of Care documented in Progress Notes

CSM 46020 E/– (03/03) DOD   Page 2 of 2

Figure 3-2, cont'd

INTENSIVE CARE UNIT DISCHARGE

When the critically ill patient is physiologically stable and is to be discharged from the ICU, a type of separation anxiety may be experienced. The patient is ready physically, but psychologically may not feel secure about the move to the new environment. New nurse-patient relationships must be developed as trusting ICU nurse-patient relationships are terminated and family members decide to terminate

Table 3-3 Differentiating Levels of Care

Acute care	Facility that provides acute and/or a specialty level of care for those who are critically ill, catastrophically injured, or otherwise medically compromised	Example: • Hospitals/trauma centers
Long-term acute care (LTAC)	Facility that provides comprehensive medical management for patients requiring diverse medical services and a longer acute stay	Examples of programs and services: • Ventilator weaning • Complex wound care • Post trauma—spinal cord injury, cerebral hemorrhage
Acute rehabilitation	Facility that provides aggressive therapies—physical, occupational, speech. The patient must be able to tolerate a minimum of 3 hours combined therapy per day.	Examples of patient/diagnoses: • Post-joint replacement • Cerebrovascular accident (CVA) • Long hospitalization
Subacute care	Facility that provides medical services such as rehabilitation services	Examples: • Long-term IV antibiotics • Therapies—physical therapy, occupational therapy, speech therapy: patient may tolerate up to $1\frac{1}{2}$ hours of therapy per day
Custodial care	Facility that provides long-term care for patients who are dependent on others for their daily care	Example of facility: • Nursing home
Home health	Agency that provides skilled services in a home setting	Examples of services: • Medication management • Home safety evaluation/therapies • Diabetic management • Wound care

Table 3-4 CRITERIA FOR UTILIZATION REVIEW

Severity of illness (SI)	Uses objective indicators related to the illness	Indicators include clinical, imaging, ECG, laboratory findings	Examples: Clinical—chief complaints, VS, diagnosis Laboratory—ABGs, chemistry, pulse oximetry, CSF analysis
Intensity of service (IS)	Uses diagnostic and therapeutic services	Indicators include treatments/ medications for which there are two types of IS criteria: nonasterisked IS treatments/ medications that generally cannot be provided at a less intensive level of care, and asterisked IS* treatments /medications that could be safely provided at a less costly level of care	Examples: Nonasterisked IS IV nitroglycerin can be provided only at the critical care level Asterisked IS* IV anti-infective given greater/equal to 3 times/24 hr
Discharge screen	Identifies the patient stability and readiness for discharge from a specified level of care	Indicators include parameters of clinical stability and relative safety for discharge or transfer to another level of care	Example: discharge criteria for Acute Cardiovascular: VS stable for past 8 hr; syncope, etiology ruled out; Pericardial effusion, resolving

ABGs, Arterial blood gases; *CSF,* cerebrospinal fluid; *ECG,* electrocardiogram; *VS,* vital signs.

their all-night vigils, thinking their relative is "out of danger." Thus the patient's anxiety may be heightened during a time when support systems are needed yet less available.

Nursing Diagnosis: RISK FOR RELOCATION STRESS SYNDROME

Outcome Criteria

Patient/family will recognize own anxiety and verbalize anxious feelings.

Patient/family will use appropriate coping mechanisms in controlling anxiety.

Interventions

1. Discuss transfer plans early in an ICU hospitalization.
2. Keep the patient and family informed of any improvement and present the transfer in a positive manner; emphasize the recovery and not the need for a bed.
3. Plan a structured pretransfer session and provide written information to explain what is expected of the patient and family in the new environment, such as what is restricted and what is not, and the floor routine.
4. During the ICU stay, identify patient and family learning needs about the illness, medications, and signs and symptoms to report.
5. Allow the patient and family to verbalize their feelings and acknowledge these feelings. Ideally, have the patient meet the new staff members before the actual transfer. Ensure a bedside introduction to the nurses on the receiving unit.
6. Reassure the patient about the skill and expertise of the nurses on the unit to which the patient is to be transferred.
7. Complete the transfer form or ICU summary form to facilitate continuity of care.
8. Transfer the patient during the day if at all possible so that the patient has time to become oriented to the new environment.
9. If the family is not present during the transfer, contact the family and inform them that their relative has been transferred.

REFERENCE

1. Cohen EL, Cesta TG: *Nursing case management: from essentials to advanced practice application,* ed 4, St Louis, 2005, Mosby.

BIBLIOGRAPHY

Appleyard ME et al: Nurse-coached interventions for the families of patients in critical care units, *Crit Care Nurse* 20:40-48, 2000.

Case Management Society of America: *Standards of practice for case management,* 2003.

Cesta TG, Tahan HA: *The case manager's survival guide,* ed 2, St Louis, 2003, Mosby.

Dantzker D: Adequacy of tissue oxygenation, *Crit Care Med* 21:S40-S43, 1993.

Guidelines Committee, American College of Critical Care Medicine, Society of Critical Care Medicine and the Transfer Guidelines Task Force, American Association of Critical-Care Nurses: guidelines for the transfer of critically ill patients, *Am J Crit Care* 2:189-195, 1993.

Harrington L: Nutrition in critically ill adults: key processes and outcomes, *Crit Care Nurs Clin North Am* 16(4):459-466, 2004.

Jeejeebhoy DN: Enteral and parenteral nutrition: evidence-based approach, *Proc Nutr Soc* 60:399-402, 2001.

Jesurum J: Tissue oxygenation and routine nursing procedures in critically ill patients, *J Cardiovasc Nurs* 11:12-30, 1997.

Johnson KL: Diagnostic measures to evaluate oxygenation in critically ill adults, *AACN Clin Issues* 15(4):506-520, 2004.

Langdon CD, Shriver R: Clinical issues in the care of critically ill diabetic patients, *Crit Care Nurs Q* 27:162-171, 2004.

Leske JS: Interventions to decrease family anxiety, *Crit Care Nurs* 22:61-65, 2002.

Long C, Greeneich D: Family satisfaction techniques: meeting family expectations, *Dimens Crit Care Nurs* 13:104-111, 1994.

Marini JJ: Principles of gas exchange. In Fink MP et al: *Textbook of critical care,* ed 5, Philadelphia, 2005, WB Saunders.

Marino P: Respiratory gas transport. In Marino P, *The ICU book,* Philadelphia, 1998, Lippincott Williams & Wilkins.

Mirr Jansen M, Schmitt N: Family-focused interventions, *Crit Care Nurs Clin North Am* 15:347-354, 2003.

Mitchell ML, Courtney M, Coyer F: Understanding uncertainty and minimizing families' anxiety at the time of transfer from intensive care, *Nurs Health Sci* 5(3):207-217, 2003.

Palazzo MO: Patient and family education in critical care. In Morton PG et al: *Critical care nursing: a holistic approach,* ed 8, Philadelphia, 2005, Lippincott Williams & Wilkins.

Rodriguiz L: Nutritional status: assessing and understanding its value in the critical care setting, *Crit Care Nurs Clin North Am* 16(4):509-514, 2004.

Roberts, SR, Hanedani B: Benefits and methods of achieving strict glycemic control in the ICU, *Crit Care Nurs Clin North Am* 16(4):537-546, 2004.

Sanford M, Pugh D, Warren N: Family presence during CPR: new decisions in the twenty-first century, *Crit Care Nurs Q* 25:61-66, 2002.

Stannard D: Individual and family response to the critical care experience. In Sole ML, Klein DG, Moseley MJ, eds: *Introduction to critical care nursing,* Philadelphia, 2005, WB Saunders.

Washington GT: Families in crisis, *Nurs Management* 32:28-32, 2001.

Witt MD, Chu LA: Infections in the critically ill. In Bongard FS, Sue DY: *Current critical care diagnosis and treatment,* New York, 2002, Lange Medical Books/McGraw-Hill.

4

Psychosocial Concerns of the Critically Ill Patient

CLINICAL BRIEF

Critically ill patients encounter myriad experiences and emotions when admitted into the dynamic and sometimes controlled chaotic world of critical care. The patient enters a complex setting and is immediately exposed to sophisticated technology, separated from significant others, and surrounded by strangers who move about the new environment with familiarity and professional expertise. Although the patient may feel secure in the hands of skilled and competent care providers, anxiety, anger, confusion, depression, hopelessness, powerlessness, sleep deprivation, and spiritual distress may be experienced during the critical illness.

Regardless of the specific behavioral manifestations, the critical care nurse's role is to protect the patient and reduce the risk of behavioral problems. The critical care nurse designs interventions to effectively manage selected behavioral needs.

ANXIETY

Anxiety, a subjective experience, is a state of apprehension or tension within a person that occurs when an interpersonal need for security and/or freedom from tension is not met. Anxiety's origin is nonspecific or unknown to the individual. Anxiety signals that a threat of some type encompasses the person's physical loss, lifestyle changes, potential death, invasive procedures, or concern about the future. Whereas mild anxiety can motivate a person to deal with the stressor, a higher level of anxiety can alter cognitive function and cause distraction, confusion, inability to concentrate, and altered memory. Higher levels of anxiety may also have physiologic consequences such as increasing oxygen consumption, reducing the immune response, and altering coagulation.

Risk Factors

Lack of control over events	Threats to self-control	Threats of illness or disease
Threats of hospital environment	Threat of critical care	Lack of knowledge
Separation from others	Role changes	Financial problems
Threat of death	Unemployment	Forced retirement
Threat of invasive procedures	Loss of status	Loss of decision-making power
Situational crisis	Obstruction of goals	Dependence

Presenting Signs and Symptoms

Regulatory	Cognitive
Palpitations	Apprehension
Nausea	Nervousness
Increased respiratory rate	Fear
Increased heart rate	Agitation
Diaphoresis	Irritability
Elevated blood pressure	Regression
Hand tremors	Inability to concentrate
Insomnia	Escape behavior
Faintness	Crying
Dry mouth	Loss of self-confidence
Paresthesia	Worry
Vomiting	Tension

Nursing Diagnosis: ANXIETY

Outcome Criteria

The patient recognizes the anxiety and communicates anxious feelings.

The patient's agitation eases in response to specific therapeutic relaxation interventions.

The patient, family, or significant other exhibits a reduction in anxiety.

The patient experiences an increase in physiologic comfort.

The patient initiates measures to decrease the onset of anxiety.

The patient uses appropriate coping mechanisms in controlling anxiety.

Interventions

1. Establish a reassuring interpersonal relationship with the patient.
2. Provide information about threatening or stressful situations, including invasive procedures and the sensations that might be expected.
3. Use simple terms and repetition to provide information regarding the current illness, the purpose of interventions, and changes in care.
4. Encourage patients to acknowledge and communicate their fears; clarify the patient's reaction to anxiety.
5. Use guided imagery through internal experience of memory to focus directly on positive thoughts allowing mental escape from information that causes stress.
6. Use music therapy to promote physiologic relaxation by listening to favorite music.
7. Help the patient establish goals, knowing that small accomplishments can promote feelings of independence and self-esteem and allow the patient a degree of control.
8. Give the patient positive feedback when alternative coping strategies are used to counteract feelings of anxiety.
9. Discuss the intensive care unit (ICU) transfer plans with the patient to keep the patient aware of his or her progress and impending discharge (see p. 62).
10. Administer antianxiety agents and monitor the patient's response, noting potential side effects.

ANGER

Anger is an emotional defense that occurs in an attempt to protect the individual's integrity and does not involve a destructive element. Anger is a relatively automatic response that occurs when the individual is threatened, and can be internalized or externalized. Anger may be manifested as the patient's illness, injury, or disease begins to stabilize. It may be expressed verbally or turned inward in the form of blame or depression. The critically ill patient who has always enjoyed good health experiences tremendous stress when confronted with an illness that leads to limitations, disability, or disfigurement.

Risk Factors

Blocked goal	Disappointment
Blow to self-concept	Illness perceived to be life-threatening

Physical dependence   Altered social integrity
Obstructed goal   Role changes

Presenting Signs and Symptoms

Regulatory	Cognitive
Increased blood pressure	Clenched muscles or fists
Increased pulse rate	Turned away body
Increased respirations	Avoidance of eye contact
Muscle tension	Tardiness
Perspiration	Silence
Flushed skin	Sarcasm
Nausea	Insulting remarks
Dry mouth	Verbal abuse

Nursing Diagnosis: INEFFECTIVE COPING: ANGER

Outcome Criteria

The patient is able to identify situations contributing to expressions of anger.

The patient monitors behavior leading to internalization or externalization of anger.

Interventions

1. Establish a reassuring interpersonal relationship and encourage the patient to acknowledge and express feelings of anger.
2. Assist the patient in identifying situations contributing to the expression of anger.
3. Explore with the patient reasons behind angry feelings and ways in which the patient's behavior can change.
4. Teach the patient to evaluate feelings that lead to either internalization or externalization of anger.
5. Encourage the family to accept the patient's behavior without judgment.
6. Encourage the patient to participate in decision making and self-care.
7. Provide diversional activities as ways to reduce stress.
8. Teach the patient to use progressive relaxation technique, meditation, or guided imagery to reduce feelings of anger and hostility.
9. Assist the patient in identifying positive aspects of the illness or injury and assist the patient in using alternative coping strategies.

CONFUSION

Confusion is a problem that can result from unit psychosis in which the person becomes distracted and unable to sleep at night. The result is confusion during the day when the patient is unable to integrate incoming stimuli. Confusion arises from a variety of pathologies involving circulation, oxygenation, and metabolism of the brain. The result can be inattention and memory deficits. The patient experiences inappropriate verbalization, disruptive behavior, noncompliance, and failure to perform activities of daily living.

Risk Factors

Medical Conditions	Surgical Conditions
Hypoxia	Anesthesia
Pulmonary disease	Pain medications
Congestive heart failure	Hypothermia
Electrolyte or fluid imbalance	Postoperative anxiety
Disorders of thyroid, parathyroid and adrenal glands	Agitation
Alcoholism	Depression
Dysrhythmias	
Alcohol intoxication or withdrawal	
Head trauma	
Cerebral anoxia	
Hypertensive encephalopathy	
Sensory-perceptual conditions	
Environmental overload	

Presenting Signs and Symptoms

Regulatory	Cognitive
Incontinence	Disorientation
Dysrhythmias	Impaired attention span
Increased heart rate	Agitation
Increased respiratory rate	Combativeness
Moist skin	Impaired memory

Nursing Diagnosis: ACUTE CONFUSION

Outcome Criteria

The patient is oriented to person, place, and time.
The patient recognizes family members.
The patient maintains appropriate responses to environmental stimuli.

The patient engages in appropriate conversation.

The patient differentiates reality from fantasy.

Interventions

1. Ask questions that encourage answers that reflect reality perception.
2. Protect the patient from injury while confused.
3. Identify situations or factors that might cause confusion.
4. Listen to the patient's confused statements and assist with reality orientation.
5. Listen to family concerns, fears, and anxieties.
6. Reassure the patient that the confusion is temporary.
7. Reduce the demand for cognitive functioning when the patient is ill or fatigued.
8. Use the presence of a family member to enhance mental status and comfort.
9. Use comforting tactile stimulation by back rub or holding hands with a family member to distract patient.
10. Use distraction when a patient focuses on a topic that leads to agitation or escalation of hyperactive behavior.
11. Help the patient use reorientation strategies by discussing the time of day, activity in the patient's day, or repeating explanations and information.
12. Provide appropriate lighting to minimize shadows and facilitate orientation.

DEPRESSION

Depression is any decrease in normal performance, such as slowing of psychomotor activity or reduction of intellectual functioning. It covers a wide range of changes in the affective state, ranging in severity from normal, everyday moods of sadness or despondency to psychotic episodes with risk of suicide. Depression also can result when feelings associated with a major loss have broken through an individual's defense. The patient's normal performance is decreased, leading to a perceived negative view of self, experiences, and the future. Depression is also a manifestation of felt hopelessness.

Risk Factors

Physiologic	Behavioral
Acute/chronic illnesses	Financial loss
Drugs	Loss of control

Electrolyte imbalances

Separation/loss from significant others
Loss of bodily function
Role or lifestyle changes

Presenting Signs and Symptoms

Regulatory	Cognitive
Constipation	Agitation
Diarrhea	Anger
Headaches	Anxiety
Indigestion	Avoidance
Insomnia	Sadness
Muscle aches	Confusion
Nausea	Crying
Tachycardia	Denial
Ulcers	Dependence
Weight loss or gain	Emptiness
Anorexia	Fatigue

Nursing Diagnosis: INEFFECTIVE COPING: DEPRESSION

Outcome Criteria

The patient will be able to communicate when feeling depressed.
The patient initiates measures to decrease feelings of depression.
The patient uses appropriate coping mechanisms in controlling depression.

Interventions

1. Assist the patient in identifying situations that contribute to feelings of depression.
2. Encourage the patient to discuss the illness, treatment, or prognosis.
3. Assist the patient in achieving a positive view of self by facilitating accurate perception of the illness, disease, or injury.
4. Assist the patient in establishing realistic goals, knowing that small accomplishments can enhance positive feelings of the future.
5. Encourage the patient to participate in self-care and to assume decision-making control in the care.
6. Assist the patient in facilitating realistic appraisal of role changes.
7. Administer antidepressive agents and monitor the patient's response, noting any potential side effects.

HOPELESSNESS

Hopelessness is an emotional state displaying the sense of impossibility, the feeling that life is too much to handle. It is a subjective state in which an individual sees limited or no alternatives or personal choices available and is unable to mobilize energy in own behalf. Hopelessness is associated with the patient's feeling of personal deficit and is an attempt to ward off feelings of despair. The critically ill patient may feel that a particular physiologic alteration is irreversible and that there are no alternatives available. Generally the patient is unable to cope and unable to mobilize energy on his or her own behalf.

Risk Factors

Threats to Internal Resources	Threats to External Resources
Autonomy	Environment
Self-esteem	Staff
Independence	Family
Strength	Abandonment
Integrity	
Biological security	

Presenting Signs and Symptoms

Regulatory	Cognitive
Weight loss	Noncompliance with treatment regimen
Appetite loss	Lack of initiative
Weakness	Decreased response to stimuli
Sleep disorder	Passivity

Nursing Diagnosis: HOPELESSNESS

Outcome Criteria

The patient will regain adequate self-care.
The patient will assess situations causing feelings of hopelessness.
The patient will identify feelings of hopelessness and goals for self.
The patient will maintain relationships with significant others.

Interventions

1. Provide an atmosphere of realistic hope.
2. Inform the patient of progress with the illness, disease, or injury.

3. Teach the patient how to identify feelings of hopelessness and encourage the patient to accept help from others.
4. Encourage the patient to express feelings about self and illness by active listening and asking open-ended questions.
5. Evaluate whether physical discomfort is causing the patient's feeling of hopelessness.
6. Create the environment to facilitate the patient's active participation in self-care.
7. Encourage physical activities that give the patient a feeling of progress and hope.
8. Provide the patient with positive feedback for successful attempts at becoming involved in self-care.
9. Assist the patient in identifying and using alternative coping mechanisms.

POWERLESSNESS

Powerlessness is the perceived lack of control over current and future physiologic, psychologic, and environmental situations. The patient feels unable to control the outcomes of the illness. In this instance, the critically ill patient feels physiologic, cognitive, environmental, and decisional powerlessness.

Risk Factors

Sensorimotor loss
Lack of knowledge or privacy
Inability to control personal care
Lack of decision-making control
Inability to communicate
Social isolation
Separation from significant others
Fear of pain

Presenting Signs and Symptoms

Regulatory	Cognitive
Tiredness	Apathy
Fatigue	Withdrawal
Dizziness	Resignation
Headache	Empty feeling
Nausea	Lack of control
	Fatalism
	Sleeplessness
	Lack of decision making
	Aggression
	Dependence on others

Nursing Diagnosis: POWERLESSNESS

Outcome Criteria

The patient identifies situations causing feelings of powerlessness.

The patient exhibits control over the illness and care.

The patient experiences an increase in physiologic control.

The patient engages in problem-solving and decision-making behaviors.

The patient seeks information about the illness, treatment, and prognosis.

The patient establishes realistic goals that foster an increased sense of control.

Interventions

1. Assign consistent health care members to provide care and information regarding the illness, treatment, and prognosis.
2. Encourage the patient to express feelings about self and illness and situations in which powerlessness is felt.
3. Encourage the use of progressive relaxation, meditation, and guided imagery techniques to achieve a sense of acceptance or uncontrol (letting go).
4. Encourage the patient to ask questions, seek information, and participate in making decisions pertaining to self-care.
5. Teach the patient how to accept the illness and potential changes in lifestyle.
6. Listen to the patient's discussion regarding possible role changes and financial concerns and assist the patient in redefining the illness situation to identify positive aspects.

SLEEP DEPRIVATION

Sleep deprivation occurs when sleep need is at its greatest level and is a significant stressor for patients in critical care. Sleep deprivation is the lack of adequate sleep or dream time related to previous or unusual sleep patterns. Sleep deprivation in critical care patients can result in decreased healing, making patients more susceptible to infection. Critically ill patients experience a lack of sleep or frequent disruption of sleep that further compounds their illness. Psychologic stressors may require more rapid eye movement (REM) sleep at a time when they have less restful sleep.

Risk Factors

Excessive noise	Stress	Lack of exercise
Pain	Illness	Depression
Anxiety	Medications	Loneliness
Disrupted sleep		

Presenting Signs and Symptoms

Regulatory	Cognitive
Non-REM sleep regulatory behaviors	Lassitude
Decreased blood pressure	Lethargy
Decreased heart rate	Hallucinations
Decreased urine volume	Disorientation
Decreased plasma volume	Confusion
Decreased metabolic rate	Restlessness
Decreased oxygen consumption	Irritability
Decreased carbon dioxide expiration	Apathy
REM sleep regulatory behaviors	Poor judgment
Increased heart rate	Memory disturbance
Increased respiratory rate	Delusions
Increased blood pressure	Paranoid ideation
Increased catecholamine level	Hostility

Nursing Diagnosis: SLEEP DEPRIVATION

Outcome Criteria

The patient sleeps through the night.
The patient identifies techniques to help induce sleep.
The patient sleeps for 90-minute segments and feels refreshed.
The patient displays no irritability, lethargy, or confusion.

Interventions

1. Evaluate the frequency and length of daytime naps.
2. Adhere to the patient's bedtime ritual.
3. Eliminate extraneous stimuli such as lights, unnecessary activities, noise, and staff verbal exchange, when realistic.
4. Provide a choice of music or music video to facilitate sleep.
5. Encourage the use of guided imagery through scenes like walking in the woods or watching a sunset.
6. Darken unit lights during normal sleep hours to maintain the circadian light cycles necessary for the patient to achieve healthy sleep.
7. Adjust room temperature and provide blankets for comfort.

8. Schedule treatments, including medications and procedures before sleep, if realistic.
9. Provide daytime activity, such as range-of-motion exercises, sitting, standing, or walking.
10. Encourage patients to increase their activity level during the day so that they can sleep at night.
11. Position patients so that they are comfortable.
12. Provide earplugs to eliminate extraneous environmental stimuli, if necessary.

SPIRITUAL DISTRESS

Critically ill patients have spiritual needs. A spiritual need is any need related to a person's beliefs, practices, habits, customs, and rituals. Spiritual distress is a situation in which individuals question the belief or value system that provides hope and meaning to their lives. Spiritual distress can result when illness causes patients to question their belief system. At this time the patient feels temporarily alone and without hope. The meaning in the patient's life is distorted by the illness.

Risk Factors

Disease or illness
Personal or family disasters
Distress related to treatments or invasive procedures
Trauma
Loss of significant others
Being embarrassed by others

Presenting Signs and Symptoms

Regulatory	Cognitive
Increased blood pressure	Sense of spiritual emptiness
Increased heart rate	Questions belief system
Increased respiratory rate	Ambivalence regarding values and beliefs

Nursing Diagnosis: SPIRITUAL DISTRESS

Outcome Criteria

The patient maintains and practices spiritual beliefs.
The patient experiences decreased feelings of abandonment or guilt.
The patient is satisfied with personal events.
The patient feels a sense of closeness to family and beliefs.

Interventions

1. Recognize own personal value and belief system.
2. Uses clergy as needed or appropriate.
3. Assist the patient with spiritual reading when requested.
4. Provide privacy so that the patient can practice spiritual rituals.
5. Allow the patient to talk about personal values and beliefs, especially when these may conflict with those of significant others.
6. Help patient identify previous sources of spiritual support resources if so desired by patient or family.
7. Encourage diet with religious restrictions when not detrimental to health.
8. Ask questions about the patient's personal past and belief systems that can be used to help her or him get through the present crisis.
9. Provide a reality base when the patient attributes pain, suffering, or illness to punishment for past wrongdoing.

BIBLIOGRAPHY

Barefoot K, Nagel C, Markie M: Use of complementary and alternative therapies to promote sleep in critically ill patients, *Crit Care Nurs Clin North Am* 15:329-340, 2003.

Evans D: The effectiveness of music as an intervention for hospital patients: a systematic review. *J Adv Nurs* 37:8-18, 2002.

Frazier SK, Moser DK, Riegel B: Critical care nurses' assessment of patients' anxiety: reliance on physiological and behavioral parameters, *Am J Crit Care* 11:52-64, 2002.

Fraiser SK, Mosier DK, Dalkey LK: Critical care nurses' belief about and reported management of anxiety, *Am J Crit Care* 12:19-27, 2003.

Guzzetta C: Critical care research: weaving a body-mind-spirit tapestry, *Am J Crit Care* 13:320-327, 2004.

Halm MH, Myers RN, Bennetts P: Providing spiritual care to cardiac patients' assessment and implications for practice, *Crit Care Nurs* 20:54-72, 2000.

Honkus UL: Sleep deprivation in critical care units, *Crit Care Nurs Quart* 26:179-191, 2003.

Jansen MJ, Schmitt N: Family-focused intervention, *Crit Care Nurs Clin North Am* 15:347-354, 2003.

Justic M: Does "ICU psychosis" really exist? *Crit Care Nurs* 20:28-37, 2000.

Keegan K: Therapies to reduce stress and anxiety, *Crit Care Nurs Clin North Am* 15:321-327, 2003.

Maclean SL, Guzzetrta C, White C: Family presence during cardiopulmonary resuscitation and invasive procedures: practices of critical care and emergency nurses, *Am J Crit Care* 12:246-257, 2003.

Paul S, Sneed NV: Strategies for behavior change in patients with heart failure, *Am J Crit Care* 13:305-313, 2004.

Riegel B, Bennett JA, Davis A: Cognitive impairment in heart failure: issues of measurement and etiology, *Am J Crit Care* 11:520-528, 2002.

Tacon AM, McComb J, Caldera Y: Mindfulness meditation, anxiety reduction, and heart disease: a pilot study, *Fam Comm Health* 16:25-33, 2003.

The Critically Ill Patient

NEUROLOGIC DISORDERS

ACUTE SPINAL CORD INJURY

Clinical Brief

Nearly 12,000 individuals sustain a spinal cord injury in the United States annually; 54% of these injuries are at the cervical spine and complete, resulting in tetraplegia. The most common cause or acute spinal cord injury is trauma: motor vehicle accidents, falls, assault-related trauma, and sports injuries. Damage to the cord also may be related to tumor; abscess; spinal artery hypoperfusion, infarction, or hemorrhage; acute disk herniation; or other pathologic conditions of the spine, such as congenital malformations, myelitis, or arthritis. There is no effective treatment in promoting recovery or repairing the damaged spinal cord.

Complete cord injuries may be acute, occurring over minutes, or subacute, occurring over hours to weeks. Typically the initial trauma involves compression and contusion of the spinal cord, leading to immediate damage of spinal neurons and blood vessels. Other mechanisms of injury include transection from a missile injury or bone fragment dislocation and distraction or traumatic stretching of the spinal column along the length of the spinal cord. Secondary injuries from hypoperfusion, hypoxia, and inflammation either systemically or at the site of injury can exacerbate the primary injury. Complete injuries are associated with total loss of all motor, sensory, and autonomic functions below the level of the injury. Cervical cord injury is associated with a loss of motor function in the upper and lower extremities (tetraplegia), whereas injuries below the cervicothoracic junction affect only the lower extremities (paraplegia).

Incomplete spinal cord injuries can result from penetrating trauma, disk or vertebral injury, and cord compression or contusion.

There is some sparing of motor and/or sensory function below the level of injury. Box 5-1 lists various syndromes associated with incomplete injuries.

Spinal shock is a state characterized by loss of reflexes and flaccid paralysis that occurs immediately after the injury. The loss of sensorimotor and autonomic function below the level of injury is temporary and usually resolves within days to several weeks. The appearance of involuntary spastic movement indicates that spinal shock has ended. Spinal shock is sequelae of cord injury and resolves over time as the initial injury resolves.

Neurogenic shock is a syndrome associated with cervical or high thoracic injury characterized by unopposed parasympathetic stimulation; sympathetic nervous system modulation may be lost with cervical spinal injury. Neurogenic shock is characterized by hypotension resulting from the vasodilation of the vascular beds below the level of injury, bradycardia, and the loss of the ability to sweat below the level of injury. Neurogenic shock is a critical care emergency and needs immediate treatment.

Presenting Signs and Symptoms

The signs and symptoms depend on the level and degree of injury (Table 5-1; see also Box 5-1).

Physical Examination

Box 5-1 and Table 5-1 describe spinal cord injuries and corresponding functional losses.
Vital signs:
  Neurogenic shock
  Blood pressure (BP): hypotension
  Heart rate (HR): bradycardia
  Temperature: hypothermia—96° to 98° F (35.5°-36.6° C)

Diagnostic Findings

A combination of tests and clinical presentation confirms the diagnosis of vertebral and/or spinal cord injury in the presence of altered mental status, abnormal neurologic examination, neck pain or tenderness, and other major injuries.

Spinal Radiography

Confirms the type and location of vertebral fracture. Three views are typically obtained immediately (e.g., cross-table lateral, anteroposterior, open-mouth odontoid spinal radiographs).

Table 5-1 COMPLETE SPINAL CORD SEGMENTAL LESION AND CORRESPONDING ACUTE FUNCTIONAL LOSS

Spinal Level	Muscles	Dermatome	Acute Dysfunction	At Risk for
C1-2	All muscles below trapezius, sternocleidomastoid	Back of head	Tetraplegia (complete); total loss of independent respiratory function; total loss of motor and sensory function from neck down	Death, hypotension, bradycardia, dysrhythmias, hypothermia, ileus, atonic bladder, skin breakdown
C3-5 C5	Diaphragm Trapezius	Ear; neckline from clavicle to wrist	Tetraplegia (complete); minimal or absent diaphragmatic function; absent intercostal respiratory effort; loss of all motor function below shoulders and sensation below clavicles	Hypotension, bradycardia, dysrhythmias, hypothermia, ileus, atonic bladder, skin breakdown
C6	Deltoid, biceps, and external rotator muscles of shoulders	Lateral third of arm, shoulder to thumb and index finger	Tetraplegia (complete); decreased respiratory function: absent intercostal respiratory effort (diaphragm intact); can move head, shoulders, with some gross arm flexion	Same as above
C7	Latissimus, serratus, pectoralis, radial wrist extensors	Dorsal and palmar midarm to first two digits	Tetraplegia (incomplete); decreased respiratory function: absent intercostal respiratory effort (diaphragm intact); can flex and extend elbow	Same as above

Continued

Table 5-1 COMPLETE SPINAL CORD SEGMENTAL LESION AND CORRESPONDING ACUTE FUNCTIONAL LOSS—cont'd

Spinal Level	Muscles	Dermatome	Acute Dysfunction	At Risk for
C8	Triceps, finger extensors and flexors	Medial third of arm, including digits three and four	Tetraplegia (incomplete); decreased respiratory function: decreased intercostal effort (diaphragm intact); some intrinsic hand function, thumb and index pincher movement present	Same as above
T1	Hand intrinsics, ulnar, wrist, and fingers	Medial arm, axilla	Paraplegia; decreased respiratory function with diaphragmatic breathing; arm function intact; finger spreading, grip and wrist flexion present	Same as above
T2-6	Upper intercostals, upper back	T4 is at nipple line	Paraplegia; some use of intercostal muscles; good upper body strength; loss of bowel and bladder function; loss of leg function; can stand with braces	Ileus, atonic bladder, skin breakdown

T6-12	Abdominals, thoracic extensors	T10 is at umbilicus; T12 is at groin	Paraplegia; no interference with respiratory function; loss of bowel and bladder function; paralysis of legs; can ambulate with braces	Atonic bladder, fecal retention
L1-4	Iliopsoas	Groin, upper thigh and knee	With injuries below L2, sensorimotor, bowel, bladder, and sexual function may be affected, depending on nerve root damage in the acute phase	—
L2-4	Quadriceps	Anterior thigh, knee, and lower leg		
L5-S2	Hamstrings, extensor digitorum, gluteus maximus, gastrocnemius	Great toe, lateral foot, sole, Achilles, posterior thigh	Injuries above the sacrum convert to reflexes, and bowel and bladder are uninhibited when reflexes return; with sacral injuries they are likely to retain atonic bowel and bladder secondary to absent reflexes	—
S3-5	Bowel and bladder sphincters	Genitals, saddle area		—

Box 5-1 Incomplete Spinal Cord Lesion and Corresponding Acute Functional Loss

Anterior Cord Syndrome

Anterior cord syndrome is caused by damage to or an infarction of the anterior two thirds of the spinal cord. Typically, hyperflexion injuries of the cervical spine cause vertebral bone fragments or disk material to compress the anterior spinal artery, which supplies two thirds of the anterior cord; the posterior portion of the spinal cord is spared.

Patient Presentation

Pain and temperature (spinothalamic function) are absent below the level of the lesion.

Complete paralysis is present below the level of the lesion. Movement (motor function) is absent below the level of the lesion.

Position, pressure, and vibration (posterior column function) is spared.

Unusual sensitivity to sensory stimuli (hyperesthesia) and lessened sensitivity to pain (hypalgesia) are present below the level of the lesion.

Central Cord Syndrome

This syndrome is caused by damage or edema to the center portion of the spinal cord in the cervical region. There is central squeezing of the cord, but the periphery of the cord is spared. A hyperextension injury can cause buckling of the ligamentum flavum, which in turn puts a "squeeze" on the cord as the column bends, interrupting the blood supply. This syndrome is usually associated with degenerative arthritis or osteophytic changes in the cervical vertebrae.

Patient Presentation

Motor loss in the upper extremities is greater than in the lower extremities, more profound in hands and fingers.

Leg function is usually intact but may be weak.

Sensory loss in upper extremities is greater than in lower extremities and more profound in hands and fingers.

Bowel and bladder problems may or may not be present; some saddle sensation is retained.

Posterior Cord Syndrome

Posterior cord syndrome is a very rare condition in which the posterior third of the spinal cord is affected. It is usually caused by a hyperextension injury or a direct penetrating mechanism, such as a knife wound.

Patient Presentation

Positional sense, vibration, and light touch are absent below the level of the lesion. Motor function, pain, and temperature sense are usually intact.

Brown-Séquard Syndrome

Brown-Séquard syndrome is usually caused by a transverse hemisection of the cord. Damage is to one side of the cord only and is usually associated with a penetrating injury, herniated disk, or bone fragment. True hemisection is rare; a partial Brown-Séquard syndrome with varying degrees of paresis and analgesia is more common.

Patient Presentation

Position, vibration, and light touch sensation on the same side of the body (ipsilateral) is absent below the level of the lesion.

Motor function on the same side of the body (ipsilateral) is absent below the level of the lesion.

Pain and temperature sensation on the opposite side of the body (contralateral) is absent below the level of the lesion.

Horner's Syndrome

This syndrome is caused by a partial cord transection at T1 or above. A lesion of either the preganglionic sympathetic trunk or the postganglionic sympathetic neurons of the superior cervical ganglion will result in this syndrome.

Patient Presentation

The pupil on the same side (ipsilateral) of the injury is smaller (miosis) than the opposite pupil.

The ipsilateral eyeball sinks (enophthalmos) and the affected eyelid droops (ptosis).

The ipsilateral side of the face does not sweat (anhidrosis).

Difficulty in speaking or hoarseness (dysphonia) may occur with hyperextension injury to the cervical cord that also causes injury to the laryngeal nerve.

Oblique, flexion, and extension views may be obtained subsequently.

May visualize tumors, arthritic changes, and congenital abnormalities

Computed Tomography (CT) Scan

Visualizes bony anatomy, fractures, and soft tissue lesions not detected on radiographs in symptomatic or unconscious patients. Some evidence that helical CT views provide superior examination of the spine

Reflects compromise of the spinal canal or nerve roots by bony fragments or extensive fractures

Magnetic Resonance Imaging (MRI)

Identifies extent of spinal cord damage, degree of cord contusion, and soft tissue lesions

Differentiates blood and edema

Demonstrates disk and soft tissue injury, subtle fractures, and chronic changes to the cord

ACUTE CARE PATIENT MANAGEMENT

Goals of Treatment

Immobilize and stabilize the spine; reduce spinal fractures.

Cervical collar or thoracic/lumbar brace

Cervical traction with Gardner-Wells tong

Halo brace

Surgery: decompression laminectomy, spinal fusion, and spinal instrumentation

Prevent secondary injury.

Avoid overdistention and rotation

Administer methylprednisolone if within 8 hours of injury

Support cardiopulmonary function.

Baseline electrocardiogram (ECG) and serum cardiac profile, if patient older than 40 years of age

Supplemental oxygen to maintain SpO_2 >95%

Intubation and mechanical ventilation

Consider fiberoptic intubation to maintain cervical alignment; avoid neck hyperextension.

Kinetic bed to aid secretion clearance.

Suction as needed to maintain airway and oxygenation.

Consider use of inhaled bronchodilator.

Crystalloid infusions to avoid hypotension.

Inotropic and/or vasopressor agents to avoid hypotension.

Atropine for bradycardia.

Deep vein thrombosis (DVT) prophylaxis.

Decrease/alleviate pain and muscle spasms.

Analgesics (e.g., ketorolac, hydromorphone, fentanyl).

Muscle relaxants (e.g., diazepam, baclofen, dantrolene sodium).

Detect/prevent clinical sequelae (Table 5-2).

Table 5-2 Clinical Sequelae of Acute Spinal Cord Injuries*

Complication	Signs and Symptoms
Respiratory insufficiency or arrest	Increasing work of breathing, NIF >−30, VC <15 mL/kg, shallow and rapid respirations, cessation of breathing
Spinal shock	Flaccid, total paralysis of all skeletal muscles, loss of spinal reflexes, loss of sensation (pain, proprioception, touch, temperature, and pressure) below the level of injury, bowel and bladder dysfunction, and possible priapism
Neurogenic shock	Symptomatic hypotension: SBP <90 mm Hg or MAP <70 mm Hg Bradycardia: HR <50 beats/min
Hypothermia	Temperature <98.6° F (<37° C) due to impaired skin innervation, responsiveness
Autonomic dysreflexia (hyperreflexia)	Occurs only in patients with injuries above the T6 level once recovered from spinal shock and reflex activity has returned; paroxysmal hypertension (SBP 240-300 mm Hg), with bradycardia, pounding headache, blurred vision, vasodilation, flushing, profuse sweating, piloerection (gooseflesh) above the level of lesion, nasal congestion, nausea, possible chest pain; if not controlled, status epilepticus, stroke, and death possible. Generally does not occur with acute injury.
Orthostatic hypotension	Dizziness, lightheadedness, loss of consciousness, drop in SBP when assuming an upright position
Immobility	Contractures, muscle wasting, mood alteration (depression)
DVT and/or PE	Related to immobility and potential for coagulopathy
Urine and fecal retention	Due to impaired innervation and immobility. Can act as a stimulus for autonomic dysreflexia
Infection	Due to invasive lines and high-dose steroid therapy
Pressure ulcer	Due to altered skin perfusion, immobility, and high-dose steroid therapy. Can act as a stimulus to autonomic dysreflexia
Gastritis and/or GI ulcer	Due to physiologic stress and high-dose steroid therapy
Ileus and/or pancreatitis	Due to unopposed parasympathetic stimulation with high thoracic and cervical injuries

DVT, Deep vein thrombosis; *GI*, gastrointestinal; *HR*, heart rate; *NIF*, negative inspiratory force; *PE*, pulmonary embolus; *SBP*, systolic blood pressure; *VC*, vital capacity.
*Above T6 level.

Priority Nursing Diagnoses and Potential Complications

Priority Nursing Diagnoses	PC: Potential Complications
Risk for injury	Ascending injury due to spinal cord hemorrhage or edema or unstable spinal cord (i.e., inadequate immobilization)
Impaired gas exchange	Acute respiratory failure, atelectasis,
Impaired spontaneous ventilation	pneumonia, aspiration, hypoxemia, pulmonary embolus
Decreased cardiac output	Hypoperfusion, bradycardia, hypotension
Ineffective breathing pattern	Atelectasis, pneumonia
Ineffective airway clearance	Hypoxemia, mucus plug
Risk for ineffective protection (see p. 48)	
Imbalanced nutrition: less than body requirements (see p. 53)	
Risk for interrupted family processes (see p. 45)	

Nursing Diagnosis: RISK FOR INJURY related to displacement of fracture, neurogenic shock, or ascending cord edema

Outcome Criteria

Absence of progressive neurologic dysfunction
Improved sensory, motor, and reflex functions

Patient Monitoring

1. Monitor mean arterial pressure (MAP), central venous pressure (CVP), and pulmonary artery (PA) pressures (if available) to evaluate fluid volume status; overhydration and dehydration can adversely affect spinal cord circulation.

Patient Assessment

1. Assess neck pain and tenderness using the patient's self-report whenever possible and evaluate the patient's response to pain interventions.
2. Determine baseline motor function (strength and tone) and conduct ongoing assessments for changes that may indicate increasing cord edema (see Box 5-1 and Table 5-1).

3. Assess baseline sensory level (pain, light touch, and positional sense) and mark level of sensation on the patient's body (Figure 5-1). Conduct ongoing assessments to determine improvement or deterioration. Also note the patient's reports of paresthesia (numbness or tingling) in extremities.

4. Observe for priapism, assess rectal tone, and note reflexive activity to evaluate course of spinal shock and/or return of neurologic function.

5. Assess the patient for clinical sequelae (see Table 5-2).

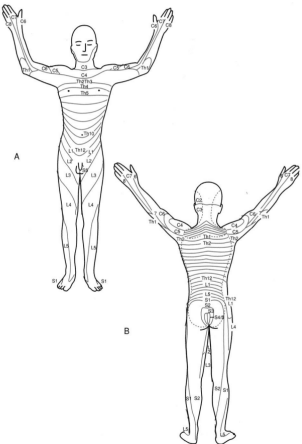

Figure 5-1 Dermstomes from anterior (A) and posterior (B) views.

Diagnostics Assessment

Review serial radiographs for proper spinal alignment.

Patient Management

1. Maintain the patient's neck in alignment until tongs or a halo ring is applied; avoid neck flexion, extension, lateral movement, or rotation.

2. Record the amount of weights necessary to achieve realignment. Ensure that the weights hang free and that the body is in proper alignment for optimal traction. If vertebral alignment of the neck is incorrect, additional weights will be applied to the tongs and follow-up lateral cervical radiographs will be taken until realignment is reached. Ensure proper body alignment, especially if a kinetic bed is used.

3. Administer methylprednisolone if ordered (this treatment is considered controversial). Generally indicated within the first 3 hours after nonpenetrating injury. Initiate with a bolus dose of 30 mg/kg intravenously (IV) over 1 hour, then start a maintenance infusion of 5.4 mg/kg/hr for the next 23 hours (or up to 48 hours if the loading dose is given between 3 and 8 hours after the initial trauma). Muscle relaxants (e.g., diazepam, baclofen) and analgesics (e.g., ketorolac, hydromorphone, fentanyl, and morphine sulfate) may be ordered to decrease pain and/or muscle spasms to facilitate spinal realignment.

4. Anticipate surgical management in patients with spinal cord compression.

Nursing Diagnoses: IMPAIRED GAS EXCHANGE related to alveolar hypoventilation; INEFFECTIVE BREATHING PATTERN secondary to paresis or paralysis of respiratory muscles; INEFFECTIVE AIRWAY CLEARANCE related to bronchial secretions and impaired cough

Outcome Criteria

Alert and oriented
O_2 sat ≥95%
Pao_2 80 to 100 mm Hg
$Paco_2$ 35 to 45 mm Hg
Vital capacity (VC) 15 mL/kg
Negative inspiratory force (NIF) greater than −30 cm H_2O
Tidal volume (V_T) >5 mL/kg
Respiratory rate (RR) 12 to 20 breaths/min, eupnea

HR 60 to 100 beats/min
Systolic blood pressure (SBP) 90 to 140 mm Hg
MAP 85 to 120 mm Hg
Lungs clear to auscultation

Patient Monitoring

1. Continuously monitor ECG because dysrhythmias such as tachycardia and bradycardia can contribute to hypoperfusion and secondary injury.
2. Continuously monitor oxygen saturation with pulse oximetry (SpO_2). Monitor interventions and patient activities that may adversely affect oxygen saturation.
3. Monitor spontaneous ventilation, NIF, V_T, and VC every 4 to 8 hours. Decreasing values suggest loss of intercostal and abdominal muscle motion and strength and are parameters for predicting impending respiratory failure that requires intubation and mechanical ventilation (hypoxemia and hypercapnia may be late findings).

Patient Assessment

1. Assess for dyspnea, breathlessness, and sensation of choking or gagging.
2. Assess RR, pattern, use of accessory muscles, and the ability to cough and strength of cough hourly (or more frequently if indicated) for the first 24 to 48 hours, then every 4 hours if the patient's condition remains stable. Inspect chest expansion for symmetry and for assessment of intercostal muscle strength, and observe epigastric area to assess diaphragmatic function. Increasing difficulty in swallowing or coughing may indicate ascending cord edema. If halo traction has been placed, check to see that the fiberglass vest does not restrict ventilatory efforts.
3. Auscultate all lung fields and record breath sounds every 2 to 4 hours. Be alert to areas of absent or decreasing breath sounds or to the development of adventitious sounds (i.e., crackles, rhonchi). Hypoventilation is common and leads to accumulation of secretions, atelectasis, and possible pneumonia.
4. Assess for signs of respiratory distress (e.g., patient's complaints of shortness of breath [SOB], shallow and rapid respirations, VC <15 mL/kg, and changes in sensorium). Evaluate speech for changes in tone or duration of sentences as a precursor to respiratory distress or failure.

5. Assess abdomen, including palpation for distention and auscultation for bowel sounds of all four quadrants. Paralytic ileus and abdominal distention can interfere with respirations and potentiates the risk for aspiration.

6. Assess the patient for clinical sequelae (see Table 5-2).

Diagnostics Assessment

1. Review serial arterial blood gases (ABGs) for adequacy of gas exchange.

2. Review serial chest radiographs to evaluate pulmonary congestion and possible development of atelectasis, consolidation, or pneumonia.

3. Review a flat plate radiograph of the abdomen (as available) if distention persists.

4. Review serial hemoglobin (Hgb) and hematocrit (Hct) levels to detect possible blood loss from internal bleeding. Oxygen carrying capacity can be adversely affected with blood loss.

Patient Management

1. Decrease factors that increase oxygen demand, such as pain, fever, and anxiety.

2. Consider use of laryngeal mask if endotracheal intubation cannot be performed. Consider use of kinetic therapy to manage secretions and enhance ventilatory effort, especially during period of early immobilization.

3. Avoid aspiration. If cervical injury is present, or has not been ruled out, do not hyperextend the patient's neck for oral intubation—use the jaw-thrust method or fiberoptic approach to intubate and prevent further cervical injury.

4. Once the spinal cord injury is stabilized, promote pulmonary hygiene: incentive spirometry, cough and deep breathing (C&DB), chest physiotherapy, and position changes every 2 hours. Position the patient in a reverse Trendelenburg at 30-degree backrest elevation to avoid ventilator-associated pneumonia. Position the patient for effective chest excursion. A kinetic bed may be used to promote mobilization of secretions. If the patient is unable to cough effectively, manually assist by placing the palm of the hand under the diaphragm (between the xiphoid and umbilicus) and push up on the abdominal muscles as the patient exhales.

NEURO

5. Administer oxygen as ordered. Mechanical ventilation may be required. (See p. 503 for information on ventilation therapies.)
6. Suction the patient's secretions if needed. Hyperoxygenate the patient's lungs before suctioning and limit pass of the suction catheter to 15 seconds or less to avoid periods of desaturation and bradycardia. Document the quality and quantity of secretions.
7. Check patency and functioning of the nasogastric (NG) tube every 2 to 4 hours because abdominal distention can impair diaphragmatic breathing.
8. Conduct passive range of motion (ROM) exercises and apply antiembolism stockings to promote venous return and decrease the risk for DVT and pulmonary embolism (PE). Sequential compression devices may be used. Measure thigh and calf circumference to detect any increase in size that may suggest DVT. Prophylactic subcutaneous heparin/low-molecular-weight heparin (LMWH) may be ordered, but it is contraindicated if internal bleeding or splenic injury is suspected.

Nursing Diagnosis: DECREASED CARDIAC OUTPUT related to relative hypovolemia and bradycardia secondary to neurogenic shock

Outcome Criteria

Alert and oriented
SBP 90 to 140 mm Hg
MAP 85 to 120 mm Hg
HR 60 to 100 beats/min
CVP 2 to 6 mm Hg
Pulmonary artery systolic (PAS) 15 to 30 mm Hg
Pulmonary artery diastolic (PAD) 5 to 15 mm Hg
Pulmonary artery wedge pressure (PAWP) 4 to 12 mm Hg
Cardiac index (CI) 2.5 to 4 L/min/m^2
Systemic vascular resistance index (SVRI) 1700 to 2600 dynes/sec/cm^{-5}/m^2
Peripheral pulses strong and equal
Urine output 30 mL/hr or 0.5 to 1 mL/kg/hr

Patient Monitoring

1. Monitor ECG rhythm and rate. Bradycardia and sinus pauses are common complications in acute cervical injuries. Hypothermia may aggravate bradycardia.

2. Continuously monitor BP and peripheral circulation because neurogenic shock or autonomic dysreflexia can cause fluctuations in BP. Note adverse changes in BP that may be related to patient position.

3. CVP and PA pressure monitoring (if available) may be used to evaluate fluid volume status. Fluid volume overload may lead to pulmonary edema. Obtain cardiac output (CO)/CI; monitor SVRI.

4. Measure intake and output (I&O) hourly and determine fluid volume balance every shift. Urinary output <30 mL/hr for 2 consecutive hours may signal decreased renal perfusion secondary to decreased CO.

Patient Assessment

1. Assess for dizziness or decreased mentation, especially with position change.

2. Assess skin temperature and color, capillary refill, and peripheral pulses as indicators of CO.

3. Evaluate orthostatic BP and HR with vertical position changes.

4. Conduct comprehensive, systematic, and consistent assessment for pressure ulcers due to hypoperfusion and immobility.

5. Assess the patient for clinical sequelae (see Table 5-2).

Diagnostics Assessment

None

Patient Management

1. Optimize venous return or decrease risk of hypotension by changing the patient's position slowly and performing passive ROM exercises every 1 to 2 hours. If necessary, elevate lower extremities to support BP. Use antiembolism hose, Ace wraps to legs, and/or abdominal binder when getting the patient out of bed.

2. Administer intravenous crystalloids (e.g., lactated Ringer's [LR] or normal saline [NS]) as ordered to maintain hydration and circulatory volume and to control mild hypotension. Monitor for mild dehydration or overhydration because both conditions can compromise spinal circulation.

3. Phenylephrine hydrochloride (Neo-Synephrine), dopamine, or dobutamine may be ordered to support BP related to compromised sympathetic outflow. Titrate infusions to desired effect.

4. Administer atropine as ordered to treat symptomatic brady-dysrhythmias.
5. Implement pressure ulcer prevention strategies.

ARTERIOVENOUS MALFORMATION (AVM)

Clinical Brief

AVMs are malformations of the cerebrovascular system in which tortuous, tangled, and malformed arterial channels drain directly into the venous system without an intervening capillary bed. The arteries supplying the AVM tend to dilate with time as a result of increased flow through the lesion. Likewise, the veins enlarge as the flow increases, creating a vicious cycle that can make these lesions increase in size. This large flow or shunting of blood through the AVM can render adjacent areas (and sometimes distal areas) of the brain ischemic. The high flow state can lead to increased pressure and eventually hemorrhage, typically into the subarachnoid space and parenchymal tissue.

Presenting Signs and Symptoms

Headache, seizures, syncope, and progressive neurologic deficits may be present. A devastating hemorrhage can result in a comatose, moribund state.

Physical Examination

Vital signs:
    BP: normotensive or hypertensive
    HR: mild tachycardia may be present
    RR: eupnea
Neurologic: depending on the area of the brain in which the AVM is located, there may be speech, motor, or sensory deficits. There also may be problems with vision, memory, and coordination.

Diagnostic Findings

CT scan without contrast identifies the location of the AVM and presence of hemorrhage or hydrocephalus.

CT scan with contrast visualizes the extent and location of the AVM and possible feeding arteries.

MRI confirms relationship of the vascular channels to the surrounding brain and the degree of surrounding hemorrhage or edema. Aids in the planning of the surgical approach.

MRA is a noninvasive diagnostic procedure that examines the brain's blood vessels, detecting presence of AVMs.

Cerebral angiography is the definitive diagnostic procedure and is essential in planning for resection of AVM. Includes the carotid and vertebral circulations to assess all possible areas of vascular supply. Essential for determining the flow dynamics of the AVM and possibility for embolization.

ACUTE CARE PATIENT MANAGEMENT

Goals of Treatment

Obliterate/excise malformation.

Embolization: for complete obliteration or, more commonly, as an adjunctive therapy

Surgical: craniotomy for complete removal, clipping, or ligation of feeding vessels

Radiotherapy: proton-beam radiation, gamma knife therapy, and linear accelerator

Prevent cerebral vascular bleed.

Subarachnoid precautions

Antihypertensives (e.g., labetalol, hydralazine hydrochloride, propranolol, sodium nitroprusside)

Stool softeners or mild laxatives

Sedatives (e.g., midazolam, phenobarbital)

Control symptoms.

Antipyretics (e.g., acetaminophen)

Anticonvulsants (e.g., phenytoin, fosphenytoin)

Analgesics (e.g., acetaminophen, acetaminophen with codeine, morphine sulfate)

Detect/prevent clinical sequelae (Table 5-3).

Table 5-3 CLINICAL SEQUELAE OF ARTERIOVENOUS MALFORMATION (AVM)

Complication	Signs and Symptoms
Intracerebral bleeding	Clinical signs vary, depending on the area involved. In general there is deterioration in consciousness, worsening headache, unilateral motor weakness, decreased EOMs, visual deficits, and changes in vital signs, particularly the respiratory pattern. Speech deficits (e.g., slurring or receptive or expressive aphasia) may be present. Meningeal signs may be present (e.g., severe headache, nuchal rigidity, fever, photophobia, lethargy, nausea, and vomiting).
Seizure	May be focal or generalized seizures

EOM, Extraocular movement.

Priority Nursing Diagnoses and Potential Complications*	
Priority Nursing Diagnoses	**PC: Potential Complications**
Ineffective tissue perfusion: cerebral	Increased intracranial pressure (ICP)
Risk for injury	Seizures
Risk for ineffective protection (see p. 48)	
Imbalanced nutrition: less than body requirements (see p. 53)	
Risk for interrupted family processes (see p. 45)	

*See also cerebrovascular accident (CVA) (p. 110)

Nursing Diagnosis: INEFFECTIVE TISSUE PERFUSION: CEREBRAL related to shunting of blood from cerebral tissue and/or intracerebral hemorrhage (ICH)

Outcome Criteria

Alert and oriented
Pupils equal and normoreactive
SBP 90 to 140 mm Hg
HR 60 to 100 beats/min
RR 12 to 20 breaths/min, eupnea
Motor function equal bilaterally
Absence of headache, nystagmus, and nausea
Intracranial pressure (ICP) <20 mm Hg
Cerebral perfusion pressure (CPP) 60 to 100 mm Hg

Patient Monitoring

1. Monitor ECG continuously because hypoxemia and cerebral bleeding are risk factors for pronounced ST segment and T-wave changes and life-threatening dysrhythmias.
2. Monitor ICP, analyze the ICP waveform, and calculate CPP every hour. (See p. 462 for ICP monitoring.)
3. Monitor BP and pulse (P) every 15 to 30 minutes initially, then hourly; obtain CVP and/or PA pressures (if available) every hour or more frequently if indicated.

Patient Assessment

1. Assess pain using the patient's self-report whenever possible. Note headache onset and severity; presence of stiff neck; and insidious onset of confusion, disorientation, decline in consciousness, and/or focal deficits (weakness of extremity, neglect, or new aphasia).

2. Assess neurologic status using Glasgow Coma Scale and assess for changes suggesting increased ICP and herniation. Be alert for subtle changes and new focal deficits.
3. Assess for factors that can cause increased ICP; evaluate the patient for restlessness, distended bladder, constipation, hypoxemia, headache, fear, or anxiety.
4. Assess the patient for clinical sequelae (see Table 5-3).

Diagnostics Assessment

Review serial ABGs for decreasing Pao_2 (<60 mm Hg) or increasing $Paco_2$ (>40 mm Hg) to identify causes for increased ICP.

Patient Management

1. Maintain patent airway and administer oxygen as ordered to prevent hypoxemia.
2. Institute measures to minimize external stimuli and maintain BP (Box 5-2).

Box 5-2 Subarachnoid Hemorrhage Precautions

Place the patient in a quiet, dimly lit private room. Television, telephone, radio, and reading may be restricted.

Complete bed rest is required, and the patient should be positioned with the head of the bed (HOB) elevated 30 to 45 degrees.

Instruct the patient to avoid Valsalva's maneuver or straining of any kind, because these activities can increase ICP. Have the patient exhale while being turned. Caution the patient against coughing, sneezing, and straining during a bowel movement. Stool softeners may be ordered.

Obtain BP, P, and RR, and assess neurologic signs at least every 30 minutes initially (may be as frequently as every 5 to 15 minutes). This schedule may be altered, depending on patient condition.

Perform activities for the patient (e.g., feeding, bathing, or shaving) that could cause the patient to overexert and raise the BP. Keep activities at a minimum, pace interventions, and provide uninterrupted rest periods.

Caution visitors against upsetting the patient in any way, because excitement or anger could increase BP and ICP. The number of visitors as well as the duration of their visits may need to be limited.

Provide analgesics for headache because pain can cause restlessness and elevated BP. Sedatives may also be required.

---

3. Administer antihypertensives as ordered (e.g., labetalol, hydralazine, or nitroprusside) to control BP. Monitor drug's effect on MAP and CPP.

4. Sedatives and stool softeners may be ordered to reduce agitation and straining.

5. Anticipate interventions such as embolization, resection, clipping, ligation of feeding vessels, proton-beam therapy, or gamma radiation.

Nursing Diagnosis: RISK FOR INJURY related to tonic-clonic movement secondary to seizures

Outcome Criteria

Patient will be seizure free.
Patient will not injure self.

Patient Monitoring

None

Patient Assessment

1. Be alert to any triggers or preseizure behaviors or sensations.

2. Observe clinical presentation during seizure activity. Note time of onset, body parts involved, and characteristics of movement; observe respiratory pattern; note pupil size, deviation, and nystagmus; note duration of seizure activity.

3. Evaluate neurologic status during postictal state and examine the patient for any injuries.

4. Assess the patient for clinical sequelae (see Table 5-3).

Diagnostics Assessment

Review serum anticonvulsant drug levels (if available) for therapeutic range.

Patient Management

1. Institute seizure precautions: pad side rails, maintain the bed in low position; keep an airway at bedside. Have suction and oxygen available.

2. Protect the patient during seizure activity: protect head from injury, avoid restraining the patient; do not force any airway into the mouth once a seizure has begun.

3. Suction the patient's secretions if necessary and maintain an adequate airway during postictal state.

4. Administer anticonvulsant medications as prescribed.
5. Be prepared to administer benzodiazepines (Valium, Ativan) as ordered if status epilepticus occurs.

CEREBRAL ANEURYSM AND SUBARACHNOID HEMORRHAGE

Clinical Brief

An aneurysm is a thin-walled, round, or saccular dilation arising from a cerebral artery. The most common site is at the bifurcation of the main cerebral vessels that make up the circle of Willis. Large aneurysms may produce focal neurologic deficits from compression of brain tissue or may lead to a stroke secondary to thrombus formation and embolization. Cerebral aneurysms are the most common source of subarachnoid hemorrhage. When a cerebral aneurysm ruptures, blood enters the subarachnoid space, ventricular system, and surrounding brain tissue. The blood acts as an irritant and causes vasospasm, a constriction of cerebral arteries. Vasospasm impairs cerebral blood flow (CBF), which can result in cerebral ischemia and infarction.

Presenting Signs and Symptoms

Often the patient will report the sudden onset of a violent headache—"the worst headache of my life"—at the time of bleeding. This usually continues as a severe headache accompanied by nausea and vomiting (N/V), photophobia, and nuchal rigidity. Specific neurologic deficits are related to the site and extent of the hemorrhage and may include a deteriorating level of consciousness (LOC), oculomotor nerve dysfunction, paralysis of extraocular muscles, and sensorimotor deficits in the patient.

Physical Examination

Vital signs:
  BP: generally hypertensive or very labile, depending on extent of hemorrhage and level of ICP
  HR: mild tachycardia, dysrhythmias
  RR: tachypnea
  Temperature: low-grade fever 24 hours after initial rupture as a result of meningeal irritation
Pulmonary: respiratory pattern changes may be present, depending on the level of ICP and area of hemorrhage (see Table 1-6).
Neurologic: as the severity of the hemorrhage increases, the LOC generally decreases, with corresponding severity of neurologic

Table 5-4 CLASSIFICATION OF CEREBRAL ANEURYSM HEMORRHAGE

Category	Criteria
Grade I	Asymptomatic or minimal headache and slight nuchal rigidity
Grade II	Moderate to severe headache
	Nuchal rigidity, no neurologic deficit other than cranial nerve palsy
Grade III	Drowsiness, confusion or mild focal deficit
Grade IV	Stupor, moderate to severe hemiparesis, possibly early decerebrate rigidity and vegetative disturbances
Grade V	Deep coma, decerebrate rigidity, moribund appearance

From Hunt W, Hess R: Surgical risk as related to time of intervention in the repair of intracranial aneurysms, *J Neurosurg* 28:14, 1968.

deficits; signs of meningeal irritation: stiff neck and positive Kernig's and Brudzinski's signs may be present. (See Table 5-4 for a classification of cerebral aneurysm hemorrhage.)

Diagnostic Findings
Computed Tomography (CT) Scan

May help predict location of aneurysm. Large aneurysms (>10 mm) may be identified.

Detects the presence of hydrocephalus and extent of subarachnoid or intracerebral hemorrhage

Cerebral Angiography

Anterior and posterior circulations are studied to document presence of aneurysm(s) and possible vasospasm. The gold standard for visualizing aneurysms.

Magnetic Resonance Angiography (MRA)

Aids in the diagnosis of large intracranial aneurysms and AVMs. MRA can yield information about the size, shape, and orientation of an aneurysm's orifice (the part of the vessel that communicates with the parent vessel).

CT Angiography (CTA)

A spiral CT scan portraying a 3-dimensional image of the brain's circulation in order to identify location of aneurysms. Also demonstrates relation of blood vessels to bony structures.

NEURO

Cerebrospinal Fluid (CSF) Studies

Performed in cases in which CT scan has been negative

Subarachnoid hemorrhage (SAH) indicated by increased opening
pressure (normal 5-15 mm Hg), increased red blood cells
(RBCs), increased CSF protein, and presence of xanthochromia.

Transcranial Doppler (TCD)

Noninvasive CBF studies to aid in diagnosing vasospasm

ACUTE CARE PATIENT MANAGEMENT

Goals of Treatment

Secure the aneurysm.

Surgery: aneurysm clipping or ligation

Endovascular coiling: detachable coils placed in aneurysm with
goal of promoting thrombosis of aneurysmal sac

Prevent rebleeding.

Subarachnoid precautions (see Box 5-2)

Antihypertensives (e.g., labetalol, hydralazine hydrochloride, propranolol, sodium nitroprusside)

Stool softeners

Anticonvulsants (e.g., phenytoin, fosphenytoin)

Control cerebral vasospasm.

Ensure hydration and normalize BP (hypervolemic/hypertension
therapy)

Calcium channel blocking agents (e.g., nimodipine)

Detect/prevent clinical sequelae (Table 5-5).

Priority Nursing Diagnoses and Potential Complications*	
Priority Nursing Diagnoses	**PC: Potential Complication**
Ineffective tissue perfusion: cerebral	Increased ICP
Risk for ineffective protection (see p. 48)	
Imbalanced nutrition: less than body requirements (see p. 53)	
Risk for interrupted family processes (see p. 45)	

*See also CVA (p. 110).

**Nursing Diagnosis: INEFFECTIVE TISSUE PERFUSION: CEREBRAL related to bleeding
and cerebral vasospasm**

Outcome Criteria

Patient alert and oriented

Pupils equal and normoreactive

Table 5-5 CLINICAL SEQUELAE OF CEREBRAL ANEURYSM RUPTURE

Complication	Signs and Symptoms
SIADH	Low serum osmolality (<280 mOsm/L), dilutional hyponatremia, decreased urinary output (400-500 mL/24 hr), generalized weight gain
CSW	Low sodium (<135mEq/L), increased hematocrit, signs of dehydration
Seizures	Tonic-clonic movements
Cerebral vasospasm	In general, progressive deterioration in consciousness, mental confusion, motor and sensory deficits; may also be visual and speech deficits
Rebleeding	Sudden, severe headache; nausea and vomiting; deterioration in LOC or comatose; new neurologic deficits
Increased intracranial pressure	Decreasing LOC, severe headache, nausea, vomiting, motor dysfunction, seizures, irregular breathing pattern (e.g., Cheyne-Stokes, central neurogenic hyperventilation, ataxia, apneustic), positive Babinski's sign, contralateral sensorimotor changes; changes in pupillary size, shape, and reaction; other cranial nerve involvement dependent upon the severity
Herniation	Comatose with no response to painful stimuli; VS changes: bradycardia, increasing systolic BP with a widening pulse pressure, cessation of respirations, absent brainstem reflexes (e.g., corneal, gag, swallow, oculocephalic, and oculovestibular), ipsilateral or bilateral pupillary dilation

BP, Blood pressure; *CSW,* cerebral salt-wasting; *LOC,* level of consciousness; *SIADH,* syndrome of inappropriate antidiuretic hormone; *VS,* vital signs.

MAP 80 to 90 mm Hg
CVP 5 to 8 mm Hg
If receiving hypervolemic, hypertensive therapy: MAP 120 to 140 mm Hg, CVP 8 to 12 mm Hg, PCWP 16 to 20 mm Hg
HR 60 to 100 beats/min
RR 12 to 20 breaths/min, eupnea
Motor function equal bilaterally
Absence of headache, papilledema, nystagmus, nausea, and seizures

ICP <20 mm Hg
CPP 60 to 100 mm Hg

Patient Monitoring

1. Continuously monitor BP and MAP. Fluctuations in BP may increase risk of aneurysm rebleeding, cerebral ischemia, or stroke.
2. Continuously monitor ECG because hypoxemia and cerebral bleeding are risk factors for pronounced ST segment and T-wave changes and life-threatening dysrhythmias.
3. Monitor ICP; analyze ICP waveform and calculate CPP every hour. (See p. 462 for ICP monitoring.)
4. Monitor VS every 15 to 30 minutes initially, then hourly and evaluate the patient's response to therapy.
5. Monitor I&O hourly and calculate hourly running totals to determine fluid volume balance.

Patient Assessment

1. Assess pain using the patient's self-report whenever possible. Note headache onset and severity; presence of stiff neck; and insidious onset of confusion, disorientation, decline in consciousness, and/or focal deficits (weakness of extremity, neglect, or new aphasia).
2. Assess neurologic status for signs/symptoms that may indicate rebleed, cerebral vasospasm, and increased ICP (see Table 5-5). Be alert for subtle changes and new focal deficits. Cerebral vasospasm peaks between days 6 and 8 after SAH; rebleeding generally occurs within the first 48 hours.
3. Assess temperature every 2 to 4 hours.
4. Assess for factors that can cause increased ICP: distended bladder, constipation, hypoxemia, hypercapnia, headache, fear, or anxiety.
5. Assess the patient for clinical sequelae (see Table 5-5).

Diagnostics Assessment

1. Review serial ABGs for decreasing PaO_2 (<60 mm Hg) or increasing $PaCO_2$ (>45 mm Hg) because these disturbances can increase ICP.
2. Review serial electrolytes for hyponatremia, which may contribute to an altered mental state or lower seizure threshold.

NEURO

3. Note trends on TCD studies; an increasing mean value may reflect vasospasm.

Patient Management

1. Maintain patent airway and administer oxygen as ordered. If the patient is intubated and mechanically ventilated, see p. 503 for information on ventilation therapies.
2. Institute subarachnoid precautions (see Box 5-2).
3. Administer antihypertensives as ordered to control sustained elevated BP (e.g., labetalol, hydralazine hydrochloride, propranolol, or sodium nitroprusside). Monitor MAP and CPP closely because a drastic reduction in BP can cause ischemia and possibly central infarction.
4. To optimize CBF during symptomatic vasospasm, hypervolemic, hypertensive, hemodilution (HHH) therapy may be ordered. Crystalloids are administered to maintain a CVP of 8 to 12 mm Hg, a PA diastolic of 14 to 16 mm Hg, and a MAP of 120 to 140 mm Hg. If neurologic deficits continue, arterial hypertension (HTN) may be induced with pharmacologic agents such as phenylephrine, dopamine, or dobutamine to raise SBP to no higher than 240 mm Hg in patients with obliterated aneurysms or no higher than 160 mm Hg in patients with untreated aneurysms. Balloon angioplasty or papaverine may be used to treat vasospasm prophylactically. Monitor BP, MAP, and CPP closely and monitor for pulmonary and cardiac congestion.
5. Calcium channel blocking agents may be ordered to reduce the severity of cerebral ischemia associated with cerebral vasospasm. Monitor the drug's effect on BP and HR.
6. Other pharmacologic agents to prevent rebleeding and increased ICP include antipyretics (e.g., acetaminophen) to keep the patient normothermic; anticonvulsants (e.g., phenytoin, fosphenytoin) to prevent or control seizures; analgesics (e.g., acetaminophen or acetaminophen with codeine, morphine sulfate) for headaches; stool softeners or mild laxatives, to prevent constipation and straining; and sedatives (e.g., midazolam) to decrease agitation.
7. Anticipate early surgical intervention for clipping or ligation of the aneurysm.
8. Endovascular coiling may be an option for aneurysms that are anatomically inoperable.

NEURO

BRAIN ATTACK: STROKE OR CEREBROVASCULAR ACCIDENT (CVA)

Clinical Brief

A stroke is a sudden loss of brain function resulting from an interference with the blood supply to the brain. The signs and symptoms of a brain attack (stroke) depend on the severity and location of the interrupted blood flow. A transient ischemic attack (TIA) produces focal neurologic deficits that resolve in less than 24 hours and does not cause tissue infarction; this may be a warning sign of an impending stroke. A stroke is characterized by symptoms persisting longer than 24 hours, and permanent neurologic deficits result. Strokes are classified as either ischemic, caused by thromboses or emboli, or hemorrhagic. Acute vascular occlusion is the central event in acute ischemic stroke. The occlusion is rarely complete. A hemorrhagic stroke is characterized by bleeding into brain tissue. The progression of a brain attack may take several hours or days; the progression of neurologic deterioration is referred to as a "stroke in evolution." A stroke is complete when symptoms have stabilized and the neurologic deficits are permanent.

Risk factors for stroke include a history of HTN, heart disease (especially valvular), cardiac dysrhythmias, cigarette smoking, diabetes mellitus, obesity, sedentary lifestyle, and age older than 65 years. In addition, patients with a strong family history of ischemic heart disease and stroke, as well as those with hyperlipidemia, appear at greater risk. Medications such as oral contraceptives, aspirin, and anticoagulants may also place patients at risk.

Thrombotic Stroke

Thrombotic stroke is the most common type of brain attack. It is associated with atherosclerosis and narrowing of the lumen of the cerebral artery with subsequent thrombosis formation as a result of the pathologic changes in the plaque.

Embolic Stroke

An embolic stroke is associated with conditions of hypercoagulability or coagulopathy such as heart disease (e.g., rheumatic heart disease with mitral stenosis, subacute bacterial endocarditis), atrial fibrillation, and cardiac or vascular surgery. Embolic strokes evolve rapidly over a few seconds or minutes and are usually without warning signs.

Hemorrhagic Stroke or Intracerebral Hemorrhage (ICH)

Bleeding into the brain tissue is frequently the result of sudden rupture of a blood vessel within the brain. The effects depend on the location of the rupture and actual size of the clot. Brain tissue adjacent to the clot is displaced and produces focal neurologic signs. The most common site for this type of hematoma is in the basal ganglia; the thalamic region is the next most common site. The usual precipitating factor of a cerebral hemorrhage is HTN. Other possible causes may include an aneurysm, AVM, tumors, trauma, or hemorrhagic disorders. In addition, illicit use of cocaine or crack may result in an ICH.

Presenting Signs and Symptoms

Signs and symptoms are directly related to the cerebral artery affected and the function of the portion of the brain that it supplies. A list of major cerebral vessels and their common correlating manifestations are listed in Box 5-3. A headache of sudden onset occasionally accompanied by N/V may accompany ICH.

Box 5-3 Correlation of Cerebral Artery Involvement and Common Manifestations

Internal Carotid Artery

Contralateral paresthesias (abnormal sensations) and hemiparesis (weakness) of arm, face, and leg
  Eventually complete contralateral hemiplegia (paralysis) and hemianesthesia (loss of sensation)
  Visual blurring or changes, hemianopsia (loss of half of visual field), repeated attacks of blindness in the ipsilateral eye
Dysphasia with dominant hemisphere involvement

Anterior Cerebral Artery

Mental impairment such as perseveration, confusion, amnesia, and personality changes
Contralateral hemiparesis or hemiplegia with decreased or loss of motor function greater in leg than arm
Sensory loss over toes, foot, and leg
Ataxia (motor incoordination), impaired gait, incontinence, and akinetic mutism

---

Continued

Box 5-3 Correlation of Cerebral Artery Involvement and Common Manifestations—cont'd

Middle Cerebral Artery

LOC varies from confusion to coma.

Contralateral hemiparesis or hemiplegia with decreased or loss of motor function greater in face and arm than leg

Sensory impairment over same areas of hemiplegia

Aphasia (inability to express or interpret speech) or dysphasia (impaired speech) with dominant hemisphere involvement

Homonymous hemianopsia (loss of vision on the same side of both visual fields), inability to turn eyes toward the paralyzed side

Posterior Cerebral Artery

Contralateral hemiplegia with sensory loss

Confusion, memory involvement, and receptive speech deficits with dominant hemisphere involvement

Homonymous hemianopsia

Vertebrobasilar Artery

Dizziness, vertigo, nausea, ataxia, and syncope

Visual disturbances, nystagmus, diplopia, field deficits, and blindness

Numbness and paresis (face, tongue, mouth, one or more limbs), dysphagia (inability to swallow), and dysarthria (difficulty in articulation)

Symptoms Related to Left versus Right Hemisphere Involvement

Left Hemisphere	Right Hemisphere
Right-sided hemiplegia or hemiparesis	Left-sided hemiplegia or hemiparesis
Expressive, receptive, or global aphasia	Spatial, perceptual deficits
Decreased performance on verbal and math testing	Denial of the disability on affected side
Slow and cautious behavior	Distractibility, impulsive behavior, and poor judgment
Defects in right visual field	
Difficulty in distinguishing left from right	Defects in left visual field

Physical Examination

Vital signs may be normal, or the following may be found:

BP: with preexisting HTN, BP may exceed 200/100 mm Hg

HR: mild tachycardia or irregular rhythm if associated with atrial fibrillation

RR: eupnea or Cheyne-Stokes respirations

Temperature: afebrile or elevated if the thermoregulation center is involved

Cardiovascular: peripheral pulses may be diminished or weak in the presence of atrial fibrillation; jugular bruits may be present with atherosclerosis of the carotid arteries.

Pulmonary: chest is clear to auscultation; some rhonchi may be present if there is a history of smoking.

Neurologic: see Box 5-3.

Diagnostic Findings

CT Scan

Visualizes areas of cerebral hemorrhage immediately and areas of ischemia or infarction beginning 3 hours after vascular occlusion

Differentiates cerebral hemorrhage from ischemia as the cause of the brain attack

Cerebral Angiogram

Usually postponed until the patient's condition is stabilized; evaluates and identifies areas of ulceration, stenosis, thrombus, and occlusion and patterns of collateral flow

Demonstrates presence of an aneurysm or AVM and any avascular zones and displaced arteries and veins from hemorrhage

Areas studied include aortic arch, carotids, and cerebral blood vessels

Magnetic Resonance Imaging (MRI)

Reflects areas of infarction as early as 8 hours after the ischemic insult

Shows early edema formation and mass effect

Magnetic Resonance Angiography (MRA)

Images the entire carotid artery from the aortic arch through the circle of Willis and provides information determining the need for carotid endarterectomy

Lumbar Puncture (LP)

Normal pressure will be seen in cerebral thrombosis, embolus, and TIA; fluid is usually clear.

In subarachnoid and intracerebral hemorrhage, the pressure is usually elevated and fluid is grossly bloody.

Total protein level may be elevated in cases of thrombosis as a result of the inflammatory process.

Echocardiogram

Rules out a cardiac source of emboli

Electrocardiogram (ECG)

Rules out the presence of a concurrent MI, possibly resulting in cerebral hypoperfusion and ischemia

Determines the presence of dysrhythmias as a source of emboli

ACUTE CARE PATIENT MANAGEMENT

Goals of Treatment

Augment blood flow.
  Euvolemia
  Thrombolytic agents, endarterectomy
Prevent additional thrombotic events.
  Anticoagulation in selected situations
  Antiplatelet agents
Protect neurons.
  Prevent hyperglycemia
  Prevent hyperthermia
Prevent further hemorrhagic events.
  Treat the cause: cerebral AVM, cerebral aneurysm, or HTN
Reduce increased ICP.
  Ventriculostomy for ICP monitoring and CSF drainage
  Corticosteroids (e.g., dexamethasone)
  Osmotic diuretics (e.g., mannitol)
  Loop diuretics (e.g., furosemide)
Detect/prevent clinical sequelae (Table 5-6).

Nursing Diagnosis: INEFFECTIVE TISSUE PERFUSION: CEREBRAL related to ICP secondary to cerebral ischemia, edema, or hemorrhage

Outcome Criteria

Patient alert and oriented
Pupils equal and normoreactive

Table 5-6 Clinical Sequelae of Brain Attack

Complication	Signs and Symptoms
Seizures	Tonic-clonic movements
Dysrhythmias/ECG changes	Change in rate and rhythm; QT prolongation, ST segment depression, T-wave inversion
Respiratory insufficiency or arrest	Shallow respirations, cessation of breathing
Increased intracranial pressure	Decreasing LOC, severe headache, nausea, vomiting, motor dysfunction, seizures, irregular breathing pattern (e.g., Cheyne-Stokes, central neurogenic hyperventilation, ataxia, apneustic), positive Babinski's sign, contralateral sensorimotor changes; changes in pupillary size, shape, and reaction; other cranial nerve involvement dependent upon the severity
Herniation	Comatose with no response to painful stimuli; VS changes: bradycardia, increasing systolic BP with a widening pulse pressure, cessation of respirations, absent brainstem reflexes (e.g., corneal, gag, swallow, oculocephalic, and oculovestibular), ipsilateral or bilateral pupillary dilation
Pain	Pain can be common in patients who have had a stroke due to disuse of limbs and spasticity. Also, those with stroke in thalamic region may suffer from postthalamic pain syndrome experiencing burning pain on some or all body parts contralateral to the side of the stroke.
Thromboembolism	Immobility due to hemiplegia or hemiparesis places a patient at risk for deep vein thrombosis or pulmonary embolism.

BP, Blood pressure; *ECG,* electrocardiogram; *LOC,* level of consciousness; *VS,* vital signs.

NEURO

Priority Nursing Diagnoses and Potential Complications

Priority Nursing Diagnoses	PC: Potential Complications
Ineffective tissue perfusion: cerebral	Increased intracranial pressure (ICP)
Ineffective airway clearance	Hypoxemia, atelectasis, pneumonia
Risk for aspiration	
Impaired verbal communication	
Risk for ineffective protection (see p. 48)	
Imbalanced nutrition: less than body requirements (see p. 53)	
Risk for interrupted family processes (see p. 45)	

Improvement in initial neurologic deficits and/or the absence of any new focal deficits

ICP <20 mm Hg

CPP 60 to 100 mm Hg

CVP 7 to 10 mm Hg

SBP <185 mm Hg and DBP <110 mm Hg—if receiving recombinant tissue plasminogen activator (rtPa)

Patient Monitoring

1. Continuously monitor ECG for changes (e.g., ventricular ectopy is common).

2. Continuously monitor oxygen saturation with pulse oximetry (SpO_2). Monitor interventions and patient activities that may adversely affect oxygen saturation.

3. If ICP monitoring is being used, calculate CPP to evaluate the patient's response to therapy. (See p. 462 for ICP monitoring.)

4. Monitor BP every 15 to 30 minutes initially and when titrating vasoactive agents. If not receiving rtPa, then generally HTN is not treated unless it exceeds 220/110 or there are signs of hypertensive emergency such as hypertensive encephalopathy, retinal hemorrhage, cardiac ischemia, congestive heart failure (CHF), or progressive renal dysfunction. Hypotension can extend the areas of infarction.

5. Monitor CVP and PA pressures (if available). Increasing pressures may signal the onset of fluid overload, which may increase cerebral edema.

6. Monitor I&O hourly and calculate fluid balance every shift to evaluate fluid volume status. Fluid overload can increase cerebral edema and further increase ICP.

Patient Assessment

1. Establish a neurologic baseline with the Glasgow Coma Scale and perform ongoing assessments to evaluate the patient for improving or deteriorating mental status, headache, and focal deficit. Assess for signs and symptoms of increased ICP: headache, nausea, vomiting, altered LOC, pupillary changes, visual defects, and sensorimotor dysfunction. Test protective reflexes (e.g., cough, gag, corneal).
2. Assess for factors that can increase ICP: hypoxemia, hypercapnia, fever, anxiety, constipation, and bladder distention.
3. Assess the patient for clinical sequelae (see Table 5-6).

Diagnostics Assessment

1. Review serial prothrombin time (PT), International Normalized Ratio (INR), and partial thromboplastin time (PTT) for therapeutic levels if the patient is receiving antico-agulant therapy. Generally 1.5 times the control is the goal of therapy.
2. Review serial electrolytes and osmolality levels, especially if diuretic therapy is employed.
3. Review serial ABGs to identify hypoxemia (Pao_2 <60 mm Hg) and hypercapnia ($Paco_2$ >45 mm Hg) because these distur-bances can cause increased ICP.
4. Review serial serum glucose values; hyperglycemia and hypo-glycemia can extend neurologic damage.

Patient Management

1. Maintain the head of the bed at 30 degrees or as ordered. Keep the patient's head in straight alignment and prevent extreme hip flexion. Pace nursing activities to allow the patient uninterrupted rest periods. Turn the patient to the lateral recumbent position to decrease the chances of aspira-tion. Instruct the patient to exhale while being turned or repositioned to prevent Valsalva-induced intracranial hyper-tension.
2. Elevated BP is generally not treated unless MAP is >130 mm Hg or SBP is >220 mm Hg. Monitor BP cautiously and

prevent a precipitous drop in BP. Anticipate use of labetalol or enalapril because they lower pressure without directly dilating cerebral vessels, which prevents vascular-induced intracranial hypertension.

3. Treat hyperglycemia according to protocol and prescribed medications; induction of postischemic hyperglycemia enhances brain injury.

4. Treat fever aggressively according to protocol and prescribed medications. Hyperthermia in the poststroke period is associated with increased morbidity and mortality.

5. Anticipate use of rtPa for ischemic stroke if the patient comes to the referral center within 3 hours of symptom onset. rtPa is contraindicated in patients with evidence of intracranial hemorrhage, with known AVM or aneurysm, with active internal bleeding within the past 14 days, with bleeding diathesis or current use of oral anticoagulants, within 3 months of intracranial surgery or stroke, and during pregnancy. Avoid use of aspirin 24 hours after rtPa use.

6. Osmotic diuretics (e.g., mannitol) may be ordered to decrease cerebral edema. Carefully monitor CPP, ICP, urine output, and BP. Alternatively, hypertonic saline (e.g., 3% NS) may be used to reduce ICP associated with cerebral edema.

7. Aspirin may be administered with ischemic stroke. Anticoagulation medications (e.g., heparin, LMWH, Warfarin) may be ordered for patients with an embolic stroke and with a completed thrombotic stroke. Antiplatelet drugs (e.g., clopidogrel [Plavix] or dipyridamole) may also be ordered. Monitor for bruising and test urine, stool, and nasogastric (NG) aspirate for occult blood. Protect the patient from injury (e.g., use soft toothbrush for oral hygiene and use electric razor).

8. Prevent constipation. Consider a bowel regimen for those with recurrent constipation.

9. Provide the patient and family with realistic information and a rationale for frequent assessments, the relationship between the patient's condition and clinical symptoms, and the treatment and care plan.

10. Maintain ventriculostomy (if present) and drain CSF according to established parameters.

Nursing Diagnoses: INEFFECTIVE AIRWAY CLEARANCE and RISK FOR ASPIRATION
related to altered consciousness or cough reflex dysfunction

Outcome Criteria

Patient will maintain a patent airway.
Absence of aspiration
RR 12 to 20 breaths/min, eupnea
Lungs clear to auscultation
O_2 sat ≥95%
Pao_2 80 to 100 mm Hg
$Paco_2$ 35 to 45 mm Hg
pH 7.35 to 7.45

Patient Monitoring

Continuously monitor oxygen saturation with pulse oximetry
(Spo_2). Monitor interventions and patient activities that may
adversely affect oxygen saturation.

Patient Assessment

1. Ongoing assessment of respiratory status at least every
   4 hours. Assess for breathlessness, note the rate, quality, and
   pattern; assess the patency of the upper airway and the
   patient's ability to handle oral secretions; assess skin color,
   nail beds, peripheral pulses, and skin temperature; and assess
   the presence and strength of gag, cough, and swallow reflexes.
2. Assess the lungs and note the presence of adventitious
   sounds. Note any restlessness or change in LOC; increased
   restlessness and deteriorating mental status may indicate
   hypoxia; new somnolence may indicate hypercarbia.

Diagnostics Assessment

1. Review serial ABGs for hypoxemia and hypercapnia because
   these disturbances can extend brain injury and increase ICP.
2. Review serial chest radiographs as indicated to evaluate for
   possible aspiration or pulmonary congestion.

Patient Management

1. Maintain a patent airway by turning and positioning the
   patient to facilitate drainage of oropharyngeal secretions, providing an oral airway if necessary and suctioning secretions.

NEURO

2. Once the patient's breathing is stabilized, provide pulmonary hygiene: deep breathing therapy every hour and as needed (PRN); provide chest physiotherapy and postural drainage if warranted and not contraindicated by increased ICP.

3. Administer oxygen with adequate humidification as ordered.

4. An NG tube may be required to prevent gastric distention and potential aspiration; check placement and patency.

5. Assist the patient with feedings if the gag and cough reflexes are intact; place the patient in an upright position and offer mechanical soft foods to avoid the risk of aspiration. Contact a speech therapist for swallowing evaluation if necessary.

Nursing Diagnosis: IMPAIRED VERBAL COMMUNICATION: DYSARTHRIA (IMPAIRED MUSCLE INVOLVEMENT), EXPRESSIVE APHASIA (INABILITY TO EXPRESS THOUGHTS VERBALLY OR IN WRITING), RECEPTIVE APHASIA (INABILITY TO UNDERSTAND THE SPOKEN OR WRITTEN WORD), OR DYSPHASIA (IMPAIRED SPEECH) related to brain attack

Outcome Criterion

Patient will be able to communicate needs.

Patient Monitoring

None

Patient Assessment

1. Assess for any deficits/decreases in communication skills and ability, articulation, and comprehension and verbalization including frustration, anger, and withdrawal at not being able to find words or to make needs known.

2. Record the following characteristics of the patient's speech: spontaneity, fluency, and context.

3. Examine the muscles used for speech, testing cranial nerves VII, IX, X, and XII (see Table 1-2).

4. Ask the patient to follow verbal then demonstrated commands.

5. Ask the patient to repeat simple phrases and sentences; test the patient for the ability to follow written commands.

6. Ask the patient to identify common objects, such as pen, scissors, and pin.

Diagnostics Assessment

Review speech therapist's evaluation of the quality and quantity of impairment if available.

Patient Management
1. Limit the amount of environmental stimuli to decrease distractions and reduce confusion for the patient.
2. Encourage the patient to focus on one task at a time; speak in a clear, calm voice. Focus on simple, basic words and short sentences, allowing time for the patient to respond. Repeat or rephrase sentences as necessary.
3. Avoid appearing rushed; anticipate the patient's needs and encourage patience when the patient is frustrated by attempts at communication.
4. Assign consistent caregivers.
5. Instruct the family about limiting stimuli to prevent confusion for the patient. Keep the family informed and involved in the plan of care.
6. For expressive aphasia, encourage the patient's present speech and encourage spontaneous attempts at speech; allow sufficient time for the patient to respond to questions and words; cue with the first syllable or give a choice of words; and provide alternate means, such as picture cards, word cards, or writing tablet.
7. For receptive aphasia, use concrete words to communicate nouns and verbs; use gestures and pictures and write messages; and use word and phrase cards. Begin introducing words to the patient in the following order: noun, verb, and pronoun.
8. Suggest referral to a speech therapist or pathologist for formal evaluation.

HEAD INJURY

Clinical Brief

Head injury involves trauma to the scalp, skull (cranium and facial bones), or brain. The severity of the injury is related to the degree of initial brain damage and associated secondary pathology. Every year, traumatic brain injury causes 52,000 deaths and permanent severe disability for another 80,000 people in the United States. Age older than 60 years increases mortality and morbidity associated with brain injury. The presence of a specific genotype associated with apolipoprotein E (which is responsible for transport of lipids in the brain) may contribute to worse outcomes in brain injury.

NEURO

Primary injury occurs with an impact from an acceleration-deceleration or rotational force, and includes fracture, concussion, contusion, and laceration. The effects of the primary injury on cerebral tissue can be focal or diffuse. Secondary injuries may begin at the time of trauma or any time thereafter. Secondary injuries include the cellular and biochemical response to trauma as well as systemic derangements that exacerbate the primary injury and contribute to additional CNS damage. Cellular secondary injuries include axonal disruption, calcium toxicity, free radical generation, and excitatory and neurotransmitter release. Other secondary injuries are intracranial hypertension, cerebral hematoma, CNS infections, hypotension, hyperthermia, hypoxemia, and hypercapnia. Every attempt must be made to prevent or control secondary injuries, which increase morbidity and mortality.

Classification of head injuries according to location and effect on the brain, as well as presenting signs and symptoms and diagnostic tests, are covered in Table 5-7.

Presenting Signs and Symptoms

Depending on the extent, degree, and location of brain injury, patients may have varying levels of consciousness and neurologic deficits (see Table 5-7).

Physical Examination

Vital signs:

BP: wide fluctuations may be seen; commonly the patient is hypertensive, which may reflect increased ICP or may also be a preexisting condition. When HTN is present with bradycardia, a widened pulse pressure, and irregular respirations (Cushing's triad), it reflects a late and possibly terminal sign of increased ICP indicative of loss of autoregulation. Hypotension from head injury alone is rare but may also indicate a terminal event.

HR: bradycardia, associated with increased ICP. Tachycardia, seen with occult hemorrhage, multitrauma, or as a terminal event.

RR: pathologic respiratory pattern will roughly correlate with the level of neurologic injury, ranging from Cheyne-Stokes, central neurogenic hyperventilation, apneustic to ataxic breathing (see Table 1-6).

Temperature: will vary widely with hypothalamic injuries. Hyperthermia with subarachnoid hemorrhage or infections.

Table 5-7 CLASSIFICATION OF HEAD INJURY ACCORDING TO LOCATION AND EFFECT ON THE BRAIN

Location	Description and Presenting Signs and Symptoms	Diagnostic Findings
SCALP INJURIES	—	Objective observation of injury is made.
Contusion	Bruise injury to the tissue of the scalp, with possible effusion of blood into the subcutaneous space without a break in the skin is seen.	CT scan or MRI may show extravascular blood in skin or subcutaneous tissue.
Abrasion	Part of the top layer of skin on the scalp is scraped away.	—
Laceration	Wound or tear in the tissue of the scalp that tends to bleed profusely is present.	—
SKULL FRACTURE INJURIES	—	Diagnosis is primarily based on CT scan or, possibly, skull radiographs; these are viewed carefully to note air in the paranasal sinuses or other areas that may indicate a basilar skull fracture.
Linear	Nondisplaced fracture of the skull at point of injury; swelling, ecchymosis, or tenderness is noted on the scalp; scalp contusion or laceration may also be present.	—
Comminuted	Multiple fragmented linear fractures are present.	—

Continued

Table 5-7 CLASSIFICATION OF HEAD INJURY ACCORDING TO LOCATION AND EFFECT ON THE BRAIN—cont'd

Location	Description and Presenting Signs and Symptoms	Diagnostic Findings
Depressed	Displacement of comminuted fragments, associated with dural laceration and brain injury; look for cerebrospinal fluid leakage from the ear (otorrhea) or nose (rhinorrhea); swelling, ecchymosis, and other scalp injuries are common.	—
Compound	May be linear, comminuted, or depressed; there is an external opening through scalp, mucous membranes of sinuses, or the tympanum (see depressed fracture).	—
Basilar skull	Linear fracture from base of temporal or frontal bone extending into the anterior, middle, or posterior fossa; it produces characteristic clinical features, depending on site of fracture (e.g., raccoon's eyes [periorbital ecchymosis], Battle's sign [mastoidal ecchymosis], otorrhea, rhinorrhea, and anosmia [impairment of the sense of smell]).	Radiograph may or may not reveal basilar fracture; CT scan and/or clinical features confirm the diagnosis; skull radiographs and CT scan confirm location and extent.
Facial	Fractures of the facial bones produce disfigurement and facial motor and sensory dysfunction.	—
MENINGEAL TEARS	Dural laceration from compound or depressed fractures or from penetrating objects; S/S of meningitis (elevated temperature, stiff neck, pain on flexion of neck, deterioration of neurologic signs, elevated WBCs) are present.	Leakage of CSF may be observed by clinician and will test positive for glucose; blood with CSF produces halo sign on porous white paper; CSF leak is confirmed by cisternography.

Continued

Diffuse cerebral injuries	—	Diagnosis is made by clinical findings in the absence of focal lesion on CT; CT scan without contrast or MRI detects presence of contusion, hematoma, hemorrhage, hydrocephalus, edema, narrowed basal cisterns, small ventricles due to edema, hemisphere or midline shift.
Concussion	Violent jarring or shaking of the brain causes transient loss of consciousness, memory loss, nausea, vomiting, dizziness, unsteady gait, headache.	—
Diffuse axonal injury	Diffuse stretching and tearing of axons that occur with acceleration–deceleration injuries, common with high-speed motor vehicle crash, often results in devastating cognitive and motor deficits, vegetative state	MRI is the preferred examination; delayed CT scan may demonstrate petechial hemorrhages, edema, or atrophy.
Hypoxic brain injury	Brain is deprived of an adequate oxygen supply resulting from cardiac arrest or a nonpenetrating head injury; varying degrees of elevated ICP, mild cognitive deficits to a vegetative state are present.	—
FOCAL CEREBRAL INJURIES		
Contusion	Bruising of the brain with perivascular hemorrhage; loss of consciousness, speech, sensory or motor disturbances, depending on site involved; and anterograde or retrograde memory loss are present.	CT scan or MRI shows local inflammation and tissue injury; extravascular blood may also be present.

Table 5-7 CLASSIFICATION OF HEAD INJURY ACCORDING TO LOCATION AND EFFECT ON THE BRAIN—cont'd

Location	Description and Presenting Signs and Symptoms	Diagnostic Findings
Laceration	Tearing of brain tissue is accompanied by focal swelling; this can lead to intracranial bleeding, brain displacement, and death. Decreased LOC, sensorimotor dysfunction, abnormal size and reaction in pupils, extraocular paralysis, other cranial nerve dysfunctions, seizures, and aphasia are observed.	—
Brainstem injury	Primary—results from direct trauma, fracture, or torsion injury; secondary—may occur as a result of compression from increased ICP and herniation of temporal lobe; and results in decreased LOC, abnormal breathing patterns, abnormal size and reaction in pupils, abnormal eye movement, motor deficits, and abnormal reflexes.	Same as cerebral injuries
HEMORRHAGE		
Subdural hematoma	Bleeding into the subdural space (between the dura mater and above the arachnoid layer); hematoma is caused by slow bleeding usually from venous vessels; S/S usually slower than epidural hematoma; altered LOC, headache, personality changes, ipsilateral dilated pupil, and contralateral weakness are found.	Same as cerebral injuries

Epidural hematoma	Extradural bleeding above the dura mater (between the periosteal lining of the skull and dura mater); usually caused by arterial bleeding from a torn middle meningeal artery and often associated with a fracture of the temporal bone; clot presses on brain and can cause rapid herniation and death; brief loss of consciousness is followed by lucid period; severe vomiting, headache, rapid deterioration with decreased LOC, ipsilateral dilated pupil, contralateral hemiparesis, and seizures may occur.	Same as cerebral injuries; brain scan is helpful with isodense hematomas; MRI may differentiate hemorrhages that occurred at different times
Subarachnoid hemorrhage and intraventricular hemorrhage	Bleeding is usually associated with ruptured aneurysm or AVM; S/S of restlessness, severe headache, nuchal rigidity; elevated temperature, positive Kernig's sign (loss of ability to extend leg when thigh is flexed on abdomen), and photophobia are present.	Same as cerebral injuries; CSF studies will reflect blood and elevated protein and pressure
Intracerebral hematoma	Bleeding is located within the brain tissue and may involve small arteries or veins; mortality is high; S/S depend on the location and size and are frequently indistinguishable from those of contusion; sudden onset of headache may be accompanied by nausea and vomiting; rapid deterioration with respiratory distress and coma is seen.	Same as cerebral injuries; CT with contrast will demonstrate presence of aneurysm, AVM, or tumor

AVM, Arteriovenous malformation; *CSF,* cerebrospinal fluid; *CT,* computed tomography; *ICP,* intracranial pressure; *LOC,* level of consciousness; *MRI,* magnetic resonance imaging; *S/S,* signs and symptoms; *WBC,* white blood cell.

Pulmonary: adventitious sounds may be present.

Cardiovascular: cardiac dysrhythmias are not uncommon and may be life threatening.

Neurologic: see Table 5-7.

Diagnostic Findings

See Table 5-7.

ACUTE CARE PATIENT MANAGEMENT

Goals of Treatment

Optimize oxygenation.
> Ensure patent airway
> Supplemental oxygen
> Intubation and mechanical ventilation
> Intravenous fluids, blood replacement
> Vasopressor, antihypertensive, and vasodilator agents

Control and/or reduce increased ICP.
> CSF drainage
> Osmotic diuretics
> Evacuation of hematoma via burr hole or craniotomy
> Mild hyperventilation therapy
> Barbiturate coma

Detect/prevent clinical sequelae (Table 5-8).

Priority Nursing Diagnoses and Potential Complications

Priority Nursing Diagnoses	PC: Potential Complications
Impaired gas exchange	Respiratory failure, hypoxemia, atelectasis, pneumonia, aspiration
Impaired spontaneous ventilation	
Ineffective tissue perfusion: cerebral	Increased intracranial pressure (ICP), decreased cerebral perfusion pressure, hypotension, seizures
Risk for ineffective protection (see p. 48)	
Imbalanced nutrition: less than body requirements (see p. 53)	
Risk for interrupted family processes (see p. 45)	

Table 5-8 CLINICAL SEQUELAE OF HEAD INJURY

Complication	Signs and Symptoms
Neurogenic pulmonary edema	Severe restlessness, anxiety, confusion, diaphoresis, cyanosis, distended neck veins, moist, rapid, and shallow respirations, crackles, rhonchi, elevated BP, thready pulse, frothy and bloody sputum
ARDS	Dyspnea, RR >30, labored breathing, decreased compliance (30-40 cm H_2O), PAWP <18 mm Hg, hypoxemia refractory to increase in Fio_2
DIC	Bleeding from areas of injury, puncture sites, mucous membranes; hematuria, ecchymoses, prolonged PT and PTT; decreased fibrinogen, platelets, factors V, VIII, XIII, II; increased FSP
DI	Serum osmolality >300 mOsm/kg, serum sodium >145 mEq/L, urine osmolality <300 mOsm/L, urine specific gravity <1.005, urine output >200 mL/hr for 2 consecutive hours
SIADH	Low serum osmolality (<275 mOsm/L), serum sodium <130 mEq/L, decreased urinary output (400-500 mL/24 hr), generalized weight gain, urine osm greater than serum osm
Myocardial ischemia	Dysrhythmias, electrographic changes

ARDS, Acute respiratory distress syndrome; *BP,* blood pressure; *DI,* diabetes insipidus; *DIC,* disseminated intravascular coagulation; *FSP,* fibrin split products; *osm,* osmolality; *PAWP,* pulmonary artery wedge pressure; *PT,* prothrombin time; *PTT,* partial thromboplastin time; *RR,* respiratory rate; *SIADH,* syndrome of inappropriate antidiuretic hormone.

Nursing Diagnoses: IMPAIRED GAS EXCHANGE related to hypoventilation secondary to altered LOC or interstitial fluid secondary to neurogenic pulmonary edema; **INEFFECTIVE BREATHING PATTERN** secondary to injury to respiratory center

Outcome Criteria

Patient alert and oriented
Pao_2 80 to 100 mm Hg
O_2 sat ≥95%
$Paco_2$ 30 to 35 mm Hg
pH 7.35 to 7.45
RR 12 to 20 breaths/min, eupnea
Absence of adventitious breath sounds
PAWP 4 to 12 mm Hg

Patient Monitoring

1. Continuously monitor oxygen saturation with pulse oximetry (SpO_2). Monitor interventions and patient activities that may adversely affect oxygen saturation. Evaluate for possible onset of acute respiratory distress syndrome (ARDS).

2. Monitor CVP and PA pressures, including PAWP (if available) to monitor fluid volume status. Hypovolemia and hypotension can extend brain injury. Increasing wedge pressure may indicate development of neurogenic pulmonary edema. Calculate pulmonary vascular resistance index (PVRI); hypoxemia can increase sympathetic tone and increase pulmonary vasoconstriction.

Patient Assessment

1. Assess the patient's ability to handle oral secretions. Assess RR, depth, and rhythm frequently. Auscultate breath sounds every 1 to 2 hours and PRN.

2. Assess for signs and symptoms of hypoxia: change in LOC, increased restlessness, confusion, disorientation, and irritability. Assess nail beds, capillary refill, and skin temperature. Cyanosis is a late sign.

3. Assess integrity of the gag and cough reflexes; the patient may need to be intubated if reflexes are not intact.

4. Assess the patient for the development of clinical sequelae (see Table 5-8).

Diagnostics Assessment

1. Review serial ABGs for hypoxemia (PaO_2 <60 mm Hg) and hypercapnia ($PaCO_2$ >45 mm Hg); these disturbances can increase ICP.

2. Monitor for peak inspiratory and plateau inspiratory pressures; ARDS in brain trauma has a very high mortality.

3. Review serial chest radiographs for pulmonary congestion.

Patient Management

1. Administer oxygen as ordered. Ensure airway patency by proper positioning of the head and neck. Keep head of bed (HOB) elevated at 30 degrees to enhance chest excursion and reduce aspiration. If cervical injury has not been ruled out, do not hyperextend the neck for oral intubation; use the jaw-thrust method. Because of the risk of direct brain trauma or infection during insertion, nasopharyngeal airways should be

avoided in the presence of rhinorrhea (a sign that may reflect a break in the integrity of the skull). An oral airway or bite block can prevent the patient from biting an endotracheal tube (ETT) if orally intubated.

2. Provide pulmonary hygiene to reduce the risk of pulmonary complications (e.g., pneumonia, atelectasis). Initiate C&DB therapy and reposition the patient to mobilize secretions, carefully monitoring for increased ICP. Avoid coughing exercises for a patient at risk of increased ICP. Position to decrease risk of aspiration and ventilator-associated pneumonia. Patients with a Glasgow Coma Scale score of 8 or less should be endotracheally intubated to protect their airway.

3. Suction secretions only as needed. Obtain an order for lidocaine to suppress the patient's cough reflex and blunt increases in ICP. Hyperoxygenate before and after suctioning and limit passes of suction catheter to two passes, each timed for 15 seconds or less to avoid prolonged intracranial hypertension. Document quality and quantity of secretions. Never use nasotracheal suctioning in the presence of rhinorrhea because of the risk of direct brain trauma or infection.

Nursing Diagnosis: INEFFECTIVE TISSUE PERFUSION: CEREBRAL related to decreased intracranial adaptive capacity secondary to space-occupying lesion or cerebral edema

Outcome Criteria

Patient alert and oriented
Pupils equal and normoreactive
Motor strength equal bilaterally
RR 12 to 20 breaths/min, eupnea
HR 60 to 100 beats/min
ICP 0 to 15 mm Hg
CPP 70 to 100 mm Hg
SBP >90 mm Hg
Absence of headache, vomiting, seizures
Normal coagulation

Patient Monitoring

1. Monitor level of consciousness. A change of two values on the Glasgow Coma Scale may require physician notification and additional CT diagnostics.

2. Monitor cerebral oxygenation using jugular venous bulb saturation, jugular venous oxygen saturation ($Sjvo_2$), transcranial cerebral oximetry (cerebral oxygen saturation) (rSo_2), or cerebral oxygen tension ($Pbto_2$), and brain tissue oxygen tension if technology is available. Maintain $Sjvo_2$ >50%, rSo_2 >65 mm Hg, and $Pbto_2$ >20 mm Hg.

3. Monitor ICP trends every hour or more often if the patient's condition warrants. Analyze the ICP waveform and calculate CPP every 30 to 60 minutes. CPP <70 mm Hg leads to decreased CBF, resulting in cerebral ischemia. (See ICP monitoring, p. 462).

4. Monitor BP frequently because hypotension and HTN can aggravate secondary brain injury. Vasopressor or vasodilator therapy may be used.

5. Monitor CVP and/or PA pressures (if available) every hour because both parameters reflect the capacity of the vascular system to accept volume and can be used to monitor for imbalances that can compromise CPP.

6. Continuously monitor ECG for changes in rate and rhythm and nonspecific ST and T-wave changes.

7. Monitor I&O hourly and calculate hourly running totals. Polyuria (5-10 L/day) may signal the onset of diabetes insipidus (DI); oliguria (400-500 mL/day) may be symptomatic of SIADH.

8. Monitor urine specific gravity in the presence of DI or SIADH. Urine specific gravity will be increased in SIADH and decreased with diuretic administration; urine specific gravity will be decreased with the diuresis associated with DI.

9. Monitor serum coagulation factors: platelets, PT and INR. Coagulopathy is common after head injury and exacerbates adverse outcomes.

Patient Assessment

1. Assess neurologic status for signs and symptoms of herniation: progressive deterioration in LOC and motor function; changes in respiratory patterns (deep sighing and yawning may signal impending herniation); ipsilateral pupil dilation; and pupils sluggish or nonreactive to light (see Table 1-6).

2. Assess for factors that are related to increased ICP, such as a distended bladder, hypoxemia, hypercapnia, pain, headache, fear, or anxiety.

3. Assess temperature; fever may reflect damage to the hypothalamus and increase metabolic demands and oxygen consump-

tion. Because of the concern of possible seizure activity, avoid oral temperature taking especially with temporal lobe injuries.

4. Assess RR and rhythm. Central neurogenic hyperventilation may occur as a compensatory mechanism to increased ICP; Cheyne-Stokes respiratory pattern often precedes herniation; ataxic or agonal respirations are associated with damage to the medulla.

5. Test cranial nerve function because nerve damage can result from craniocerebral trauma (see Table 1-2). Table 5-9 identifies conditions that may have cranial nerve involvement.

6. Assess the patient for clinical sequelae (see Table 5-8).

Table 5-9 CRANIAL NERVE FUNCTIONS AND CLINICAL CORRELATIONS

Nerve	Function	Clinical Correlation
I Olfactory	Smell	Anterior fossa or cribriform plate fracture, frontal lobe or pituitary lesion, tumor, or meningitis
II Optic	Vision	Anterior fossa or orbital plate fracture, direct eye trauma, vascular disruption via carotid system and cerebral lesion
III Oculomotor	Elevates lid, moves eyeball, constricts pupil	Orbital plate fracture, temporal lobe swelling, increased ICP, aneurysm compression, or damage to midbrain
IV Trochlear	Moves eyeball	Inflammation or aneurysm
V Trigeminal	Muscles of mastication, facial sensation	Fractures of skull and face, pontine tumors, trauma
VI Abducens	Moves eyeball	Trauma, increased ICP, aneurysms, inflammation
VII Facial	Muscles of facial movement and taste	Temporal bone or middle fossa fracture, tumors, stroke, Bell's palsy, pons and medulla damage
VIII Acoustic	Hearing and balance	Temporal bone or middle fossa fractures, tumors, infection

Continued

Table 5-9   CRANIAL NERVE FUNCTIONS AND CLINICAL CORRELATIONS—Cont'd

Nerve	Function	Clinical Correlation
IX Glossopharyngeal	Sensation for gag, swallow	Dysfunction, usually seen with vagus nerve
X Vagus	Innervation of pharynx and thoracoabdominal viscera	Surgery (e.g., endarterectomy); unopposed action with cervical spine injuries, medulla damage
XI Accessory	Turns head	Neck surgery or trauma
XII Hypoglossal	Tongue movement	Brainstem involvement or higher

Modified from Hickey JV: *Neurological and neurosurgical nursing,* ed 5, Philadelphia, 2003, Lippincott Williams & Wilkins; Plum F, Posner J: *The diagnosis of stupor and coma,* ed 3, Philadelphia, 1980, FA Davis.
ICP, Intracranial pressure.

Diagnostics Assessment

1. Review serial ABGs for hypoxemia (PaO_2 <60 mm Hg) and hypercapnia ($PaCO_2$ >45 mm Hg); these disturbances can increase ICP.
2. Review serial serum glucose values; hyperglycemia can extend brain injury. Institute tight glycemic control protocol.
3. Review serum osmolality to maintain normal range, especially when using diuretics to manage intracranial hypertension.
4. Review serial electrolyte studies, serum and urine osmolality, and specific gravity for imbalances secondary to diuretic use and/or development of DI or SIADH.
5. Review serial Hgb and Hct levels for anemic states; WBC counts to evaluate the inflammatory process; fibrin degradation products (FDP), PT, and PTT to identify coagulopathy.
6. Review baseline and serial CT or MRI reports.

Patient Management

1. Administer oxygen as ordered to maximize cerebral oxygenation.
2. Reduce or minimize fluctuations in ICP by maintaining the patient's head and neck in neutral position, elevating the

HOB to 30 degrees to promote CSF drainage, and avoiding extreme flexion of hips. Some patients may have improved ICP and CPP with the HOB flat. Avoid taping or tying the ETT around the patient's neck.

3. Space nursing activities to avoid prolonging increased ICP. Calculate CPP before and after all nursing activities. If an increase in ICP is observed or the CPP falls below 70 mm Hg, stop the activity and all interactions until the ICP and CPP return to the previous reading.

4. Administer intravenous fluids carefully to minimize fluctuations in systemic and cerebral perfusion pressures and ICP. Hypotonic fluids (5% dextrose in water [D_5W]) are usually avoided to reduce the risk of cerebral edema. Hypertonic fluids may improve ICP.

5. Antihypertensive and vasopressor agents may be ordered to maintain BP and CPP. Monitor BP and CPP carefully. Even brief episodes of hypotension in the initial phase of resuscitation are significantly associated with mortality in brain injury.

6. Osmotic diuretics (e.g., mannitol) may be used to reduce edema. Monitor serum osmolality closely; an increased osmolality (>310 mOsm/kg) may disrupt the blood-brain barrier and actually increase edema. Monitor for hypotension and decreased CPP and increased ICP, which may occur up to 12 hours after osmotic diuresis. If loop diuretics are used, monitor urine output and electrolytes.

7. Consider use of fosphenytoin or phenytoin for prophylaxis to seizure activity; acetaminophen, to maintain normothermia; codeine or morphine sulfate for pain; propofol or midazolam for sedation; and paralytics to control agitation and/or assist with optimal ventilation. Seizures, fever, pain, agitation and hypoxemia may increase mortality and morbidity in the presence of severe brain injury.

8. Mild hyperventilation therapy (see p. 495) and barbiturate coma may be employed (see p. 487).

9. Mild hypothermia may be employed: use cooling blanket to maintain patient core temperature at 89.6° to 91.4° F (32°-33° C) within 3 to 4 hours of injury for 24 hours with gradual rewarming over the next 2 days.

10. Surgical intervention, such a decompression craniectomy or hematoma removal, may be required to evacuate the hematoma (see p. 491).

SEIZURES—STATUS EPILEPTICUS

NEURO

Clinical Brief

Seizures represent intermittent, sudden, massive discharge of abnormal activity from a group of neurons within the brain. Status epilepticus is a neurologic emergency in which two or more sequential seizures occur without full recovery of consciousness between seizures, or more than 30 minutes of continuous seizure activity occurs. Sustained seizures cause selective neuronal loss and functional decline; therefore it is reasonable to intervene when a seizure lasts more than 5 minutes, rather than waiting for the full 30 minutes that defines status epilepticus. Status epilepticus can present in a variety of clinical manifestations: repeated, generalized convulsions; focal motor or sensory disturbances with a variable change in the patient's LOC (partial complex or partial simple status epilepticus [SE]); or subtle myoclonus or ocular movements with electroencephalogram (EEG) signs of continuous abnormal CNS discharge (nonconvulsive SE). Status epilepticus should be suspected in patients who do not begin to wake up within 20 minutes after a seizure; an EEG can confirm ongoing seizure activity.

Causes of status epilepticus include sudden and total suppression of anticonvulsants (withdrawal), subtherapeutic levels of anticonvulsants, meningitis, encephalitis, cortical brain tumors, metabolic and toxic encephalopathies (e.g., nonketotic hyperglycemia), subarachnoid and intracerebral hemorrhage, stroke, and severe head injury. Drug toxicities (e.g., theophylline, cyclosporine, gamma-aminobutyric acid [GABA] antagonists), hypoxia (e.g., carbon monoxide poisoning, drowning) and withdrawal from alcohol use may also initiate status epilepticus.

Presenting Signs and Symptoms

The patient is comatose. Tonic-clonic epilepticus is characterized by generalized, repetitive tonic-clonic motor activity. Onset of symptoms may be partial (localized) or generalized. Nonconvulsive status epilepticus is characterized by fluctuating abnormal mental status, confusion, impaired responsiveness, and automatism as a result of absence (petite mal) and complex partial seizures.

Physical Examination

Vital signs:

   BP: mild HTN initially; hypotension with circulatory collapse

HR: tachycardia

RR: apnea during tonic phase; irregular gasping respiration during clonic phase

Temperature: mild to moderately elevated

Pulmonary: hypoxia and cyanosis during seizure activity

Cardiovascular: with sustained seizure activity, cardiovascular collapse possible

Neurologic: recurring, impaired consciousness, focal or generalized tonic-clonic movements without the patient regaining consciousness; incontinence, perspiration, salivation, and emesis may occur; pupils are often fixed and dilated; and eyes may be deviated or dysconjugate

Diagnostic Findings

Clinical manifestations are the basis for diagnosis. Diagnostic tests are performed to identify the cause of the seizure.

ACUTE CARE PATIENT MANAGEMENT

Goals of Treatment

Maintain oxygenation.

Establish an airway

Supplemental oxygen

Intubation

Mechanical ventilation

Maintain hemodynamic stability.

IV fluids

Vasopressor or vasodilator agents

Control seizure activity.

IV 50% dextrose in case hypoglycemia is responsible for seizure

Fast-acting anticonvulsant therapy (e.g., IV lorazepam, diazepam, midazolam)

Long-acting anticonvulsant therapy (e.g., IV fosphenytoin or phenytoin, pentobarbital)

Neuromuscular blockade (e.g., paraldehyde, lidocaine, general anesthesia)

Identify and treat cause.

Implementation of appropriate therapy

Detect/prevent clinical sequelae (Table 5-10).

Table 5-10   CLINICAL SEQUELAE OF SEIZURES

Complication	Signs and Symptoms
Respiratory arrest due to obstructed airway or changes in respiratory status during a seizure	Cessation of breathing
Trauma/falls incurred during the seizure	Musculoskeletal trauma
Cardiopulmonary arrest	Nonpalpable pulse, absent respirations

Priority Nursing Diagnoses and Potential Complications

Priority Nursing Diagnoses	PC: Potential Complications
Risk for injury	Musculoskeletal trauma, hypoxemia, CNS ischemia
Risk for ineffective protection (see p. 48)	
Imbalanced nutrition: less than body requirements (see p. 53)	
Risk for interrupted family processes (see p. 45)	

Nursing Diagnosis: RISK FOR INJURY related to increased metabolic demand secondary to continuous seizure activity

Outcome Criteria

Patient alert and oriented
Pupils equal, round, and normoreactive
Motor strength equal in all extremities
SBP 90 to 140 mm Hg
HR 60 to 100 beats/min
RR 12 to 20 breaths/min, eupnea
Normothermic
Pao_2 80 to 100 mm Hg
$Paco_2$ 35 to 45 mm Hg
O_2 sat ≥95%
pH 7.35 to 7.45
HCO_3 22 to 25 mEq/L
Absence of musculoskeletal trauma
Urine output 30 mL/hr or 0.5 to 1 mL/kg/hr

Patient Monitoring

1. Continuously monitor for cardiac dysrhythmias, which may occur as a result of hypoxemia, acidosis, or anticonvulsant drug administration.
2. Continuously monitor oxygen saturation with pulse oximetry (SpO_2).
3. Monitor CPP if ICP monitoring is available.
4. Monitor the compressed spectral analysis (CSA) if available for continued EEG trends and effectiveness of medications.
5. Monitor I&O; myoglobinuria may occur with prolonged seizure activity and lead to renal failure.

Patient Assessment

1. Assess and document information detailing seizure activity: length of tonic and clonic phases, motor characteristics and body involvement, and deviation of eyes and pupil reaction. Note: use room light to assess pupils because a direct flashing light may elicit or cause progression of seizure. Note any automatic behavior (e.g., lip smacking, chewing), incontinence, or cyanosis.
2. Assess respiratory status, including airway patency; rate, depth, and rhythm of respirations; breath sounds; use of accessory muscles; and color of skin, lips, and nail beds. Monitor ability to handle secretions; and assess gag, cough, and swallow reflexes.
3. Assess peripheral pulses, skin, and urinary output at least every hour to evaluate tissue perfusion.
4. During seizure activity and during the administration of anticonvulsant drugs, monitor VS. Respiratory depression, decreased BP, and dysrhythmias can occur with rapid infusion of diazepam, phenytoin, and phenobarbital.
5. Perform baseline and serial neurologic assessments after status is interrupted. During the postictal phase of the seizure, assessment should include LOC, motor response to stimuli, and speech every 15 minutes for the first hour, then every 30 minutes for 2 hours. Patient responses should improve with each assessment. Be alert to the presence of focal findings suggestive of an expanding lesion and signs of increased ICP.
6. After the seizure, assess skin integrity for bruises, lacerations, or shearing injuries. Assess tongue, lips, and mouth for evidence of bite injuries.

7. Assess IV insertion sites for patency and extravasation of anticonvulsants.
8. Assess patients for development of clinical sequelae (see Table 5-10).

Diagnostics Assessment

1. Review EEG recording and maintain communication with the physician regarding the results.
2. Review electrolyte and blood glucose levels because electrolyte imbalance and hypoglycemia may precipitate seizures or occur as a result of prolonged seizure activity.
3. Review serum anticonvulsant drug levels for therapeutic ranges.
4. Review ABGs for hypoxemia and acidosis; both abnormalities can precipitate seizures or can occur as a result of prolonged seizure activity.
5. Review LP results if available.
6. Review CT, MRI for presence of CNS tumors, infections, inflammation, injury, or infarction. Review chest radiographs for indications of pulmonary complications (e.g., infiltrates, aspiration).

Patient Management

1. Pad side rails and keep them up at all times; maintain the bed in its lowest position.
2. Keep an oral airway at the bedside with suction equipment.
3. Protect the patient during the seizure (e.g., do not restrain the patient, and guide extremity movement during the seizure to prevent injury and protect the patient's head).
4. Maintain airway and ventilation to ensure maximum delivery of oxygen to the brain cells. Administer an oxygen concentration of 100% via mask or bag-mask during seizure activity. An oral airway may help maintain airway patency, but do not force an airway during seizure activity.
5. Position the patient on one side to facilitate drainage of oral secretions, and suction as necessary. Do not simply turn the patient's head to the side; this position promotes aspiration of emesis or secretions, occludes the airway, and interferes with venous return, which increases ICP. Maintain a suction setup at all times.
6. Be prepared to assist with intubation and mechanical ventilation if necessary. (See p. 503 for information on ventilation therapies.)

7. An NG tube may be required to prevent vomiting and aspiration.

8. Maintain a large-bore IV line for fluids and medication administration. Assess IV insertion sites for patency, especially after seizure activity, and be particularly careful to avoid extravasation of anticonvulsants.

9. Administer anticonvulsants such as lorazepam or diazepam as ordered: doses will vary and should be administered slow intravenous push (IVP). Monitor the patient for respiratory depression and hypotension.

    Fosphenytoin (rapidly converted to phenytoin in the body; fewer cardiovascular events) or *phenytoin* 500 to 1000 mg (18-20 mg PE [phenytoin equivalents]/kg) IV may be ordered. IV line must be flushed with NS before and after administration. Rate of phenytoin should not exceed 50 mg/min and fosphenytoin should not exceed 150 mg/min; administer at a setting equipped to provide advanced cardiac life support with continuous monitoring of LOC, HR, and BP. If fosphenytoin or phenytoin is not effective, *valproic acid* (10-15 mg/kg/day, divided dose) or *pentobarbital* 5 mg/kg loading dose, followed by a maintenance infusion of 1 to 3 mg/kg/hr for 6 to 48 hours may be ordered.

    Other pharmacologic therapy may include thiamine (100 mg), midazolam, propofol, phenobarbital, paraldehyde, lidocaine, general anesthesia, or neuromuscular blockade to stop the seizure activity. If neuromuscular blocking agents are used, the tonic-clonic motor activity will stop but the abnormal cerebral electrical activity will not.

10. After the seizure, stay with the patient, reassuring and reorienting the patient as necessary.

11. Keep the patient in a side-lying position to facilitate drainage of oral secretions; suction the secretions as needed.

PULMONARY DISORDERS

ACUTE RESPIRATORY FAILURE (ARF)

Clinical Brief

Respiratory failure results from the inability of the lungs to adequately oxygenate the blood to meet the metabolic needs of the body. The impaired gas exchange results in hypoxemia. The causes of ARF (Table 5-11) involve one of four following mechanisms, or a combination of the mechanisms.

1. *Alveolar hypoventilation* occurs in disorders of the CNS or neuromuscular system, causing less oxygen to be supplied and less carbon dioxide to be removed.

2. *Intrapulmonary shunting* occurs when blood moves past alveoli that are fluid filled or collapsed. This shunted blood, which is poorly oxygenated, mixes with oxygenated blood, lowering the PaO_2.

3. *Ventilation-perfusion mismatch* occurs when there is blood flow to the underventilated areas of the lung or when there is

Table 5-11 CAUSES OF ACUTE RESPIRATORY FAILURE

System	Disorder	Example
Central nervous	Overdose	Opioids, sedatives, anesthetics, barbiturates
	Head trauma	Brainstem injury
	Infections	Meningitis, encephalitis
Neuromuscular	Infections	Polio
	Trauma	Spinal cord injury
	Neurologic condition	Myasthenia gravis, Guillain-Barré syndrome
Respiratory	Airway obstruction	Epiglottitis, fractured trachea, laryngeal edema, laryngospasm, asthma
	Pulmonary	Flail chest, pneumothorax, hemothorax, COPD exacerbation, pneumonia, pulmonary edema, ARDS, SARS

ARDS, Acute respiratory distress syndrome; *COPD,* chronic obstructive pulmonary disease; *SARS,* severe acute respiratory syndrome.

adequate ventilation but blood flow is decreased or absent in that area.

4. *Diffusion abnormalities* occur when gas exchange across the alveolar capillary membrane is disrupted, such as in pulmonary edema or pulmonary fibrosis.

PULM

Presenting Signs and Symptoms

The patient may have an increased or decreased RR, shallow respirations, use of accessory muscles, and an altered LOC. Chronic obstructive pulmonary disease (COPD) patients may exhibit increased cough and dyspnea.

Physical Examination

Appearance: diaphoretic, agitated, restless
Vital signs:
BP: $\uparrow$ caused by hypoxemia or $\downarrow$ in shock
HR: tachycardia
RR: >30 breaths/min (<10/min if CNS depression)
Temperature: normal or $\uparrow$ with infectious process
Skin: cool and dry to diaphoretic
Neurologic: restlessness, deteriorating mental status
Pulmonary: use of accessory muscles, paradoxical motion of abdomen; crackles, rhonchi, diminished breath sounds or wheezing on auscultation

Diagnostic Findings

Room air ABGs: decreased PaO_2 (<60 mm Hg), usually with an increased $PaCO_2$ (>50 mm Hg) and decreased pH (<7.35).
When ARF develops in patients with COPD, there is a low to normal pH, elevated bicarbonate level, and decreased serum chloride level.

ACUTE CARE PATIENT MANAGEMENT

Goals of Treatment

Optimize oxygenation.
Patent airway
Oxygen therapy
Bronchodilator therapy
Mechanical ventilation
Treatment of underlying problem
Detect/prevent clinical sequelae (Table 5-12).

Table 5-12 CLINICAL SEQUELAE OF ACUTE RESPIRATORY FAILURE

Complication	Signs and Symptoms
Tissue hypoxia	Restlessness, decreased level of consciousness, dysrhythmias, angina, myocardial infarction, right-sided heart failure, decreased urine output
Cardiopulmonary arrest	Absence of palpable pulses, no spontaneous respirations (nonventilated patients)

Priority Nursing Diagnoses and Potential Complications

Priority Nursing Diagnoses	PC: Potential Complications
Impaired gas exchange	Hypoxemia, respiratory alkalosis (early), respiratory acidosis (late)
Ineffective tissue perfusion	Dysrhythmias, metabolic acidosis
Ineffective protection (see p. 48)	Atelectasis, pneumonia
Imbalanced nutrition: less than body requirements (see p. 53)	Negative nitrogen balance, electrolyte imbalances
Risk for interrupted family process (see p. 45)	

Nursing Diagnosis: IMPAIRED GAS EXCHANGE related to hypoventilation, increased pulmonary shunt, ventilation-perfusion mismatch, or diffusion disturbances

Outcome Criteria

Alert and oriented
Relaxed accessory muscles in neck and shoulders
Lungs clear to auscultation
PaO_2 80 to 100 mm Hg (or baseline for a patient with COPD)
pH 7.35 to 7.45
$PaCO_2$ 35 to 45 mm Hg (or baseline for a patient with COPD)
O_2 sat ≥95%
SvO_2 60% to 80%
SBP 90 to 120 mm Hg
MAP 70 to 105 mm Hg
HR 60 to 100 beats/min
RR 12 to 20 breaths/min

Patient Monitoring

1. Continuously monitor oxygen saturation with pulse oximetry (SpO_2). If SvO_2 monitoring is available, continuously

monitor readings. Carefully monitor nursing interventions and patient activities that may adversely affect oxygenation status.

2. Monitor PAS pressure (if available) because hypoxemia can increase sympathetic tone and increase pulmonary vasoconstriction.

3. Continuously monitor ECG for changes in HR, ischemic changes, and development of dysrhythmias.

4. Monitor arterial BP, PA pressures, CO/CI, and CVP because hypoxemia can produce deleterious effects on the cardiovascular system.

Patient Assessment

1. Assess LOC. Note if the patient becomes restless, agitated, or complains of a headache; these signs may signal decreased cerebral oxygenation.

2. Assess for signs of respiratory distress, signaling the need for intubation and mechanical ventilation: intercostal retractions, RR >30 breaths/min, and paradoxical breathing.

3. Assess for adventitious lung sounds.

4. Assess the patient for signs of heart failure (HF): jugular venous distention (JVD), peripheral edema, cough, crackles, S_3, and tachycardia.

5. Assess the patient for clinical sequelae (see Table 5-12).

Diagnostics Assessment

1. Review ABGs for decreasing Pao_2, increasing $Paco_2$, and acidosis. In COPD patients, $Paco_2$ levels are normally high and are not the sole factor on which to base the decision to intubate and mechanically ventilate the patient's lungs.

2. Review Hgb and Hct levels because adequate hemoglobin is needed to carry oxygen.

Patient Management

1. Administer oxygen therapy as ordered.

2. Assist the patient to assume a position that improves chest excursion. Correlate the effects of position changes on oxygen saturation to determine which position improves oxygenation.

3. Anticipate noninvasive positive pressure ventilation for acute hypoxemic respiratory failure, acute cardiogenic pulmonary edema, or acute-on-chronic respiratory failure. This therapy may prevent intubation. It is useful in patients who have

limited secretions, are hemodynamically stable, and have a cause of respiratory failure that can be quickly reversed.

4. If the patient's lungs are mechanically ventilated, see p. 503 for more information on ventilation therapies.

5. Inhaled β-agonists (albuterol) may be prescribed to relieve bronchoconstriction.

6. Anticholinergic agents (ipratropium bromide) may be administered by inhalation to relieve bronchoconstriction.

7. Corticosteroids may be prescribed to reduce an inflammatory response in patients with lung disease.

8. Proceed in a calm manner and reassure the anxious and fearful patient because anxiety and fear may increase feelings of dyspnea and tissue oxygen demands.

9. Reduce oxygen demands by pacing activities and scheduling rest periods. Relieve anxiety, pain, and fever. Sedate the patient as needed, closely monitoring respiratory function.

10. Provide pulmonary hygiene: chest physiotherapy, postural drainage, and C&DB. Suction secretions if the patient's cough is ineffective.

ACUTE RESPIRATORY DISTRESS SYNDROME (ARDS)

Clinical Brief

ARDS is a syndrome of lung inflammation and increased pulmonary capillary permeability caused by acute injury. ARDS is usually associated with sepsis, aspiration, pneumonia, or trauma. The three criteria that define ARDS are bilateral lung infiltrates, PaO_2/FIO_2 ≤200 mm Hg, and PAWP ≤18 mm Hg. Noncardiogenic pulmonary edema, decreased lung compliance, and hypoxemia refractory to supplemental oxygen characterize ARDS.

Presenting Signs and Symptoms

The patient may exhibit dyspnea, tachypnea, tachycardia, restlessness, and anxiety. As ARDS progresses, the patient may exhibit multiorgan dysfunction.

Physical Examination

Vital signs:

BP: ↑ or ↓ in response to hypoxemia or hemodynamic compromise

HR: ↑ or ↓ in response to hypoxemia

RR: >30 breaths/min

Neurologic: restlessness, agitation, decrease in sensorium
Pulmonary: cough, fine inspiratory crackles, use of accessory muscles

Diagnostic Findings

Arterial Blood Gases (ABGs)

Pao_2 <60 mm Hg, unresponsive to oxygen therapy

Chest Radiograph

May be normal for the first 12 to 24 hours after the respiratory distress occurs. The earliest abnormalities seen are patchy, bilateral, interstitial, and alveolar infiltrates. If the patient improves, the radiographic appearance may return to normal. When the disease progresses, the alveolar infiltrates advance to a diffuse consolidation (see Figure 1-11 on p. 21).

Pulmonary Function

Compliance <50 mL/cm H_2O
Shunt fraction (Qs/Qt) >5%
Alveolar-arterial gradient (P[A-a]o_2)
P(a/A)o_2 ratio <0.6
Pao_2/Fio_2 ≤200 mm Hg
PAWP ≤18 mm Hg (implies that alveolar infiltrates are not related to fluid volume excess)

ACUTE CARE PATIENT MANAGEMENT

Goals of Treatment

Optimize tissue oxygenation as for ARF, then add:
  PEEP
  Pressure control ventilation
  Inverse ratio ventilation
  Prone positioning
  High-frequency ventilation
  Extracorporeal membrane oxygenation (ECMO)
Maintain hemodynamic stability.
  Careful fluid volume management
  Vasopressor agents
  Inotropic agents
In clinical trials: surfactant replacement
  Antioxidants
  Liquid ventilation

PULM

Inhaled nitric oxide

Prostaglandin E_1

Antiinflammatory agents

Detect/prevent clinical sequelae (Table 5-13).

PULM

Table 5-13 CLINICAL SEQUELAE OF ACUTE RESPIRATORY DISTRESS SYNDROME

Complication	Signs and Symptoms
Dysrhythmias	Changes in rate, rhythm
	Change in LOC or syncope
Pneumonia	Purulent sputum, fever
GI bleeding	Coffee-ground emesis, guaiac-positive emesis and stool
DIC	Bleeding from any orifice, mucous membranes; petechiae, hematuria, hematemesis; prolonged PT/PTT; ↑ fibrin split products; ↓ platelets
Renal failure	Decreased urine output; ↑ BUN and Cr
Respiratory arrest	Cessation of breathing

BUN, Blood urea nitrogen; *Cr*, creatinine; *DIC*, disseminated intravascular coagulation; *GI*, gastrointestinal; *LOC*, level of consciousness; *PT*, prothrombin time; *PTT*, partial thromboplastin time.

Priority Nursing Diagnoses and Potential Complications

Same as for ARF, see p. 144

Nursing Diagnoses: IMPAIRED GAS EXCHANGE related to interstitial and alveolar fluid accumulation; INEFFECTIVE BREATHING PATTERN related to decreased respiratory compliance

Outcome Criteria

Patient alert and oriented

O_2 sat ≥95%

PaO_2 >60 mm Hg

SvO_2 60% to 80%

RR 12 to 20 breaths/min, eupnea

Lung sounds clear to auscultation

HR 60 to 100 beats/min

P(a/A)O_2 ratio >0.60

PaO_2/FIO_2 ≥200 mm Hg

Patient Monitoring

1. Continuously monitor ECG for dysrhythmias that may be related to hypoxemia or acid-base imbalances.

2. Continuously monitor oxygen saturation with pulse oximetry (SpO_2). Carefully monitor interventions and patient activities that may adversely affect oxygen saturation.

3. Continuously monitor SvO_2 (if available); carefully monitor interventions and patient activities that may adversely affect oxygenation.

4. Monitor pulmonary function by evaluating serial vital capacities and tidal volumes. Monitor airway pressures and compliance every 8 hours.

5. Monitor PA systolic because hypoxia can increase sympathetic tone and increase pulmonary vasoconstriction. Calculate PVRI.

6. Obtain CO/CI readings because oxygen delivery depends on adequate CO.

7. Calculate $P(a/A)O_2$ ratio and PaO_2/FiO_2 to evaluate oxygenation.

8. Monitor fluid volume status: measure I&O hourly, determine fluid balance every 8 hours. Compare serial weights for changes (1 kg is approximately 1000 mL of fluid). Fluid excess may cause cardiogenic pulmonary edema.

9. If the patient's lungs are mechanically ventilated, see p. 503 for information on ventilation therapies.

Patient Assessment

1. Assess respiratory status every 2 hours or more often, depending on patient condition. Note RR, rhythm, depth, and use of accessory muscles. Observe for paradoxical breathing pattern, increased restlessness, increased complaints of dyspnea, and changes in LOC. Cyanosis is a late sign of respiratory distress.

2. Assess the patient for clinical sequelae (see Table 5-13).

Diagnostics Assessment

1. Review serial ABGs to evaluate oxygenation and acid-base balance.

2. Review serial chest radiographs to evaluate improving or worsening condition.

3. Review serial Hgb and Hct levels; a reduced Hgb can adversely affect oxygen-carrying capacity.

PULM

1. Administer oxygen as ordered; intubation and mechanical ventilation are usually required. Use lung protective ventilation with positive end-expiratory pressure (PEEP) and small tidal volumes of 6 to 10 mL/kg. Pressure control and inverse ratio ventilation may also be used. (See p. 503 for information on ventilation therapies.)

2. Reposition the patient to improve oxygenation, mobilize secretions, and decrease the risk of aspiration and ventilator-acquired pneumonia. Evaluate the patient's response to position changes with ABGs or SpO_2 to determine the best position for oxygenation.

3. Consider placing the patient in the prone position for 6 to 12 hours/day in the early phase of ARDS to improve gas exchange. Ensure good patient alignment; secure airway and invasive lines with a minimum of four staff members assisting to prevent patient or staff injury. Use turning sheets and slideboard or a commercial proning device. Pad bony prominences for pressure relief while prone. Avoid pressure on eyes and abdomen. Partially reposition for pressure relief every 1 to 2 hours. Have team prepared to return patient to supine position rapidly in case of hemodynamic instability or cardiac arrest.

4. Suction the patient's secretions as needed to maintain airway patency. Preoxygenate the patient's lungs with an FIO_2 of 1 to prevent a decrease in oxygen saturation. Assess hemodynamic response to suctioning. Note the characteristics of the sputum.

5. Administer antibiotics as ordered to treat the identified organism.

6. Replace fluids judiciously to maintain intravascular volume without contributing to alveolar edema.

7. Decrease oxygen consumption by limiting and pacing activities, providing uninterrupted rest, decreasing anxiety, controlling pain, and decreasing fever.

8. Sedation may be needed to provide adequate ventilation.

9. Therapeutic paralysis with the administration of a neuromuscular blocking agent may be required for patient-ventilator synchrony or to decrease oxygen needs. (See p. 595 for information on neuromuscular blockade.)

10. High-frequency ventilation or ECMO may be used to improve gas exchange when other methods of ventilatory

support have failed. (See p. 503 for information on ventilation therapies.)

11. NG intubation may be required to decompress the stomach
    and decrease the risk of aspiration.

12. Nutritional support will be required to prevent respiratory
    muscle dysfunction and to maintain immunologic defense
    mechanisms.

PULM

**Nursing Diagnoses: INEFFECTIVE TISSUE PERFUSION related to hypoxia and/or
decreased cardiac output secondary to decreased venous return with PEEP**

Outcome Criteria

Alert and oriented
Peripheral pulses strong
SBP 90 to 120 mm Hg
MAP 70 to 105 mm Hg
HR 60 to 100 beats/min
CI 2.5 to 4 L/min/m^2
Urine output 30 mL/hr or 0.5 to 1 mL/kg/hr
PAWP 4 to 12 mm Hg
CVP 2 to 6 mm Hg
SVRI 1700 to 2600 dynes/sec/cm^{-5}/m^2
PVRI 200 to 450 dynes/sec/cm^{-5}/m^2

Patient Monitoring

1. Obtain PA, arterial BP, and CVP readings hourly or more
   often if titrating pharmacologic agents or increasing PEEP
   levels. Monitor MAP; a MAP <60 mm Hg can adversely affect
   cerebral and renal perfusion. Obtain CO/CI with each change
   in PEEP. Monitor SVRI and PVRI.

2. Monitor fluid volume status: measure I&O hourly and determine fluid balance every 8 hours. Compare serial weights for
   changes (1 kg is approximately 1000 mL of fluid). Decrease in
   urinary output may be related to decreased renal perfusion
   secondary to decreased CO or to development of SIADH in
   the patient undergoing mechanical ventilation therapy.

3. Continuously monitor ECG for signs of myocardial ischemia
   or the onset of dysrhythmias.

Patient Assessment

1. Assess LOC, skin, peripheral pulses, and capillary refill as
   indicators of CO and tissue perfusion.

2. With increasing levels of PEEP, assess for development of pneumothorax.

3. Assess skin for pressure ulcer development related to hypoperfusion.

4. Assess the patient for clinical sequelae (see Table 5-13).

Diagnostics Assessment

1. Review serial ABGs; hypoxemia and acidosis can adversely affect myocardial contractility and contribute to decreasing CO.

2. Review serial Hgb and Hct levels; adequate hemoglobin is necessary to maintain normal oxygen transport.

3. Review lactate levels, which are an indicator of anaerobic metabolism. Increased levels may signal decreased O_2 delivery.

Patient Management

1. Administer crystalloids or colloids as ordered to maintain adequate preload. Monitor fluid status carefully because excessive fluid can increase hydrostatic pressure and worsen pulmonary edema.

2. Titrate positive inotropic agents to improve myocardial contractility and increase CO. Vasopressor agents may be required to maintain SBP ≥90 mm Hg.

3. Institute pressure ulcer prevention strategies.

CHEST TRAUMA

Clinical Brief

Injuries to the structures of the thorax can be caused by blunt or penetrating trauma such as motor vehicle accidents, falls, gunshot wounds, and stab wounds. Tissue hypoxia is a major concern because the intrathoracic organs are highly vascular and hemorrhagic shock is common. Hypercarbia may result from hypoventilation. Respiratory acidosis may be caused by inadequate ventilation, depressed LOC, or changes in intrathoracic pressure relationships. Pleural pressure changes can lead to collapsed lungs or mediastinal shift; ventilation-perfusion mismatch can also occur as a result of the injury. Dysrhythmias can occur with myocardial injury secondary to trauma to the sternum. According to the American College of Surgeons, approximately 25% of all trauma deaths are a result of chest injuries. (Table 5-14 has a summary of chest injuries.)

Table 5-14 SUMMARY OF CHEST INJURIES

Injury	Clinical Brief	Signs and Symptoms
Flail chest	Instability of chest wall as a result of multiple rib or sternal fractures Diagnostic findings: chest radiograph confirms fractures; abnormal respiratory motion and crepitus aids diagnosis	Paradoxical chest motion, labored shallow respirations
Pneumothorax	Accumulation of air in the pleural space; partial or total lung collapse Diagnostic findings: chest radiograph visualizes air between visceral and parietal pleura	Dyspnea, decreased or absent breath sounds, asymmetric chest movement, subcutaneous emphysema Open pneumothorax: wound present, often sucking in nature Closed pneumothorax: no opening to external environment
Tension pneumothorax	Accumulation of air without a means of escape, causing complete collapse of the lung and mediastinal shift; immediate decompression necessary Diagnostic findings: clinical, not radiologic, findings are the basis for diagnosis	Severe dyspnea, cyanosis, restlessness, distended neck veins, absence of breath sounds on affected side, tracheal shift to the unaffected side, hypotension, distant heart sounds, tachycardia

Continued

Table 5-14 SUMMARY OF CHEST INJURIES—cont'd

Injury	Clinical Brief	Signs and Symptoms
Hemothorax	Accumulation of blood in the pleural space Diagnostic findings: chest radiograph visualizes blood accumulation	Cool, clammy skin; hypotension, decreased capillary refill, tachycardia, decreased or absent breath sounds on affected side
Pulmonary contusion	Injury to lung tissue that can cause respiratory failure, potentially lethal Diagnostic findings: chest radiograph shows local or diffuse patchy infiltrates, poorly outlined densities, or irregular linear infiltrates (changes may not be evident until 12-24 hours after injury); ABGs: hypoxemia and hypercarbia	Dyspnea, restlessness, hemoptysis, tachycardia, ineffective cough, crackles, decreased lung compliance
Tracheobronchial tear	Injury to tracheobronchial tree that can result in airway obstruction and tension pneumothorax Diagnostic findings: clinical findings are the basis of diagnosis: CT scan, endoscopic procedures or bronchoscopy confirms the tear	Fractured larynx: hoarseness, subcutaneous emphysema, palpable fracture Tracheal injury: noisy breathing, depressed LOC, labored respiratory effort Bronchial injury: hemoptysis, subcutaneous emphysema, possible S/S of tension pneumothorax
Myocardial contusion	Injury to cardiac muscle that may result in dysrhythmias, muscle damage, cardiac rupture	Chest discomfort, bruising, abnormal ECG changes: multiple PVCs, unexplained sinus tachycardia, atrial fibrillation, ST segment; hypotension

PULM

Injury		Diagnostic findings	Signs and symptoms
		Diagnostic findings: no single diagnostic test is used; echocardiogram is helpful to evaluate abnormal wall motion; ECG monitoring for PVCs, atrial fibrillation, ST segment abnormalities; serial CKs or troponin levels to evaluate myocardial damage are of questionable value	
Diaphragm rupture	Tear in the diaphragm that may allow abdominal contents to herniate into thorax	Diagnostic findings: chest radiograph with contrast confirms tear; NG tube may be observed curled in lower left chest; appearance of peritoneal lavage fluid in chest tube drainage confirms the diagnosis	Chest pain referred to shoulder, dyspnea, decreased breath sounds, bowel sounds auscultated in chest, possible rhonchi
Esophageal rupture	Perforation of the esophagus that allows gastric and esophageal contents to contaminate the mediastinum and pleura	Diagnostic findings: chest radiograph visualizes mediastinal air on the left side, pleural effusion, pneumothorax; contrast studies and/or esophagoscopy confirms tear	Left pneumothorax or hemothorax without rib fracture; history of blow to lower sternum or epigastrium and pain or shock out of proportion to injury; particulate matter in chest tube

ABG, Arterial blood gas; *CK,* creatine kinase; *CT,* computed tomography; *ECG,* electrocardiogram; *LOC,* level of consciousness; *NG,* nasogastric; *PVC,* premature ventricular contraction; *S/S,* signs and symptoms.

Presenting Signs and Symptoms and Diagnostic Findings

See Table 5-14.

ACUTE CARE PATIENT MANAGEMENT

Goals of Treatment

Improve ventilation and gas exchange.

Provide a patent airway

Oxygen therapy

Intubation and mechanical ventilation

Chest tube insertion

Hemothorax: Chest tube, thoracotomy

Pulmonary contusion: diuretics, methylprednisolone (controversial), unilateral lung ventilation, ECMO

Tracheobronchial tear: thoracotomy

Esophageal rupture: NG intubation, surgical repair

Maintain hemodynamic stability.

Crystalloid infusion

Blood products, autotransfusion

Tension pneumothorax: needle decompression, chest tube insertion

Myocardial contusion: antidysrhythmic agents

Decrease/alleviate pain.

Opioids

Patient-controlled analgesia (PCA)

Intercostal nerve block

Epidural analgesia

Detect/prevent clinical sequelae (Table 5-15).

Priority Nursing Diagnoses and Potential Complications	
Priority Nursing Diagnoses	**PC: Potential Complications**
Impaired gas exchange	Hypoxemia, pneumothorax, dysrhythmias, respiratory acidosis
Ineffective tissue perfusion	Decreased cardiac output, dysrhythmias
Decreased cardiac output	Metabolic acidosis, dysrhythmias
Acute pain	
Risk for ineffective protection (see p. 48)	Sepsis
Imbalanced nutrition: less than body requirements (see p. 53)	Negative nitrogen balance, electrolyte imbalances
Risk for interrupted family processes (see p. 45)	

PULM

Table 5-15 Clinical Sequelae of Chest Trauma

Complication	Signs and Symptoms
Hypoxemia	Restlessness, RR >30 breaths/min, HR >120 beats/min, labored breathing, increase in PAP
Hemothorax/shock	Decrease in sensorium; cool, clammy skin; HR >120 beats/min, SBP <90 mm Hg; urine output <0.5 mL/kg/hr
Tension pneumothorax	Severe dyspnea, tracheal deviation toward unaffected side, absence of breath sounds, distended neck veins, unequal chest symmetry (chest is larger on side of pneumothorax), cyanosis, hypotension
Pulmonary contusion	Chest wall abrasions, ecchymosis, hemoptysis; history of blunt chest trauma
Pulmonary edema	Tachypnea, cough, frothy sputum, crackles
ARDS	Dyspnea, RR >30, labored breathing, tachycardia, decreased compliance (30-40 cm H_2O), PAWP ≤18 mm Hg, hypoxemia refractory to increase in FiO_2
Pneumonia	Temperature >101.3° F (38.5° C), purulent secretions, ineffective cough, diminished breath sounds

ARDS, Acute respiratory distress syndrome; *HR,* heart rate; *PAP,* pulmonary artery pressure; *PAWP,* pulmonary artery wedge pressure; *RR,* respiratory rate; *SBP,* systolic blood pressure.

Nursing Diagnosis: IMPAIRED GAS EXCHANGE related to ventilation-perfusion mismatch, decreased compliance, inadequate ventilation

Outcome Criteria

Patient alert and oriented
RR 12 to 20 breaths/min, eupnea
PaO_2 80 to 100 mm Hg
pH 7.35 to 7.45
$PaCO_2$ 35 to 45 mm Hg
O_2 sat ≥95%
$P(a/A)O_2$ 0.75 to 0.90
Minute ventilation <10 L/min

PULM

1. Continuously monitor ECG because hypoxemia is a risk factor for dysrhythmias.

2. Continuously monitor oxygen saturation with pulse oximetry (Sp_{O_2}). Be alert for interventions and patient activities that may adversely affect oxygen saturation.

3. Continuously monitor end-tidal CO_2 with capnography (if available) to evaluate adequacy of ventilation.

4. Monitor pulmonary function by reviewing serial minute ventilation, calculating physiologic shunt (Qs/Qt), or calculating arterial-alveolar oxygen tension ratio $P(a/A)_{O_2}$.

5. Monitor PAS (if available) because hypoxemia can increase sympathetic tone and increase pulmonary vasoconstriction. Monitor PVRI.

6. Monitor the chest drainage system, which is used to drain air or fluid from the pleural space. Record drainage hourly; consult with physician if drainage is >200 mL/hr. If drainage suddenly ceases, check the patient and system—a tension pneumothorax can develop. (See p. 497 for more information on chest drainage.)

7. If the patient is undergoing mechanical ventilation therapy, see p. 503 for more information.

1. Assess respiratory status and observe for respiratory distress and increased patient effort: RR >30 breaths/min; paradoxical motion of the rib cage and abdomen; and presence of intercostal and supraclavicular retraction. Auscultate lungs and note adventitious or diminished lung sounds.

2. Assess for signs and symptoms of hypoxia: increased restlessness, increased complaints of dyspnea, and changes in LOC. Cyanosis is a late sign.

3. Assess the patient for clinical sequelae (see Table 5-15).

1. Review ABGs for decreasing trend in Pa_{O_2}, despite increasing FI_{O_2}. This may suggest ARDS, which can develop with lung injury (e.g., flail chest, pulmonary contusion).

2. Review serial chest radiographs or CT scans to evaluate patient progress or worsening lung condition and to verify the placement of CT and other invasive catheters.

3. Review Hgb and Hct levels because oxygen carrying capacity can be adversely affected with decreased Hgb.

Patient Management

1. Administer supplemental oxygen. Oxygen percentage and delivery system are based on ABGs, SpO_2, and the patient's respiratory status.
2. Promote pulmonary hygiene with incentive spirometry, chest physiotherapy, C&DB therapy, and position changes every 2 hours. Note sputum color and consistency. Patients with impaired breathing patterns who are immobilized and have an ineffective cough are at risk for atelectasis and secretion retention. Anticipate antibiotic therapy for pulmonary infections.
3. If the patient develops respiratory distress, be prepared for intubation and mechanical ventilation. Unconventional modes of ventilation may be employed if ventilation and gas exchange do not improve. (See p. 503 for information on ventilation therapies.) If mechanically ventilated, position patient to decrease the risk of aspiration and ventilator-acquired pneumonia.
4. Flail chest: positive pressure ventilation with PEEP or pressure support ventilation may be required to splint the chest wall internally.
5. Open pneumothorax: place a sterile dressing on the wound, taping only three sides. This type of dressing will allow air to escape but not reenter the pleural space. Continue to assess the patient for tension pneumothorax.
6. Diaphragmatic and esophageal rupture: anticipate NG insertion to decompress the stomach and reduce the risk of contaminating the thorax. Anticipate antibiotic therapy.
7. Prepare the patient for surgical repair of the injured structures.

Nursing Diagnosis: INEFFECTIVE TISSUE PERFUSION related to decreased cardiac output secondary to blood loss, development of tension pneumothorax, dysrhythmias, cardiac contusion

Outcome Criteria

Patient alert and oriented
  Skin warm and dry
  Peripheral pulses strong

HR 60 to 100 beats/min

Absence of life-threatening dysrhythmias

SBP 90 to 120 mm Hg

MAP 70 to 105 mm Hg

RR 12 to 20 breaths/min, eupnea

Urine output 30 mL/hr or 0.5 to 1 mL/kg/hr

O_2 sat ≥95%

Hgb 13 to 18 g/dL (males); 12 to 16 g/dL (females)

CVP 2 to 6 mm Hg

CI 2.5 to 4 L/min/m²

$\dot{D}o_2I$ 500 to 600 mL/min/m²

$\dot{V}o_2I$ 115 to 165 mL/min/m²

Patient Monitoring

1. Measure hemodynamic pressure (as appropriate to patient's clinical condition). Obtain PA pressures and CVP hourly or more frequently if the patient's condition is unstable. Obtain CO/CI, and note trends or the patient's response to therapy.

2. Measure arterial oxygen delivery ($\dot{D}o_2I$) and consumption ($\dot{V}o_2I$) to monitor indicators of tissue perfusion.

3. Obtain BP hourly or more frequently if the patient's condition is unstable, monitor MAP and pulse pressure, and note trends and the patient's response to therapy.

4. Monitor hourly urine output to evaluate effects of decreased CO and/or pharmacologic intervention. Determine fluid volume balance every 8 hours (1 kg is approximately 1000 mL of fluid).

5. Continuously monitor ECG for dysrhythmia development that may further compromise CO and tissue perfusion.

6. Continuously monitor oxygen saturation with pulse oximetry (Spo_2). Carefully monitor patient activities and nursing interventions that may adversely affect oxygen saturation.

7. Monitor the chest drainage system that is used to drain air or fluid from the pleural space. Record drainage hourly; consult with the physician if drainage is >200 mL/hr. If drainage suddenly ceases, check the patient and the system; a tension pneumothorax can develop. (See p. 497 for more information on chest drainage.)

8. If patient's lungs are being mechanically ventilated, see p. 503 for more information on ventilation therapies.

Patient Assessment

1. Assess the patient's mentation, peripheral pulses, and skin and note urine output at least hourly as indicators of tissue perfusion. Assess for pressure ulcer development related to hypoperfusion.
2. Obtain BP, HR, and RR hourly or more frequently if the patient's condition is unstable.
3. Check the patient for tracheal deviation, severe dyspnea, unilateral absence of breath sounds, and distended neck veins, which are highly suggestive of tension pneumothorax and must be treated immediately with CT insertion or needle decompression.
4. Assess the patient for clinical sequelae (see Table 5-15).

Diagnostics Assessment

1. Review ABGs (if available) for hypoxemia (Pao_2 <60 mm Hg) and acidosis (pH <7.35) because both conditions compromise CO and tissue perfusion.
2. Review Hgb and Hct levels to evaluate blood loss. Oxygen carrying capacity can be adversely affected with blood loss.

Patient Management

1. Insert large-bore IV catheters to administer crystalloids and blood products as ordered to maintain intravascular volume and replace blood loss. Autotransfusion may be performed in patients with bleeding into the thorax. Measure PA pressures, CVP (if available), and BP to evaluate effectiveness of fluid resuscitation.
2. Pulmonary contusion: limit IV fluids unless the patient is in shock. Rapid fluid administration can increase hydrostatic pressure and cause pulmonary edema. Blood products may be given to replace blood loss and maintain oncotic pressure.
3. If tension pneumothorax is suspected, immediate treatment is required with needle decompression and CT insertion.
4. Be alert for dysrhythmia risk factors: anemia, hypovolemia, hypotension, hypothermia, hypokalemia, hyperkalemia, hypomagnesemia, acidosis, and decreased coronary perfusion pressure. Treat life-threatening dysrhythmias according to advanced cardiac life support (ACLS) algorithms.
5. Implement pressure ulcer prevention strategies.

PULM

Nursing Diagnosis: ACUTE PAIN related to injured thoracic structures

Outcome Criterion

Patient communicates decreased pain.

Patient Monitoring

None

Patient Assessment

1. Perform systematic initial and ongoing pain assessment (intensity, location, quality, aggravating and relieving factors). Use a self-report pain rating scale, such as the 0-to-10 numerical pain rating scale, to assess pain intensity in patients who are awake and oriented.
2. Assess for behaviors such as grimacing, groaning, grunting, sobbing, crying, irritability, withdrawing, or hostility because they may be signs of pain. However, the absence of these behaviors does not necessarily mean the absence of pain.
3. Assess for physiologic indicators, such as increased RR, HR, and BP; dilated or constricted pupils; and pallor, which may be signs of pain. However, the absence of these physiologic indicators does not necessarily mean the absence of pain. *Note that some of these symptoms can also indicate other conditions such as hypoxia.*
4. Assess respiratory status and LOC before administering analgesics.

Diagnostics Assessment

None

Patient Management

1. See section on acute pain (p. 35).
2. Administer medication as ordered, evaluating its effects on pain control and respiration.
3. Administer medication before initiating pulmonary hygiene or other procedures; patients with chest trauma are reluctant to participate because of the pain.
4. Epidural analgesia, intercostal nerve blocks, or PCA may be used to control pain.
5. Consult with the physician if the medication proves ineffective.

PNEUMONIA

Clinical Brief

Pneumonia is an inflammation of the lung parenchyma caused by infectious agents or toxins via aspiration, inhalation, or translocation of organisms. Critically ill patients are at increased risk for nosocomial pneumonia because normal defense mechanisms are disrupted. Table 5-16 summarizes pathogens and risk factors for pneumonia.

Presenting Signs and Symptoms

The patient may have fever, chills, cough with purulent or rust-colored sputum, recent influenza, and SOB.

Physical Examination

Vital signs:
    HR: >100 beats/min
    RR: >24 breaths/min
    Temperature: >101.3° F (38.5° C)
Pulmonary: tachypnea, crackles, bronchial breath sounds, nasal flaring, or intercostal retractions may be present; dullness to percussion over the affected area may also be present.

Table 5-16   PATHOGENS AND RISK FACTORS ASSOCIATED WITH PNEUMONIA

Type	Pathogen	Risk Factors
Bacterial	*Streptococcus pneumoniae*	COPD, alcoholism, advanced age, multiple myeloma, recent influenza
	Staphylococcus aureus	Alcoholism, DM
	Haemophilus influenzae	COPD, alcoholism
	Pseudomonas aeruginosa	Mechanical ventilation
	Escherichia coli	Mechanical ventilation
	Klebsiella pneumoniae	Advanced age, nosocomial infection
	Legionella pneumophila	Immunodeficiency
Viral	Cytomegalovirus	AIDS, lymphomas, organ transplantation
Fungal	*Candida* species	AIDS, immunosuppression
Protozoal	*Pneumocystis jiroveci*	AIDS, immunosuppression

AIDS, Acquired immunodeficiency syndrome; *COPD,* chronic obstructive pulmonary disease; *DM,* diabetes mellitus.

PULM

Diagnostic Findings

Routine Sputum Specimen

Characteristics: purulent or rust colored. Gram stain is used to rapidly identify the pathogen. Specialized testing techniques are available for tuberculosis, fungi, and protozoa identification. Electron microscopy can be helpful to identify viruses. Cultures for precise identification take approximately 2 to 3 days.

Bronchoalveolar Lavage (BAL)

The established method for diagnosing opportunistic pneumonia in immunosuppressed patients is bronchoscopy with BAL.

Chest Radiograph

Patchy, ill-defined, fluffy opacification; lobar or segmental infiltrates; cavitation; air bronchograms; or reticular shadows

ACUTE CARE PATIENT MANAGEMENT

Goals of Treatment

Optimize oxygenation.
  Oxygen therapy
  Mechanical ventilation
  Hydration
Treat infectious process.
  Antibiotics
  Antipyretics
Detect/prevent clinical sequelae (Table 5-17).

Table 5-17 CLINICAL SEQUELAE OF PNEUMONIA

Complication	Signs and Symptoms
Respiratory failure	Restlessness, increased RR, Pao_2 <50 mm Hg, $Paco_2$ >50 mm Hg, pH <7.35
Septic shock	T >38° C or <36° C (101.3° F or 96.8° F) SBP <90 mm Hg, HR >90 beats/min, RR >20 breaths/min or $Paco_2$ <32 mm Hg, Pao_2/Fio_2 <280, altered mental status, plasma lactate >2 mmol/L, urine output <0.5 mL/kg/hr, WBCs >12,000/mm³ or <4000/mm³ or >10% neutrophils

HR, Heart rate; *RR,* respiratory rate; *SBP,* systolic blood pressure; *WBC,* white blood cell.

Priority Nursing Diagnoses and Potential Complications

Priority Nursing Diagnoses	PC: Potential Complications
Impaired gas exchange	Hypoxemia
Hyperthermia	Sepsis
Ineffective protection (see p. 48)	
Imbalanced nutrition: less than body requirements (see p. 53)	Negative nitrogen balance, electrolyte imbalances
Risk for interrupted family processes (see p. 45)	

PULM

Nursing Diagnosis: IMPAIRED GAS EXCHANGE related to ventilation-perfusion mismatch

Outcome Criteria

Alert and oriented
Lungs clear to auscultation
RR 12 to 20 breaths/min, eupnea
pH 7.35 to 7.45
PaO_2 80 to 100 mm Hg
$PaCO_2$ 35 to 45 mm Hg
O_2 sat ≥95%

Patient Monitoring

1. Continuously monitor oxygen saturation with pulse oximetry (SpO_2). Carefully monitor patient activities and nursing interventions that may adversely affect oxygen saturation.
2. Continuously monitor ECG because hypoxemia is a risk factor for dysrhythmias.
3. Monitor PAS pressure (if available) because hypoxemia can increase sympathetic tone and increase pulmonary vasoconstriction.

Patient Assessment

1. Assess respiratory status: auscultate breath sounds; and note rate, rhythm, depth, and use of accessory muscles. Observe for paradoxical breathing, increased restlessness, increased complaints of dyspnea, RR >30 breaths/min, and changes in LOC.
2. Assess for the presence of protective reflexes (e.g., gag and cough) because a loss of these increases the risk for aspiration.
3. Assess the patient for clinical sequelae (see Table 5-17).

Diagnostics Assessment

1. Review ABGs to evaluate oxygenation status and acid-base balance.
2. Review serial chest radiographs to evaluate improving or worsening condition.

Patient Management

1. Administer oxygen therapy as ordered and assist the patient to a position of comfort.
2. Reposition the patient to improve oxygenation and mobilize secretions. Evaluate the patient's response to position changes with ABGs or SpO$_2$ to determine the best position for oxygenation.
3. Provide chest physiotherapy and postural drainage to mobilize secretions, followed by deep breathing and coughing or suctioning. Perform endotracheal suctioning when rhonchi are present in the intubated patient and nasopharyngeal suctioning in patients unable to expectorate secretions. Document the color and consistency of sputum.
4. If the patient is mechanically ventilated, see p. 503 for more information on ventilation therapies.
5. Kinetic therapy or continuous lateral rotational therapy (via specialty bed) may be used to treat pneumonia by changing the patient's position and draining pulmonary secretions.
6. Minimize risk for aspiration by elevating HOB ≤30 degrees. Adequately inflate endotracheal or tracheostomy tube cuff. However, even properly inflated cuffs do not prevent aspiration. Carefully monitor patients receiving tube feedings.
7. Reduce oxygen demand: pace patient activities, relieve anxiety and pain, and decrease fever.
8. Reduce risk of ventilator-associated pneumonia: use strict handwashing and adherence to barrier precautions; prevent contamination of respiratory equipment; suction only when indicated and avoid use of normal saline (NS) lavage; prevent inadvertent lavage of ventilator tubing condensate down ETT; provide oral and nasal hygiene; prevent aspiration of gastric contents and subglottic secretions; and prevent rise in gastric pH.

Nursing Diagnosis: HYPERTHERMIA

Outcome Criterion

Temperature: 97.7° to 100.9° F (36.5°–38.3° C)

Patient Monitoring

1. Monitor temperature every 4 hours; obtain temperature 1 hour after antipyretics have been administered. If a hypothermia blanket is being used, continuously monitor core temperature and frequently assess skin integrity. (See p. 605 for more information on thermal regulation.)
2. Monitor BP, CO/CI, PA pressures, PVRI, SVRI, pulse pressure, and MAP because hemodynamic changes occur in the presence of sepsis.

Patient Assessment

1. Assess for chills, rigors, and diaphoresis.
2. Assess the patient for development of clinical sequelae. (See Table 5-17.)

Diagnostics Assessment

1. Review culture reports for identification of the infecting pathogen.
2. Review serial WBC count to monitor infective process.

Patient Management

1. Consult with the physician when temperature is >101.3° F (>38.5° C). Obtain cultures before initiating antibiotics whenever possible.
2. Administer acetaminophen as ordered and monitor patient response. A hypothermia blanket may be required to decrease temperature. (See p. 605 for more information on thermal regulation.)
3. Prevent the patient from shivering by covering with a light blanket or using pharmacologic agents if necessary because shivering can cause an increase in oxygen demand.

PULMONARY EMBOLUS (PE)

Clinical Brief

A PE is an occlusion in pulmonary vasculature that occurs from a fibrin or blood clot. Most commonly emboli are detached thrombi from the deep veins of the legs. Predisposing factors include Virchow's triad: acute injury to blood vessel walls, venous stasis, and hypercoagulable states. Air emboli usually result from air entering the circulatory system through intravascular catheters. Fat emboli occur with long-bone fractures.

Presenting Signs and Symptoms

The signs and symptoms are nonspecific. The hemodynamic effects depend on the size of the embolus, presence of cardiopulmonary disease, and the neurohormonal response to the embolus. The patient may be apprehensive and exhibit dyspnea, pleuritic pain, hemoptysis, tachycardia, tachypnea, crackles, cough, diaphoresis, and syncope.

Physical Examination

Appearance: restless, anxious
Vital signs:

BP: normal or ↑ BP as a result of anxiety

HR: normal or ↑ HR >100 beats/min

RR: ↑ rate

Cardiovascular: increased intensity of pulmonic S_2, S_4
Pulmonary: SOB, localized crackles, pleural rub may develop later
Massive PE: cyanosis, altered LOC, sudden shock
DVT symptoms: calf swelling, warmth, and tenderness

Diagnostic Findings

History of Risk Factors

Immobility; paralysis; traumatic injury; major surgery; fracture of hip, leg, or pelvis; malignancy; pregnancy; use of oral contraceptives; obesity; atrial fibrillation; CHF; and prior venous thromboembolism

ABGs

Pao_2 ≤80 mm Hg, $Paco_2$ <35 mm Hg, pH >7.45, and increased alveolar-arterial oxygen tension gradient

Chest Radiograph

Initially normal; later findings include pleural effusions, wedge collapse, focal oligemic lung, and enlarged descending right PA

ECG

Usually nonspecific; right-axis deviation, ST-segment depression in V_1-V_4, new right bundle branch block (BBB), and tachycardic rhythms are suggestive.

Ventilation-Perfusion Lung Scan

Results are suggestive of PE if a perfusion defect is found with normal ventilation.

Pulmonary Angiography

Pulmonary angiography is the most definitive test for PE, showing an abrupt cutoff of a vessel or a filling defect. PA pressures may be elevated; PVR may be increased.

Helical CT scan

Helical CT may identify PE, particularly chronic multiple PE.

Ultrasound/Impedance Plethysmography of the Lower Extremities

Presence of DVT is a significant risk factor for the development of PE.

ACUTE CARE PATIENT MANAGEMENT

Goals of Treatment

Optimize tissue oxygenation.
  Oxygen therapy
  Mechanical ventilation
  Pulmonary embolectomy or thrombolytic therapy for massive PE that compromises cardiac output
  Analgesia
Prevent embolic phenomenon.
  Sequential compression devices
  Antithromboembolism stockings
  Anticoagulation
  Filter or ligation of vena cava
Detect/prevent clinical sequelae (Table 5-18).

Table 5-18   CLINICAL SEQUELAE OF PULMONARY EMBOLI

Complication	Signs and Symptoms
Pulmonary infarction	Pleuritic pain, friction rub, hemoptysis, elevated temperature, cyanosis, shock, death
Pleural effusions	On affected side: decreased respiratory excursion and breath sounds, dullness on percussion
Right ventricular failure	Jugular venous distention; increased CVP, RAP, and RV pressure; Kussmaul's sign

CVP, Central venous pressure; *RAP*, right atrial pressure; *RV*, right ventricular.

Priority Nursing Diagnoses and Potential Complications

Priority Nursing Diagnoses	PC: Potential Complications
Impaired gas exchange	Hypoxemia, atelectasis, pneumonia
Ineffective tissue perfusion: cardiopulmonary	Decreased cardiac output, dysrhythmias
Risk for ineffective protection (see p. 48)	Anticoagulant therapy adverse effects
Imbalanced nutrition: less than body requirements (see p. 53)	Negative nitrogen balance, electrolyte imbalances
Risk for interrupted family processes (see p. 45)	

Nursing Diagnosis: **IMPAIRED GAS EXCHANGE** related to ventilation-perfusion mismatch and/or hypoventilation secondary to pain

Outcome Criteria

Alert and oriented
RR 12 to 20 breaths/min, eupnea
Absence of adventitious breath sounds
PaO_2 80 to 100 mm Hg
O_2 sat ≥95%
$P(a/A)O_2$ ratio >0.60

Patient Monitoring

1. Continuously monitor oxygen saturation with pulse oximetry (SpO_2). Carefully monitor patient activities and interventions that may adversely affect oxygen saturation.
2. Continuously monitor ECG for dysrhythmias or ischemic changes.
3. Calculate $P(a/A)O_2$ ratio to evaluate intrapulmonary shunt.

Patient Assessment

1. Assess respiratory status: note rate and depth of respirations; observe for dyspnea and restlessness. Hypoxia may be manifested as increased restlessness or change in LOC and RR >30 breaths/min. Auscultate breath sounds; crackles and pleuritic rub may be present.
2. Perform systematic initial and ongoing pain assessment (intensity, location, quality, aggravating and relieving factors). Use a self-report pain rating scale, such as 0-to-10 numerical pain rating scale, to assess pain intensity in patients who are awake and oriented.

3. Assess for behaviors such as grimacing, groaning, grunting, sobbing, crying, irritability, withdrawing, or hostility because they may be signs of pain. However, the absence of these behaviors does not necessarily mean the absence of pain.

4. Assess for physiologic indicators, such as increased RR, HR, and BP; dilated or constricted pupils; and pallor, which may be signs of pain. However, the absence of these physiologic indicators does not necessarily mean the absence of pain. *Note that some of these symptoms can also indicate other conditions such as hypoxia.*

5. Assess the patient for clinical sequelae (see Table 5-18).

Diagnostics Assessment

Review ABGs for changes in SaO_2 and PaO_2 to evaluate improvement or deterioration in the patient's pulmonary status.

Patient Management

1. Place the patient on bed rest initially and assist the patient to assume a comfortable position.

2. Administer supplemental oxygen as ordered. Intubation and mechanical ventilation may be required. (See p. 503 for information on ventilation therapies.)

3. Pace activities to decrease the patient's oxygen demand, allowing adequate time for patient recovery.

4. Assist the patient with turning and coughing and deep breathing exercises; note the color and character of sputum.

5. Administer analgesics as ordered to prevent splinting and improve chest excursion.

Nursing Diagnosis: INEFFECTIVE TISSUE PERFUSION: CARDIOPULMONARY related to embolic phenomenon

Outcome Criteria

Patient alert and oriented
RR 12 to 20 breaths/min, eupnea
Lungs clear to auscultation
Peripheral pulses strong
Skin warm and dry
Absence of JVD
PaO_2 80 to 100 mm Hg
O_2 sat ≥95%
SBP 90 to 120 mm Hg

HR 60 to 100 beats/min
CI 2.5 to 4 L/min/m^2
PVRI 200 to 450 dynes/sec/cm^{-5}/m^2

Patient Monitoring

1. Continuously monitor oxygen saturation with pulse oximetry (SpO$_2$). Carefully monitor patient activities and interventions that may adversely affect oxygen saturation.
2. Continuously monitor ECG for dysrhythmias and ischemic changes. Tachycardia may reflect compensation to maintain CI.
3. Monitor CO/CI, PA pressure (if available), CVP, arterial BP, and PVRI. PE can cause an increase in right ventricular (RV) workload or afterload and ultimately reduce CO.

Patient Assessment

1. Assess for thrombophlebitis: warmth, redness, tenderness, and swelling of lower extremities.
2. Assess the patient for manifestations of RV failure: JVD and peripheral edema.
3. Assess respiratory status: auscultate breath sounds and note increased work of breathing (e.g., increased RR, use of accessory muscles, and dyspnea).
4. Be alert for emboli in other body systems. Assess LOC and muscle strength to monitor for cerebral infarction; note any abdominal pain, nausea, or vomiting or decreased or absent bowel sounds to monitor for GI infarction; check for decreased urinary output and hematuria to monitor for renal infarction.
5. Assess patient for development of clinical sequelae (see Table 5-18).

Diagnostics Assessment

1. Review serial ABGs to evaluate oxygenation status.
2. Review cardiac profile (if available) for evidence of myocardial infarction (MI).
3. Review serial blood urea nitrogen (BUN) and creatinine studies to evaluate renal function.

Patient Management

1. Assist the patient to a position that will promote chest excursion and ease of breathing.

2. Administer oxygen therapy as ordered.
3. Administer anticoagulants as ordered (unfractionated heparin or low-molecular-weight heparin [LMWH]). Unfractionated heparin requires monitoring PTT to titrate therapy (therapeutic range 1.5-2.5 times control). It has a shorter half-life than LMWH and can be reversed with protamine. LMWH provides more predictable anticoagulation and less risk of thrombocytopenia and does not require laboratory monitoring (except in patients who weigh less than 50 kg, are morbidly obese, or have renal insufficiency).
4. Placement of an inferior vena cava filter may be indicated for patients with recurrent DVT or PE or for patients with contraindications to anticoagulant therapy.
5. Anticipate thrombolytic therapy as a treatment option for massive PE or in the face of hemodynamic instability. (See p. 545 for information on thrombolytic therapy.)
6. Surgical embolectomy may be required for hemodynamically significant PE or when other therapy has been unsuccessful.
7. Reduce risk factors: conduct ROM exercises to extremities; avoid sharp flexion at knees and groin; apply antithromboembolism stockings and sequential compression devices on admission. Remove devices every 8 hours to assess skin and to prevent skin breakdown. Mobilize the patient as soon as possible. (Do not implement these interventions if DVT is already suspected because thromboembolism can occur.)

Nursing Diagnosis: RISK FOR INEFFECTIVE PROTECTION: BLEEDING related to anticoagulant or thrombolytic agents

Outcome Criteria

Absence of bleeding
Hct 40% to 54% (males); 37% to 47% (females)
Hgb 14 to 18 g/dL (males); 12 to 16 g/dL (females)
PTT within therapeutic range
SBP 90 to 120 mm Hg
HR 60 to 100 beats/min

Patient Assessment

1. Assess the patient for bleeding from puncture sites, wounds, gums, or any body orifice. Note any altered LOC or abdominal pain that may indicate internal bleeding.

PULM

2. Test NG aspirate, emesis, urine, stool, and sputum for occult blood.

Diagnostics Assessment

1. Review serial Hgb and Hct levels for decreasing trend that may suggest bleeding.
2. Review serial PTT results (heparin); INR (warfarin). If results are greater than two times the control, consult with the physician.
3. Review serial platelet counts to monitor for heparin-induced thrombocytopenia (HIT).

Patient Management

1. Reposition the patient at least every 2 hours to prevent high-pressure areas. Handle the patient gently to prevent bruising.
2. An arterial or central line should be used to obtain specimens if available. If venipuncture is necessary, apply direct pressure to the puncture site for 10 to 15 minutes and then apply a pressure dressing. When discontinuing intravenous or arterial catheters apply pressure for 20 to 30 minutes, then apply a pressure dressing to ensure hemostasis. Reassess sites within 30 minutes for further bleeding or hematoma formation.
3. H_2 antagonists may be ordered to prevent gastric bleeding. Monitor gastric pH.
4. Stool softeners should be administered to prevent straining and rectal bleeding.
5. Avoid aspirin or aspirin-containing products, which may contribute to bleeding.

SEVERE ASTHMA

Clinical Brief

Asthma is a chronic inflammatory disorder of the airways characterized by recurrent episodes of acute airflow obstruction. Acute exacerbations of asthma can be triggered by exposure to allergens (dust mites, mold, pollen, animal dander, sulfites), irritants (smoke, pollution, chemical fumes), medications (aspirin, nonsteroidal antiinflammatory drugs [NSAIDs], beta blockers), viral infections, exercise, or gastroesophageal reflux disease. These triggers produce a cascade of cellular reactions that lead to bronchoconstriction, airway edema, and mucus plug formation. The chronic inflammation of asthma causes airway remodeling, which is a result of tissue injury and cellular changes. Asthma exacerbations are classified as being mild, moderate, or severe. Severe acute asthma that is unresponsive to treatment may be referred to as status asthmaticus.

Presenting Signs and Symptoms

The patient may complain of chest tightness, dyspnea, and cough. Diffuse wheezing is audible on inspiration and expiration. There is often a history of recent upper respiratory infection, worsening of asthma symptoms, and increased use of inhalers.

Physical Examination

Vital signs:
  BP: ↑ (anxiety, hypoxemia), or ↓ (hemodynamic compromise)
  HR: tachycardia
  RR: >30 breaths/min
  Pulsus paradoxus
Neurologic: agitation and restlessness, progressing to confusion and lethargy
Pulmonary: cough, use of accessory muscles, paradoxical movement, inspiratory and expiratory wheezing

Diagnostic Findings

Arterial Blood Gases (ABGs)

  PaO_2 <60 mm Hg on room air
  $PaCO_2$ ≥42 mm Hg
  SaO_2 <91% on room air

Chest Radiograph

  Hyperinflation, pulmonary hypertension, possible atelectasis

Pulmonary Function

  Forced expiratory volume in 1 second (FEV_1) <50% of predicted or patient's personal best. Peak expiratory flow (PEF) <50% of predicted or patient's personal best.

ACUTE CARE PATIENT MANAGEMENT

Goals of Treatment

Improve ventilation and gas exchange.
  Oxygen therapy
  Bronchodilator therapy

Steroid therapy
Intubation and mechanical ventilation
Detect/prevent clinical sequelae (Table 5-19).

Priority Nursing Diagnoses and Potential Complications

Priority Nursing Diagnoses	PC: Potential Complications
Impaired gas exchange	Hypoxemia, dysrhythmias, respiratory acidosis
Ineffective breathing pattern	Hypoxemia, pneumothorax, decreased cardiac output
Risk for ineffective protection (see p. 48)	
Risk for interrupted family processes (see p. 45)	

Nursing Diagnoses: IMPAIRED GAS EXCHANGE related to inflammation, airway edema, and mucus plugging; INEFFECTIVE BREATHING PATTERN related to bronchospasm

Outcome Criteria

Alert and oriented
RR 12 to 20 breaths/min, eupnea
Lungs clear to auscultation
pH 7.35 to 7.45
Pao_2 80 to 100 mm Hg

Table 5-19 CLINICAL SEQUELAE OF SEVERE ASTHMA

Complication	Signs and Symptoms
Tension pneumothorax	Tachycardia, hypotension, worsening gas exchange, severe dyspnea, tracheal deviation toward affected side, diminished or absent breath sounds on affected side, asymmetric chest expansion
Respiratory arrest	Absence of respirations
Dysrhythmias	Changes in heart rate, rhythm; change in LOC or syncope; hypotension
Cardiac arrest	Absence of palpable pulses

LOC, Level of consciousness.

Paco$_2$ 35 to 45 mm Hg
O$_2$ sat ≥95%
P(a/A)o$_2$ ratio 0.75 to 0.95

Patient Monitoring

1. Continuously monitor ECG for dysrhythmias that may be related to hypoxemia or acid-base imbalances.
2. Continuously monitor oxygen saturation with pulse oximetry (Spo$_2$). Carefully monitor interventions and patient activities that may adversely affect oxygen saturation.
3. Calculate P(a/A)o$_2$ ratio and Pao$_2$/Fio$_2$ to evaluate oxygenation.
4. If the patient's lungs are mechanically ventilated, see the information about ventilation therapies on p. 503.

Patient Assessment

1. Assess respiratory status hourly or more often, depending on patient condition. Note RR, rhythm, depth, and use of accessory muscles. Observe for paradoxical breathing pattern, increased complaints of dyspnea, and inability to complete sentences as a result of breathlessness. Auscultate breath sounds for increasing wheezing. Diminished breath sounds or a silent chest is an ominous sign and indicates impending respiratory failure.
2. Assess neurologic status; note increase in agitation or restlessness or decrease in LOC.
3. Assess the patient for clinical sequelae (see Table 5-19).

Diagnostics Assessment

1. Review ABGs to evaluate oxygenation status and acid-base balance.
2. Use peak flow meter to follow PEF readings; decreasing flow readings indicate increasing airflow obstruction.

Patient Management

1. Administer oxygen therapy as ordered and assist the patient to a position of comfort. Minimize oxygen demand by limiting activities and reducing anxiety.
2. Administer β$_2$-agonists (albuterol) by nebulizer as ordered for bronchodilation. Monitor the drug's effect on HR. May require hourly or continuous administration for severe exacerbation.

3. Nebulized anticholinergics (ipratropium bromide) may also be given to enhance bronchodilator effects of β_2-agonists.

4. Administer intravenous corticosteroids (methylprednisolone) as ordered to reduce airway inflammation. Monitor blood glucose levels for glucocorticoid-induced hyperglycemia, particularly for patients known to have diabetes.

5. Heliox, a mixture of helium and oxygen, may be given to improve gas flow through narrowed airways and to lower airway resistance.

6. Prepare for possible intubation and mechanical ventilation. Anticipate lung protective strategies to prevent complications of mechanical ventilation. (See p. 503 for information on ventilation therapies.) Position patient to decrease risk of aspiration and ventilator-acquired pneumonia.

7. Provide sedation in mechanically ventilated patients to decrease anxiety, improve comfort, and decrease oxygen consumption.

8. Therapeutic paralysis with the administration of a neuromuscular blocking agent may be required to achieve patient-ventilator synchrony and decrease oxygen demands. Avoid use in patients receiving corticosteroids because of the risk of prolonged paralysis. (See p. 595 for information on neuromuscular blockade.)

9. During mechanical ventilation, assess for the development of auto-PEEP, which is a result of incomplete alveolar emptying at the end of exhalation. This may increase work of breathing, increase the risk for pneumothorax, and decrease venous return to the heart.

10. In conditions refractory to conventional therapy, permissive hypercapnia may be used. This is a mechanical ventilation technique that uses very small tidal volumes (as low as 5 mL/kg) to reduce distending pressure. $Paco_2$ levels slowly increase, and pH is lowered to 7.2.

11. After extubation, develop a plan for teaching the patient about asthma management techniques (Table 5-20).

Table 5-20 ASTHMA EDUCATION

Topic	Education Points
Basic facts	Asthma is a chronic illness that can be controlled.
	Good control means few or no symptoms, participation in normal activities, no missed work/school days, and fewer or no hospital visits.
Triggers	Discuss substances that precipitate symptoms.
	Develop strategies for elimination, avoidance, or control of triggers.
Skills	Demonstrate accurate monitoring of peak flowmeter readings.
	Demonstrate proper use of metered-dose inhaler.
	Demonstrate correct use of spacer.
Medications	Differentiate between medications for long-term control and quick relief (rescue).
	Teach about long-term control: medication name, dose, frequency, side effects, and importance of uninterrupted use.
	Explain about quick relief: medication name, dose, frequency, and side effects.
	Inform about medications to use before exercise or exposure to triggers.
Action plan	Explain importance of monitoring signs and symptoms, PEF readings.
	Explain what medications to consider and actions to take when PEF <50% of personal best and when PEF <80% of personal best.
	Instruct how to seek help if symptoms worsen.
	Review importance of follow-up medical visits.

PEF, Peak expiratory flow.

PULM

CARDIOVASCULAR DISORDERS

ACUTE CORONARY SYNDROME (ACS)

Acute coronary syndrome is a continuum of a disease process that includes unstable angina, non-ST segment elevation myocardial infarction (NSTEMI), and ST elevation MI (STEMI). This differentiation is a result of the treatment modalities specific for these conditions.

ANGINA

Clinical Brief

Angina is a subjective experience of chest discomfort resulting from an imbalance in myocardial oxygen supply and demand. Etiologic factors in angina are usually related to the atherosclerotic disease process (coronary artery disease [CAD]), whereby the coronary arteries lose their ability to dilate and to increase blood flow in the presence of increased oxygen consumption. Angina may be classified as (1) stable angina, which typically results from atherosclerotic vessel changes; (2) unstable angina, which usually results from accelerated or multivessel disease; (3) Prinzmetal's angina, which usually results from coronary artery vasospasm; and (4) syndrome X which is angina with normal coronary arteries. Prolonged myocardial ischemia may ultimately result in an MI.

Risk Factors

Risk factors mirror those for CAD: cigarette smoking, hyperlipidemia, HTN, diabetes, obesity, sedimentary lifestyle and stress; angina occurs most often in men, especially those older than 50 years, or in postmenopausal women. Metabolic syndrome, which includes central obesity, atherogenic dyslipidemia, insulin resistance, prothrombotic state, elevated blood pressure, and proinflammatory state, also is a risk factor that is an increasing problem in the United States. A positive family history of cardiovascular disease predisposes an individual to angina.

Presenting Signs and Symptoms

Stable angina (classic exertional): chest discomfort that can be predicted by the patient; usually follows exertion, meals, or increased activity levels; is relieved by rest and/or nitroglycerin (NTG); and manifests as ST segment depression (subendocardial ischemia) or T-wave inversion on ECG during the episode of discomfort.

Unstable angina (crescendo or preinfarction angina): chest discomfort that is new onset or has changed in character and is now more severe, lasts longer, is more difficult to relieve, and occurs with less exertion than previously.

Prinzmetal's angina (variant angina): chest discomfort that is nontypical and occurs with rest, is not relieved with NTG or rest, and manifests as ST segment elevation on ECG during the episode of discomfort.

Physical Examination

Appearance: anxious
Vital signs:
    BP: may be elevated secondary to pain or decreased secondary to hemodynamic compromise and/or pharmacologic therapy
    HR: may be elevated secondary to pain
Cardiovascular: S_4 may be present.
Pulmonary: dyspnea and tachypnea may be present.

Diagnostic Findings

ECG changes: ST segment depression or T-wave inversion (classic and unstable) or ST segment elevation (Prinzmetal)

ACUTE CARE PATIENT MANAGEMENT

Goals of Treatment

Improve myocardial oxygen supply.
    Supplemental oxygen
    NTG
    Aspirin or antiplatelet inhibitors
    Possible percutaneous transluminal coronary angioplasty (PTCA) and stent placement
    Coronary artery bypass graft (CABG)
Decrease myocardial oxygen demand.
    Bed rest
    NTG
    Morphine sulfate
    β-Adrenergic blocking agents
    Angiotensin-converting enzyme (ACE) inhibitors (especially with left ventricular [LV] dysfunction)
    Calcium channel blocking agents

Priority Nursing Diagnoses

Acute pain
Risk for interrupted family processes (see p. 45)
Deficient knowledge (see p. 58)

Nursing Diagnosis: ACUTE PAIN related to imbalance of myocardial oxygen supply and demand

Outcome Criteria

Patient communicates pain relief.
ST segment returns to baseline, or T wave returns to upright.

Patient Monitoring

Continuously monitor ECG for indications of ischemia (ST, T-wave changes), injury (ST elevation), or infarction (pathologic Q wave).

Patient Assessment

1. Assess pain using PQRST acronym (Table 5-21) to validate ischemic origin (Table 5-22). Assess pain using a patient's self-report whenever possible. See p. 35 for information on acute pain. A visual analog scale can be found on p. 3.
2. Check VS and SpO_2 frequently during anginal episode and with administration of antianginal agents. Hypotension and reflex tachycardia can occur with these agents.

Diagnostics Assessment

1. Review serial 12-lead ECGs to evaluate patterns of ischemia, injury, and infarction.
2. Review laboratory results of cardiac markers (if available) for characteristic changes of MI (Table 5-23).

Table 5-21 EVALUATING CHEST PAIN

	Assessment/Documentation
P	Precipitating events and Placement (location)
Q	Quality of discomfort
R	Radiation
S	Severity (0 to 10 scale) and associated Signs and Symptoms
T	Timing since onset and response to Treatment

Table 5-22 ORIGIN OF ISCHEMIA, DIFFERENTIATING CHEST PAIN

Type	Symptoms	Signs	Pain Relief
CARDIAC ISCHEMIA	Substernal "crushing" chest pain: may radiate to left upper extremity and/or jaw (common) or right upper extremity or back	Anxiety; pale, diaphoretic	Depends on specific ischemic conditions
Stable angina	Predictable: follows exertion, meals, or increased activity	ECG changes: inverted T wave, ST segment depression	Rest, NTG, O_2, morphine sulfate
Unstable or crescendo or preinfarction angina	Less predictable: occurs with less exertion and lasts longer	ECG changes: inverted T wave, ST segment depression	Rest, NTG, O_2, morphine sulfate
Prinzmetal's or variant angina	Unpredictable: may occur at rest or during the night	ECG changes: ST segment elevation	Rest, NTG, O_2, morphine sulfate, Ca channel blockers
MYOCARDIAL INFARCTION	Has all the symptoms of angina but lasts longer and may be more severe; SOB, nausea	ECG changes: new significant Q waves, ST segment elevation or depression, inverted T waves, elevated cardiac markers, crackles S_3, S_4	Thrombolytics, PCI, rest, NTG, O_2, morphine sulfate

Continued

CV

Table 5-22 Origin of Ischemia, Differentiating Chest Pain—cont'd

Type	Symptoms	Signs	Pain Relief
NONISCHEMIC			
Pericarditis	Severe, sharp, precordial pain that may radiate to LUE	Patient appears restless; pericardial friction rub, pulsus paradoxus, dyspnea, ↑ RR, ECG changes; diffuse, nonspecific ST segment elevation, T-wave inversion	NSAIDs (indomethacin, ibuprofen), steroids, leaning forward, shallow breaths
GASTROINTESTINAL			
Gastric reflux	May report substernal pressure or burning	Anxiety Skin: diaphoretic, pale Hx of peptic ulcer, hiatal hernia	Antacids, H₂ blockers, viscous lidocaine, GI cocktail, remain upright after eating
MUSCULOSKELETAL			
Costochondritis	Chest pain that may/may not be discrete; ↑ when ribs/sternum are palpated and on deep inspiration	Anxiety Skin: diaphoretic, pale Shallow respirations, ↑ ESR, ↑ WBCs	Position changes, NSAIDs (ibuprofen, indomethacin), analgesic medication

Chest wall trauma	Chest pain that may/may not be discrete; ↑ on deep inspiration	Anxiety Skin: diaphoretic, pale May see bruises/laceration/distortions, possible crepitus/subcutaneous emphysema Hx of trauma	Position changes, depends on causes, analgesic medication
PULMONARY			
Pulmonary embolism	Severe, sharp, often unilateral/specific chest pain; breathlessness	Anxiety Skin: diaphoretic, pale Dyspnea/tachypnea ABGs: ↓ O_2 sat, ↓ Pao_2, ↓ $Paco_2$ early and as patient tires will climb May see hemoptysis	Analgesic medication, thrombolytics, anticoagulation to prevent further clots, possible inferior vena cava filter

Continued

CV

Table 5-22 Origin of Ischemia, Differentiating Chest Pain—cont'd

Type	Symptoms	Signs	Pain Relief
Pleurisy	Sudden onset Stabbing chest pain that may/may not be discrete; increases with inspiration	Anxiety Rapid, shallow respirations	ASA, antiinflammatory drug (ibuprofen); position changes, use analgesic (e.g., codeine) with caution
Pneumothorax	Dyspnea, anxiety, may complain of chest pressure	Absent breath sounds in affected area, possible $\downarrow$ O$_2$ sat/Pao$_2$, $\uparrow$ peak airway pressures, tachycardia	Decompression using needle (emergently) or pleural chest tube

ABG, Arterial blood gas; *ASA,* aspirin; *ECG,* electrocardiogram; *ESR,* erythrocyte sedimentation rate; *GI,* gastrointestinal; *Hx,* history; *LUE,* left upper extremity; *NSAID,* nonsteroidal antiinflammatory drug; *NTG,* nitroglycerin; *PCI,* primary coronary intervention; *RR,* respiratory rate; *SOB,* shortness of breath; *WBC,* white blood cell.

Table 5-23 CARDIAC MARKERS

Marker	Onset	Peak	Return to Normal
Myoglobin	1-2 hr	4-12 hr	24 hr
Troponin I	4-6 hr	14-18 hr	5-7 days
Troponin T	3-4 hr	4-6 hr	14-21 days
CK	2-5 hr	~24 hr	2-3 days
CK-MB	4-8 hr	16-24 hr	2-3 days
LDH	6-12 hr	48-72 hr	7-10 days
LDH_1	6-12 hr	24-48 hr	Variable

CK, Creatine kinase; *CK-MB*, creatine kinase–myocardial bound; *LDH*, lactate dehydrogenase.

3. Review results of echocardiography or cardiac catheterization (if available) for ventricular function and degree of CAD involvement.

Patient Management

1. Stay with the patient, providing a calm, quiet environment. Assess for level of anxiety and other factors that increase myocardial oxygen demand, such as fever, dysrhythmias, stress and emotion, HTN, and hypoxemia.
2. Provide oxygen at 2 to 6 L/min to maintain or improve oxygenation. Keep SpO_2 >92%.
3. Initiate and maintain intravenous line(s) for emergent drug and fluid resuscitation.
4. Administer aspirin as ordered to reduce risk of thrombus formation. If patient is allergic to aspirin, use clopidogrel (Plavix).
5. Administer NTG as indicated to decrease preload, decrease myocardial oxygen demand, and increase myocardial oxygen supply: sublingual, 1 tablet (0.4 mg) every 5 minutes × 3; IV, start with an infusion of 5 mcg/min, titrate to desired response maintaining SBP >90 mm Hg, and increase dosage every 5 to 10 minutes by 5 to 10 mcg/min. If hypotension or reflex tachycardia occurs, raise the patient's legs and reduce the dose to keep SBP >90 mm Hg.
6. Administer morphine sulfate as ordered. Give IVP in 2-mg increments every 5 minutes to relieve chest discomfort. Monitor the patient's respirations because morphine is a respiratory depressant. Notify the physician if pain is not

relieved despite pharmacologic intervention or if pain has subsided but recurs.

7. Administer β-blockers, such as atenolol or metoprolol (Lopressor), as ordered to decrease myocardial oxygen demand. Monitor drug effects on HR and BP. Note: contraindicated with pulmonary disease secondary to risk of bronchospasm.

8. Administer anticoagulants (heparin or LMWH) and antiplatelet drugs (IIb/IIIa inhibitors) as ordered to decrease chance of thrombus formation.

9. Administer lipid-lowering agent to reduce disease progression and lower total cholesterol and low-density lipoproteins (LDLs)

10. Administer calcium channel blockers to slow accelerated heart rate as needed to increase coronary perfusion time and reduce O_2 consumption.

11. Angiogram with cardiac intervention may be indicated.

ACUTE MYOCARDIAL INFARCTION (MI)

Clinical Brief

Myocardial infarction can be classified as non–ST segment elevation myocardial infarction (NSTEMI), and ST elevation MI (STEMI). The death of myocardial tissue is a result of decreased blood supply to the myocardium. An MI can go unnoticed (silent MI) or produce major hemodynamic consequences and death. It may result from atherosclerosis, from coronary artery spasm, or more commonly from coronary thrombosis.

Risk Factors

Risk factors mirror the risk factors for CAD: cigarette smoking, hyperlipidemia, HTN, diabetes, obesity, sedentary lifestyle, and stress. Men, especially those older than 50 years, are predisposed to MI as are postmenopausal women and African Americans. A positive family history of cardiovascular disease also places one at risk.

Presenting Signs and Symptoms

Signs and symptoms are chest discomfort lasting longer than 30 minutes that is unrelieved by NTG and rest, anxiety, feelings of impending doom, nausea and vomiting, dyspnea, weakness, diaphoresis, and palpitations.

Physical Examination

Appearance: anxious, pale

Vital signs:

    BP: may be ↑ in response to pain or ↓ secondary to hemodynamic compromise

    HR: may be ↑ as a compensatory response or secondary to pain or ↓ secondary to ischemia and/or pharmacologic therapy; may be irregular secondary to dysrhythmias

Cardiovascular: S_3, S_4, murmur, and/or rubs may be present

Pulmonary: SOB, tachypnea, crackles

Right Ventricular Infarction

Cardiovascular: distended jugular veins, hypotension, heart block may be present.

Pulmonary: clear lungs

Diagnostic Findings

Cardiac markers: characteristic elevations are evident within expected time frame (see Table 5-23).

Isoenzymes: creatine kinase–myocardial bound (CK-MB) is cardiac specific; positive MB, troponin, and myoglobin can all be diagnostic for MI; LDH_1 and LDH_2 are cardiac specific, an LDH "flip" (LDH_1 greater than LDH_2) is diagnostic for MI.

ECG changes: usually occur from hours to within 7 days (Table 5-24).

Table 5-24 ELECTROCARDIOGRAM CHANGES ASSOCIATED WITH MYOCARDIAL INFARCTION

Type	Indicative Changes	Reciprocal Changes
Anterior	V_2-V_4	II, III, aV_F
Anteroseptal	V_1-V_4	—
Anterolateral	I, aV_L, V_3-V_6	—
Lateral	I, aV_L, V_5-V_6	II, III, aV_F
Inferior	II, III, aV_F	I, aV_L, V_1-V_4
Posterior	—	Tall R waves and ST depression in V_1-V_3
Right ventricle	ST segment elevation in V_{3R}, V_{4R}	—

ST elevation infarction: pathologic Q waves (≥0.04 sec or 25% of the height of the R wave), ST segment elevation with reciprocal ST depression in opposite leads; T-wave changes are initially positive, then become negative in leads facing the infarcted area.

Non-ST elevation infarction: ST depression and inverted T waves in leads facing the epicardial surface overlying the infarction; ST elevation and upright T waves in opposite leads.

ACUTE CARE PATIENT MANAGEMENT

Goals of Treatment

Salvage myocardium/limit infarction size.
  Thrombolytic therapy
  Glycoprotein IIb/IIIa inhibitors
  Intraaortic balloon pump (IABP) counterpulsation
  PTCA, primary coronary intervention (PCI)
  Stent placement—drug eluding and non–drug eluding
  CABG
Improve myocardial oxygen supply.
  Supplemental oxygen
  Aspirin
  Heparin or LMWH
  IABP counterpulsation
Decrease myocardial oxygen demand.
  Mechanical assist devices
  Bed rest
  Nothing by mouth (NPO), liquid or soft diet
  β-Adrenergic blocking agents
Decrease preload (except RV infarction).
  Morphine sulfate
  NTG
  Diuretic agents
Decrease afterload.
  Morphine sulfate
  NTG
  Calcium channel blocking agents
  ACE inhibitors
  IABP counterpulsation
Increase contractility.
  Positive inotropes (dobutamine, milrinone [Primacor])
Maintain electrophysiologic stability.
  Lidocaine
  Amiodarone

β-Adrenergic blocking agents

Calcium channel blocking agents

Magnesium sulfate, calcium gluconate/chloride and/or potassium chloride

Maintain hemodynamic stability.

Volume loading to provide adequate filling pressure (especially RV infarction)

Vasoactive medications (dopamine, nitroprusside)

Detect/prevent clinical sequelae (Table 5-25).

Table 5-25 CLINICAL SEQUELAE ASSOCIATED WITH MYOCARDIAL INFARCTION

Complications	Signs and Symptoms
Right heart failure	JVD, peripheral edema, fatigue, increased HR
Left heart failure	S_3, crackles, increased HR
Pulmonary edema	Worsening HF, breathlessness, moist cough, frothy sputum, diaphoresis, cyanosis, ↓ Pao_2, ↑ RR, ↓ BP, PAWP >25 mm Hg
Reinfarction/ extension of infarction	Recurrence of chest pain, ST and T-wave changes, hemodynamic changes
Cardiogenic shock	↓ Mentation, ↓↑ HR, SBP <90 mm Hg, CI <2 L/min/m², urine output <20 mL/hr, cool, clammy, mottled skin
Dysrhythmias/sudden death	Change in rate or rhythm, change in LOC, syncope, chest discomfort, ↓ BP
Pericarditis	Chest discomfort aggravated by supine position or on deep inspiration, diffuse nonspecific ST segment elevation, intermittent friction rub may be present, fever
Papillary muscle rupture	Abrupt-onset holosystolic murmur, sudden left ventricular failure, S_3, S_4, midsystolic ejection click, crackles
Ventricular aneurysm	Paradoxical pulse, ventricular ectopy, MAP <80 mm Hg, possible atrial fibrillation with BP changes, change in HR, outward bulging of precordium
Ventricular septal rupture	Sudden onset of palpable thrill, holosystolic murmur at LSB, sudden left ventricular failure, SOB, cough

BP, Blood pressure; *CI,* cardiac index; *HF,* heart failure; *HR,* heart rate; *JVD,* jugular venous distention; *LOC,* level of consciousness; *LSB,* left sternal border; *MAP,* mean arterial pressure; *PAWP,* pulmonary artery wedge pressure; *RR,* respiratory rate; *SBP,* systolic blood pressure; *SOB,* shortness of breath.

Priority Nursing Diagnoses and Potential Complications	
Priority Nursing Diagnoses	**PC: Potential Complications**
Acute pain	
Decreased cardiac output	Dysrhythmias
Ineffective tissue perfusion	Dysrhythmias, renal insufficiency, hypoxemia
Risk for ineffective protection (see p. 48)	
Risk for interrupted family processes (see p. 45)	

Nursing Diagnosis: ACUTE PAIN related to impaired myocardial oxygenation

Outcome Criteria

Patient communicates pain relief.
Absence of ST segment, T-wave changes.

Patient Monitoring

Continuously monitor ECG to evaluate ST segment and T-wave changes, which may indicate ischemia, injury, or infarction (extension or new onset) and to detect the onset of dysrhythmias or conduction problems.

Patient Assessment

1. Assess pain to validate ischemic origin (see Table 5-22). Use patient's self-report whenever possible to evaluate the severity of the pain.
2. Check VS frequently during pain episode and with administration of antianginal agents. Hypotension and reflex tachycardia can occur with these agents.
3. Assess the patient for clinical sequelae (see Table 5-25).

Diagnostics Assessment

1. Obtain 12-lead ECG and compare with previous ECGs, if available.
2. Review cardiac marker results, if ordered.

Patient Management

1. Stay with the patient, providing a calm, quiet environment.
2. Maintain O_2 therapy and assist the patient to a position of comfort.
3. Administer NTG: sublingual, 1 tablet (0.4 mg) every 5 minutes × 3; as an infusion, start at 5 mcg/min, titrate to desired

response to maintain SBP >90 mm Hg, and increase dosage every 5 to 10 minutes by 5 to 10 mcg/min. If hypotension or reflex tachycardia occurs, raise the patient's legs and reduce dose to keep SBP >90 mm Hg.

4. Administer morphine sulfate as ordered. Give IVP in 2-mg increments every 5 minutes to relieve chest discomfort. Monitor respirations and oxygen saturations.

5. Administer aspirin if not already received to prevent platelet adherence in coronary arteries. If patient is allergic to aspirin, use clopidogrel (Plavix).

6. Administer β-adrenergic blocking agents such as atenolol, metoprolol, or propranolol as ordered. These pharmacologic agents decrease sympathetic nervous system (SNS) tone, reduce cardiac demand, and have been shown to improve outcomes and reduce mortality. Monitor the drug's effect on HR and BP.

7. Administer a calcium channel blocking agent, such as diltiazem (Cardizem), as ordered to reduce coronary vasospasm; these agents may also be used to reduce afterload and control tachydysrhythmias. Monitor the drug's effect on HR and BP.

8. Administer glycoprotein IIb/IIIa inhibitor agents to prevent platelet adherence in coronary arteries.

9. Administer an anticoagulant, such as heparin or LMWH as ordered. These agents may be given prophylactically or with thrombolytic therapy to prevent further clot formation. Monitor the patient for overt and covert bleeding and check daily aPTT for therapeutic anticoagulation (1.5-2.5 times normal). Note: therapeutic levels may vary depending on the facility's aPTT reagent.

10. IABP insertion may be required. (See p. 524 for information on IABP.)

11. Consider thrombolytic therapy. (See p. 545 for information on thrombolytic therapy.) PCI may be considered. (See p. 531 for information on PTCA/stent.)

Nursing Diagnosis: DECREASED CARDIAC OUTPUT related to electrophysiologic instability and impaired inotropic state

Outcome Criteria

Patient alert and oriented
Skin warm and dry
Pulses strong and equal bilaterally

Capillary refill <3 sec

SBP 90 to 120 mm Hg

MAP 70 to 105 mm Hg

Pulse pressure 30 to 40 mm Hg

HR 60 to 100 beats/min

Absence of life-threatening dysrhythmias

Urine output 30 mL/hr or 0.5 to 1 mL/kg/hr

CVP 2 to 6 mm Hg

PAS 15 to 30 mm Hg

PAD 5 to 15 mm Hg

PAWP 4 to 12 mm Hg

CI 2.5 to 4 L/min/m^2

SVRI 1700 to 2600 dynes/sec/cm^{-5}/m^2

PVRI 200 to 450 dynes/sec/cm^{-5}/m^2

Svo_2 60% to 80%

$\dot{D}o_2I$ 500 to 600 mL/min/m^2

$\dot{V}o_2I$ 115 to 165 mL/min/m^2

Patient Monitoring

1. Monitor (in the lead appropriate for infarction and vessel) for ischemia or dysrhythmia identification. Place in lead II to monitor for supraventricular tachycardia (SVT) and axis deviation. Place in lead MCL_1 to differentiate between ventricular ectopy and aberrantly conducted beats, to determine types of BBB, or to verify RV pacemaker beats (paced QRS beat should be negative). (Table 5-26 lists the sites of infarction and related conduction problems.)

2. Analyze ECG rhythm strip at least every 4 hours and note rate; rhythm; and PR, QRS, and QT intervals (prolonged QT is associated with torsades de pointes). Note ST segment, T wave, or Q-wave changes, which may indicate ischemia, injury, or infarction. Note occurrence of premature atrial contractions (PACs) or premature ventricular contractions (PVCs) because premature beats are often the forerunner of more serious dysrhythmias. Second-degree heart block type II (Mobitz II) may progress to complete heart block. (See p. 441 for information on the dysrhythmia interpretation.)

3. Obtain PA pressures, PAWP and CVP (right atrium [RA]) hourly (if available) or more frequently if titrating pharmacologic agents. Obtain CO/CI as ordered and as patient condition indicates. Note trends in CI, PVRI, and SVRI and the patient's response to therapy. Note left ventricular stroke

Table 5-26 INFARCTIONS AND RELATED CONDUCTION PROBLEMS

Site	ECG Changes
Anterior MI	BBB as a result of septal involvement; check widened QRS
	RBBB = rSR′ in V_1, Rs in V_6
	LBBB = rS in V_1, large monophasic R wave in V_6
	Left anterior hemiblock: LAD greater than −45°; negative QRS in II, III, aV_F
	Second-degree AV block, type II
	Complete heart block
Inferior MI	Bradycardia, second-degree AV block, type I
	Complete heart block
Posterior MI	See inferior MI
Right ventricular infarction	Second degree AV block

AV, Atrioventricular; *BBB,* bundle branch block; *ECG,* electrocardiogram; *LAD,* left anterior descending; *LBBB,* left bundle branch block; *MI,* myocardial infarction; *RBBB,* right bundle branch block.

work index (LVSWI) and right ventricular stroke work index (RVSWI) to evaluate contractility.

4. Monitor $\dot{D}o_2I$ and $\dot{V}o_2I$ as indicators of tissue perfusion.
5. Obtain BP hourly; note trends in MAP and pulse pressure, and the patient's response to therapy.
6. Monitor urine output as an indicator of adequate CO and/or of pharmacologic intervention. Determine fluid balance each shift and obtain daily weight. Compare serial weights for rapid changes (0.5-1 kg/day) suggesting fluid gain or loss.
7. Continuously monitor Svo_2 (if available) to evaluate oxygen supply and demand; a downward trend can indicate decreased supply or increased demand.

Patient Assessment

1. Obtain HR, RR, and BP every 15 minutes during the acute phase and when titrating vasoactive drugs. Obtain temperature every 4 hours.
2. Assess the patient's mentation, skin color and temperature, capillary refill, and peripheral pulses at least hourly to monitor adequacy of CO.
3. Assess the patient for clinical sequelae (see Table 5-25).

Diagnostics Assessment

1. Review serial 12-lead ECGs to identify ECG changes.
2. Review serial electrolyte levels; a disturbance in potassium, calcium, or magnesium is a risk factor for dysrhythmias.
3. Review serial cardiac markers to identify elevations—a sign of myocardial tissue damage.
4. Review serial ABGs (if ordered) for hypoxemia and acidosis because these conditions increase the risk for dysrhythmias and decreased contractility.

Patient Management

1. Provide oxygen at 2 to 6 L/min to maintain or improve oxygenation.
2. Minimize oxygen demand: eliminate pain, decrease anxiety, keep the patient NPO or provide a liquid diet in the acute phase.
3. Maintain the patient on bed rest to decrease myocardial oxygen demand during the acute phase.
4. Initiate intravenous line to ensure emergency vascular access.
5. Administer intravenous fluids as ordered to provide adequate filling pressures that maintain CO/CI. A PAD of approximately 15 to 20 mm Hg may be required in patients with right ventricular infarction.
6. Be alert for dysrhythmia risk factors: anemia, hypovolemia, hypokalemia, hypomagnesemia, acidosis, administration of beta blockers and antidysrhythmic agents, pain, pulmonary artery or pacemaker catheter misplacement. Treat life-threatening dysrhythmias according to ACLS algorithms.
7. If the patient is bradycardic, consider transcutaneous (TCP) or transvenous pacing and/or be prepared to administer atropine 0.5 mg IV *if* the patient manifests the following: SBP <90 mm Hg, decreased mentation, PVCs, chest discomfort, or dyspnea. Pacemaker insertion may be required.
8. If the patient is tachycardic, assess BP, mentation, skin temperature etc. Drug therapy depends on the origin of tachydysrhythmia. Be prepared to countershock or defibrillate if patient is very symptomatic. Note: rapid HR increases oxygen consumption, decreases oxygen supply, and increases oxygen demand.

9. Administer NTG and calcium channel blocking agents as ordered to reduce preload and afterload. Monitor drug effects on BP and HR.

10. Administer diuretics (e.g., furosemide) as ordered to decrease preload. Monitor urine output, electrolytes, and daily weights. Inotrope therapy (e.g., dobutamine) may be required to enhance contractility. Dopamine or nesiritide may be ordered to increase renal blood flow although dopamine's efficacy is controversial.

11. Invasive therapeutic modalities may be required or considered: thrombolytic therapy, counterpulsation (IABP), PCI, stent placement, or revascularization surgery.

Nursing Diagnosis: INEFFECTIVE TISSUE PERFUSION related to inadequate cardiac output

Outcome Criteria

Patient alert and oriented
Skin warm and dry
Pulses strong and equal bilaterally
Capillary refill <3 sec
Urine output 30 mL/hr or 0.5 to 1 mL/kg/hr
HR 60 to 100 beats/min
Absence of symptomatic bradycardia
Absence of life-threatening dysrhythmias
SBP 90 to 120 mm Hg
Pulse pressure 30 to 40 mm Hg
MAP 70 to 90 mm Hg
CI 2.5 to 4 L/min/m^2
$\dot{D}o_2I$ 500 to 600 mL/min/m^2
$\dot{V}o_2I$ 115 to 165 mL/min/m^2
Svo_2 60% to 80%
O_2 sat ≥95%

Patient Monitoring

1. Obtain PA pressures, PAWP and CVP (RA) hourly or as patient condition indicates (if available). Obtain CO and monitor CI as patient condition indicates; note trends and the patient's response to therapy.

2. Monitor Svo_2, $\dot{D}o_2I$ and $\dot{V}o_2I$ as indicators of tissue perfusion.

3. Monitor BP hourly or more frequently if the patient's condition is unstable; note trends in MAP and pulse pressure and the patient's response to therapy.

4. Monitor hourly urine output to evaluate effective CO and/or pharmacologic intervention.

5. Continuously monitor oxygen status with pulse oximetry (SpO_2) or SvO_2 (if available). Monitor patient activities and nursing interventions that may adversely affect oxygenation.

Patient Assessment

1. Obtain HR, RR, and BP every 15 minutes during acute phase and when titrating vasoactive drugs.

2. Assess mentation, skin temperature and color, capillary refill, and peripheral pulses as indicators of tissue perfusion. Assess skin for pressure ulcer development secondary to hypoperfusion.

3. Assess chest discomfort to validate ischemic origin (see Table 5-22). Assess pain using patient's self-report whenever possible. (See p. 35 for information about acute pain.)

4. Assess the patient for clinical sequelae. (See Table 5-25.)

Diagnostics Assessment

1. Review serial ABGs for hypoxemia (<60 mm Hg), acidosis (pH <7.35), and metabolic acidosis (base excess [BE] <2), which may further compromise tissue perfusion.

2. Review lactate levels (if ordered) as an indicator of anaerobic metabolism.

3. Review serial BUN and creatinine levels to evaluate renal function; BUN >20 mg/dL and creatinine >1.5 mg/dL suggest renal insufficiency, which may be a result of decreased renal perfusion.

4. Review echocardiography or cardiac catheterization results (if available) to review ventricular function (ejection fraction and wall motion).

Patient Management

A progressive reduction in CO/CI leading to decreased tissue perfusion in the patient with MI may be a result of heart failure (see p. 237), cardiogenic pulmonary edema (see p. 206), or cardiogenic shock (see p. 213).

AORTIC DISSECTION

Clinical Brief

Aortic dissection involves a tear in the medial layer of the aortic wall, causing blood to extravasate into the media and thus compromising blood flow to the brain, heart, and other organs. Usually the causative factor is an underlying disease of the media. Dissection can be classified by the site(s) involved: (1) DeBakey type I—ascending aorta beyond arch, (2) DeBakey type II—ascending aorta, and (3) DeBakey type III—descending aorta.

Demographic risk factors include being male, African American, and in the fifth to seventh decade of life. Medical risk factors include HTN, aortic valve disease, coarctation of the aorta, Marfan's syndrome, recent deceleration injury, cocaine use, and/or complications from invasive procedures such as angiography or intraaortic balloon.

Presenting Signs and Symptoms

The patient experiences abrupt, severe, tearing pain that may be localized in the anterior chest, intrascapular, abdominal, or lumbar area. The pain is usually nonprogressive and most intense at its onset.

Physical Examination

Appearance: anxiety, paleness, restless
Vital signs:
    ↑ BP, diastolic BP may be >150 mm Hg.
    ↓ BP, if hypovolemic (aortic rupture) or cardiac tamponade develops.
Neurologic: intermittent lightheadedness, LOC changes, weakness, CVA symptoms
Cardiovascular:
    Diastolic murmurs (aortic insufficiency) may be present.
    Pulse deficits and BP differences between right and left or upper and lower limbs may be noted.

Diagnostic Findings

Chest radiographs: changes seen may include a widened mediastinum, enlarged ascending aorta, blurring of the aortic knob, and/or a left-sided effusion.
MRI is the gold standard for definite identification of location and vessels involved.

Transesophageal echocardiography (TEE): identifies presence and
location of tear; may also identify degree of aortic insufficiency
present.

Aortography: confirms presence and location of tear.

ACUTE CARE PATIENT MANAGEMENT

Goals of Treatment

Reduce BP and HR to prevent further dissection of aorta and relieve
pain.
Antihypertensive agents: sodium nitroprusside, labetalol
β-Adrenergic blockers: atenolol, esmolol, propranolol
Relief of stress/anxiety: morphine sulfate
Correct problem.
Surgical repair of aorta and aortic valve
Percutaneous intraluminal stent graft insertion

Priority Nursing Diagnoses and Potential Complications	
Priority Nursing Diagnoses	**PC: Potential Complications**
Ineffective tissue perfusion	Decreased cardiac output, hypoxemia, renal insufficiency
Acute pain	
Risk for ineffective protection (see p. 48)	
Risk for interrupted family processes (see p. 45)	

Nursing Diagnosis: INEFFECTIVE TISSUE PERFUSION related to compromised arterial
blood flow secondary to blood extravasation via aortic dissection

Outcome Criteria

Patient alert and oriented
Skin warm and dry
SBP 80 to 100 mm Hg or as low as can possibly maintain systemic
perfusion
Urine output 30 mL/hr or 0.5 to 1 mL/kg/hr
Pulses strong and equal bilaterally
Capillary refill <3 sec in all extremities
Pupils equal and normoreactive
Motor strength strong and equal bilaterally

Patient Monitoring

1. Continuously monitor arterial BP during acute phase to evaluate the patient's response to therapy.
2. Monitor hourly urine output because a drop in output may indicate renal artery dissection or a decrease in arterial blood flow.
3. Continuously monitor ECG for dysrhythmia formation, ST segment or T-wave changes, suggesting coronary sequelae or a decrease in arterial blood flow.

Patient Assessment

1. Assess neurologic status to evaluate the course of dissection. Confusion or changes in sensation and motor strength may indicate compromised cerebral blood flow (CBF).
2. Auscultate for changes in heart sounds and signs and symptoms of HF (e.g., sustained tachycardia, S_3, crackles), which may indicate that the dissection involves the aortic valve.
3. Compare BP and pulses in both arms and legs to determine differences.

Diagnostics Assessment

1. Review serial BUN and creatinine levels to evaluate renal function.
2. Review cardiac enzymes because a dissection involving coronary arteries may result in MI.
3. Review the ECG for patterns of ischemia, injury, and infarction.
4. Review results of radiology tests: CT scan, MRI, TEE, aortogram.

Patient Management

1. Administer oxygen therapy as ordered to keep SpO_2 >92%.
2. Keep the patient on bed rest to prevent further dissection.
3. Nitroprusside may be ordered to lower BP. Titrate the infusion to desired BP. The dose may range from 0.5 to 6 mcg/kg/min. Monitor for signs and symptoms of cyanide toxicity: tinnitus, blurred vision, delirium, and muscle spasm. Refer to specific facility policy/procedure regarding the administration of nitroprusside.

4. A β-adrenergic blocking agent such as atenolol, esmolol, or propranolol may be ordered to reduce stress on the aortic wall.

5. Anticipate surgical intervention. Surgery typically consists of resection of the torn portion of the aorta and replacement with a prosthetic graft. With severe aortic regurgitation, valve replacement may also be indicated.

Nursing Diagnosis: ACUTE PAIN related to aortic dissection

Outcome Criterion

Patient communicates that pain is relieved or tolerable.

Patient Monitoring

Monitor VS for evidence of pain and anxiety (e.g., increased HR, SBP, and RR). Be sure to differentiate these signs of pain from signs of hypovolemic shock.

Patient Assessment

Note facial expression and evidence of guarding. However, absence of these behaviors does not necessarily mean absence of pain. Increased severity may indicate increasing dissection. Note BP because an increased BP can cause further dissection and increase pain.

Diagnostics Assessment

None specific

Patient Management

1. If BP permits, morphine sulfate may be given as ordered. This will decrease the catecholamine response, thus reducing HR and BP.

2. Administer antihypertensive agents to control BP. Nitroprusside infusion to be titrated to 0.5 to 6 mcg/kg/min. Monitor for signs and symptoms of cyanide toxicity: tinnitus, blurred vision, delirium, and muscle spasm. Refer to specific facility policy/procedure regarding the administration of nitroprusside.

3. Alleviate anxieties by providing realistic assurances and providing family support as indicated. Administer antianxiety agents as ordered.

CARDIAC TAMPONADE

Clinical Brief

Cardiac tamponade is the accumulation of excess fluid within the pericardial space, resulting in impaired cardiac filling, reduction in SV, and epicardial coronary artery compression with resultant myocardial ischemia. Clinical signs of cardiac tamponade depend on the rapidity of fluid accumulation and on the fluid volume. The acute accumulation of 200 mL of blood within the pericardium as a result of blunt or penetrating trauma to the thorax will result in rapid evidence of decompensation, whereas an insidious effusion may not evidence decompensation until as much as 2000 mL of fluid have slowly accumulated.

Risk factors include recent cardiac trauma such as open trauma to the thorax (gunshot wounds and stabs), closed trauma to the thorax (impact of the chest on a steering wheel during a motor vehicle accident), cardiac surgery, and iatrogenic causes (cardiac catheterization or pacemaker electrode perforation); nontraumatic factors include metastatic neoplasm, tuberculosis, acute infectious or idiopathic pericarditis, renal failure, and hemopericardium from anticoagulant therapy.

Presenting Signs and Symptoms

Symptoms reflect the loss of CO/CI like restlessness, agitation, weakness, anorexia, chest discomfort, SOB, and a feeling of impending doom. However, decreased CO/CI and poor tissue perfusion are the net result.

Physical Examination

Pulsus paradoxus >10 mm Hg (hallmark)
Narrowed pulse pressure (<30 mm Hg)
Hypotension
Neurologic: anxiety, confusion, obtunded if decompensation is
    advanced
Cardiovascular:
    JVD
    Reflex tachycardia
    Muffled, distant heart sounds
    Pericardial rub may be present
    Equalizing of all PA and CVP pressures
Skin: cool, pale, may be clammy

Diagnostic Findings

Cardiac tamponade should be suspected if there is a rise in CVP and PAWP, fall in arterial pressure, and a muffling of heart tones.

ECG changes: usually nonspecific; may note electrical alternans and/or diffuse low voltage of QRSs.

Chest radiograph: in acute cases is rarely diagnostic, but widened mediastinum may be observed. Chronic effusions may result in a "water bottle" appearance of the cardiac silhouette.

Echocardiography: usually shows widespread compression of the heart and inferior and superior vena cava congestion; evidence of pericardial effusion.

Hemodynamics: as cardiac tamponade progresses, RA pressure begins to approximate PAWP (pressure plateau), ↑ SVRI.

ACUTE CARE PATIENT MANAGEMENT

Goals of Treatment

Maintain hemodynamic stability.

     Supplemental oxygen

     Volume expanders (↑ preload)

     β-Adrenergic agents: epinephrine

Relieve cardiac compression.

     Pericardiocentesis/pericardiectomy to drain fluid from around the heart.

     Possible thoracotomy to repair traumatic defect

Priority Nursing Diagnoses and Potential Complications

Priority Nursing Diagnoses	PC: Potential Complications
Decreased cardiac output	Dysrhythmias
Risk for ineffective protection (see p. 48)	
Risk for interrupted family processes (see p. 45)	

Nursing Diagnosis: DECREASED CARDIAC OUTPUT related to reduced ventricular filling secondary to increased intrapericardial pressure

Outcome Criteria

     Patient alert and oriented

     Skin warm and dry

     Pulses strong and equal bilaterally

     Capillary refill <3 sec

HR 60 to 100 beats/min
SBP 90 to 120 mm Hg
Pulse pressure 30 to 40 mm Hg
MAP 70 to 105 mm Hg
CVP 2 to 6 mm Hg
PAWP 4 to 12 mm Hg
CO 4 to 8 L/min
CI 2.5 to 4 L/min/m^2
SVRI 1700 to 2600 dynes/sec/cm^{-5}/m^2
Urine output 30 mL/hr or 1 mL/kg/hr

Patient Monitoring

1. Continuously monitor ECG for dysrhythmia formation, which may be a result of myocardial ischemia secondary to epicardial coronary artery compression. Electrical alternans, a waxing and waning of the R wave, may be evident.

2. Monitor the BP every 5 to 15 minutes during the acute phase. Monitor for pulsus paradoxus via arterial tracing or during manual BP reading. A drop in SBP >10 mm Hg during the inspiratory phase of a normal respiratory cycle confirms the presence of pulsus paradoxus.

3. Monitor PA pressures and CVP (if available) for pressure plateau. Right atrial and wedge pressures will equalize as fluid accumulates in the pericardial space.

4. Monitor MAP, SVRI, and pulse pressure to evaluate the patient's response to increasing intrapericardial pressure and/or therapy. As the pressure increases, MAP will fall, pulse pressure will narrow, and SVRI will increase.

5. Monitor urine output hourly; a drop in urine output may indicate decreased renal perfusion as a result of decreased SV secondary to cardiac compression.

Patient Assessment

1. Assess cardiovascular status: monitor for JVD and presence of Kussmaul's sign. Note skin temperature, color, and capillary refill. Assess amplitude of femoral pulse during quiet breathing. Pulse amplitude that decreases or disappears may indicate pulsus paradoxus. Auscultate the anterior chest for muffled or distant heart sounds.

2. Assess LOC for changes that may indicate decreased cerebral perfusion.

Diagnostics Assessment

1. Review ECG for electrical alternans.
2. Review echocardiogram report if available.
3. Review chest radiographs for enlarged cardiac silhouette and "water bottle" appearance.

Patient Management

1. Provide supplemental oxygen as ordered.
2. Initiate two large-bore intravenous lines for fluid administration to maintain filling pressure.
3. Pharmacologic therapy may include dobutamine to enhance myocardial contractility and decrease peripheral vascular resistance. This is a temporary measure to maintain CO/CI and tissue perfusion until the tamponade can be relieved. Monitor for cardiac dysrhythmias and hypotension.
4. Pericardiocentesis may be performed. Monitor the patient for dysrhythmias, coronary artery laceration (chest discomfort suggestive of ischemia), or hemopneumothorax (dyspnea, decreased or absent ipsilateral breath sounds, contralateral tracheal shift).
5. Surgical intervention to identify and repair bleeding site, to evacuate clots in the mediastinum, to resect or open the pericardium.

CARDIOGENIC PULMONARY EDEMA

Clinical Brief

Pulmonary edema is an abnormal accumulation of extravascular fluid in the lung parenchyma that interferes with adequate gas exchange. This is a life-threatening situation that needs immediate treatment. The most common cause of cardiogenic pulmonary edema is left ventricular failure exhibited by increased left atrial ventricular pressures. Risk factors include ischemic heart disease, cardiomyopathy, valvular disease, MI, and acute septal defects.

Presenting Signs and Symptoms

Signs and symptoms include SOB, orthopnea, moist cough with pink frothy sputum, chest discomfort, palpitations, fatigue, syncope, cyanosis, and respiratory distress.

Physical Examination

Appearance: anxious, diaphoretic, clammy
Vital signs:

HR: sustained tachycardia
SBP: <90 mm Hg
RR: >30 breaths/min
Falling O_2 saturations

Cardiovascular:

Tachydysrhythmias with possible ectopy
Laterally displaced point of maximal impulse (PMI)
Murmur—mitral valve regurgitation
S_3 with possible S_4

Pulmonary:

Respiratory distress, respiratory failure
Orthopnea
Coarse bilateral crackles, wheezing, and/or rhonchi
Cough, frothy sputum

Diagnostic Findings

ABGs: acidosis (pH <7.35) with hypoxemia (PaO_2 <60 mm Hg)
Elevation in pro BNP or BNP
Chest radiograph:

Increased heart shadow
Kerley B lines—onset of interstitial edema
Pulmonary venous congestion
Diffuse infiltrates and intra-alveolar fluid

Echocardiogram: left ventricular enlargement
PAWP: >25 mm Hg, CI <2 L/min/m^2

ACUTE CARE PATIENT MANAGEMENT

Goals of Treatment

Reduce preload and afterload.

Diuretics (e.g., furosemide)
ACE inhibitors (e.g., captopril)
Nitrates
Morphine sulfate
Other vasodilators (e.g., nesiritide)
IABP
Continuous renal replacement therapy (CRRT)

Improve LV function and contractility.
    Inotropes: dobutamine, milrinone, dopamine, digoxin
    IABP
    Left ventricular assist device (LVAD)
Improve oxygenation/ventilation.
    Bed rest
    Supplemental oxygen
    Endotracheal intubation and mechanical ventilation

Priority Nursing Diagnoses and Potential Complications	
Priority Nursing Diagnoses	**PC: Potential Complications**
Impaired gas exchange	Hypoxemia
Decreased cardiac output	Dysrhythmias
Risk for ineffective protection (see p. 48)	
Risk for interrupted family processes (see p. 45)	

Nursing Diagnosis: IMPAIRED GAS EXCHANGE related to increased pulmonary congestion secondary to increased left ventricular end diastolic pressure (LVEDP)

Outcome Criteria

RR 12 to 20 breaths/min
Eupnea
Lungs clear to auscultation
pH 7.35 to 7.45
PaO_2 80 to 100 mm Hg
$PaCO_2$ 35 to 45 mm Hg
O_2 sat ≥95%
SvO_2 60% to 80%
$P(a/A)O_2$ ratio 0.75 to 0.95

Patient Monitoring

1. Obtain PA pressures (if available) including PAWP to evaluate course of pulmonary edema and/or the patient's response to therapy. Obtain hemodynamic profile (if available) as an indicator of contractility, preload, and afterload.
2. Continuously monitor oxygenation status with pulse oximetry (SpO_2) or SvO_2 monitoring. Note patient activities and nursing interventions that may adversely affect oxygen saturation.
3. Continuously monitor ECG for dysrhythmia development that may be related to hypoxemia, acid-base imbalance, or ventricular irritability.

4. Calculate arterial-alveolar oxygen tension ratio ($P[a/A]o_2$) as an index of gas exchange efficiency.

5. Document hourly I&O to monitor fluid status. Obtain daily weights. Rapid (0.5-1 kg/day) changes in weight suggest fluid gain or loss.

Patient Assessment

1. Measure HR, RR, and BP every 15 minutes to evaluate the patient's response to therapy and to detect cardiopulmonary deterioration.

2. Assess the patient for changes that may indicate respiratory compromise, necessitating intubation and mechanical ventilation: frequent assessment of lung sounds and observation of air hunger; acute onset of pink, frothy sputum; diaphoresis; and cyanosis.

Diagnostics Assessment

1. Review ABGs for hypoxemia (Pao_2 <60 mm Hg) and acidosis (pH <7.35), which may further compromise tissue perfusion and/or indicate need for mechanical ventilation.

2. Review serial chest radiographs for worsening or resolving pulmonary congestion.

3. Review lactate levels as an indicator of anaerobic metabolism.

4. Review changes in BNP or pro BNP.

Patient Management

1. Provide supplemental oxygen via mask; consider continuous positive airway pressure (CPAP), bilevel positive airway pressure (BiPAP), PEEP or pressure support. Be prepared to intubate and provide mechanical ventilation. PEEP will most likely be employed to facilitate adequate oxygen exchange. Pressure support will reduce the work of breathing. (See p. 503 for information on ventilation therapies.)

2. Administer diuretic agents or nesiritide to reduce circulating volume, which will improve gas exchange. Monitor urine output and electrolytes. Nesiritide is given in a bolus of 2 mcg/kg over 10 minutes followed by an infusion of 0.01 mcg/kg/min to assist with diuresis and vasodilation.

3. Administer vasodilating agents (e.g., nitrates, morphine, dobutamine) to redistribute fluid volumes, which will facilitate gas exchange.

4. Morphine sulfate may be ordered to promote preload and afterload reduction and to decrease anxiety.

5. Minimize oxygen demand: maintain bed rest, decrease anxiety, keep the patient NPO in the acute phase, pace nursing interventions, and provide uninterrupted rest periods.

6. Position the patient to maximize chest excursion; evaluate the patient's response to position changes with SpO_2 or SvO_2 monitoring. Encourage frequent patient repositioning.

7. Once the patient's condition is stabilized, promote pulmonary and oral hygiene to reduce risk of pneumonia and atelectasis: assist the patient to C&DB, encourage incentive spirometry, and reposition the patient frequently. If mechanically ventilated, position patient to reduce the risk of aspiration and ventilator-acquired pneumonia.

Nursing Diagnosis: DECREASED CARDIAC OUTPUT related to impaired left ventricular function

Outcome Criteria

Patient alert and oriented
Skin warm and dry
Pulses strong and equal bilaterally
Capillary refill <3 sec
SBP 90 to 120 mm Hg
MAP 70 to 105 mm Hg
Pulse pressure 30 to 40 mm Hg
HR 60 to 100 beats/min
Absence of life-threatening dysrhythmias
Urine output 30 mL/hr or 0.5 to 1 mL/kg/hr
CVP 2 to 6 mm Hg
PAS 15 to 30 mm Hg
PAD 5 to 15 mm Hg
PAWP 4 to 12 mm Hg
SVRI 1700 to 2600 dynes/sec/cm^{-5}/m^2
PVRI 200 to 450 dynes/sec/cm^{-5}/m^2
CI 2.5 to 4 L/min/m^2
SvO_2 60% to 80%

Patient Monitoring

1. Obtain PA pressures and CVP (RA) hourly (if available) or more frequently if titrating pharmacologic agents. Obtain complete hemodynamic profile as patient condition indicates; monitor CI, SVRI, and PVRI; and note trends or the patient's response to therapy.

2. Obtain BP hourly or more frequently if the patient's condition is unstable. Note trends in MAP and pulse pressure and the patient's response to therapy.
3. Monitor hourly urine output as an indicator of CO/CI and/or response to pharmacologic intervention.
4. Analyze ECG rhythm strip at least every 4 hours and note rate; rhythm; and PR, QRS, and QT intervals. Note ST segment and T-wave changes, which may indicate ischemia or injury.

Patient Assessment

1. Obtain HR, RR, and BP every 15 minutes during acute phase and when titrating vasoactive drugs.
2. Assess skin for warmth, color, and capillary refill time. Assess distal pulses bilaterally for strength, regularity, and symmetry.
3. Assess heart and lung sounds every 4 hours and as clinically indicated to evaluate the course of pulmonary edema.
4. Assess for chest discomfort because myocardial ischemia may result from poor perfusion secondary to decreased CO/CI.
5. Assess for changes in neurologic function hourly and as clinically indicated; note orientation to person, place, and time; arousability to verbal and/or tactile stimuli; and bilateral motor and sensory responses.
6. Assess for pressure ulcer formation related to hypoperfusion.

Diagnostics Assessment

1. Review serial BUN and creatinine levels to evaluate renal function; BUN >20 mg/dL and creatinine >1.5 mg/dL suggest renal impairment, which may be a result of decreased renal perfusion.
2. Review echocardiography or cardiac catheterization results (if available) for ventricular function (ejection fraction and wall motion) and valvular function.
3. Review BNP and pro BNP to assess the degree of heart failure.

Patient Management

1. Multiple intravenous sites may be necessary to maintain vasoactive drips.
2. Administer diuretic agents (e.g., furosemide, bumetanide) to reduce preload and afterload. Administer furosemide 20 mg/min IVP as ordered. Doses as high as 120 mg may be

required. Administer bumetanide 0.5 to 1 mg IVP over 1 minute. A common effect of furosemide and bumetanide administration is potassium depletion; therefore, monitor serum potassium before and after administration of loop diuretics. Administer potassium supplements orally or intravenous piggyback as ordered. Signs and symptoms of symptomatic hypokalemia (potassium <4 mEq/L) include ECG/rhythm changes (flattened T wave, prolonged PR interval, ventricular tachyarrhythmias) and muscle weakness. Consider monitoring magnesium levels.

3. Administer vasodilators as ordered to reduce preload and afterload. Administer morphine sulfate as ordered. Give IVP in 2-mg increments every 5 minutes to relieve symptoms. NTG may be ordered: sublingual, 1 tablet (0.4 mg) every 5 minutes × 3; IV, start with an infusion of 5 mcg/min, titrate to desired response or to maintain SBP >90 mm Hg, and increase dosage every 5 to 10 minutes by 5 to 10 mcg/min. If hypotension or reflex tachycardia occurs, raise the patient's legs and reduce the dose as needed for SBP >90 mm Hg. Nesiritide dose is given in a bolus of 2 mcg/kg followed by an infusion of 0.01 mcg/kg/min to assist with diuresis and vasodilation. Sodium nitroprusside (0.01-6 mcg/kg/min) may be ordered to reduce afterload for patients whose SBP is >100 mm Hg. Monitor for signs and symptoms of cyanide toxicity: tinnitus, blurred vision, delirium, and muscle spasm. Refer to facility policy/procedure on the administration of nitroprusside.

4. Titrate inotropic agents as ordered to enhance contractility (e.g., dobutamine, amrinone, milrinone, dopamine, and digoxin). Dobutamine can be administered at 2.5 to 10 mcg/kg/min. Milrinone is administered as a 50-mcg/kg bolus over 10 minutes, followed by an infusion of 0.375 to 0.75 mcg/kg/min. Use lower doses with renal impairment. Dopamine administered at low doses (1-5 mcg/kg/min) increases renal and mesenteric blood flow; at moderate doses (2-10 mcg/kg/min), contractility is enhanced. Use caution when using higher doses of dopamine because of the vasoconstrictive and tachycardic effects. Monitor for signs and symptoms of digitalis toxicity: dysrhythmia formation (blocks, bradycardias, PSVT), nausea, vomiting, diarrhea, and blurred or yellow vision. Signs and symptoms of digitalis toxicity will be exhibited earlier if the patient is hypokalemic.

5. Institute pressure ulcer prevention strategies because of hypoperfusion/low cardiac output state.

CARDIOGENIC SHOCK

Clinical Brief

Cardiogenic shock is the inability to meet the metabolic needs due to severely impaired contractility of either ventricle. That leads to decreased tissue perfusion and a shocklike state. Risk factors include prior MI, advanced age, female, diabetes, or anterior wall MI. The most common causes of cardiogenic shock are acute MI, ventricular septal defect, acute mitral regurgitation, cardiac tamponade, aortic dissection, massive pulmonary infarct, and severe dysrhythmias.

Presenting Signs and Symptoms

The patient's skin will be pale, cool, and clammy. Pulmonary congestion and hypoxemia worsen as the ventricles fail to eject adequate volume and the blood backs up into the lung. Tissue hypoperfusion continues because the oxygen does not meet the metabolic needs.

Physical Examination

Appearance:
    Restlessness progressing to unresponsiveness
    Chest pain
    Dysrhythmias
Vital signs:
    HR: >100 beats/min
    SBP: <80 mm Hg
    RR: >20 breaths/min
    UOP: <0.5 mL/kg/hr
Neurologic: agitation, restlessness progressing to unresponsiveness, and changes in LOC
Cardiovascular: weak, thready pulses; decreased CO/CI; rhythm may be irregular; S_3, S_4; diminished heart tones; and JVD
Pulmonary: orthopnea, crackles, cough with increased secretions, dyspnea, and tachypnea
Skin: cool, clammy skin; pale; delayed capillary refill time; and cyanosis

Diagnostic Findings

Clinical manifestations and hemodynamic findings are the basis for diagnosis.
CI <2 L/min/m^2

PAWP >18 mm Hg
SVRI increasing trend
Pulse pressure narrowed
SV decreased
LVSWI decreasing trend
↑ CVP if right HF
Urine output <0.5 mL/kg/hr

ACUTE CARE PATIENT MANAGEMENT

Goals of Treatment

Optimize oxygen delivery.
    Supplemental oxygen
    Intubation and mechanical ventilation
    Coronary artery vasodilating agents
    Morphine sulfate
    Nitrates
Optimize cardiac output and reduce myocardial oxygen demand
    Inotropes: dopamine, dobutamine, milrinone
    Vasopressors: norepinephrine, epinephrine, phenylephrine, dopamine
    Mechanical support: IABP, RVAD, LVAD
    ECMO
    Thrombolytics
    PCI and CABG
Reduce oxygen demand.
    Morphine sulfate
    Diuretics: furosemide, bumetanide
    Vasodilators: NTG
    Mechanical support: IABP, ventricular assist device (VAD)
Detect/prevent clinical sequelae (Table 5-27).

Priority Nursing Diagnoses and Potential Complications	
Priority Nursing Diagnoses	**PC: Potential Complications**
Ineffective tissue perfusion	Dysrhythmias, renal insufficiency
Impaired gas exchange	Hypoxemia
Ineffective protection (see p. 48)	
Risk for interrupted family processes (see p. 45)	
Imbalanced nutrition: less than body requirements (see p. 53)	

Table 5-27 CLINICAL SEQUELAE ASSOCIATED WITH CARDIOGENIC SHOCK

Complication	Signs and Symptoms
Cardiopulmonary arrest	Nonpalpable pulse, absent respirations
Extension of MI	Cardiac pain, ST/T-wave changes involving more leads
Pulmonary edema	Dyspnea, cough, frothy sputum, cyanosis, ↓ Pao_2, ↑ RR, ↓ BP, PAWP >25 mm Hg
Renal failure	Urine output <0.5 mL/kg/hr, steady rise in creatinine
GI dysfunction/bleeding	Blood in NG aspirate, emesis or stool; absent bowel sounds, distention
Multisystem organ dysfunction syndrome (MODS)	Renal, respiratory, hepatic, and/or hematologic failure

BP, Blood pressure; *GI,* gastrointestinal; *MI,* myocardial infarction; *NG,* nasogastric; *PAWP,* pulmonary artery wedge pressure; *RR,* respiratory rate.

Nursing Diagnosis: INEFFECTIVE TISSUE PERFUSION related to decreased cardiac output secondary to decreased contractility

Outcome Criteria

Patient alert and oriented
Skin warm and dry
Peripheral pulses strong
HR 60 to 100 beats/min
Absence of life-threatening dysrhythmias
Urine output 30 mL/hr or 0.5 to 1 mL/kg/hr
SBP 90 to 120 mm Hg
MAP 70 to 105 mm Hg
CI 2.5 to 4 L/min/m^2
SVRI 1700 to 2600 dynes/sec/cm^{-5}/m^2
PVRI 200 to 450 dynes/sec/cm^{-5}/m^2
O_2 sat ≥95%
Svo_2 60% to 80%
$\dot{D}o_2I$ 500 to 600 mL/min/m^2
$\dot{V}o_2I$ 115 to 165 mL/min/m^2

Patient Monitoring

1. Monitor BP continuously via arterial cannulation (if available) because cuff pressures are less accurate in shock states.

Monitor MAP, an indicator that accurately reflects tissue perfusion. MAP <60 mm Hg adversely affects cerebral and renal perfusion.

2. Continuously monitor ECG to detect life-threatening dysrhythmias or HR greater than 140 beats/min, which can adversely affect SV. Monitor for ischemia (ST segment, T-wave changes) associated with decreased coronary perfusion.

3. Monitor PA pressures and CVP (if available) hourly or more frequently to evaluate the patient's response to treatment. These parameters can be used to monitor for fluid overload and pulmonary edema.

4. Obtain a complete hemodynamic profile every 8 hours or more frequently. Monitor CO/CI to evaluate the patient's response to changes in therapy. Note trends in LVSWI/RVSWI to evaluate myocardial contractility. An increase reflects improved contractility. Monitor trends in SVRI and PVRI. An increasing trend reflects increased afterload and increased myocardial oxygen consumption, which can further compromise myocardial function.

5. Monitor trends in $\dot{D}o_2I$ and $\dot{V}o_2I$ to evaluate effectiveness of therapy. Inadequate oxygen delivery or consumption produces tissue hypoxia.

6. Continuously monitor Svo_2 (if available). A decreasing trend may indicate decreased CO and increased tissue oxygen extraction (inadequate perfusion).

7. Monitor hourly urine output to evaluate renal perfusion.

Patient Assessment

1. Obtain HR, RR, and BP every 15 minutes to evaluate the patient's response to therapy and to detect cardiopulmonary deterioration.

2. Assess mentation, skin temperature/color/condition, peripheral pulses, and the presence of cardiac or abdominal pain to evaluate CO and state of vasoconstriction.

3. Assess the patient for clinical sequelae (see Table 5-27).

Diagnostics Assessment

1. Review ABGs for hypoxemia and metabolic or respiratory acidosis because these conditions can precipitate dysrhythmias, affect myocardial contractility, or indicate the need to be mechanically ventilated. O_2 saturation should be ≥95%.

2. Review serial ECGs to evaluate myocardial ischemia, injury, or infarction.

3. Review Hgb and Hct levels and note trends. Decreased red blood cells (RBCs) can adversely affect oxygen carrying capacity.

4. Review lactate levels, an indicator of anaerobic metabolism. Increased levels may signal decreased oxygen delivery.

5. Review BUN, creatinine, and electrolytes and note trends to evaluate renal function.

Patient Management

1. Administer supplemental oxygen and reduce oxygen consumption by minimizing oxygen demands (e.g., limit activities, bed rest). Anticipate intubation and mechanical ventilation if oxygen status deteriorates or cardiopulmonary arrest ensues.

2. Administer inotropes such as dobutamine and dopamine to increase contractility, increase SV, and improve CO.

3. Administer vasodilators such as NTG (mainly venous effects) and nitroprusside (mainly arterial effects) to reduce preload and afterload, improve SV, and reduce myocardial oxygen consumption. Monitor BP closely to prevent hypotension. NTG may have more beneficial effects with myocardial ischemia or infarction than nitroprusside secondary to coronary vasodilation.

4. Administer low-dose morphine sulfate as ordered to promote venous pooling and decrease dyspnea, anxiety, and pain.

5. Administer colloids as ordered if the patient is hypovolemic (CVP <6 mm Hg; PAWP <18 mm Hg). Cardiac patients, especially with RV infarction, generally require a higher filling pressure (preload). Monitor PAWP closely, >25 mm Hg is associated with pulmonary edema.

6. Administer diuretics (furosemide, bumetanide) as ordered to decrease circulating volume and to decrease preload as necessary. Monitor CVP and PAWP for decreasing trends that could suggest hypovolemia. Monitor for electrolyte imbalance secondary to diuresis. Electrolyte replacement therapy may be indicated.

7. Correct acidosis, which can block or diminish responsiveness to drug therapy and reduce contractility. If sodium bicarbonate administration is necessary, monitor pH and potassium levels because hypokalemia may result.

8. Treat dysrhythmias (see Appendix E).

9. Consider preparing the patient for IABP, VAD, or ECMO.

10. Anticipate administration of thrombolytics or prepare for PCI and/or open-heart surgery to restore myocardial perfusion or to repair valvular dysfunction.

11. Other surgical interventions (e.g., ventricular septal defect [VSD] repair, aneurysm resection) may be required.

12. Institute pressure ulcer prevention strategies and frequently monitor for damaged skin and tissue on bony prominences.

Nursing Diagnosis: IMPAIRED GAS EXCHANGE related to increased left ventricular end diastolic pressure (LVEDP) and pulmonary edema associated with severe left ventricular (LV) dysfunction

Outcome Criteria

Patient alert and oriented

PaO_2 80 to 100 mm Hg

pH 7.35 to 7.45

$PaCO_2$ 35 to 45 mm Hg

O_2 sat ≥95%

RR 12 to 20 breaths/min, eupnea

Lungs clear to auscultation

PAWP 4 to 12 mm Hg (<18 mm Hg)

Patient Monitoring

1. Continuously monitor oxygenation status with pulse oximetry. Monitor for desaturation in response to nursing interventions and patient activity.

2. Continuously monitor ECG for dysrhythmias caused by hypoxemia, electrolyte imbalances, or ventricular dysfunction.

3. Continuously monitor PAS pressure because hypoxia can increase pulmonary vascular tone, leading to increased PAS.

4. Note trends in PAD and PAWP; increasing values may indicate LV dysfunction and pulmonary congestion.

5. Monitor fluid volume status; measure hourly I&O and measure serial weights (1 kg weight gain reflects approximately 1000 mL fluid retention).

Patient Assessment

1. Obtain HR, RR, and BP every 15 minutes to evaluate the patient's response to therapy and detect cardiopulmonary deterioration.

2. Assess the patient's respiratory status: RR >28 breaths/min, use of accessory muscles, inability to speak in sentences, and presence of adventitious breath sounds suggest worsening pulmonary congestion and impending respiratory dysfunction.

3. Assess for signs and symptoms of hypoxemia: increased restlessness, increased complaints of dyspnea, and changes in LOC. Cyanosis is a late sign.

4. Assess for excess fluid volume, which can further compromise myocardial function: note pulmonary congestion, increased JVD, peripheral edema, and positive hepatojugular reflex.

5. Assess the patient for clinical sequelae (see Table 5-27).

Diagnostics Assessment

1. Review ABGs for decreasing trends in PaO_2 (hypoxemia) or pH (acidosis). These conditions can adversely affect myocardial contractility, SV, and tissue perfusion. O_2 sat should be ≥95%.

2. Review serial chest radiographs to evaluate the patient's progress or a worsening lung condition.

3. Review Hgb and Hct levels and note trends. Decreased RBCs can adversely affect oxygen carrying capacity.

4. Review ventilation/perfusion $\dot{V}/\dot{Q}$ scan results (if ordered) to determine probability of PE.

Patient Management

1. Provide supplemental oxygen as ordered. If the patient develops respiratory distress, be prepared for intubation and mechanical ventilation. (See p. 503 for information on ventilation therapies.)

2. Administer low-dose morphine sulfate as ordered to reduce preload in an attempt to decrease pulmonary congestion.

3. Minimize oxygen demand by maintaining bed rest and decreasing anxiety, fever, and pain.

4. Position the patient for maximum chest excursion and comfort.

5. Administer diuretics and/or vasodilators as ordered to reduce circulating volume and decrease preload.

6. When the patient is hemodynamically stable: promote pulmonary hygiene with cough, deep breathing, incentive spirometry, and position changes every 2 hours.

CARDIOMYOPATHY

Clinical Brief

Cardiomyopathy is a dysfunction of cardiac muscle that can be associated with CAD, HTN, cardiotoxic agents, valvular disorders, and vascular or pulmonary diseases. Cardiomyopathies are classified into three groups by etiology and the abnormal physiology of the left ventricle.

Dilated or congestive cardiomyopathy (DC) is characterized by ventricular dilation and impaired systolic contractile function. Emboli may occur because of blood stasis in the dilated ventricles. This is the most common type of cardiomyopathy. Categories of causes include toxic, metabolic, familial, inflammatory, abnormal cardiac microvasculature, and idiopathic.

Hypertrophic cardiomyopathy (HC) is characterized by inappropriate myocardial hypertrophy without ventricular dilation. Obstruction to left ventricular outflow may or may not be present. Ventricular compliance is decreased and diastolic filling is impaired (diastolic dysfunction).

Restrictive cardiomyopathy (RC) is characterized by abnormally rigid ventricles with decreased diastolic compliance. The ventricular cavity is decreased, and clinical manifestations are similar to constrictive pericarditis. This is the least common type of cardiomyopathy, which is classified by primary or secondary.

Presenting Signs and Symptoms

Signs and symptoms of cardiomyopathy include manifestations of HF such as dyspnea and fatigue, dysrhythmias, or conduction disturbances. Onset may be insidious or exhibited by sudden death.

Physical Examination

Vital signs:
    HR: increased, irregular rhythm
    BP: ↑ or ↓, depending on underlying disease or degree of HF
    RR: may be ↑, depending on degree of HF
Cardiovascular:
    Murmurs
    S_3 and/or S_4
    Ectopy
    JVD or peripheral edema

Pulmonary:
  Crackles
  Dry cough

Diagnostic Findings

ECG changes: supraventricular and ventricular dysrhythmias, LV and/or RV hypertrophy, and/or strain, and abnormal Q waves without infarction

Chest radiograph: evidence of HF, enlarged cardiac silhouette, possibly pleural effusion

Echocardiogram:
  Four-chamber cardiac enlargement (DC)
  LV hypertrophy
  RV hypertrophy
  ↓ EF
  ↓ CO
  Mitral or tricuspid regurgitation
  Possible area of hypokinesia

Hemodynamics:
  ↓ PAWP and CVP
  ↓ SVRI
  ↓ CO/CI

ACUTE CARE PATIENT MANAGEMENT

Goals of Treatment

Maximize CO.
  Inotropic drugs: dobutamine, amrinone, milrinone, digoxin*
  Antidysrhythmic agents, automatic implantable cardioverter defibrillator (AICD)
  β-Blockers: propranolol (consider ejection fraction)
  Surgery: heart transplant (DC), transmyocardial revascularization (DC), and myotomy/myectomy (HC)

Decrease myocardial work.
  Bed rest
  Supplemental oxygen
  Diuretics: furosemide, bumetanide*
  Nitrates: NTG, nitroprusside*

---

*Note: Inotropic, diuretic, and vasodilator agents are contraindicated in the early stages of HC.

ACE inhibitors: (to prevent dilation) captopril

β-Blockers: propranolol

Detect/prevent clinical sequelae (Table 5-28).

Table 5-28 CLINICAL SEQUELAE ASSOCIATED WITH CARDIOMYOPATHY

Complication	Signs and Symptoms
Pulmonary edema	Worsening HF: breathlessness, moist cough, frothy sputum, crackles, ↓ Pao₂, ↑ RR, ↓ BP
Cardiogenic shock	↓ Mentation, ↓ or ↑ HR, SBP <90 mm Hg, CI <2 L/min/m², urine output <0.5 mL/kg/hr; cool, clammy, mottled skin
Dysrhythmias/sudden death	Change in rate and/or rhythm, change in LOC, syncope, chest discomfort, cardiac arrest
Thrombus with embolic events	Change in LOC, hemiparesis, ECG changes indicative of ischemia, dysrhythmias, renal failure, GI ileus, abdominal pain, SOB, changes in CMS of the extremities, ↓ Pao₂, crackles

BP, Blood pressure; *CI,* cardiac index; *CMS,* color, movement, sensation; *ECG,* electrocardiogram; *GI,* gastrointestinal; *HF,* heart failure; *HR,* heart rate; *LOC,* level of consciousness; *RR,* respiratory rate; *SBP,* systolic blood pressure; *SOB,* shortness of breath.

Priority Nursing Diagnoses and Potential Complications

Priority Nursing Diagnoses	PC: Potential Complications
Decreased cardiac output	Dysrhythmias
Ineffective tissue perfusion	Renal insufficiency
Impaired gas exchange	Hypoxemia
Excess fluid volume	Pulmonary edema, electrolyte imbalance
Risk for ineffective protection (see p. 48)	
Risk for interrupted family processes (see p. 45)	
Imbalanced nutrition: less than body requirements (see p. 53)	

Nursing Diagnosis: DECREASED CARDIAC OUTPUT related to left ventricular dysfunction and dysrhythmias

<u>Outcome Criteria</u>

Patient alert and oriented
Skin warm and dry
Pulses strong and equal bilaterally
Capillary refill <3 sec
SBP 90 to 120 mm Hg
MAP 70 to 105 mm Hg
Pulse pressure 30 to 40 mm Hg
HR 60 to 100 beats/min
Absence of life-threatening dysrhythmias
Urine output 30 mL/hr or 0.5 to 1 mL/kg/hr
CVP 2 to 6 mm Hg
PAS 15 to 30 mm Hg
PAD 5 to 15 mm Hg
PAWP 4 to 12 mm Hg
SVRI 1700 to 2600 dynes/sec/cm^{-5}/m^2
PVRI 200 to 450 dynes/sec/cm^{-5}/m^2
CI 2.5 to 4 L/min/m^2

<u>Patient Monitoring</u>

1. Obtain PA pressures and CVP (RA) hourly (if available) or more frequently if titrating pharmacologic agents. Obtain CO/CI as patient condition indicates and as ordered. Monitor HR, CI, SVRI, PVRI, RVSWI, and LVSWI, noting trends or the patient's response to therapy.
2. Obtain BP hourly or more frequently if the patient's condition is unstable. Note trends in MAP and pulse pressure and the patient's response to therapy.
3. Monitor $\dot{D}o_2I$ and $\dot{V}o_2I$ as indicators of tissue perfusion.
4. Monitor hourly urine output to evaluate effects of decreased CO and/or pharmacologic intervention.
5. Analyze ECG rhythm strip at least every 4 hours and note rate; rhythm; and PR, QRS, and QT intervals. Note ST segment and T-wave changes, which may indicate ischemia or injury.
6. Continuously monitor oxygen status with pulse oximetry (SpO$_2$). Monitor patient activities and nursing interventions that may adversely affect oxygenation.

CV

Patient Assessment

1. Obtain HR, RR, and BP every 15 minutes during acute phase and when titrating vasoactive drugs.
2. Assess for changes in neurologic function hourly and as clinically indicated; note orientation to person, place, and time; arousability to verbal and/or sensory stimuli; and bilateral motor responses.
3. Assess skin for warmth, color, and capillary refill time. Assess distal pulses bilaterally for strength, regularity, and symmetry.
4. Assess for chest discomfort because myocardial ischemia may result from poor perfusion secondary to decreased CO.
5. Assess heart and lung sounds to evaluate the degree of HF.
6. Assess for pressure ulcer development secondary to hypoperfusion
7. Assess the patient for clinical sequelae (see Table 5-28).

Diagnostics Assessment

Review signal-averaged ECG, echocardiography, or cardiac catheterization results (if available) and note ventricular function (ejection fraction and wall motion) and valve function.

Patient Management

1. Provide oxygen at 2 to 4 L/min to maintain or improve oxygenation.
2. Minimize oxygen demand: maintain bed rest, decrease anxiety, and keep the patient NPO or provide a liquid diet in acute phase.
3. Administer diuretic agents (e.g., furosemide, bumetanide) to reduce preload and afterload. Administer furosemide 20 mg/min IVP as ordered. Doses as high as 120 mg may be ordered. Administer bumetanide 0.5 to 1 mg IVP over 1 minute. Bumetanide doses are not to exceed 10 mg in 24 hours. A common effect of furosemide and bumetanide administration is potassium depletion; therefore, monitor serum potassium before and after administration of loop diuretics. Administer potassium supplements orally or intravenous piggyback as ordered. Signs and symptoms of symptomatic hypokalemia (potassium <4 mEq/L) include ECG/rhythm changes (flattened T wave, prolonged PR interval,

ventricular tachydysrhythmias) and muscle weakness. Consider monitoring magnesium levels.

4. Administer vasodilators to reduce preload and afterload in patients with DC. Vasodilators are contraindicated in HC. Administer morphine sulfate as ordered. Give IVP in 2-mg increments every 5 minutes to relieve symptoms. NTG may be ordered; start the infusion at 5 mcg/min, and titrate to desired response or to maintain SBP >90 mm Hg. Increase dosage every 5 to 10 minutes by 5 to 10 mcg/min. If hypotension or reflex tachycardia occurs, raise the patient's legs and reduce the dose as needed for SBP >90 mm Hg. Sodium nitroprusside may be ordered to reduce afterload for patients whose SBP is >100 mm Hg. Do not administer more than 10 mcg/kg/min. Monitor for signs and symptoms of cyanide toxicity: tinnitus, blurred vision, delirium, and muscle spasm. Refer to facility policy/procedure for the administration of nitroprusside.

5. Titrate inotropic agents as ordered to enhance contractility (e.g., dobutamine, amrinone, milrinone, dopamine, and digoxin). Note drug effects on HR, CI, SVRI, PVRI, MAP, and pulse pressure. Dobutamine can be administered at 2.5 to 10 mcg/kg/min. Amrinone is typically administered via initial intravenous bolus of 0.75 mcg/kg over 2 to 3 minutes, followed by a maintenance drip titrating the dose at 5 to 10 mcg/kg/min to the desired effects. Total 24-hour dose should not exceed 10 mg/kg. Milrinone is administered as a 50-mcg/kg bolus over 10 minutes, followed by an infusion of 0.375 to 0.75 mcg/kg/min. Dopamine administered at low doses (1 to 2 mcg/kg/min) increases renal and mesenteric blood flow; at moderate doses (2 to 10 mcg/kg/min), contractility is enhanced. Use caution when using higher doses of dopamine because of the vasoconstrictive effects. Monitor for signs and symptoms of digitalis toxicity, which may include dysrhythmia formation (blocks, bradycardias, PSVT), nausea, vomiting, diarrhea, and blurred or yellow vision. Signs and symptoms of digitalis toxicity will be exhibited earlier if the patient is hypokalemic.

6. Prophylactic heparin or LMWH may be ordered to prevent thromboembolus formation secondary to venous pooling.

7. Institute pressure ulcer prevention strategies secondary to hypoperfusion/vasoconstrictor agents.

Nursing Diagnosis: INEFFECTIVE TISSUE PERFUSION related to decreased oxygen supply secondary to outflow tract obstruction (HC) or impaired systolic function (DC) resulting in decreased cardiac output

Outcome Criteria

Patient alert and oriented
Skin warm and dry
Peripheral pulses strong
HR 60 to 100 beats/min
Absence of life-threatening dysrhythmias
Urine output 30 mL/hr or 0.5 to 1 mL/kg/hr
SBP 90 to 120 mm Hg
MAP 70 to 105 mm Hg
CI 2.5 to 4 L/min/m^2
SVRI 1700 to 2600 dynes/sec/cm^{-5}/m^2
PVRI 200 to 450 dynes/sec/cm^{-5}/m^2
O$_2$ sat ≥95%
Svo$_2$ 60%-80%
Ḋo$_2$I 500 to 600 mL/min/m^2
V̇o$_2$I 115 to 165 mL/min/m^2

Patient Monitoring

1. Monitor BP continuously via arterial cannulation (if available) because cuff pressures are less accurate in shock states. Monitor MAP, an indicator that accurately reflects tissue perfusion. MAP <60 mm Hg adversely affects cerebral and renal perfusion.

2. Continuously monitor ECG to detect life-threatening dysrhythmias or HR >140 beats/min, which can adversely affect SV. Monitor for ischemia (ST segment, T-wave changes) associated with decreased coronary perfusion.

3. Monitor PA pressures and CVP (if available) hourly or more frequently to evaluate the patient's response to treatment. These parameters can be used to monitor for fluid overload and pulmonary edema.

4. Obtain a complete hemodynamic profile every 8 hours or more frequently. Monitor CO/CI to evaluate the patient's response to changes in therapy. Note trends in LVSWI/RVSWI to evaluate myocardial contractility. An increase reflects improved contractility. Monitor trends in SVRI and PVRI. An increasing trend reflects increased afterload and increased myocardial oxygen consumption, which can further compromise myocardial function.

5. Monitor trends in $\dot{D}o_2I$ and $\dot{V}o_2I$ to evaluate effectiveness of therapy. Inadequate oxygen delivery or consumption produces tissue hypoxia.

6. Continuously monitor Svo_2 (if available). A decreasing trend may indicate decreased CO and increased tissue oxygen extraction (inadequate perfusion).

7. Monitor hourly urine output to evaluate renal perfusion.

Patient Assessment

1. Obtain HR, RR, and BP every 15 minutes to evaluate the patient's response to therapy and detect cardiopulmonary deterioration.

2. Assess mentation, skin temperature/color/condition, and peripheral pulses and the presence of cardiac or abdominal pain to evaluate CO and state of vasoconstriction.

3. Assess the patient for clinical sequelae (see Table 5-28).

Diagnostics Assessment

1. Review ABGs for hypoxemia and metabolic or respiratory acidosis because these conditions can precipitate dysrhythmias, affect myocardial contractility, or indicate the need to be mechanically ventilated.

2. Review serial ECGs to evaluate myocardial ischemia, injury, or infarction.

3. Review Hgb and Hct levels, and note trends. Decreased RBCs can adversely affect oxygen carrying capacity.

4. Review lactate levels, an indicator of anaerobic metabolism. Increased levels may signal decreased oxygen delivery.

5. Review BUN, creatinine, and electrolytes and note trends to evaluate renal function.

6. Review echocardiogram as an indicator of ventricular and valvular function and dysfunction.

Patient Management

1. Administer supplemental oxygen and reduce oxygen consumption by minimizing oxygen demands (e.g., limit activities, bed rest). Anticipate intubation and mechanical ventilation if oxygen status deteriorates or cardiopulmonary arrest ensues. (See p. 503 for intubation and ventilation therapies.)

2. Administer inotropes such as dobutamine and dopamine to increase contractility, increase SV, and improve CO, when systolic dysfunction exists (DC).

3. Administer vasodilators such as NTG (mainly venous effects) and nitroprusside (mainly arterial effects) to reduce preload and afterload, improve SV, and reduce myocardial oxygen consumption. Monitor BP closely to prevent hypotension. As a result of the coronary vasodilatory effects, NTG may have more beneficial effects with myocardial ischemia or infarction than nitroprusside. Note: vasodilators and diuretics may be contraindicated with HC because reductions in preload may enhance obstruction to left ventricular outflow.

4. Administer low-dose morphine sulfate as ordered to promote venous pooling and decrease dyspnea, anxiety, and pain.

5. Administer colloids as ordered if the patient is hypovolemic (CVP <6 mm Hg; PAWP <18 mm Hg). Cardiac patients, especially with RV infarction, generally require a higher filling pressure (preload). Monitor PAWP closely, >25 mm Hg is associated with pulmonary edema.

6. Administer diuretics (furosemide, bumetanide) as ordered to decrease circulating volume and decrease preload as necessary. Monitor CVP and PAWP for decreasing trends that could suggest hypovolemia. Monitor for electrolyte imbalance secondary to diuresis. Electrolyte replacement therapy may be indicated. Note: vasodilators and diuretics may be contraindicated with HC because reductions in preload may enhance obstruction to left ventricular outflow.

7. Correct acidosis because acidosis can block or diminish responsiveness to drug therapy and reduce contractility. If sodium bicarbonate administration is necessary, monitor pH and potassium levels because hypokalemia may result.

8. Treat dysrhythmias.

9. Consider preparing the patient for IABP, VAD, or ECMO.

10. Institute pressure ulcer prevention strategies secondary to hypoperfusion or vasoactive drugs.

Nursing Diagnosis: IMPAIRED GAS EXCHANGE related to increased pulmonary congestion secondary to increased left ventricular end diastolic pressure (LVEDP) associated with ventricular failure

Outcome Criteria

Pao_2 80 to 100 mm Hg
pH 7.35 to 7.45
$Paco_2$ 35 to 45 mm Hg

O_2 sat $\geq$95%
RR 12 to 20 breaths/min, eupnea
Lungs clear to auscultation

Patient Monitoring

1. Continuously monitor oxygenation status with pulse oximetry (SpO_2) or SvO_2 monitoring. Note patient activities and nursing interventions that may adversely affect oxygen saturation.

2. Obtain PA and CVP pressures hourly (if available). Obtain complete hemodynamic profile every 4 hours or more frequently and note PAWP. Increasing PAWP may signal development of pulmonary edema. Increasing PAS pressure may signal hypoxia. Monitor PVRI.

3. Continuously monitor ECG for dysrhythmias that may be related to hypoxemia or acid-base imbalance.

4. Calculate arterial-alveolar oxygen tension ratio ($P[a/A]O_2$ ratio) as an index of gas exchange efficiency.

5. Measure I&O hourly. Determine fluid balance each shift. Compare serial weights. Rapid (0.5 to 1 kg/day) changes in weight suggest fluid gain or loss. Fluid gains may be suggestive of worsening failure.

Patient Assessment

1. Assess respiratory status frequently during the acute phase. RR >30 breaths/min, increasing complaints of dyspnea, inability to speak in sentences, increasing restlessness, cough, and use of accessory muscles may indicate respiratory distress and increased patient effort. Cyanosis is a late sign.

2. Assess lung sounds for adventitious sounds and to evaluate the course of pulmonary congestion.

3. Assess the patient for the development of clinical sequelae (see Table 5-28).

Diagnostics Assessment

1. Review serial ABGs for hypoxemia (PaO_2 <60 mm Hg) and acidosis (pH <7.35), signs of poor gas exchange, which may further compromise tissue perfusion.

2. Review lactate levels if ordered, an indicator of anaerobic metabolism.

3. Review serial chest radiographs for pulmonary congestion.

Patient Management

1. Provide supplemental oxygen as ordered to maintain or improve oxygenation. Consider CPAP or BiPAP. If the patient develops respiratory distress, be prepared for intubation and mechanical ventilation. (See p. 503 for information on intubation and ventilation therapies.)

2. Minimize oxygen demand: maintain bed rest, decrease anxiety, keep the patient NPO or provide a liquid diet in the acute phase, treat pain, limit patient activities, pace activities and nursing interventions, and provide uninterrupted rest periods.

3. Position the patient to maximize chest excursion; evaluate the patient's response to position changes with SpO_2 or SvO_2 monitoring.

4. Low-dose morphine sulfate may be ordered to promote venous pooling and decrease dyspnea. This may effectively decrease anxiety.

5. Diuretic agents may be ordered to reduce circulating volume. Monitor urine output, electrolytes, and daily weights.

6. Promote pulmonary hygiene to reduce the risk of pneumonia and atelectasis; assist the patient to C&DB, encourage incentive spirometry, and reposition the patient frequently.

Nursing Diagnosis: EXCESS FLUID VOLUME related to fluid retention secondary to decreased renal perfusion

Outcome Criteria

Absence of peripheral edema
Lungs clear to auscultation
PAWP 4 to 12 mm Hg or not to exceed 18 mm Hg
PAS 15 to 30 mm Hg
PAD 5 to 15 mm Hg
CVP 2 to 6 mm Hg
Urine output 30 mL/hr or 0.5 to 1 mL/kg/hr

Patient Monitoring

1. Obtain PA pressures and CVP readings (if available) hourly or more frequently, depending on patient condition. These parameters can be used to monitor for fluid overload and pulmonary edema.

2. Monitor fluid volume status; measure I&O hourly and determine fluid balance each shift. Compare serial weights. Rapid

(0.5-1 kg/day) changes in weight suggest fluid gain or loss (note: 1 kg is approximately 1000 mL fluid).

Patient Assessment

1. Assess fluid volume status: note JVD, peripheral edema, tachycardia, S_3, and adventitious breath sounds.
2. Assess for pressure ulcer development.
3. Assess the patient for clinical sequelae (see Table 5-28).

Diagnostics Assessment

Review serial BUN and creatinine levels to evaluate renal function. BUN >20 mg/dL and creatinine >1.5 mg/dL suggest renal impairment.

Patient Management

1. Administer diuretics (furosemide, bumetanide) as ordered to decrease circulating volume and decrease preload as necessary. Monitor CVP and PAWP for decreasing trends that could suggest hypovolemia. Monitor for electrolyte imbalance secondary to diuresis. Electrolyte replacement therapy may be indicated.
2. Provide meticulous skin care and reposition the patient frequently to enhance tissue perfusion. Relieve pressure points.
3. Titrate pharmacologic agents as ordered to improve CO to kidneys.

ENDOCARDITIS

Clinical Brief

Endocarditis is an inflammation of the endocardium; it is usually limited to the membrane lining and the valves. The cause of endocarditis may be viral, fungal or most commonly, bacterial. The most common organism is *Streptococcus viridans*. Vegetations (growths or lesions) may cause valvular dysfunction, with mortality from endocarditis being as high as 25%.

Risk factors include any high-risk individual as a patient with valvular disease or mitral valve prolapse; undergoing any type of invasive procedure, especially dental surgery; any chronically ill individual, especially one who is immunosuppressed; any individual with previously damaged or congenitally malformed valves; any individual with prosthetic valves; and illicit drug users.

Presenting Signs and Symptoms

Signs and symptoms may be nonspecific. Fever and flulike symptoms are the most common early manifestation. Fatigue, weight loss, malaise, or night sweats are also seen in this population.

Physical Examination

Physical findings are nonspecific. The hallmark for endocarditis is a fever and a new murmur. Signs and symptoms of HF may be present.

Diagnostic Findings

History and physical examination: high index of suspicion in individuals with fever of unknown origin, who are anemic, and who have the presence of a new murmur

Blood cultures and sensitivity, aerobic and anaerobic, may isolate the organism.

Sedimentation rate may be elevated.

Chest radiograph: findings consistent with HF

    Possible enlargement of heart shadow

    Redistribution of fluid to upper lobes

    Kerley B lines

    Pleural effusion

    Dilated aorta

    Left atrial enlargement

Transthoracic or transesophageal echocardiogram is the gold standard for diagnosis of valvular disease or vegetations.

ACUTE CARE PATIENT MANAGEMENT

Goals of Treatment

Eliminate infection.

    Antibiotic therapy

Maintain valvular integrity or improve myocardial function.

    Supplemental oxygen

    Inotropic drugs: digoxin, dobutamine, amrinone, milrinone

    Vasodilators: NTG, nitroprusside

    Surgical valve repair and/or replacement

Reduce myocardial work.

    Bed rest

    Vasodilators: NTG

Reduce circulating volume.

    Diuretics: furosemide, bumetanide

    Vasodilators: NTG

Priority Nursing Diagnoses and Potential Complications	
Priority Nursing Diagnoses	**PC: Potential Complications**
Decreased cardiac output	Dysrhythmias
Ineffective tissue perfusion	Hypoxemia, renal insufficiency
Risk for ineffective protection (see p. 48)	
Risk for interrupted family processes (see p. 45)	
Imbalanced nutrition: less than body requirements (see p. 53)	

Nursing Diagnosis: DECREASED CARDIAC OUTPUT secondary to valvular dysfunction from infective process

Outcome Criteria

Patient alert and oriented
Skin warm and dry
Pulses strong and equal bilaterally
O_2 sat ≥95%
Capillary refill <3 sec
SBP 90 to 120 mm Hg
MAP 70 to 105 mm Hg
Pulse pressure 30 to 40 mm Hg
HR 60 to 100 beats/min
Absence of life-threatening dysrhythmias
Urine output 30 mL/hr or 0.5 to 1 mL/kg/hr
CVP 2 to 6 mm Hg
PAS 15 to 30 mm Hg
PAD 5 to 15 mm Hg
PAWP 4 to 12 mm Hg
CI 2.5 to 4 L/min/m^2
SVRI 1700 to 2600 dynes/sec/cm^{-5}/m^2
PVRI 200 to 450 dynes/sec/cm^{-5}/m^2

Patient Monitoring

1. Monitor PA pressure and CVP (if available) hourly or more frequently if titrating pharmacologic agents. Obtain complete hemodynamic profile as patient condition indicates. Note trends in CO/CI and the patient's response to therapy.
2. Obtain BP hourly or more frequently if the patient's condition is unstable. Note trends in MAP, pulse pressure, and the patient's response to therapy.

3. Monitor hourly urine output to evaluate for responses to pharmacologic intervention and to use as an indicator of CO/CI.

4. Analyze ECG rhythm strip at least every 4 hours and note rate; rhythm; and PR, QRS, and QT intervals. Note ST segment and T-wave changes, which may indicate ischemia.

5. Continuously monitor SpO_2 or SvO_2 (if available) to evaluate oxygen supply and demand; a downward trend can indicate decreased supply or increased demand.

Patient Assessment

1. Obtain HR, RR, and BP every hour or more frequently if the patient is exhibiting signs and symptoms of HF and vasoactive drugs are being administered. Obtain temperature every 4 hours.

2. Assess for changes in neurologic function hourly and as clinically indicated; note orientation to person, place, and time; arousability to verbal and/or tactile stimuli; and bilateral motor and sensory responses.

3. Assess skin for warmth, color, and capillary refill time. Assess distal pulses bilaterally for strength, regularity, and symmetry.

4. Assess for chest discomfort; myocardial ischemia may result from poor perfusion secondary to decreased CO.

5. Assess heart and lung sounds every 4 hours and as clinically indicated for signs of progressive valvular dysfunction. Note any murmurs, degree of JVD, dyspnea, sustained tachycardia, and crackles.

Diagnostics Assessment

1. Review BUN and creatinine levels to evaluate renal function; BUN >20 mg/dL and creatinine >1.5 mg/dL suggest renal impairment, which may be a result of decreased renal perfusion.

2. Review echocardiography findings (if available) for valvular and ventricular function (ejection fraction and wall motion) and presence of vegetations.

3. Review WBC counts to evaluate course of infection.

Patient Management

1. Provide supplemental oxygen at 2 to 4 L/min to maintain or improve oxygenation.

2. Minimize oxygen demand: decrease anxiety, maintain the patient on bed rest if in acute HF, and keep NPO or on a clear liquid diet as tolerated during the acute phase.

3. Administer multi-IV antibiotic regimen as ordered and obtain serum antibiotic peak and trough levels as ordered to determine therapeutic serum levels.

4. Administer antipyretics as ordered and as needed.

5. If the patient is in acute HF, administer diuretic agents (e.g., furosemide, bumetanide) to reduce preload and afterload. Administer furosemide 20 mg/min IVP as ordered. Doses as high as 120 mg may be ordered. Administer bumetanide 0.5 to 1 mg IVP over 1 minute. Bumetanide drip may be infused a 0.5 to 2 mg/hr. A common effect of furosemide and bumetanide administration is potassium depletion; therefore, monitor serum potassium before and after administration of loop diuretics. Administer potassium supplements orally or intravenous piggyback as ordered. Signs and symptoms of symptomatic hypokalemia include ECG/rhythm changes (flattened T wave, prolonged PRI, ventricular tachydysrhythmias) and muscle weakness. Consider monitoring magnesium levels also.

6. Administer vasodilators as ordered. Nitrates (NTG) may be administered to decrease preload. Start the infusion at 5 mcg/min and titrate to desired response or to maintain SBP >90 mm Hg. Increase dosage every 5 to 10 minutes by 5 to 10 mcg/min. If hypotension or reflex tachycardia occurs, raise the patient's legs and reduce the dose as needed for SBP >90 mm Hg.

7. Titrate inotropic agents as ordered to enhance contractility (e.g., dobutamine, amrinone, milrinone, dopamine, and digoxin). Monitor drug effects on hemodynamic status (e.g., CI, SVRI, PVRI, pulse pressure, HR, and MAP). Dobutamine can be administered at 2.5 to 10 mcg/kg/min. Milrinone is administered as a 50-mcg/kg bolus over 10 minutes, followed by an infusion of 0.375 to 0.75 mcg/kg/min. Use lower doses with renal impairment. Dopamine administered at low doses (1-2 mcg/kg/min) increases renal and mesenteric blood flow; at moderate doses (2-10 mcg/kg/min), contractility is enhanced. Use caution when using higher doses of dopamine because of the vasoconstriction effects. Monitor for signs and symptoms of digitalis toxicity, which may include dysrhythmias (blocks, bradycardias, PSVT), nausea, vomiting, diarrhea, and blurred or yellow vision. Signs and symptoms of digitalis toxicity are exhibited earlier if the patient is hypokalemic.

8. Prepare the patient for anticipated surgical intervention to repair or replace affected valve(s). In stable patients, this will usually occur 6 to 8 weeks after the completion of antibiotic

therapy. In patients with acute HF, valve replacement surgery may be performed emergently.

Nursing Diagnosis: INEFFECTIVE TISSUE PERFUSION secondary to embolic event

Outcome Criteria

Patient alert and oriented and able to move all four extremities equally

Vision unchanged

RR 12 to 20 breaths/min, regular and nonlabored

Urine output 30 mL/hr or 0.5 mL/kg/hr and clear yellow

Skin intact, warm, and dry

No reports of pain to flank, left upper quadrant (LUQ), or periphery

Peripheral pulses strong and equal all four extremities

Patient Monitoring

Monitor hourly urine output for volume and clarity. Check for hematuria.

Patient Assessment

1. Assess neurologic status: note any change in LOC or change in motor or sensory responses.
2. Assess for chest discomfort that may signal MI or PE.
3. Note skin color and temperature of extremities. Check pulses and capillary refill for development of peripheral emboli.
4. Assess respiratory status for increasing dyspnea, restlessness, tachypnea, pleuritic chest pain, and tachycardia suggesting a PE.
5. Investigate complaints of abdominal pain, which may suggest decreased perfusion to the bowel or kidney.
6. Assess for pressure ulcer development secondary to hypoperfusion.

Diagnostics Assessment

1. Review results of echocardiogram for presence of vegetations and extent of myocardial compromise.
2. Review ABGs to evaluate oxygenation and acid-base status.
3. Monitor serial BUN and creatinine levels to evaluate renal function; BUN >20 mg/dL and creatinine >1.5 mg/dL suggest renal impairment, which may be a result of decreased renal perfusion.

Patient Management

1. Administer antibiotics as ordered in a timely fashion.
2. Protect intravenous site because antibiotic therapy may be required over several weeks. Observe the site for redness, tenderness, or infiltration. Consider long-term intravenous access.
3. If the patient has a prosthetic valve, continue anticoagulant therapy throughout the acute phase.
4. Assist with ROM exercises while the patient is maintained on bed rest.
5. Institute pressure ulcer prevention strategies.

HEART FAILURE

Clinical Brief

HF is the inability of the heart to maintain adequate CO to meet the metabolic and oxygen demands of the tissues despite adequate venous return. It is measured by the ejection fraction (EF). Conditions that produce abnormal cardiac muscle contraction and/or relaxation (cardiomyopathies), conditions that lead to pressure or volume overload (increased preload or increased afterload), and conditions or diseases that greatly increase demands on the heart are associated with the development of HF. Heart failure can be classified as diastolic or systolic. Systolic heart failure is defined by the presence of impaired contractility of the left ventricle as seen in metabolic alterations (thyroid disease, anemia), systemic conditions (scleroderma), or toxins (chemotherapy, alcohol). Right-sided HF may be precipitated by RV dysfunction or left-sided HF.

Risk Factors

Risk factors for HF include ischemic heart disease, valvular disease, cardiomyopathies, and high CO.

Presenting Signs and Symptoms

Left-Sided HF	Right-Sided HF
Cardiomegaly	JVD
S_3, S_4	Weight gain
Crackles	Hepatojugular reflex
Dyspnea	Ascites
Orthopnea	Hepatomegaly

Nocturia and night cough

Paroxysmal nocturnal dyspnea

Dependent edema

Right upper quadrant (RUQ)
  pain/abdominal pain

Anorexia, bloating

Nocturia

Venous distention

Both Right- and Left-Sided HF

Fatigue

Increased RR and HR

Decreased pulses

Pulsus alternans

S_3

Cheyne-Stokes respirations (associated with advanced failure)

Physical Examination

See presenting signs and symptoms.

Diagnostic Findings

ECG: may have evidence of LV or RV hypertrophy and ischemia, atrial fibrillation, tachydysrhythmias, and low voltage

Chest radiograph:

　　Heart shadow may be enlarged

　　Redistribution of fluid to upper lobes

　　Pulmonary infiltrates

　　Pulmonary venous congestion

　　Kerley B lines

　　Pleural effusion

　　Dilated aorta

　　Left atrial enlargement

　　Chest radiograph findings may lag clinical presentation by 24 hours

ACUTE CARE PATIENT MANAGEMENT

Goals of Treatment

Improve myocardial function.

　　Supplemental oxygen

　　Inotropes: dobutamine, milrinone, digoxin

　　ACE inhibitors

　　Cardiomyoplasty

　　Biventricular pacer

Reduce myocardial work.
  Bed rest
  Vasodilators: NTG, hydralazine, nitroprusside
  ACE inhibitors captopril, lisinopril (angiotensin receptor blockers [ARBs]) may be used as alternatives.
  β-Blocker (use cautiously with EF <40%): pindolol
  IABP
Reduce circulating volume (caution with right HF).
  Diuretics: furosemide, bumetanide
  Nesiritide
  Aldosterone antagonist: spironolactone
  Vasodilators: NTG, captopril, hydralazine, prazosin
Detect/prevent clinical sequelae (Table 5-29).

Table 5-29 CLINICAL SEQUELAE ASSOCIATED WITH HEART FAILURE

Complication	Signs and Symptoms
Pulmonary edema	Worsening HF, dyspnea, ↑ RR, ↓ BP, moist cough, frothy sputum, diaphoresis, crackles, cyanosis, ↓ Pao_2
Acute myocardial infarction	ECG and cardiac enzyme changes consistent with AMI, dysrhythmias, ↓ BP, hemodynamic compromise, chest pain
Cardiogenic shock	↓ LOC, ↑ HR, SBP <90 mm Hg, CI <2 L/min/m², urine output <20 mL/hr; cool, clammy, and mottled skin
Embolic events	
Spleen	Sharp LUQ pain, splenomegaly, local tenderness, abdominal rigidity
Kidneys	Flank pain, hematuria, increasing BUN and creatinine, ↓ UOP
Small, peripheral vessels	Mottled, cool skin, peripheral pain, ↓ pulses
CNS	Changes in LOC, focal signs, changes in vision, motor impairment
Lungs	↑ RR, SOB, ↓ Pao_2, pleuritic chest pain

AMI, Acute myocardial infarction; *BP,* blood pressure; *BUN,* blood urea nitrogen; *CI,* cardiac index; *CNS,* central nervous system; *ECG,* electrocardiogram; *HF,* heart failure; *HR,* heart rate; *LOC,* level of consciousness; *LUQ,* left upper quadrant; *RR,* respiratory rate; *SBP,* systolic blood pressure; *SOB,* shortness of breath; *UOP,* urine output.

Priority Nursing Diagnoses and Potential Complications

Priority Nursing Diagnoses	PC: Potential Complications
Decreased cardiac output	Dysrhythmias
Ineffective tissue perfusion	Hypoxemia, renal insufficiency
Risk for ineffective protection (see p. 48)	
Risk for interrupted family processes (see p. 45)	
Imbalanced nutrition: less than body requirements (see p. 53)	

CV

Nursing Diagnosis: DECREASED CARDIAC OUTPUT related to impaired inotropic state of the myocardium

Outcome Criteria

Patient alert and oriented
Skin warm and dry
Pulses strong and equal bilaterally
Capillary refill <3 sec
O_2 sat ≥95%
SBP 90 to 120 mm Hg
MAP 70 to 105 mm Hg
Pulse pressure 30 to 40 mm Hg
HR 60 to 100 beats/min
Absence of life-threatening dysrhythmias
Urine output 30 mL/hr or 0.5 to 1 mL/kg/hr
CVP 2 to 6 mm Hg
PAS 15 to 30 mm Hg
PAD 5 to 15 mm Hg
PAWP 4 to 12 mm Hg
SVRI 1700 to 2600 dynes/sec/cm^{-5}/m^2
PVRI 200 to 450 dynes/sec/cm^{-5}/m^2
CI 2.5 to 4 L/min/m^2

Patient Monitoring

1. Obtain PA pressures and CVP (RA) hourly (if available) or more frequently if titrating pharmacologic agents. Obtain complete hemodynamic profile as ordered and as patient condition indicates. Note trends in CO/CI and the patient's response to therapy.
2. Obtain BP hourly or more frequently if the patient is unstable; note trends in MAP and pulse pressure and the patient's response to therapy.

3. Monitor hourly urine output to evaluate effects of decreased CO and/or of pharmacologic intervention.

4. Analyze ECG rhythm strip at least every 4 hours and note rate, rhythm, and PR, QRS, and QT intervals. Note ST segment and T-wave changes, which may indicate ischemia or injury.

5. Continuously monitor SpO_2 or SvO_2 (if available). A decreasing trend may indicate reduced CO and increased tissue oxygen extraction (indicates inadequate perfusion).

Patient Assessment

1. Obtain HR, RR, and BP every hour or more frequently during acute phase and when titrating vasoactive drugs.

2. Assess for changes in neurologic function hourly and as clinically indicated; note orientation to person, place, and time; arousability to verbal and/or tactile stimuli; and bilateral motor and sensory responses.

3. Assess skin for warmth, color, and capillary refill time. Assess distal pulses bilaterally for strength, regularity, and symmetry.

4. Assess for chest discomfort: myocardial ischemia may result from poor perfusion secondary to decreased CO.

5. Assess heart sounds every 4 hours and as clinically indicated. S_3 is a hallmark of HF. Note degree of JVD and presence of peripheral edema.

6. Assess for pressure ulcer development secondary to hypoperfusion.

7. Assess the patient for clinical sequelae (see Table 5-29).

Diagnostics Assessment

1. Review ABGs for hypoxemia and metabolic or respiratory acidosis because these conditions can precipitate dysrhythmias, affect myocardial contractility, or indicate the need to be mechanically ventilated.

2. Review serial ECGs to evaluate myocardial ischemia, injury, or infarction.

3. Review serial BUN and creatinine levels to evaluate renal function. BUN >20 mg/dL and creatinine >1.5 mg/dL suggest renal impairment that may be a result of decreased renal perfusion.

4. Review echocardiography or cardiac catheterization results (if available) to assess ventricular function (ejection fraction and wall motion) and valvular function.

Patient Management

1. Provide supplemental oxygen at 2 to 4 L/min to maintain or improve oxygenation.

2. Minimize oxygen demand: maintain bed rest, decrease anxiety, keep the patient NPO or provide a liquid diet in the acute phase, and decrease pain.

3. Administer diuretic agents (e.g., furosemide, bumetanide) to reduce preload and afterload. Administer furosemide 20 mg/min IVP as ordered. Doses as high as 120 mg may be ordered. Administer bumetanide 0.5 to 1 mg IVP over 1 minute every 4 to 8 hours, or infuse bumetanide drip at 0.5 to 2 mg/hour. A common effect of furosemide and bumetanide administration is potassium depletion; therefore, monitor serum potassium before and after administration of loop diuretics. Administer potassium supplements orally or intravenous piggyback as ordered. Signs and symptoms of symptomatic hypokalemia include ECG/rhythm changes (flattened T wave, prolonged PR interval, ventricular tachydysrhythmias) and muscle weakness. Consider monitoring magnesium levels.

4. Administer vasodilators (e.g., captopril, hydralazine, nitroprusside) to reduce preload and afterload. NTG may be administered emergently: sublingual, 1 tablet (0.4 mg) every 5 minutes × 3; IV, start with an infusion of 5 mcg/min and titrate to desired response or to maintain SBP >90 mm Hg. Increase dosage every 5 to 10 minutes by 5 to 10 mcg/min. If hypotension or reflex tachycardia occurs, raise the patient's legs and reduce the dose as needed for SBP >90 mm Hg. Nesiritide is started with a loading dose of 2 mg/kg followed by an infusion of 0.01 mg/kg/min. Administer morphine sulfate as ordered. Give IVP in 2-mg increments to relieve symptoms.

5. Titrate inotropic agents as ordered to enhance contractility (e.g., dobutamine, amrinone, milrinone, dopamine, and digoxin). Monitor drug effects on hemodynamic states. Note CI, SVRI, PVRI, MAP, and pulse pressure. Dobutamine can be administered at 2.5 to 10 mcg/kg/min. Amrinone is typically administered via initial intravenous bolus of 0.75 mcg/kg over 2 to 3 minutes, followed by a maintenance drip, titrating the dose at 5 to 10 mcg/kg/min to the desired effects. Total 24-hour dose should not exceed 10 mg/kg. Milrinone is administered as a 50-mcg/kg bolus over 10 minutes, followed

by an infusion of 0.375 to 0.75 mcg/kg/min. Dopamine administered at low dose (1-2 mcg/kg/min) increases renal and mesenteric blood flow; at moderate doses (2-10 mcg/kg/min), contractility is enhanced. Use caution when using higher doses of dopamine because of the vasoconstrictive effects. Monitor for signs and symptoms of digitalis toxicity, which may include dysrhythmia formation (blocks, bradycardias, PSVT), nausea, vomiting, diarrhea, and blurred or yellow vision. Signs and symptoms of digitalis toxicity are exhibited earlier if the patient is hypokalemic.

6. Prophylactic heparin or LMWH may be ordered to prevent thromboembolus formation secondary to venous pooling.
7. Institute pressure ulcer prevention strategies secondary to hypoperfusion or vasoactive agents.

Nursing Diagnosis: IMPAIRED GAS EXCHANGE related to increased pulmonary congestion secondary to increased left ventricular end diastolic pressure (LVEDP)

Outcome Criteria

PaO_2 80 to 100 mm Hg
pH 7.35 to 7.45
$PaCO_2$ 35 to 45 mm Hg
O_2 sat ≥95%
SvO_2 60% to 80%
RR 12 to 20 breaths/min
Lungs clear to auscultation
PAWP 4 to 12 mm Hg
$P(a/A)O_2$ ratio 0.75 to 0.90

Patient Monitoring

1. Continuously monitor oxygenation status with pulse oximetry (SpO_2) or SvO_2 monitoring. Note patient activities and nursing interventions that may adversely affect oxygen saturation.
2. Obtain PA pressures and CVP hourly (if available). Obtain complete hemodynamic profile every 4 hours or more frequently. Note increasing PAWP may signal development of pulmonary edema. Increasing PAS pressure may signal hypoxia. Monitor PVRI.
3. Continuously monitor ECG for dysrhythmia development, which may be related to hypoxemia or acid-base imbalance.
4. Calculate $P(a/A)O_2$ ratio as an index of gas exchange efficiency.

5. Measure I&O hourly. Determine fluid balance each shift. Compare serial weights. Rapid (0.5-1 kg/day) changes in weight suggest fluid gain or loss. Fluid gain can be suggestive of worsening failure.

Patient Assessment

1. Assess respiratory status frequently during the acute phase. RR >28 breaths/min, increasing complaints of dyspnea, inability to speak in sentences, increasing restlessness, cough, and use of accessory muscles indicate respiratory distress and increased patient effort. Cyanosis is a late sign.
2. Assess lung sounds for adventitious sounds and to evaluate the course of pulmonary congestion.
3. Assess the patient for clinical sequelae (see Table 5-29).

Diagnostics Assessment

1. Review serial ABGs for hypoxemia (Pao_2 <60 mm Hg) and acidosis (pH <7.35), signs of poor gas exchange, which may further compromise tissue perfusion.
2. Review lactate levels if ordered, an indicator of anaerobic metabolism.
3. Review serial chest radiographs for pulmonary congestion.

Patient Management

1. Provide supplemental oxygen as ordered to maintain or improve oxygenation. If the patient develops respiratory distress, be prepared for intubation and mechanical ventilation. (See p. 503 for information on ventilation therapies.)
2. Minimize oxygen demand: maintain bed rest, decrease anxiety, keep the patient NPO or provide liquid diet in the acute phase, treat pain, limit patient activities, pace activities and nursing interventions, and provide uninterrupted rest periods.
3. Position the patient to maximize chest excursion. Evaluate the patient's response to position changes with Spo_2 or Svo_2 monitoring.
4. Low-dose morphine sulfate may be ordered to promote venous pooling and decrease dyspnea. This may effectively reduce anxiety.
5. Diuretic agents may be ordered to reduce circulating volume. Monitor urine output, electrolytes, and daily weights.
6. Promote pulmonary hygiene to reduce risk of pneumonia and atelectasis; assist the patient to C&DB, encourage incentive spirometry, and reposition the patient frequently.

Nursing Diagnosis: EXCESS FLUID VOLUME related to fluid retention secondary to decreased renal perfusion

Outcome Criteria

Absence of peripheral edema
Lungs clear to auscultation
PAWP 4 to 12 mm Hg or not to exceed 18 mm Hg
PAS 15 to 30 mm Hg
PAD 5 to 15 mm Hg
CVP 2 to 6 mm Hg
Urine output 30 mL/hr or 0.5 to 1 mL/kg/hr

Patient Monitoring

1. Obtain PA pressures, PAWP, and CVP readings hourly or more frequently, depending on patient's condition. These parameters can be used to monitor for fluid overload and pulmonary edema.
2. Monitor fluid volume status; measure I&O hourly, and determine fluid balance each shift. Compare serial weights. Rapid (0.5-1 kg/day) changes in weight suggest fluid gain or loss (note: 1 kg is approximately 1000 mL fluid).

Patient Assessment

1. Assess fluid volume status: note JVD, peripheral edema, tachycardia, S_3, and adventitious breath sounds.
2. Assess for pressure ulcer development secondary to hypoperfusion/edema
3. Assess the patient for clinical sequelae (see Table 5-29).

Diagnostics Assessment

1. Review serial BUN and creatinine levels to evaluate renal function. BUN >20 mg/dL and creatinine >1.5 mg/dL suggest renal impairment.
2. Review B-type natriuretic peptide levels to assess severity of heart failure. BNP is a cardiac hormone produced by the heart ventricles in response to ventricular volume expansion and pressure overload.

Patient Management

1. Administer diuretics (furosemide, bumetanide) as ordered to decrease circulating volume and decrease preload as necessary. Monitor CVP and PAWP for decreasing trends that could suggest hypovolemia. Monitor for electrolyte imbalance secondary to diuresis. Electrolyte replacement therapy may be indicated.

   2. Institute pressure ulcer prevention strategies, e.g., provide meticulous skin care and reposition the patient frequently to enhance tissue perfusion. Relieve pressure points.

   3. Titrate pharmacologic agents (e.g., dopamine, dobutamine) as ordered to improve CO to kidneys.

HYPERTENSIVE CRISIS

Clinical Brief

Hypertensive crisis is an emergent situation in which a marked elevation in DBP can cause end-organ damage. Severe HTN (usually a diastolic reading >120 mm Hg) can cause irreversible injury to the brain, heart, and kidneys and can rapidly lead to death. Hypertensive crisis can occur in patients with either essential HTN (cause unknown) or secondary HTN (which can be a result of renal or endocrine disease). Emergencies include HTN in association with acute CNS events, acute aortic dissection, pulmonary edema, pheochromocytoma crisis, eclampsia, and nonadherence to medical therapy.

Presenting Signs and Symptoms

Signs and symptoms depend on the underlying disease and end-organ damage. Headache, nausea, dizziness, visual disturbances, and altered LOC may be present.

Physical Examination

DBP >120 mm Hg. (See Presenting Signs and Symptoms, previously.) Other findings may be the result of damage to end organs (Table 5-30).

Priority Nursing Diagnoses and Potential Complications	
Priority Nursing Diagnoses	**PC: Potential Complications**
Ineffective tissue perfusion	Dysrhythmias, renal insufficiency
Risk for ineffective protection (see p. 48)	
Risk for interrupted family processes (see p. 45)	
Imbalanced nutrition: less than body requirements (see p. 53)	

Table 5-30 CLINICAL SEQUELAE ASSOCIATED WITH HYPERTENSIVE CRISIS

Complication	Signs and Symptoms
Heart failure	Sustained elevated HR, cough, S_3, crackles, PAWP >20 mm Hg
Pulmonary edema	Worsening heart failure, breathlessness, ↑ RR, ↑ HR, moist cough, frothy sputum, diaphoresis, cyanosis, PAWP >25 mm Hg
Acute myocardial infarction	Chest pain, ECG and cardiac enzyme changes indicative of ischemia/infarct, hemodynamic compromise
CVA	Change in LOC, change in focal neurologic signs, pupil changes
Renal failure	Urine output <0.5 mL/kg/hr, edema
Aortic dissection	Severe pain to chest, abdomen, or lumbar area; pulse and BP differentials between RUE and LUE; murmur; initial ↑ BP followed by drop in BP and tachycardia
Hypertensive encephalopathy	Change in LOC, ↑ ICP, retinopathy with papilledema, seizures

BP, Blood pressure; *CVA,* cerebrovascular accident; *ECG,* electrocardiogram; *HR,* heart rate; *ICP,* intracranial pressure; *LOC,* level of consciousness; *LUE,* left upper extremity; *PAWP,* pulmonary artery wedge pressure; *RUE,* right upper extremity.

Diagnostic Findings

Diagnostic tests are used to evaluate the effects of increased BP on target organs or to determine the cause of secondary HTN.

ACUTE CARE PATIENT MANAGEMENT

Goals of Treatment

Reduce BP (SBP <140 mm Hg, MAP <120 mm Hg, DBP <90 mm Hg).
  Vasodilators: nitroprusside, diazoxide, NTG
  β-Blockers: labetalol, esmolol
  Calcium channel blocking agents: diltiazem, verapamil, nicardipine
  Diuretics: furosemide, bumetanide
  Surgical intervention
Detect/prevent clinical sequelae (see Table 5-30).

Nursing Diagnosis: INEFFECTIVE TISSUE PERFUSION related to compromised blood flow secondary to severe hypertension resulting in end-organ damage

Outcome Criteria

Patient alert and oriented
Skin warm and dry
Pulses strong and equal bilaterally
Capillary refill <3 sec
SBP <140 mm Hg
DBP <90 mm Hg
MAP 70 to 120 mm Hg
HR 60 to 100 beats/min
Absence of life-threatening dysrhythmias
Urine output 30 mL/hr or 0.5 to 1 mL/kg/hr
BUN <20 mg/dL, creatinine <1.5 mg/dL

Patient Monitoring

1. Monitor arterial BP continuously (arterial line if available) and note sudden increases or decreases in readings. A precipitous drop in BP can cause reflex ischemia to the heart, brain, kidneys, and/or the GI tract. Note trends in MAP and the patient's response to therapy.
2. Monitor hourly urine output and note any presence of blood in the urine.
3. Continuously monitor the ECG for dysrhythmias or ST segment and T-wave changes associated with ischemia or injury.

Patient Assessment

Assess the patient for clinical sequelae (see Table 5-30).

Diagnostics Assessment

1. Review BUN and creatinine to evaluate the effect of BP on kidneys. BUN >20 mg/dL and creatinine >1.5 mg/dL suggest renal impairment.
2. Review serial chest radiography for pulmonary congestion.
3. Review serial 12-lead ECGs for patterns of injury, ischemia, and infarction.

Patient Management

1. Provide oxygen at 2 to 4 L/min to maintain or improve oxygenation.

2. Minimize oxygen demand: maintain bed rest, decrease anxiety, and keep the patient NPO or provide a liquid diet in the acute phase.

3. Administer nitrates as ordered to reduce preload and afterload. NTG may be ordered: sublingual, 1 tablet (0.4 mg) every 5 minutes × 3; IV, start with an infusion of 5 mcg/min and titrate to desired response or to maintain SBP >90 mm Hg. Increase dosage every 5 to 10 minutes by 5 to 10 mcg/min. If hypotension or reflex tachycardia occurs, raise the patient's legs and reduce the dose as needed for SBP >90 mm Hg. Sodium nitroprusside may be ordered to reduce afterload for patients whose SBP is >100 mm Hg. Do not administer more than 10 mcg/kg/min. Cyanide toxicity can be prevented with the use of thiosulfate. Monitor for signs and symptoms of cyanide toxicity: tinnitus, blurred vision, delirium, and muscle spasm.

4. Administer β-blockers as ordered. Labetalol may be given as 20- to 80-mg bolus every 10 to 15 minutes to rapidly lower BP. Miniboluses or an infusion may be ordered. Esmolol may be given as a bolus of 500 mcg/kg/min over 1 minute followed by infusion of 50 to 200 mcg/kg/min.

5. Prepare the patient and family for surgical intervention to correct the underlying cause, if this is indicated.

HYPOVOLEMIC SHOCK

Clinical Brief

Hemorrhage is a major cause of hypovolemic shock. However, plasma loss/dehydration and interstitial fluid accumulation (third spacing) adversely reduce circulating volume by decreasing tissue perfusion. The primary defect is decreased preload.

There are four classifications of hypovolemic shock based on the amount of fluid and blood loss:

Class I: <750 mL, or ≤15% total circulating volume
Class II: 750 to 1000 mL, or 15% to 30% total circulating volume
Class III: 1500 to 2000 mL, or 30% to 40% total circulating volume
Class IV: >2000 mL, or >40% total circulating volume. The patient's compensatory response intensifies as the percent of blood loss is increased.

Presenting Signs and Symptoms

Signs and symptoms depend on the degree of blood loss and compensatory response.

Physical Examination

Appearance: anxiety progressing to coma
Vital signs:
    BP normal to unobtainable
    Palpable radial pulse reflects SBP of 80 mm Hg
    Palpable femoral pulse reflects SBP of 70 mm Hg
    Palpable carotid pulse reflects SBP of 60 mm Hg
    HR normal to >140 beats/min
    RR normal to >35 breaths/min
Cardiovascular: weak, thready pulse
Pulmonary: deep or shallow rapid respirations, lungs usually clear
Skin:
    Cool, clammy skin, pale color
    Delayed/absent capillary refill
    Lips cyanotic (late sign)

Diagnostic Findings

Clinical findings are the basis for diagnosis. Other findings include
the following:
    CI <2 L/min/m^2
    Lactate >2 mmol/L
    Svo$_2$ <60%
    MAP <80 mm Hg
    PA pressures declining trend
    CVP declining trend
    PAWP declining trend
    SVR increasing trend

ACUTE CARE PATIENT MANAGEMENT

Goals of Treatment

Reestablish intravascular volume.
    Blood and blood products
    Autotransfusion
    Colloids (e.g., hetastarch, plasma protein fraction)
    Crystalloids (e.g., normal saline [NS], lactated Ringer's [LR])
Optimize oxygen delivery.
    Oxygen therapy, intubation, and mechanical ventilation
    Blood transfusion
    Vasopressors (e.g., dopamine, norepinephrine, epinephrine)
Treat underlying problem.
    Surgery
Detect/prevent clinical sequelae (Table 5-31).

Table 5-31 CLINICAL SEQUELAE ASSOCIATED WITH HYPOVOLEMIC SHOCK

Complication	Signs and Symptoms
Cardiopulmonary arrest	Absent respiration and absent pulse
ARDS	Dyspnea, tachycardia, labored breathing, tachypnea, hypoxemia refractory to increase in F_{IO_2}, PAWP $\leq$18 mm Hg, decreased lung compliance, $\uparrow$ peak airway pressures
Acute tubular necrosis (ATN)/renal failure	Urine output <0.5 mL/kg/hr, steady rise in creatinine
GI dysfunction/bleeding	Blood in NG aspirate, emesis and/or stool; absent bowel sounds, abdominal pain, nausea and vomiting, jaundice
DIC	Bleeding from puncture sites, mucous membranes; hematuria, ecchymosis; labs: prolonged PT, ACT, and aPTT; $\downarrow$ fibrinogen, platelets, factors V, VIII, XIII, and II; $\uparrow$ FSP (FDP); + D-dimer

ACT, Activated clotting time; *aPTT,* activated partial thromboplastin time; *ARDS,* acute respiratory distress syndrome; *ATN,* acute tubular necrosis; *DIC,* disseminated intravascular coagulation; *FDP,* fibrin degradation products; *FSP,* fibrin split products; *GI,* gastrointestinal; *NG,* nasogastric; *PAWP,* pulmonary artery wedge pressure; *PT,* prothrombin time.

Priority Nursing Diagnoses and Potential Complications

Priority Nursing Diagnoses	PC: Potential Complications
Ineffective tissue perfusion	Dysrhythmias, hypovolemia, renal insufficiency
Risk for ineffective protection (see p. 48)	
Imbalanced nutrition: less than body requirements (see p. 53)	
Risk for interrupted family processes (see p. 45)	

Nursing Diagnosis: INEFFECTIVE TISSUE PERFUSION related to blood loss and hypotension

Outcome Criteria

Patient alert and oriented
Skin warm and dry
Peripheral pulses strong

Urine output 30 mL/hr or 0.5 to 1 mL/kg/hr

Hct ~32%

SBP 90 to 120 mm Hg

MAP 70 to 105 mm Hg

CI 2.5 to 4 L/min/m^2

O_2 sat $\geq$95%

Svo$_2$ 60% to 80%

$\dot{D}o_2I$ 500 to 600 mL/min/m^2

$\dot{V}o_2I$ 115 to 165 mL/min/m^2

Oxygen extraction ratio (ERo$_2$) 25%

Patient Monitoring

1. Monitor BP continuously via arterial cannulation because cuff pressures are less accurate in shock states. Monitor MAP, an indicator that accurately reflects tissue perfusion. MAP <60 mm Hg adversely affects cerebral and renal perfusion.

2. Obtain CO/CI at least every 8 hours or more frequently to evaluate the patient's response to changes in therapy.

3. Monitor trends in $\dot{D}o_2I$ and $\dot{V}o_2I$ to evaluate effectiveness of therapy. Inadequate oxygen delivery or consumption produces tissue hypoxia. Calculate ERo$_2$; a value >25% suggests increased oxygen consumption, decreased oxygen delivery, or both.

4. Monitor PA pressures and CVP (if available) hourly or more frequently to evaluate the patient's response to treatment. These parameters reflect the volume status of the vascular system and can be used to monitor for degree of hypovolemia or fluid overload.

5. Continuously monitor Svo$_2$. A decreasing trend may indicate decreased CO/CI and increased tissue oxygen extraction.

6. Continuously monitor ECG to detect life-threatening dysrhythmias or HR >140 beats/min, which can adversely affect SV.

7. Monitor hourly urine output to evaluate renal perfusion.

8. Measure blood loss (if possible) to quantify the loss and evaluate progression or improvement of the problem.

Patient Assessment

1. Obtain HR, RR, and BP every 15 minutes to evaluate the patient's response to therapy and to detect cardiopulmonary deterioration.

2. Assess LOC, mentation, skin temperature, and peripheral pulses to evaluate tissue perfusion.
3. Assess for pressure ulcer development secondary to hypoperfusion/vasoactive drugs.
4. Assess the patient for clinical sequelae(see Table 5-31).

Diagnostics Assessment

1. Review Hgb and Hct levels and note trends. Decreased RBCs can adversely affect oxygen carrying capacity.
2. Review lactate levels, an indicator of reduced tissue perfusion and anaerobic metabolism. Increased levels may signal decreasing oxygen delivery or utilization.
3. Review ABGs for hypoxemia and respiratory or metabolic acidosis because these conditions can precipitate dysrhythmias, affect myocardial contractility, and indicate reduced tissue perfusion. O_2 sat should be ≥92%.
4. Review BUN, creatinine, and electrolytes and note trends to evaluate renal function.

Patient Management

1. Use a large-bore (16- to 18-gauge) cannula for intravenous lines to replace volume rapidly.
2. Administer blood products or autotransfuse as ordered to reestablish intravascular volume. (See p. 585 for information on blood administration.)
3. Administer colloids (hetastarch or plasma protein fraction) and crystalloids (LR or NS) in addition to blood products as ordered. Monitor CVP and PAWP to evaluate response to fluid resuscitation. A PAWP >25 mm Hg is associated with pulmonary edema.
4. Avoid dextran infusions and platelet inhibition drugs for hypovolemia secondary to hemorrhage because coagulation problems can occur and enhance the bleeding problem.
5. Pharmacologic agents may be used to improve hemodynamic parameters if intravascular volume is replaced. Vasopressors (dopamine or norepinephrine) may be used to increase preload and to maintain an adequate MAP for cerebral and coronary perfusion.
6. Provide oxygen therapy as ordered. Anticipate intubation and mechanical ventilation if oxygenation status deteriorates or cardiopulmonary arrest ensues. Correct acidosis because

acidosis blocks or diminishes responsiveness to drug therapy, oxygen delivery, and cardiac function.

7. If the site of bleeding is known (e.g., GI bleeding), anticipate appropriate treatment.
8. A pneumatic antishock garment or military antishock trousers may be used in addition to other therapy, although controversy in their use still exists.
9. Prepare the patient for surgical intervention if required.
10. Institute pressure ulcer prevention strategies, e.g., meticulous skin care, repositioning, relieving pressure points.

CV

PERICARDITIS

Clinical Brief

Pericarditis is an inflammation and/or infectious process of the pericardium, the sac that contains the heart. It may be an acute or chronic (constrictive) condition that can lead to pericardial effusion or tamponade. It can lead to atrial and ventricular dysrhythmias, limit the cardiac chamber's ability to fill, and affect CO/CI. Risk factors include bacterial and viral infections, vasculitis–connective tissue disease, MI, uremia, neoplasms, and trauma; or can be iatrogenic (after cardiac surgery, drugs, cardiac resuscitation) or idiopathic.

Presenting Signs and Symptoms

Chest pain and fever are the most common manifestations. A pericardial friction rub is a clinical hallmark. Typically, the pain begins suddenly, is severe and sharp, and is aggravated by inspiration and deep breathing. Pain is usually anterior to the precordium, radiates to the left shoulder, and is generally relieved by sitting up and leaning forward.

Physical Examination

Appearance:
Restlessness
Irritability
Weakness
Pallor
Vital signs:
HR: increased
Temperature: normal or increased
RR: increased

Cardiovascular:
   Friction rub
   Pulsus paradoxus if a pericardial effusion accompanies pericarditis
   JVD
Pulmonary: dyspnea

Diagnostic Findings

ECG: early phase—diffuse ST segment elevation with concave curvature representing injury caused by inflammation, present in all leads except aV_R and V_1; several days later, ST segments return to normal; T wave may flatten or become inverted
Cardiac enzymes: normal, but are increased with underlying acute MI
Echocardiogram: may indicate presence of pericardial effusion

---

ACUTE CARE PATIENT MANAGEMENT

Goals of Treatment

Treat underlying disease and relieve pain.
   Antiinflammatory agents: indomethacin, ibuprofen, aspirin, and corticosteroids
   Antibiotic or antifungal therapy
   Surgery to drain pericardial fluid or make pericardial window
   Supplemental oxygen
Maintain CO/CI.
   Bed rest
   Surgical intervention (pericardiocentesis or pericardiectomy)
Detect/prevent clinical sequelae (Table 5-32).

Table 5-32   CLINICAL SEQUELAE ASSOCIATED WITH PERICARDITIS

Complication	Signs and Symptoms
Cardiac tamponade	↓ SBP, narrowed pulse pressure; pulsus paradoxus, ↑ CVP, ↑ JVP, ↑ HR (if left untreated will precipitate bradycardia), ↑ RR, possible friction rub, muffled heart sounds, low-voltage ECG, electrical alternans, rapidly enlarging cardiac silhouette, anxiety, chest pain. If PA line in place, RAP = PAD = PAWP (equalization of pressure in all chambers)

CVP, Central venous pressure; *ECG,* electrocardiogram; *HR,* heart rate; *JVP,* jugular venous pressure; *PA,* pulmonary artery; *PAD,* pulmonary artery diastolic; *PAWP,* pulmonary artery wedge pressure; *RAP,* right atrial pressure; *RR,* respiratory rate; *SBP,* systolic blood pressure.

Priority Nursing Diagnoses and Potential Complications	
Priority Nursing Diagnoses	**PC: Potential Complications**
Acute pain	
Ineffective breathing pattern	Hypoxemia, atelectasis, pneumonia
Risk for ineffective protection (see p. 48)	
Risk for interrupted family processes (see p. 45)	

CV

Nursing Diagnosis: INEFFECTIVE BREATHING PATTERN related to acute pain secondary to inflammation and aggravated by position and inspiration

Outcome Criteria

Patient communicates pain relief.
Patient breathes with comfort.
O_2 sat ≥92%.
RR 12 to 20 breaths/min, eupnea.

Patient Monitoring

1. Monitor temperature every 4 hours to evaluate the course of inflammatory process.
2. Monitor for changes in ECG to validate reduction in inflammatory process.

Patient Assessment

1. Assess pain using patient's self-report when possible. A self-report rating scale to assess intensity of pain can be found on p. 3. Validate inflammation-type chest pain versus ischemic pain (see Table 5-22).
2. Auscultate the anterior chest to determine the quality of the friction rub.
3. Assess respiratory status because the patient may hypoventilate as a result of pain. Note RR and depth and ease of breathing.
4. Assess the patient for clinical sequelae (see Table 5-32).

Diagnostics Assessment

1. Review ABGs to evaluate oxygenation and acid-base status.
2. Review results of echocardiogram and chest x-ray if available. Pleural and pericardial effusion can be identified with echocardiography or chest x-ray.

3. Review serial ECGs for changes. ST segments generally return to baseline within 7 days, followed by T-wave inversion within 1 to 2 weeks from the onset of pain.

4. Review CBC, leukocyte counts, and cultures if applicable.

Patient Management

1. Administer pharmacologic agents, such as ibuprofen and indomethacin, as ordered to reduce inflammation and pain. If NSAIDs are unsuccessful, corticosteroids may be ordered. Other agents may be ordered for pain relief; note the patient's response to therapy. Note: post-MI patient should be treated with aspirin only.

2. Stay with the patient, providing a calm, quiet environment.

3. Assist the patient to maintain a position of comfort (leaning forward may help).

4. Ensure activity restrictions while the patient is symptomatic, febrile, or if a friction rub is present.

5. Promote pulmonary hygiene to prevent risk of atelectasis: encourage incentive spirometry, assist the patient to C&DB, and reposition the patient frequently.

SUDDEN CARDIAC DEATH

Clinical Brief

Sudden cardiac death (SCD) is unexpected cardiopulmonary collapse. SCD can occur as a primary manifestation of ischemic heart disease.

Risk factors mirror the risk factors for coronary artery disease (CAD): cigarette smoking, hyperlipidemia, HTN, diabetes, obesity, stress, and a positive family history of cardiovascular disease. Men, especially those older than 50 years, and postmenopausal women are susceptible. Additional risk factors include patients who (1) are known sudden cardiac death survivors, (2) have had an acute MI within the past 12 months, (3) have cardiomyopathies that have demonstrated left ventricular ejection fractions <40%, or (4) have prolonged QT intervals.

Presenting Signs and Symptoms

A previously normal-appearing adult will suddenly collapse with cardiopulmonary arrest not associated with accidental or traumatic causes. There are commonly no prodromal symptoms, although there may be a brief period of anxiousness or chest discomfort.

Physical Examination

Full cardiopulmonary arrest
Pulselessness
No respirations

Diagnostic Findings

Clinical findings are the basis for diagnosis of sudden cardiac death.
ECG: ventricular tachycardia/ventricular fibrillation (VT/VF),
  asystole

CV

ACUTE CARE PATIENT MANAGEMENT

Goals of Treatment

Provide adequate cardiopulmonary support.
  Cardiopulmonary resuscitation (CPR) and ACLS protocols
  Supplemental oxygen
Restore cardiopulmonary function.
  Supplemental oxygen
  Morphine sulfate
  Antidysrhythmic agents
  Biventricular pacemaker
  Implantable cardioverter defibrillator (ICD)
Detect/prevent clinical sequelae (Table 5-33).

Table 5-33 CLINICAL SEQUELAE ASSOCIATED WITH SUDDEN CARDIAC DEATH

Complication	Signs and Symptoms
Cardiopulmonary arrest	Pulselessness, absence of respirations
Acute myocardial infarction	ECG and cardiac enzyme changes indicative of MI (see Tables 5-23 and 5-24) dysrhythmias, ↓ BP
Dysrhythmias	Change in rate and rhythm, change in LOC, syncope, chest discomfort, ↓ SBP (<90 mm Hg)
HF	Sustained elevated HR, cough, S_3, PAWP >20 mm Hg
Pulmonary edema	Worsening HF, breathlessness, moist cough, frothy sputum, diaphoresis, cyanosis ↓ Pao_2, ↑ RR, ↓ SBP (<90 mm Hg)

AMI, Acute myocardial infarction; *BP,* blood pressure; *ECG,* electrocardiogram; *HF,* heart failure; *HR,* heart rate; *LOC,* level of consciousness; *PAWP,* pulmonary artery wedge pressure; *RR,* respiratory rate; *SBP,* systolic blood pressure.

Priority Nursing Diagnoses and Potential Complications	
Priority Nursing Diagnoses	PC: Potential Complications
Decreased cardiac output Risk for interrupted family processes (see p. 45)	Dysrhythmias, renal insufficiency, hypoxemia

Nursing Diagnosis: DECREASED CARDIAC OUTPUT related to electrophysiologic
instability after resuscitation

Outcome Criteria

Patient alert and oriented
Skin warm and dry
HR 60 to 100 beats/min
Absence of lethal dysrhythmias
SBP 90 to 120 mm Hg
MAP 70 to 105 mm Hg
Urine output 30 mL/hr or 0.5 to 1 mL/kg/hr
CI 2.5 to 4 L/min/m^2

Patient Monitoring

1. Monitor in the lead appropriate for ischemia or dysrhythmia
   identification. Place in lead II to monitor for SVT and axis
   deviation. Place in lead MCL$_1$ to differentiate between ventricular ectopy and aberrantly conducted beats, to determine
   types of BBB, or to verify RV pacemaker beats (paced QRS
   beat should be negative). Recurrence of dysrhythmias is most
   common within the first 72 hours.
2. Analyze ECG rhythm strip at least every 4 hours and note
   rate, rhythm; PR, QRS, and QT intervals (prolonged QT is
   associated with torsades de pointes). Note ST and T-wave
   changes, which may indicate ischemia, injury, or infarction.
   Note occurrence of PACs or PVCs because premature beats
   are frequently the forerunner of more serious dysrhythmias.
   Second-degree type II heart block (Mobitz II) may progress
   to complete heart block. (See p. 441 for information on dysrhythmia interpretation.)
3. Obtain PA pressures and CVP (RA) hourly (if available) or
   more frequently if titrating pharmacologic agents. Obtain
   complete hemodynamic profile as patient condition indicates. Note trends in CO/CI, PVRI, and SVRI and the

patient's response to therapy. Note LVSWI and RVSWI to evaluate contractility.

4. Continuously monitor Svo_2 (if available) to evaluate oxygen supply and demand; a downward trend can indicate decreased supply or increased demand.

5. Monitor arterial oxygen delivery ($\dot{D}o_2$) and oxygen consumption ($\dot{V}o_2$) as indicators of tissue perfusion.

6. Obtain BP hourly; note MAP, pulse pressure, and the patient's response to therapy.

7. Monitor hourly urine output to evaluate effects of decreased CO and/or of pharmacologic intervention. Perform I&O balances each shift. Compare serial weights. A rapid (0.5-1 kg/day) change in weight suggests fluid gain or loss (1 kg is approximately 1 L of fluid).

Patient Assessment

1. Obtain HR, RR, and BP every 15 minutes during acute phase and when titrating vasoactive drugs. Obtain temperature every 4 hours.

2. Assess the patient's mentation, skin temperature and color, and peripheral pulses at least hourly to monitor adequacy of CO.

3. Be alert to the development of dysrhythmias (i.e., change in rate or rhythm, change in LOC, syncope, chest discomfort, hypotension, and/or pulselessness).

4. Assess the patient for clinical sequelae (see Table 5-33).

Diagnostics Assessment

1. Review serial 12-lead ECGs and cardiac enzymes to determine whether ischemia, injury, or infarct has occurred.

2. Review signal-averaged ECG, Holter monitor, and echocardiogram (if available) to identify the high-risk patient for sudden death.

3. Review serial electrolyte levels because a disturbance in potassium or magnesium is a risk factor for dysrhythmias.

4. Review ABGs for hypoxemia and acidosis because these conditions increase the risk for dysrhythmias, decreased contractility, and decreased tissue perfusion.

Patient Management

1. Provide supplemental oxygen to maintain or improve oxygenation. The patient may be intubated and mechanically ventilated. (See p. 503 for information on ventilation therapies.)

2. Minimize oxygen demand: maintain bed rest, decrease anxiety, keep the patient NPO or provide a liquid diet in the acute phase, and decrease pain.

3. Be alert for dysrhythmia risk factors: anemia, hypovolemia, hypokalemia, hypomagnesemia, acidosis, administration of digitalis and other antidysrhythmic agents, pain, and CVP/PA catheter or pacemaker lead misplacement. Treat life-threatening dysrhythmias according to ACLS algorithms. Be prepared to cardiovert or defibrillate the patient.

4. Amiodarone, lidocaine, and possibly magnesium sulfate may be used prophylactically to prevent ventricular dysrhythmias. Administer amiodarone with a bolus dose of 150 mg over 10 minutes (300 mg IVP for cardiopulmonary arrest). The infusion starts with 360 mg over 6 hours (1 mg/min), followed by 540 mg over 18 hours (0.5 mg/min). Administer lidocaine with a bolus dose of 1 to 1.5 mg/kg, follow with infusion of 1 to 4 mg/min. Do not exceed 4 mg/min. The recommended dose of magnesium sulfate is 1 to 2 g in 50 to 100 mL of D_5W administered IV over 5 to 60 minutes an infusion of 0.5 to 1 g/hr should follow for up to 24 hours.

5. Because most sudden cardiac death occurrences are secondary to a lethal dysrhythmia, 24-hour Holter monitoring and possible electrophysiologic study (EPS) may be done to determine the effectiveness of a pharmacologic regimen. Cardiac catheterization may be indicated to determine underlying disease.

6. Anticipate ICD insertion. (See p. 522 for information on ICD.)

VALVULAR DISORDERS

Clinical Brief

Valvular disorders may be congenital or acquired. Common causes of acquired valvular heart disease include rheumatic heart disease (which is declining in incidence), infective endocarditis, ischemia (which usually affects the mitral valve), aging, traumatic damage (commonly caused by blunt chest trauma), and syphilitic disease (aortic valvular disease). When valve leaflets fail to close properly, blood leaks from one chamber back into another; this is called a regurgitant valve. When the valve orifice is restricted and is not allowed to open properly, forward blood flow is obstructed and the valve is described as stenotic. All valves can be diseased; however, the mitral and aortic valves are most commonly affected. Murmurs and related valvular disorders are listed in Table 5-34.

Presenting Signs and Symptoms

Symptoms reflect left ventricular or biventricular failure. (See Heart Failure, p. 237.) Atrial dysrhythmias can also be present.

Physical Examination

Table 5-34 lists physical examination for valvular disorders.

Diagnostic Findings

See Table 5-34.

ACUTE CARE PATIENT MANAGEMENT

See Cardiac Surgery, p. 515, and Heart Failure, p. 237.

Table **5-34** VALVULAR DISORDERS

Type	Physical Examination	Diagnostic Study Findings
Mitral stenosis	Diastolic heart murmur Weakness Fatigue Predisposition to respiratory infections Orthopnea Paroxysmal nocturnal dyspnea Palpitations (from atrial fibrillation) Hemoptysis Hepatomegaly JVD Peripheral edema	ECG: Left atrial enlargement Prolonged, notched P wave (P mitrale) or atrial fibrillation Right ventricular hypertrophy Chest radiograph: Left atrial enlargement Pulmonary venous congestion Interstitial pulmonary edema Right ventricular enlargement Cardiac catheterization: ↑ Pressure across mitral valve ↑ Left atrial pressure ↑ PAWP ↓ CO/CI

CV

Table 5-34 Valvular Disorders—cont'd

Type	Physical Examination	Diagnostic Study Findings
		Echocardiogram: Abnormal leaflet movement Enlarged LA
Mitral regurgitation (mitral insufficiency)	Murmur throughout systole Weakness Fatigue DOE Palpitations (if atrial fibrillation) LV failure, S_3, S_4 Crackles May present with S/S of emboli secondary to stagnation of blood and mural thrombi development	ECG: Left atrial enlargement (P mitrale) Left ventricular hypertrophy Atrial fibrillation, sinus tachycardia Chest radiograph: Left atrial enlargement Left ventricular enlargement Pulmonary vascular congestion/infiltrates (acute) Cardiac catheterization: Angiography used to identify and quantify regurgitation ↑ LVEDP ↓ CO/CI
Aortic stenosis	Systolic murmur Syncope (especially on exertion) Angina pectoris Left ventricular failure Fatigue Dyspnea	Echocardiogram: Left atrial enlargement Hyperdynamic left ventricle ECG: Left ventricular hypertrophy Left atrial enlargement (P mitrale) Chest radiograph: Poststenotic aortic dilation Aortic valve calcification Left ventricular enlargement

Continued

Table 5-34 VALVULAR DISORDERS—cont'd

CV

Type	Physical Examination	Diagnostic Study Findings
		Cardiac catheterization: Left ventricular dysfunction Abnormal aortic pressure gradient ↑ LVEDP Normal or ↑ left atrial and pulmonary pressures (secondary to severity of stenosis) ↓ Size of aortic valve orifice
		Echocardiogram: Restricted movement of stenotic valve
Aortic regurgitation (aortic insufficiency)	Diastolic and systolic murmurs Water-hammer pulse Palpitations Syncope DOE, orthopnea Angina pectoris Heart failure Hepatomegaly JVD Edema	ECG: Left ventricular hypertrophy Chest radiograph: Left ventricular enlargement Dilation of ascending aorta Cardiac catheterization: ↑ Pulse pressure ↑ LAP/PAWP ↑ Pulmonary pressures Angiography used to identify and quantify regurgitation Echocardiogram: ↑ Volume in left ventricle during diastole

CO/CI, Cardiac output/cardiac index; *DOE*, dyspnea on exertion; *ECG*, electrocardiogram; *JVD*, jugular venous distention; *LA*, left atrium; *LAP*, left atrial pressure; *LV*, left ventricular; *LVEDP*, left ventricular end diastolic pressure; *S/S*, signs and symptoms; *PAWP*, pulmonary artery wedge pressure.
NOTE: symptoms will vary depending on chronic versus acute problem and/or degree of valvular disorder.

GASTROINTESTINAL DISORDERS

ACUTE PANCREATITIS

Clinical Brief

Pancreatic autodigestion is the hallmark of acute pancreatitis. The zymogen (e.g., enzyme precursor) trypsinogen becomes inappropriately activated to trypsin within the pancreatic acinar cells, thereby causing widespread enzymatic destruction of parenchymal and ductal cells within the pancreas. This incites a continued morbid cascade of events that causes activation of other proteolytic enzymes and mobilization of inflammatory biochemical mediators that may ultimately result in ischemic necrosis and hemorrhage. Alcohol abuse and biliary tract disease account for 80% of the cases of acute pancreatitis. Other causes include trauma or surgery, pharmacologic agents (sulfonamides, tetracycline, lipids, procainamide, enalapril, furosemide), hyperlipidemia, endoscopic retrograde cholangiopancreatography (ERCP) examination, and infection. The exact events that trigger the rapid sequence of enzymatic reactions that initiate acute pancreatitis remain unknown, however.

Subtypes of acute pancreatitis include edematous or interstitial pancreatitis and necrotizing or hemorrhagic pancreatitis. Necrotizing pancreatitis is the most lethal and less common subtype. Severe metabolic alterations are common in both subtypes, and tend to include hypocalcemia, hyperglycemia, hypertriglyceridemia, and acidosis. Hypotension and shock also can occur secondary to hemorrhage in cases of necrotizing pancreatitis and secondary to abdominal fluid sequestration in all subtypes.

Chronic pancreatitis presents with a more insidious onset of clinical signs and symptoms than acute pancreatitis. The pancreatic tissue is calcified in chronic pancreatitis rather than acutely inflamed as it appears in cases of acute pancreatitis. Calcification of the pancreas occurs over time as a result of continued exposure of the pancreas to a variety of toxins, alcohol being the most common culprit. Patients with chronic pancreatitis present less acutely ill than patients with acute pancreatitis and have varying degrees of loss of pancreatic exocrine and endocrine function.

Presenting Signs and Symptoms

The hallmark of acute pancreatitis is a steady, dull, or boring pain in the epigastrium or left upper abdominal quadrant that may radiate to the flank and rapidly increases in intensity. Nausea and vomiting (N/V) generally accompany the pain. The patient may be in respiratory distress and complain of thirst.

Physical Examination

Vital signs:

    HR: may be elevated as a result of acute pain

    BP: narrow pulse pressure as a result of hypovolemia and peripheral vasodilation to frank hypotension (SBP <90 mm Hg) if grossly hypovolemic from abdominal fluid sequestration

    Temperature: mildly elevated

    RR: tachypnea

Neurologic: restlessness

Pulmonary:

    Dyspnea

    Crackles may be present.

Abdominal:

    Distended, ascites may be present if concomitant history of alcoholic cirrhosis

    Cullen's sign (bluish brown discoloration periumbilically)

    Bowel sounds decreased or absent

    Left upper quadrant or epigastric tenderness with deep palpation; initially no abdominal wall rigidity or rebound tenderness

Skin:

    Grey Turner's sign (bluish brown discoloration of flanks)

    Jaundice may be present.

    Decreased turgor

Diagnostic Findings

Diagnostic findings depend on the clinical examination: acute non-colicky epigastric pain, history of risk factors, and laboratory findings (i.e., hyperamylasemia, hyperlipasemia, hyperglycemia, and hypocalcemia). Contrast CT scan is invaluable in the diagnosis of pancreatitis. ERCP is only diagnostically important in suspected biliary pancreatitis. According to Ranson's criteria, the number of signs present during the first 48 hours after admission is directly related to the patient's chances for significant morbidity and mortality (Table 5-35).

Table 5-35 RANSON'S CRITERIA

Criteria	Alcoholic	Nonalcoholic
Age	>55 years	>70 years
WBCs	>16,000/mm^3	>18,000/mm^3
LDH	>300 international units/L	>400 international units/L
AST (SGOT)	>250 international units/L	>250 international units/L
Blood glucose	>200 mg/dL	>220 mg/dL
Within 48 hours		
Hematocrit drop	>10% points	>10% points
Base deficit	>4 mEq/L	>5 mEq/L
Serum calcium	<8 mg/dL	<8 mg/dL
Serum BUN rise	>5 mg/dL	>2 mg/dL
Arterial Pao$_2$	<60 mm Hg	<60 mm Hg
Fluid sequestration	>6 L	>4 L

AST, Aspartate aminotransferase; *BUN,* blood urea nitrogen; *LDH,* lactate dehydrogenase; *SGOT,* serum glutamic-oxaloacetic transaminase; *WBC,* white blood cell.

GI

ACUTE CARE PATIENT MANAGEMENT

Goals of Treatment

Restore fluid and electrolyte balance.
    Crystalloids, colloids
    Electrolyte replacement
Maintain adequate oxygenation.
    Supplemental oxygen
    Intubation/mechanical ventilation
Alleviate the pain.
    Opioid analgesics
Minimize pancreatic exocrine function.
Support diminished pancreatic endocrine function by administering insulin as needed.
Provide early metabolic support.
    Enteral nutrition or parenteral nutrition (PN) if enteral access not possible
Treat the cause.
    Appropriate therapy
Administration of octreotide or glucagon to inhibit pancreatic secretions (controversial therapy)
Detect/prevent clinical sequelae (Table 5-36).

Table 5-36　CLINICAL SEQUELAE ASSOCIATED WITH ACUTE PANCREATITIS

Complication	Signs and Symptoms
Shock	Tachycardia; hypotension; altered mentation; cool, clammy skin
Respiratory insufficiency	Dyspnea, hypoxemia, tachypnea, crackles, use of accessory muscles
Acute tubular necrosis	Oliguria, increased BUN and creatinine levels, urine sodium >30 mEq/L; urine casts, red cells, and protein
Sepsis	Two or more of the following: HR >90 beats/min, RR >20 breaths/min or $Paco_2$ <32 mm Hg, T >100.4° F or <96.8° F (38° C or <36° C), WBCs >12,000/mm^3 or <4000/mm^3 or >10% neutrophils; infection
Coagulopathies	Thrombocytopenia, delayed thrombin time, decreased fibrinogen, elevated fibrin degradation products
Diabetes	Elevated serum glucose, glycosuria
Pancreatic abscess	Increasing temperature, elevated WBC count, abdominal distention, pain
Pancreatic cutaneous fistula	Drainage through skin tract
Pseudocysts	Seen on CT, ultrasound evaluation

BUN, Blood urea nitrogen; *CT,* computed tomography; *HR,* heart rate; *RR,* respiratory rate; *T,* temperature; *WBC,* white blood cell.

Priority Nursing Diagnoses and Potential Complications

Priority Nursing Diagnoses	PC: Potential Complications
Deficient fluid volume	Hypovolemia, decreased cardiac output, electrolyte imbalances, abdominal fluid sequestration, pancreatic pseudocysts
Impaired gas exchange	Hypoxemia, atelectasis, pneumonia
Acute pain	
Imbalanced nutrition: less than body requirements (see p. 53)	Negative nitrogen balance, hyperglycemia
Risk for infection (see p. 48)	Sepsis, pancreatic abscess
Risk for interrupted family processes (see p. 45)	

Nursing Diagnosis: DEFICIENT FLUID VOLUME related to fluid sequestration to retroperitoneum and interstitium, intraperitoneal bleeding, pseudocyst formation, vomiting, or nasogastric suction

Outcome Criteria

CVP 2 to 6 mm Hg
PAS 15 to 30 mm Hg
PAD 5 to 15 mm Hg
SBP 90 to 120 mm Hg
MAP 70 to 105 mm Hg
Serum sodium 135 to 145 mEq/L
Serum potassium 3.5 to 4.5 mEq/L
Serum calcium 8.5 to 10.5 mg/dL
HR 60 to 100 beats/min
Hgb 12 to 16 g/dL (females); 13.5 to 17.5 g/dL (males)
Hct 37% to 47% (females); 40% to 54% (males)
Moist mucous membranes
Elastic skin turgor
Urine output 30 mL/hr or 0.5 to 1 mL/kg/hr

Patient Monitoring

1. Obtain CVP, PA pressures (if available), and BP every hour or more frequently during rapid fluid resuscitation. Monitor MAP, an indicator of tissue perfusion. MAP <60 mm Hg adversely affects renal and cerebral perfusion.
2. Monitor fluid volume status: measure urine output hourly and other bodily drainage to determine fluid balance every 8 hours. Compare serial weights for rapid (0.5-1 kg/day) changes that suggest fluid imbalances (1 kg is approximately 1000 mL of fluid).
3. Continuously monitor ECG for dysrhythmias secondary to electrolyte imbalance associated with NG suction.

Patient Assessment

1. Assess tissue perfusion: note level of mentation, skin color and temperature, peripheral pulses, and capillary refill.
2. Assess hydration status: note skin turgor on inner thigh or forehead, condition of buccal membranes, and development of edema or crackles. Fever increases fluid loss.
3. Assess abdomen: measure abdominal girth once each shift to determine the degree of ascites or increasing fluid sequestration either retroperitoneally or interstitially.

4. Assess for signs and symptoms of electrolyte imbalance.
5. Assess the patient for clinical sequelae (see Table 5-36).

Diagnostics Assessment

1. Review serial serum electrolytes to evaluate degree of imbalance or the patient's response to therapy.
2. Review serial serum Hgb and Hct because intraperitoneal bleeding may occur.
3. Review serum albumin and protein levels because these will be decreased with third spacing of fluid.
4. Review trends in serum amylase, lipase, and pancreatic isoamylase over time to partially determine effectiveness of therapy.
5. Review trends in serum creatinine and BUN that may suggest onset of acute tubular necrosis.

Patient Management

1. Administer crystalloids for fluid resuscitation as ordered. Albumin may be required in hypoproteinemic patients to pull fluid back into the intravascular space. Blood or blood products may be required in case of bleeding or coagulopathies.
2. Calcium, magnesium, or potassium supplements may be needed to restore serum levels. (See pp. 348-375 for information on electrolyte imbalances.)
3. Vasopressors, such as dopamine or norepinephrine, may be necessary if hypotension persists despite fluid resuscitation.
4. See the information on hypovolemic shock, p. 249.

Nursing Diagnosis: IMPAIRED GAS EXCHANGE related to pulmonary complications: infiltrates, atelectasis, diaphragmatic elevation, pleural effusion secondary to toxic effects of pancreatic enzymes on pulmonary membranes

Outcome Criteria

RR 12 to 20 breaths/min, eupnea
PaO_2 80 to 100 mm Hg
$PaCO_2$ 35 to 45 mm Hg
pH 7.35 to 7.45
O_2 sat ≥95%
Lungs clear to auscultation
HR 60 to 100 beats/min

Patient Monitoring

1. Continuously monitor ECG for dysrhythmias and ischemic changes (ST segment and T-wave changes) secondary to hypoxemia.
2. Continuously monitor oxygen saturation with pulse oximetry (SpO_2). Monitor interventions and patient activities that may adversely affect oxygen saturation.
3. Continuously monitor PAS pressure (if available) because hypoxia can increase sympathetic tone and pulmonary vasoconstriction.

Patient Assessment

1. Assess respiratory status: note RR and depth and use of accessory muscles; auscultate breath sounds and note onset of adventitious sounds or decreased breath sounds. Signs and symptoms of hypoxemia include restlessness, dyspnea, RR >30 breaths/min, and altered mental status. ARDS may develop.
2. Assess the patient for clinical sequelae (see Table 5-36).

Diagnostics Assessment

1. Review serial ABGs; note trends of PaO_2 because pulmonary complications are associated with pancreatitis, and abdominal pain and distention may compromise ventilation. A decreasing trend in PaO_2, despite increases in FIO_2 administration, is indicative of ARDS.
2. Review serial chest radiographs for development or resolution of pleural effusions (left side most common), infiltrates, and atelectasis.
3. Review serum ionized calcium and magnesium levels and triglyceride levels. Hypocalcemia and hypertriglyceridemia (>1000 mg/dL) are risk factors for ARDS in patients with pancreatitis.
4. Review serum amylase and lipase levels to evaluate pancreatic function.

Patient Management

1. Administer supplemental oxygen; anticipate intubation and mechanical ventilation. (See p. 503 for information on ventilation therapies.)
2. Elevate HOB if at all possible to improve chest excursion.
3. Reposition the patient every 2 hours; assist the patient to C&DB hourly to prevent atelectasis and encourage incentive

spirometry. If mechanically ventilated, position patient to decrease risk of aspiration and ventilator-acquired pneumonia.
4. Administer morphine sulfate as the preferential opioid agent for pain relief.
5. Assist the patient in assuming a position of comfort, provide a calm environment, and explore alternative means of pain control (e.g., distraction, imagery).
6. A peritoneal lavage may be performed to remove toxic substances and fluid and to decrease the pressure on the diaphragm.

Nursing Diagnosis: ACUTE PAIN related to edema/distention of pancreas, peritoneal irritation, and interruption of blood supply

Outcome Criterion

Patient will communicate pain relief.

Patient Monitoring

None specific

Patient Assessment

1. Assess pain intensity level using the patient self-report rating scale whenever possible. Reassess pain intensity after each pain intervention for effectiveness of therapy. See the information on acute pain, p. 35.
2. Assess for anxiety and fear, which may increase the release of enzymes and increase pain.
3. Note changes in HR, BP, and RR that may suggest SNS stimulation, which may signal pain. However, absence of changes in HR, BP, and RR does not necessarily mean absence of pain.
4. Observe for cues such as grimacing, grunting, splinting, guarding, sobbing, irritability, withdrawal, or hostility, which may signal pain. However, absence of these behaviors does not necessarily mean absence of pain.

Diagnostics Assessment

None specific

Patient Management

1. Anticipate early enteral feedings via jejunum; slowly advance feedings as indicated. Monitor for increased pain with

advancement of feedings from untoward increased pancreatic enzyme activity.

2. Anticipate NG intubation if ileus or significant abdominal distention is present. Connect the NG tube to suction to decompress the stomach and prevent gastric stimulation of the pancreatic enzymes.

3. Administer octreotide or glucagon as indicated to diminish pancreatic exocrine activity (controversial therapy).

4. Ensure bed rest and limit activities to decrease the metabolic rate and the production of pancreatic enzymes.

5. Assist the patient to assume a position of comfort, provide a restful environment, and explore alternate means of pain relief (e.g., distraction, imagery).

6. Administer morphine sulfate as the preferential opioid agent for pain relief.

7. See the information on acute pain, p. 35.

Nursing Diagnosis: IMBALANCED NUTRITION: LESS THAN BODY REQUIREMENTS related to nausea, vomiting, hypermetabolic state, pancreatic β-cell destruction, and NPO status

Outcome Criteria

Absence of nausea and vomiting
Positive nitrogen balance
Serum albumin 3.5 to 5 g/dL
Transferrin >230 mg/dL
Serum glucose 100 to 120 mg/dL

Patient Monitoring

1. Monitor I&O and caloric intake. Daily weights in acutely ill are poor indicators of lean body mass gain or loss, but excellent indicators of fluid balance.

2. Monitor serial serum albumin, prealbumin, and total protein levels.

3. Monitor serum glucose levels four times a day and as needed.

Patient Assessment

1. Assess GI status: auscultate bowel sounds and evaluate abdominal distention; assess for nausea, vomiting, and anorexia.

2. Assess the patient for clinical sequelae (see Table 5-36).

Diagnostics Assessment

1. Review serum glucose levels because pancreatic β-cells become inflamed during acute pancreatitis, resulting in diminished insulin production. In addition, pancreatitis-associated hyperglycemia can be aggravated once enteral or PN is initiated.

2. Review nutritional panel (e.g., albumin, serum transferrin, total lymphocytes, and creatinine height index) to evaluate nutritional status.

3. Review results of 24-hour urine urea nitrogen (UUN); increased levels indicate that protein loss is taking place.

Patient Management

1. An NG tube may be required to reduce vomiting and abdominal distention.

2. Consult with a dietitian or nutritional support team for a formal nutritional workup.

3. Administer enteral nutrition as ordered. Preferred route of administration is nasojejunal. Administer PN if enteral access is not possible. Lipids are generally avoided because they increase pancreatic exocrine secretion, particularly in the presence of elevated serum triglycerides. See p. 561 for information on nutrition.

4. Monitor serum glucose levels at least four times a day and as indicated via laboratory analysis and/or glucometer readings. Maintain tight glycemic control with sliding-scale insulin as ordered.

5. Administer pharmacologic agents as ordered to reduce gastric acidity and pancreatic juices.

6. Oral feedings may be instituted once pain has subsided and GI function returns. Provide small feedings high in carbohydrates and low in proteins and fat. Note patient tolerance (i.e., absence of vomiting, abdominal distention, and pain).

7. Administer antiemetic as ordered and before meals if necessary. Supplemental nourishment may be needed. Provide good mouth care to enhance appetite.

8. Decrease metabolic demands: allow rest periods between nursing activities, reduce anxiety, and control fever and pain.

HEPATIC FAILURE

Clinical Brief

Hepatic failure can result from acute liver injury, causing acute liver failure (ALF) or fulminant hepatic failure (FHF), or progressive chronic liver disease (e.g., cirrhosis). An alteration in hepatocyte functioning affects liver metabolism, detoxification processes, protein synthesis, manufacture of clotting factors, and preservation of immunocompetence. FHF occurs when severe hepatic injury results in encephalopathy and severe coagulopathy within 28 days of the onset of symptoms in patients without a history of chronic liver disease. Liver transplant is the only viable treatment option for patients with FHF. The most commonly identified cause of FHF is drug induced, with acetaminophen the most common culprit, followed by viral hepatitis. Other causes include infection (cytomegalovirus [CMV], adenovirus), metabolic disorders (Wilson's disease, acute fatty liver of pregnancy), and severe ischemic insult (shock).

Cirrhosis is caused by chronic alcohol-induced toxicity (most common); biliary stasis; severe long-term right-sided HF; or necrotic damage resulting from hepatotoxins, chemicals, infection, or metabolic disorders. It is generally categorized by presentation and causative agent (i.e., alcoholic, biliary, postnecrotic, or cardiac cirrhosis). Generally, patients with cirrhosis are admitted to the intensive care unit (ICU) as a result of GI bleeding (severe coagulopathy or variceal bleeding), spontaneous bacterial peritonitis, hepatic encephalopathy (HE), and/or hepatorenal syndrome. Hepatorenal syndrome is a type of prerenal acute renal failure observed in severe liver disease in the absence of other known causes of renal failure. Hepatorenal syndrome is almost always fatal unless the patient receives a liver transplant. The worst prognostic indicator for patients with hepatic failure is a rising creatinine level, indicative of hepatorenal syndrome.

Presenting Signs and Symptoms

Manifestations depend on the complications associated with the liver dysfunction. Patient behavior may range from agitation to frank coma. Evidence of GI bleeding, renal failure, or respiratory distress may also be present. The initial manifestation in FHF is most commonly bleeding from coagulopathy.

Physical Examination

Vital signs:
    SBP: <90 mm Hg (with shock)
    HR: >120 beats/min (with shock)
    Temperature: may be mildly elevated
    RR: tachypnea initially progressing to respiratory depression associated with encephalopathy

Neurologic:
    Mildly confused to coma
    Personality changes
    Asterixis
Pulmonary:
    Crackles
    Labored respirations
Gastrointestinal:
    Hematemesis and melena
    Ascites
    Hepatomegaly may be present.
    Splenomegaly may be present.
    Fetor hepaticus
    Diarrhea (if given a cathartic for treatment to cleanse colon of
        bacteria)
Skin:
    Jaundice and spider nevi may be present.
    Ecchymosis and petechiae
    Pruritus
    Edema

Diagnostic Findings

The following laboratory findings reflect hepatocellular dysfunction:
Serum bilirubin >1.2 mg/dL
Prolonged PT (e.g., 10 seconds greater than normal) or INR (e.g.,
    >2) suggests massive liver necrosis
Aspartate aminotransferase (AST) >40 units/mL
Alanine aminotransferase (ALT) >40 units/mL
    Other laboratory findings vary, depending on the severity of the
disease and its effect on other bodily functions.

ACUTE CARE PATIENT MANAGEMENT

Goals of Treatment

Restore fluid volume and electrolyte balance.
    Crystalloids, colloids
    Electrolyte therapy
    Shunting procedures
    Diuretic therapy
Maintain adequate oxygenation.
    Supplemental oxygen or intubation/mechanical ventilation
    Blood products

Decrease circulating ammonia and toxins.
    Bowel evacuations
    Neomycin or metronidazole
    Lactulose
    Protein-restricted diet
Maintain coagulation factors.
    Fresh frozen plasma
    Vitamin K
Decrease ICP (FHF).
    Head/bed positioning
    Control Pao_2 and Pco_2 levels
    Mannitol
Detect/prevent clinical sequelae (Table 5-37).

Table 5-37 CLINICAL SEQUELAE ASSOCIATED WITH HEPATIC FAILURE

Complication	Signs and Symptoms
Hepatorenal syndrome mmol/L	Oliguria, azotemia, BUN/Cr ratio >30:1, urine osmolality >400 mOsm, urinary Na <10
Gastrointestinal hemorrhage	Frank bleeding from the upper or lower GI tract
Hepatic encephalopathy	Alterations in mentation advancing to coma
DIC	Prolonged bleeding from all sites, skin bruising, intracerebral bleeding
Septic shock	SBP <90 mm Hg, HR >90 beats/min, RR >20 breaths/min or $Paco_2$ <32 mm Hg, Pao_2/Fio_2 <280, T >100.4° F or <96.8° F (38° C or <36° C), WBCs >12,000/mm³ or <4000/mm³ or >10% neutrophils; altered mental status, urine output <0.5 mL/kg/hr, plasma lactate >2 mmol/L
Hypoglycemia	Headache, impaired mentation, hunger, irritability, lethargy
Respiratory failure	Restlessness, Pao_2 <50 mm Hg, $Paco_2$ >50 mm Hg, pH <7.35
Spontaneous bacterial peritonitis	Fever, abdominal pain, leukocytosis

BUN, Blood urea nitrogen; *Cr,* creatinine; *DIC,* disseminated intravascular coagulation; *GI,* gastrointestinal; *HR,* heart rate; *Na,* sodium; *RR,* respiratory rate; *SBP,* systolic blood pressure; *T,* temperature; *WBC,* white blood cell.

Priority Nursing Diagnoses and Potential Complications

Priority Nursing Diagnoses	PC: Potential Complications
Deficient fluid volume	GI bleeding, hypovolemia, electrolyte imbalances
Impaired gas exchange	Hypoxemia; atelectasis, pneumonia
Risk for injury	Hepatic encephalopathy
Risk for ineffective protection (see p. 48)	Sepsis, spontaneous bacterial peritonitis
Risk for interrupted family processes (see p. 45)	
Risk for imbalanced nutrition: less than body requirements (see p. 53)	Negative nitrogen balance

Nursing Diagnosis: DEFICIENT FLUID VOLUME related to ascites secondary to hypoalbuminemia, bleeding secondary to decreased clotting factors or variceal hemorrhage, and diuretic therapy

Outcome Criteria

SBP 90 to 120 mm Hg
MAP 70 to 105 mm Hg
CVP 2 to 6 mm Hg
PAS 15 to 30 mm Hg
PAD 5 to 15 mm Hg
PAWP 4 to 12 mm Hg
Serum albumin 3.5 to 5 mg/dL
Hgb 12 to 16 g/dL (females); 13 to 17.5 g/dL (males)
Hct 37% to 47% (females); 40% to 54% (males)
Platelet count >50,000/mm^3
Urine output 30 mL/hr or 0.5 to 1 mL/kg/hr
Serum sodium 135 to 145 mEq/L
Serum potassium 3.5 to 5 mEq/L
Intake approximates output

Patient Monitoring

1. Obtain PA pressures, CVP, and BP continuously until the patient's condition is stable, then hourly. Monitor pulse pressure, MAP, PAWP, and CI to evaluate effectiveness of fluid resuscitation. Increased abdominal pressure secondary to ascitic fluid accumulation can compress the inferior vena cava, decreasing venous return and lowering the CO.

2. Continuously monitor ECG for lethal dysrhythmias that may result from electrolyte and acid-base imbalances.

3. Monitor fluid volume status: measure intake and urine output hourly; determine fluid balance every 8 hours; compare serial weights to determine rapid (0.5-1 kg/day) changes indicating fluid imbalances.

Patient Assessment

1. Assess hydration status: note skin turgor on inner thigh or forehead, condition of buccal membranes, and development of edema or crackles.

2. Assess for signs and symptoms of bleeding: bleeding from gums or puncture sites and bruising or petechiae; test urine, stool, and gastric aspirate for occult blood and note changes in mentation.

3. Measure abdominal girth once each shift to determine progression of ascites. Percuss and palpate abdomen because dullness is representative of fluid accumulation.

4. Assess respiratory status: note rate and depth of respirations or complaints of dyspnea; ascites may impair ventilation. Auscultate lungs for adventitious sounds.

5. Assess the patient for clinical sequelae (see Table 5-37).

Diagnostics Assessment

1. Review serial serum ammonia, albumin, bilirubin, AST (SGOT), ALT (SGPT), lactate dehydrogenase (LDH), platelet count, PT, PTT, and INR results to evaluate hepatic function.

2. Review serial serum electrolytes. Hypokalemia and other electrolyte imbalances can precipitate hepatic encephalopathy.

3. Review serial serum Hgb and Hct for decreasing values suggesting blood loss.

4. Review urine electrolytes, BUN, and creatinine to evaluate renal function.

Patient Management

1. Administer intravenous crystalloids as ordered: dextrose solutions will be needed in acute FHF because the patient is at risk for hypoglycemia; colloids may be given to increase oncotic pressure and pull ascitic fluid into the intravascular space. Blood and blood products may be required to replace RBCs and clotting factors. Carefully monitor the patient for fluid volume overload during fluid resuscitation.

2. Administer potassium as ordered. Validate adequate urine output before potassium administration.

3. Sodium restriction of 0.5 g/day and fluid restriction to 1000 mL/day may be ordered.

4. Vitamin K or fresh frozen plasma (FFP) may be required to promote the clotting process. Protect the patient from injury; pad side rails, keep the bed in low position, and minimize handling; avoid injections or invasive procedures if at all possible if results of clotting studies are abnormal.

5. Institute bleeding precautions: avoid razor blades and use soft-bristled toothbrushes. Minimize needlesticks.

6. In patients with ascites, diuretic agents may be required. Rapid diuresis (>2000 mL/day) can precipitate renal failure. Carefully monitor the patient for hypovolemia, electrolyte imbalances, and increasing BUN and creatinine.

7. Ascites refractory to pharmacologic therapy may necessitate placement of a transjugular intrahepatic portosystemic shunt (TIPS) (see p. 571) to shunt blood within the liver's vasculature, thereby alleviating portal hypertension. Monitor the patient for adverse affects: infection, clotting, or bleeding.

8. Paracentesis may be performed if abdominal distention is severe. Note amount, color, and character of fluid. Send samples to the laboratory for analysis as appropriate, including Gram stain and culture and sensitivity. Monitor the patient for shock and hepatorenal syndrome.

9. Prepare the patient and family for a liver transplant, as indicated.

10. See the information about hypovolemic shock, p. 249.

Nursing Diagnosis: IMPAIRED GAS EXCHANGE related to intrapulmonary and portopulmonary shunt, hyperventilation secondary to ascites, pulmonary edema secondary to circulating toxic substances, or respiratory depression secondary to encephalopathy

Outcome Criteria

PaO_2 80 to 100 mm Hg
$PaCO_2$ 35 to 45 mm Hg
pH 7.35 to 7.45
O_2 sat ≥95%
RR 12 to 20 breaths/min, eupnea
Lungs clear to auscultation

Patient Monitoring

1. Continuously monitor oxygen saturation with pulse oximetry (SpO_2). Monitor interventions and patient activities that may adversely affect oxygen saturation.
2. Continuously monitor ECG for dysrhythmias: hypoxemia is a risk factor for dysrhythmias.

Patient Assessment

1. Assess respiratory status: note RR and depth; RR >30 breaths/min or <12 breaths/min suggests impending respiratory dysfunction. Auscultate breath sounds every 2 hours or more frequently during fluid resuscitation; note development of crackles or other adventitious sounds suggesting pulmonary congestion. Note dyspnea and cough, which may suggest pulmonary edema. Cyanosis is a late sign.
2. Assess the patient for clinical sequelae (see Table 5-37).

Diagnostics Assessment

1. Review ABGs for decreasing trend in SaO_2, PaO_2 (hypoxemia), or pH (acidosis).
2. Review serial chest radiographs to evaluate a worsening lung condition. Right-sided pleural effusions are common in chronic liver disease.

Patient Management

1. Administer supplemental oxygen as ordered to prevent hypoxemia. Anticipate intubation and mechanical ventilation. See p. 503 for information on mechanical ventilation.
2. Reposition and assist the patient to C&DB every 2 hours to prevent atelectasis. If necessary, suction secretions gently, being careful to avoid trauma to the mucosa, which can increase the risk for bleeding.
3. Elevate HOB to promote adequate chest excursion. A paracentesis may be performed to remove excess fluid from the abdomen and ease the work of breathing.

Nursing Diagnosis: RISK FOR INJURY related to brain exposure to toxic substances (hepatic encephalopathy)

Outcome Criteria

Patient alert and oriented
Serum ammonia 12 to 55 mmol/L
Patient will not injure self

Patient Monitoring
_____

Monitor LOC using Glasgow Coma Scale.

Patient Assessment
_____

1. Assess the patient's LOC at least hourly. A decreased awareness of the environment is an early manifestation of
   encephalopathy. Note any personality changes and slurred or
   slow speech. In ALF, the mental impairment progresses to
   coma rapidly and includes a period of agitation, whereas the
   encephalopathy in chronic liver disease progresses gradually
   to coma without a phase of agitation.
2. Assess the patient for asterixis (flapping tremors of the
   wrist when hand extended), an early manifestation of
   encephalopathy.
3. Assess sleep pattern because a reversal of day-night sleep pattern is an early indicator of encephalopathy.
4. Assess for other etiologies of encephalopathy (e.g., hypoglycemia, hypoxemia, hemorrhage, sepsis, sedatives/hypnotics,
   electrolyte imbalance, acid-base disturbance, hypotension).
5. Assess the patient for clinical sequelae (see Table 5-37).

Diagnostics Assessment
_____

1. Monitor serum ammonia levels in patients with cirrhosis
   because increasing ammonia levels correlate with increased
   manifestations of encephalopathy.
2. Monitor serum glucose levels; hypoglycemia is a common
   finding in acute liver failure and may further impair cerebral
   functioning.
3. Monitor serum sodium and potassium levels because imbalances can contribute to hepatic encephalopathy.

Patient Management
_____

1. Administer ammonia-reducing medications as ordered (e.g.,
   lactulose, neomycin, or metronidazole). The goal of therapy
   is three or four soft stools per day. If diarrhea occurs, hypovolemia and electrolyte imbalances may ensue. Avoid lactulose use in patients with FHF because it may increase the
   formation of colonic gas, which could hinder subsequent
   liver transplantation.
2. Maintain a safe environment; restrain the patient only if all
   alternatives have been exhausted.

3. Restrict dietary protein to 20 to 40 g/day until normal mentation returns. If the patient is receiving total parenteral nutrition (TPN) or enteral feedings, see pp. 563 and 566 for patient care management guidelines. Formulas rich in branched-chain amino acids (BCAA) may be preferred.

4. NG intubation may be required to decompress the stomach, reduce absorption of protein breakdown products, and reduce the risk of aspiration in an unconscious patient.

5. Avoid sedatives if at all possible or use with extreme caution because respiratory depression and circulatory collapse can result.

6. Patients with FHF may develop cerebral edema and increased ICP and may require mannitol 20%, 0.5 to 1 g/kg/hr if adequate renal function. If renal failure is present, ultrafiltration may be required. Calculate serum osmolality; the goal is an osmolality <310 mOsm/L but in high normal range. Keep head and neck in neutral position, elevate HOB, and be alert to factors that may increase ICP (e.g., hypoxemia, fluid overload). (See p. 462 for information on increased ICP.)

PERITONITIS

Clinical Brief

Acute peritonitis is an inflammatory process within the peritoneal cavity most commonly caused by a bacterial infection. Types of acute peritonitis include primary and secondary. Primary peritonitis, otherwise known as spontaneous bacterial peritonitis, most commonly occurs in patients with cirrhosis and clinically significant ascites. Secondary peritonitis most commonly occurs as a result of spillage of intestinal, biliary, or urinary tract contents into the peritoneal space as a result of perforation, suppuration, or ischemic injury. Patients at risk for developing secondary peritonitis include those with recent abdominal surgery, a perforated ulcer or colon, a ruptured appendix or viscus, a bowel obstruction, a gangrenous bowel, or ischemic bowel disease. These complications cause what is called a "surgical abdomen." The resultant inflammatory response causes vascular dilation and an increase in vascular permeability. These changes mobilize antiinflammatory cells as well as biochemical mediators that promote fluid shifts from the extracellular compartment into the peritoneum, producing hypovolemia.

Presenting Signs and Symptoms

Signs and symptoms include a patient assuming a flexed-knee position and complaining of severe localized (parietal) or generalized (visceral) abdominal pain, nausea, and vomiting.

Physical Examination

Vital signs:
  HR: tachycardia
  BP: hypotension
  RR: increased and shallow
  Temperature: elevated
Neurologic: normal to decreased mentation
Skin: pale, flushed, or diaphoretic
Cardiovascular: pulse thready or weak or may be bounding in presence of fever
Pulmonary: breath sounds may be diminished secondary to shallow breathing
Abdominal:
  Rebound tenderness with guarding
  May have referred pain to the shoulder
  Rigid, distended abdomen
  Bowel sounds decreased to absent

Diagnostic Findings

Diagnostic findings are based on clinical manifestations of fever, abdominal pain, and rebound tenderness along with a history of precipitating factors. Cultures of peritoneal fluid will yield positive results.

In addition, the following may be found:
WBC >10,000 mm^3
Serum protein <6 g/dL
Serum amylase >160 U/L

ACUTE CARE PATIENT MANAGEMENT

Goals of Treatment

Restore fluid and electrolyte balance.
  Crystalloid, colloid, blood, and blood products
  Electrolyte replacement
Eradicate infection.
  Cultures, antibiotic therapy
Control pain.

Analgesics

Rest GI tract.

NPO, NG intubation

Correct the underlying problem.

Surgery

Detect/prevent clinical sequelae (Table 5-38).

Table 5-38 CLINICAL SEQUELAE ASSOCIATED WITH PERITONITIS

Complication	Signs and Symptoms
Septic shock	SBP <90 mm Hg, HR >90 beats/min, RR >20 breaths/min or $Paco_2$ <32 mm Hg, Pao_2/Fio_2 <280, T >100.4° F or <96.8° F (>38° C or <36° C), WBCs >12,000/mm^3 or <4000/mm^3 or >10% neutrophils; altered mental status, urine output <0.5 mL/kg/hr, plasma lactate >2 mmol/L
Paralytic ileus	Absent bowel sounds, abdominal distention
Respiratory failure	Restlessness, RR >30 breaths/min, labored breathing, Pao_2 <50 mm Hg, $Paco_2$ >50 mm Hg, pH <7.35
Acute renal failure	Urinary output <30 mL/hr after fluid replacement, increasing BUN and creatinine
Acute liver failure	Jaundice, elevated AST, ALT
Dysrhythmias	Irregular rhythm, decreased mentation

AST, Aspartate aminotransferase; *ALT,* alanine aminotransferase, BUN, blood urea nitrogen; *HR,* heart rate; *RR,* respiratory rate; *SBP,* systolic blood pressure; *T,* temperature; *WBC,* white blood cell.

Priority Nursing Diagnoses and Potential Complications

Priority Nursing Diagnoses	PC: Potential Complications
Deficient fluid volume	Hypovolemia, decreased cardiac output, electrolyte imbalances
Acute pain	
Ineffective breathing pattern	Hypoxemia, atelectasis, pneumonia
Risk for ineffective protection (see p. 48)	Sepsis
Risk for interrupted family processes (see p. 45)	
Risk for imbalanced nutrition: less than body requirements (see p. 53)	Paralytic ileus

Nursing Diagnosis: DEFICIENT FLUID VOLUME related to intravascular fluid shift to the peritoneal space and inability to ingest oral fluids

Outcome Criteria

CVP 2 to 6 mm Hg
SBP 90 to 120 mm Hg
MAP 70 to 105 mm Hg
PAS 15 to 30 mm Hg
PAD 5 to 15 mm Hg
HR 60 to 100 beats/min
Urine output 30 mL/hr or 0.5 to 1 mL/kg/hr

Patient Monitoring

1. Obtain PA pressures and CVP (if available) and monitor MAP hourly or more frequently if the patient's hemodynamic status is unstable. Note the patient's response to therapy. A MAP <60 mm Hg adversely affects cerebral and renal perfusion.
2. Monitor fluid volume status: measure urine output hourly and measure NG and other bodily drainage. Determine fluid balance every 8 hours. Urine output <0.5 mL/kg/hr may indicate renal insufficiency. Compare serial weight (1 kg is approximately 1000 mL of fluid) to evaluate for rapid (0.5-1 kg/day) changes, which suggests fluid imbalance.
3. Continuously monitor ECG for dysrhythmias resulting from electrolyte disturbances.

Patient Assessment

1. Assess tissue perfusion: note LOC, skin color and temperature, pulses, and capillary refill.
2. Assess hydration status: note skin turgor on inner thigh or forehead, condition of buccal membranes, and development of edema or crackles.
3. Assess abdomen: note resolution of rigidity, rebound tenderness, and distention; auscultate bowel sounds.
4. Assess the patient for clinical sequelae (see Table 5-38).

Diagnostics Assessment

1. Review serum sodium and potassium levels, which may become depleted with NG suctioning or fluid shifts.
2. Review serial WBC count and differential to evaluate the course of infection.

Patient Management

1. Administer crystalloid or colloid solutions to improve intravascular volume. CVP and PA pressures reflect the capacity of the vascular system to accept volume and can be used to monitor fluid volume status.

2. Replace potassium as ordered; validate adequate urine output before administration.

3. Keep the patient NPO during acute phase and before evaluation by a surgeon. NG intubation with suction may be required to decompress the stomach and prevent aspiration. When vomiting and ileus resolve, provide the patient with oral fluids as tolerated.

4. Provide nutritional support as indicated; most patients will benefit from postpyloric delivery of early enteral nutrients at a minimal hourly rate to prevent bacterial translocation and sepsis.

5. Administer antibiotics as prescribed after appropriate cultures obtained. Most patients will require surgery to treat the cause of peritonitis.

Nursing Diagnosis: ACUTE PAIN related to inflammation of the peritoneal cavity

Outcome Criterion

Patient will communicate pain relief.

Patient Monitoring

None specific

Patient Assessment

1. Assess pain using the patient self-report rating scale whenever possible. Observe for nonverbal cues of increased pain intensity, including grimacing, guarding, diaphoresis, and irritability. However, absence of these behaviors does not necessarily mean absence of pain.

2. Assess abdomen for increasing girth, rigidity, or change in bowel sounds.

3. Obtain BP and HR; elevated values may reflect the presence of pain. However, absence of these does not necessarily mean absence of pain.

Diagnostics Assessment

None specific

Patient Management

1. Administer pain medication as ordered and evaluate its effectiveness and safety (use a sedation scale to monitor sedation level and prevent opioid-induced respiratory depression; see scale on p. 41.
2. Administer antibiotics as ordered to eradicate the infecting organism.
3. Provide a relaxed environment to alleviate anxiety.
4. Place the patient in a position of comfort. Elevating the HOB will help enhance chest excursion.
5. Administer analgesics preemptively, around the clock via PCA device to keep pain tolerable. Instruct the patient to self-bolus opioids using PCA or to request additional analgesics as necessary if pain increases to levels intolerable to the patient.
6. Explore alternative methods of pain relief with the patient (e.g., distraction, imagery).
7. See discussion of acute pain, p. 35.

Nursing Diagnosis: INEFFECTIVE BREATHING PATTERN related to abdominal distention and pain

Outcome Criteria

RR 12 to 20 breaths/min, eupnea
PaO_2 80 to 100 mm Hg
$PaCO_2$ 35 to 45 mm Hg
pH 7.35 to 7.45
Lungs clear to auscultation

Patient Monitoring

1. Continuously monitor oxygen saturation with pulse oximetry (SpO_2). Monitor interventions and patient activities that can adversely affect oxygen saturation.
2. Monitor PAS pressure (if available) because hypoxia can increase sympathetic tone and pulmonary vasoconstriction.

Patient Assessment

Assess respiratory status: note rate and depth of respirations. Rate >30 breaths/min, labored breathing, dyspnea, and restlessness suggest respiratory distress. Auscultate lungs; the onset of crackles may suggest fluid volume overload. Diminished lung sounds may be associated with shallow breathing, atelectasis, or pleural effusion.

Diagnostics Assessment

1. Review serial ABGs to identify decreasing trends in PaO_2, SaO_2, (hypoxemia), and pH (acidosis).
2. Review serial chest radiographs to identify improvement or worsening of the condition.

Patient Management

1. Administer supplemental oxygen as ordered. See p. 503 for information on ventilation therapies.
2. Elevate HOB to enhance chest excursion. Assist the patient to C&DB hourly to prevent atelectasis. Encourage slow, deep inspirations because patients have a tendency to take short, shallow breaths.
3. Ensure NG tube patency to prevent gastric secretion accumulation, which might increase the risk for aspiration or might increase abdominal distention and interfere with diaphragmatic motion.
4. Administer pain medication to promote deep breathing and improved pulmonary function. Assess level of sedation and respiratory status. Combine nonopioid analgesics (e.g., ketorolac, ibuprofen) with opioid analgesics (morphine sulfate, hydromorphone, oxycodone) to provide pain relief with lower doses than would be possible with one drug alone. This approach will produce fewer adverse effects, such as increased sedation, ileus, urinary retention, and respiratory depression.

UPPER GASTROINTESTINAL BLEEDING

Clinical Brief

Upper GI bleeding is characterized by the sudden onset of bleeding from the GI tract at a site (or sites) proximal to the ligament of Treitz. Most upper GI bleeds are a direct result of peptic ulcer erosion, stress-related mucosal disease, that may evidence as superficial erosive gastric lesions to frank ulcerations, erosive gastritis (secondary to use or abuse of NSAIDs, oral corticosteroids, or alcohol) or esophageal varices (secondary to hepatic failure). In addition to these, Mallory-Weiss tears can cause gastroesophageal bleeding as a result of severe retching and vomiting, but the bleeding tends to be less severe than in other types. Hospitalized critically ill patients are at heightened risk for stress-related mucosal disease, particularly if they are intubated and mechanically ventilated and/or evidencing coagulopathies.

Presenting Signs and Symptoms

Signs and symptoms depend on the amount and rapidity of blood loss; however, melena and hematemesis are usually present. Pain may be present with peptic ulcer disease, whereas the patient will be pain free if esophageal varices are the source of bleeding, but hemorrhaging rapidly. Patients may have signs and symptoms of hypovolemic shock: cool, clammy skin; pallor; apprehension to unresponsiveness; weak, thready pulse; and hypotension.

Physical Examination

Vital signs:

SBP: <90 mm Hg recumbent (>30% volume loss) or orthostatic BP (15%-30% volume loss)

HR: >100 beats/min

RR: tachypnea

Temperature: may be elevated

Other: obvious blood: hematemesis, melena, bloody stool with a fetid odor, coffee ground gastric aspirate

Neurologic: syncope, lightheadedness, altered mentation, apprehension

Skin:

Pale, diaphoretic

Cool, clammy

Jaundice, petechiae, or hematomas may be present with liver disease.

Cardiovascular:

Weak, thready pulse

Capillary refill >3 sec (shock)

Abdominal:

May be tender with guarding

Bowel sounds hyperactive or absent

Diagnostic Findings

BUN >20 mg/dL (newly elevated)

Emesis and/or stool positive for occult blood

Decreasing trend in Hgb and Hct

Endoscopy and angiography may be used to diagnose the site of bleeding.

ACUTE CARE PATIENT MANAGEMENT

Goals of Treatment

Optimize tissue oxygenation.

Supplemental oxygenation

Intubation/mechanical ventilation
Blood transfusion therapy
Stabilize the hemodynamic status.
   Crystalloids, colloids, blood administration
Arrest/prevent bleeding and locate the source.
   Gastric lavage
   Octreotide therapy (first-line agent) and/or vasopressin therapy
   Esophageal tamponade (varices)
   Sclerotherapy (varices)
   Band ligation (varices)
   Electrocoagulation
   Transjugular intrahepatic portosystemic shunt (TIPS) (varices)
   Surgical intervention
   Proton pump inhibitors (first-line agent) and/or H$_2$-receptor
      antagonists and/or antacids, and/or cytoprotective agents
Detect/prevent clinical sequelae (Table 5-39).

Table 5-39   CLINICAL SEQUELAE ASSOCIATED WITH GASTROINTESTINAL
              BLEEDING

Complication	Signs and Symptoms
GENERAL	
Hypovolemic shock	SBP <90 mm Hg; HR >120 beats/min; cool, clammy skin
Aspiration pneumonia	↑ Temperature, decreased breath sounds, ↓ Pao$_2$ and Sao$_2$
Myocardial, cerebral ischemia	ST segment, T-wave changes, chest pain, decreased LOC
DIC	Abnormal clotting factors, uncontrolled bleeding from all orifices
PEPTIC ULCER DISEASE	
Perforation of stomach or intestine	Profound shock, sudden change in the character of the pain to include back pain and boardlike abdominal pain, rebound tenderness, absent bowel sounds
Gastric outlet obstruction	Protracted vomiting, visual peristaltic waves
Peritonitis	↓ Temperature, abdominal pain, ↓ WBCs

DIC, Disseminated intravascular coagulation; *HR*, heart rate; *LOC*, level of consciousness; *SBP*, systolic blood pressure; *WBC*, white blood cell.

Priority Nursing Diagnoses and Potential Complications

Priority Nursing Diagnoses	PC: Potential Complications
Deficient fluid volume	Continued or recurrent GI bleeding, decreased cardiac output
Risk for aspiration	Hypoxemia, pneumonia
Risk for imbalanced nutrition: less than body requirements (see p. 53)	Negative nitrogen balance
Risk for ineffective protection (see p. 48)	
Risk for interrupted family processes (see p. 45)	

GI

Nursing Diagnosis: DEFICIENT FLUID VOLUME related to blood loss from hemorrhage

Outcome Criteria

Patient alert and oriented
Skin, pink, warm, and dry
CVP 2 to 6 mm Hg
PAS 15 to 30 mm Hg
PAD 5 to 15 mm Hg
SBP 90 to 120 mm Hg
MAP 70 to 105 mm Hg
HR 60 to 100 beats/min
Urine output 30 mL/hr or 0.5 to 1 mL/kg/hr
Hct ≥25% in males and females during initial fluid resuscitation, then:
Hgb 12 to 16 g/dL (females); 13.5 to 17.5 g/dL (males)
Hct 37% to 47% (females); 40% to 54% (males)

Patient Monitoring

1. Obtain PA pressures (if available), CVP, and BP every 15 minutes during acute episodes to evaluate fluid needs and the patient's response to therapy. Monitor MAP, an indicator of tissue perfusion. MAP <60 mm Hg adversely affects cerebral and renal perfusion. Orthostatic VS, a narrowed pulse pressure, and delayed capillary refill time indicate a loss of 15% to 30% of circulating blood volume.

2. Monitor fluid volume status: measure intake and urine output hourly to evaluate renal perfusion; measure blood loss if possible; determine fluid balance every 8 hours. Compare serial weights to evaluate rapid (0.5-1 kg/day) changes suggesting fluid volume imbalance.

3. Continuously monitor ECG for dysrhythmias and myocardial ischemia (ST and T-wave changes) associated with reduced oxygen carrying capacity associated with blood loss.

Patient Assessment

1. Assess the patient for increased restlessness, apprehension, or altered consciousness, which may indicate decreased cerebral perfusion.
2. Assess hydration status: note skin turgor on inner thigh or forehead, condition of buccal membranes, and development of edema or crackles.
3. Be alert for recurrence of bleeding.
4. Assess the patient for clinical sequelae (see Table 5-39).

Diagnostics Assessment

1. Review Hgb and Hct levels to determine the effectiveness of treatment or worsening of the patient's condition. The Hct should rise two or three points for each unit of packed red blood cells (PRBCs) given.
2. Review clotting factors and serum calcium levels if multiple transfusions have been given.
3. Review serial BUN levels; elevated BUN (with a normal creatinine) can provide information about the degree of hypovolemia.
4. Review serial ABGs to evaluate oxygenation and acid-base status. Hypoxia can lead to lactic acidosis.
5. Review the results of endoscopic evaluation or arteriogram if available.

Patient Management

1. Maintain a patent airway; administer supplemental oxygen as ordered; intubation and mechanical ventilation may be required. See p. 503 for information on ventilation therapies.
2. Administer NS, LR, or colloids as ordered to restore intravascular volume. Intravenous fluids should contain multivitamins, magnesium, and thiamine with dextrose in patients with alcohol abuse after the hemodynamic status is stabilized and bleeding has stopped. Carefully monitor patient response: note CVP, PA pressures, and BP.
3. Type and crossmatch for anticipated blood products. Transfuse the patient with blood or blood products to improve tissue oxygenation and correct coagulation deficiencies. Use

uncrossmatched (e.g., O negative) packed RBCs until cross-matched blood is available, as needed. May need to use fast infusers to deliver blood rapidly. Observe for transfusion reaction. (See Blood Administration, p. 585.)

4. Evacuate the stomach contents with a nasogastric tube and initiate lavages with room temperature water or saline to clear blood clots from the stomach. Keep HOB elevated to reduce the risk of aspiration. Remove NG tube after irrigation.

5. Continue to monitor the patient closely once stabilized; rebleeding can occur even up to 1 week after the initial bleeding. Test all gastric secretions and stools for occult blood.

6. Vitamin K and/or fresh-frozen plasma (FFP) may be ordered to correct coagulation deficiencies. Ensure that administration of any anticoagulants (e.g., warfarin, heparin, clopidogrel) is stopped. If patient was receiving heparin before the bleeding episode, anticipate administration of protamine sulfate.

7. Administer proton pump inhibitors (PPIs) (e.g., omeprazole, pantoprazole) as first-line agents to decrease gastric acid secretion rapidly; may supplement with H_2-receptor antagonists (e.g., ranitidine, cimetidine, famotidine); cytoprotection may be provided with sucralfate to prevent mucosal lesion development; antacids should be used cautiously because they may stimulate secretion of hydrochloric acid and promote electrolyte imbalances. Gastric pH should be kept >3.5 or the value established by physician.

8. Explain all procedures and tests to the patient to help alleviate anxiety and decrease tissue oxygen demands.

9. Anticipate endoscopy, hemostatic therapy, and possible arteriography. Anticipate GI surgery (e.g., pyloroplasty, vagotomy, gastrectomy) if medical therapy is unsuccessful.

Management of Esophageal Varices

1. Administer fluids conservatively and monitor CVP (keep pressure <8 mm Hg) because rapid volume expansion can increase portal and variceal pressures, causing further rupture and bleeding.

2. Administer octreotide as ordered to control esophageal bleeding. Intravenous octreotide causes rapid reduction of portal pressure. Dose with a 50- to 100-mcg bolus, followed by a 5- to 50-mcg/hr infusion. A secondary agent that may be tried is intravenous vasopressin. The effects of vasopressin

are similar to octreotide, but this agent has a worrisome adverse effect profile that includes myocardial and/or bowel ischemia. NTG may be given along with vasopressin to reduce the likelihood of these effects. Dose at 0.3 units/min and titrate to desired effect but do not administer more than 0.9 units/min; keep SBP >90 mm Hg.

3. Anticipate balloon tamponade to temporarily control esophageal bleeding if vasopressin and sclerotherapy are unsuccessful. (See Sengstaken-Blakemore tube, p. 552.)

4. Anticipate endoscopic band ligation to obliterate the varices.

5. Anticipate portosystemic shunting (TIPS or surgery) if medical treatment is unsuccessful. (See Transjugular Intrahepatic Portosystemic Shunt [TIPS], p. 571.)

GI

Nursing Diagnosis: RISK FOR ASPIRATION related to vomiting, esophageal tamponade, ileus, increased intragastric pressure, and altered mentation

Outcome Criteria

Lungs clear to auscultation
PaO_2 80 to 100 mm Hg
O_2 sat ≥95%
Afebrile
Absence of vomiting

Patient Monitoring

1. Monitor temperature every 4 hours; elevation may indicate aspiration pneumonia.

2. Continuously monitor oxygen saturation with pulse oximetry (SpO_2). Monitor interventions and patient activities that may adversely affect oxygen saturation.

Patient Assessment

1. Assess LOC; the patient may not be able to protect the airway if mentation is altered.

2. Assess respiratory status: auscultate lungs for excessive secretions or absence of breath sounds that may indicate pneumonia.

3. Assess abdomen: auscultate bowel sounds; absence of intestinal peristalsis can cause increased intragastric pressure and vomiting.

4. If present, assess placement of nasogastric and/or Sengstaken-Blakemore tube.

Diagnostics Assessment

1. Review serial chest radiographs to evaluate placement of nasogastric and Sengstaken-Blakemore tubes and assess lung fields.
2. Review serial ABGs because aspiration can decrease gas exchange.

Patient Management

1. Elevate HOB if the patient is hemodynamically stable; a right side-lying position may enhance gastric emptying if the patient can tolerate this position.
2. If present, maintain patency of the NG tube to promote adequate decompression of the stomach.
3. Secure all tubes to prevent dislodgment and excessive movement that can cause gastric irritation.
4. Restrain or sedate the patient if necessary to prevent tubes from being inadvertently pulled out. Administer sedation cautiously in patients with underlying liver dysfunction.
5. Maintain esophageal tamponade with Sengstaken-Blakemore–type tubes (see p. 552).

ENDOCRINE DISORDERS

ADRENAL CRISIS

Clinical Brief

Acute adrenal insufficiency (AI) is a potentially life-threatening condition related to insufficient synthesis, release, or use of the hormones produced by the adrenal glands. These include the glucocorticoids (e.g., cortisol) and the mineralocorticoids (e.g., aldosterone). Primary adrenal insufficiency (a problem within the adrenal gland) may be idiopathic, but is most often caused by autoimmune injury. It may also be related to a bacterial infection (e.g., tuberculosis or pneumonia), infiltrative disease (e.g., sarcoidosis or amyloidosis), neoplasms, adrenal hemorrhage/infarction, medications, and congenital/hereditary factors. Secondary adrenal insufficiency may be related to reduced adrenocorticotropic (ACTH) hormone release (pituitary insufficiency or irradiation, hypothalamic insufficiency, head trauma, or sepsis) or blunted cortisol production. In secondary AI, aldosterone levels usually are adequate due to the actions of the renin-angiotensin-aldosterone system regulated by the kidneys. Functional adrenal insufficiency may occur secondary to a reduction in ACTH release when exogenous steroids, particularly glucocorticoids, are stopped abruptly.

Aldosterone is one of the key regulators of sodium and water balance. Insufficient amounts of aldosterone may profoundly affect the patient's fluid and electrolyte balance. It may also result in a reduction of the patient's regulation of vascular tone, leading to hypotension. Cortisol is involved in the stress response, as well as immune defenses and glucose regulation. Insufficiency is likely to impair the stress response and alter glucose metabolism, resulting in infection and hypoglycemia.

Presenting Signs and Symptoms

Signs and symptoms of AI may not occur until 80% to 90% of adrenal gland function has been altered. These include GI symptoms: anorexia, nausea, vomiting, weight loss, nonspecific abdominal pain, and diarrhea. The patient may complain of extreme fatigue, muscle pain, and salt craving. Depending on the severity of the fluid and electrolyte imbalance, the patient may present with hypotension or altered LOC.

Physical Examination

Vital signs:

BP: low or orthostatic hypotension (primary AI)

ENDO

HR: tachycardia (primary AI)
RR: increased
Skin:
Pale
Hyperpigmentation (primary AI)
Dehydrated, decreased turgor
Neurologic: confusion, lassitude progressing to unresponsiveness
Gastrointestinal: nausea, vomiting, abdominal pain

Diagnostic Findings

There should be a high index of suspicion if unexplained hypotension (or hypotension unresponsive to vasopressors or inotropes), hypoglycemia, hyperkalemia, and hyponatremia are present. Serum potassium levels may be normal in the presence of diarrhea. A lack of a response to intravenous cosyntropin confirms AI. (A normal response is an increase in the cortisol level of at least 7 mcg/dL over the basal level and a serum cortisol level to at least 20 mcg/dL.)

ACUTE CARE PATIENT MANAGEMENT

Goals of Treatment

Replace glucocorticoids and sometimes mineralocorticoids.
Hydrocortisone
Dexamethasone
Fludrocortisone
Restore fluid, glucose, and electrolyte balance.
Crystalloids
Dextrose
Electrolyte therapy
Reduce stress.
Stress-free environment
Detect/prevent clinical sequelae (Table 5-40).

Table 5-40 CLINICAL SEQUELAE ASSOCIATED WITH ACUTE ADRENAL CRISIS

Complication	Signs and Symptoms
Shock	CI <2.5 L/min/m^2; SBP <90 mm Hg; HR >120 beats/min; change in mental status; cool, clammy skin; oliguria
Electrolyte imbalances	Life-threatening dysrhythmias

CI, Cardiac index; *HR*, heart rate; *SBP*, systolic blood pressure.

Priority Nursing Diagnoses and Potential Complications

Priority Nursing Diagnoses	PC: Potential Complications
Deficient fluid volume	Hypovolemia, decreased cardiac output, electrolyte imbalance
Ineffective protection (see p. 48)	Sepsis
Risk for imbalanced nutrition: less than body requirements (see p. 53)	Negative nitrogen balance
Risk for interrupted family processes (see p. 45)	

Nursing Diagnosis: DEFICIENT FLUID VOLUME related to increased sodium and water excretion secondary to insufficient mineralocorticoids

ENDO

Outcome Criteria

Patient alert and oriented
CVP 2 to 6 mm Hg
PAS 15 to 30 mm Hg
PAD 5 to 15 mm Hg
CI 2.5 to 4 L/min/m^2
SBP 90 to 120 mm Hg
MAP 70 to 105 mm Hg
HR 60 to 100 beats/min
Serum sodium 135 to 145 mEq/L
Urine output 30 mL/hr or 0.5 to 1 mL/kg/hr
Intake approximates output
Elastic skin turgor
Moist mucous membranes

Patient Monitoring

1. Obtain CVP, PA pressures (if available), and BP hourly or more frequently to evaluate hypovolemia and the patient's response to therapy. Monitor CI and MAP; MAP <60 mm Hg adversely affects cerebral and renal perfusion.
2. Monitor fluid volume status: measure urine output hourly; determine fluid balance every 8 hours; compare serial weights for a rapid decrease (0.5-1 kg/day), which suggests fluid loss.
3. Continuously monitor ECG for dysrhythmias secondary to electrolyte imbalance.

Patient Assessment
_____

1. Assess hydration status: thirst, skin turgor on inner thigh or forehead, condition of buccal membranes, and pulse pressure.
2. Assess indicators of tissue perfusion: note LOC, skin color and temperature, peripheral pulses, and capillary refill.
3. Assess the patient for clinical sequelae (see Table 5-40).

Diagnostics Assessment
_____

1. Review serial serum sodium and potassium levels to evaluate the patient's response to therapy.
2. Review serial serum glucose levels; neurologic symptoms of hypoglycemia usually appear when level is <50 mg/dL.

Patient Management
_____

1. Administer D_5NS rapidly to restore volume and provide a glucose source, because the patient may be hypoglycemic. Carefully monitor CVP, PA pressures, BP, and CI to determine fluid needs and signs of fluid volume overload.
2. Administer glucocorticoids (hydrocortisone) as ordered, usually 100 mg IV every 6 hours initially, then tapering the dose as patient condition allows to an oral maintenance dosage of 20 mg every morning and 10 mg every evening. If a diagnosis is not established, dexamethasone 1 to 4 mg IV may be required while results of the cosyntropin stimulation test are pending. Long-term replacement therapy may include glucocorticoid preparations such as prednisone, methylprednisolone, or hydrocortisone.
3. Colloids may be required if fluids and steroid administration do not improve intravascular volume. Sympathomimetic agents will not be effective without glucocorticoid replacement.
4. Fludrocortisone may be required in patients with primary AI to help maintain sodium and potassium balance and control postural hypotension.
5. If the patient is able to take oral fluids, encourage fluids high in sodium to combat excessive sodium excretion.

Nursing Diagnoses: INEFFECTIVE PROTECTION related to decreased immune response, insufficient adrenocorticoids, and electrolyte imbalance

Outcome Criteria
_____

Serum glucose 80 to 110 mg/dL
Serum sodium 135 to 145 mEq/L

Patient alert and oriented
Absence of aspiration
Patient will not injure self

Patient Monitoring

None specific

Patient Assessment

1. Assess LOC because fluid and electrolyte imbalance can alter mentation, which increases the risk of patient injury.
2. Assess respiratory status because a patient with altered mentation may be unable to protect the airway and is at risk for aspiration and respiratory distress. Note rate and depth of respirations; auscultate lungs for decreased or adventitious breath sounds.
3. Assess response to activity and monitor for fatigue because muscle strength may be affected.
4. Assess level of anxiety because added stressors may further compromise patient condition.

Diagnostics Assessment

1. Review serum glucose levels. Neurologic signs of hypoglycemia generally manifest at glucose levels <50 mg/dL.
2. Review sodium levels. Neurologic signs generally manifest at sodium levels <125 mEq/L and become more severe at levels <115 mEq/L.

Patient Management

1. Protect the patient from stimuli or stressors; maintain a quiet, dimly lit room; control room temperature to avoid extremes; screen visitors to allow only those who promote patient relaxation.
2. Explain all procedures and ICU routine so that the patient is not unnecessarily stressed.
3. Maintain bed rest and limit activities until the patient's condition stabilizes.
4. Maintain a patent airway and supply supplemental oxygen as ordered, especially with activity.
5. Increase activity gradually. Terminate activity if there are signs and symptoms of intolerance.
6. Keep the patient NPO until nausea and vomiting (N/V) resolve and patient mentation improves.

ENDO

7. Maintain sterile technique when performing invasive procedures to prevent infection.

DIABETES INSIPIDUS (DI)

Clinical Brief

DI is a disorder characterized by impaired renal conservation of water resulting from a deficiency in antidiuretic hormone (ADH) secretion or renal resistance to ADH. Excessive water loss, hyperosmolality, and hypernatremia result. DI is classified as neurogenic, nephrogenic, dipsogenic, or gestagenic. DI may be transitory or permanent, depending on the cause; however, profound diuresis regardless of the cause will occur. Neurogenic DI (decreased ADH production or release) may be idiopathic or result from pituitary surgery or conditions that disturb the hypothalamus (e.g., head trauma, infection, cancerous brain tumors, or anoxic brain death). Nephrogenic DI occurs if the renal receptors are insensitive or resistant to circulating ADH. Causes include diseased kidneys or drug therapy (lithium carbonate, demeclocycline). Dipsogenic DI occurs with compulsive water consumption. Gestagenic DI is caused by an accelerated breakdown of ADH during pregnancy from a transient increase in vasopressinase, the enzyme that degrades ADH. In all types of DI, patients can excrete from 4 to 24 L/day. As long as patients are able to respond to the thirst mechanism, serum osmolality will remain normal and dehydration will be prevented.

Presenting Signs and Symptoms

The alert patient will complain of polydipsia, polyuria, and fatigue as a result of lack of sleep from nocturia. Unresponsive patients will have profound dehydration or hypovolemic shock.

Physical Examination

Vital signs:
    BP: postural hypotension
    HR: tachycardia
    RR: eupneic
    Temperature: normothermic
Cardiovascular:
    Cool, clammy skin
    Capillary refill >3 sec

Pulse weak, thready

Skin: decreased turgor; dry, sticky mucous membranes

Diagnostic Findings

Water deprivation test demonstrates the following:
    Serum osmolality >300 mOsm/kg
    Serum sodium >145 mEq/L
    Urine osmolality <200 mOsm/L
In addition:
    Decreased serum ADH (normal = 1-5 pg/mL)
    Urine specific gravity <1.005

ACUTE CARE PATIENT MANAGEMENT

ENDO

Goals of Treatment

Restore fluid balance.
    Hypotonic fluid replacement
    Vasopressin
    Treatment of the cause
Detect/prevent clinical sequelae (Table 5-41)

Table 5-41 CLINICAL SEQUELAE ASSOCIATED WITH DIABETES INSIPIDUS

Complication	Signs and Symptoms
Circulatory collapse	Tachycardia, decreasing trend in BP, decreasing trend in urine output, diminished pulse, decreased sensorium, cool clammy skin, restlessness

BP, Blood pressure.

Priority Nursing Diagnoses and Potential Complications

Priority Nursing Diagnoses	PC: Potential Complications
Deficient fluid volume	Hypovolemia, decreased output, electrolyte imbalances
Risk for ineffective protection (see p. 48)	
Risk for interrupted family processes (see p. 45)	
Risk for imbalanced nutrition: less than body requirements (see p. 53)	

Nursing Diagnosis: DEFICIENT FLUID VOLUME related to excessive diuresis of dilute urine secondary to inadequate antidiuretic hormone secretion/response

Outcome Criteria

Patient alert and oriented
Moist buccal membranes
Elastic skin turgor
CVP 2 to 6 mm Hg
PAS 15 to 30 mm Hg
PAD 5 to 15 mm Hg
SBP 90 to 120 mm Hg
MAP 70 to 105 mm Hg
Intake approximates output
Urine osmolality 300 to 1400 mOsm/L
Serum osmolality 275 to 295 mOsm/L
Urine specific gravity 1.001 to 1.030
Serum sodium 135 to 145 mEq/L

Patient Monitoring

1. Monitor CVP and PA pressures (if available) hourly or more frequently to evaluate volume status. Hypovolemic shock can occur.

2. Monitor MAP; MAP <60 mm Hg adversely affects cerebral and renal perfusion.

3. Monitor urine output hourly and determine fluid balance each shift. Urine output can exceed 1 L/hr. Compare daily weights; dramatic weight loss can occur if fluid replacement is inadequate. Neurosurgical patients (neurohypophysis destruction) may develop polyuria immediately after surgery, which lasts for approximately 24 to 48 hours, followed by oliguria for approximately 3 to 4 days before developing permanent polyuria and polydipsia.

Patient Assessment

1. Obtain VS hourly or more often if the patient's condition is unstable; hypovolemic shock can occur. Signs and symptoms include restlessness; cool, clammy skin; tachycardia; and SBP <90 mm Hg.

2. Assess hydration status to evaluate the patient's response to therapy. Note skin turgor on inner thigh or forehead, condition of buccal membranes, complaints of thirst, and resolution of postural hypotension.

3. Assess LOC; mental status changes can be caused by decreased perfusion or dehydration.
4. Assess the patient for clinical sequelae (see Table 5-41).

Diagnostics Assessment

Monitor serum sodium, potassium, and osmolality and urine specific gravity and osmolality to evaluate water deficiency and the patient's response to therapy. Serum osmolality can be calculated:

$$2Na + K + BUN/3 + Glucose/18$$

Patient Management

1. Administer hypotonic fluids as ordered to reduce serum hyperosmolality and prevent circulatory collapse. Fluids are usually titrated to hourly urine output. Monitor the patient for fluid volume overload. NS may be used if signs of circulatory collapse are present.
2. Recognize risk factors that may potentiate osmolality problems such as the administration of TPN or enteral feedings.
3. ADH replacement is required in neurogenic DI. Desmopressin (DDAVP) is the preferred vasopressin agent for ADH replacement therapy and may be administered 2 to 4 mcg daily subcutaneously (subQ) or IV in two divided doses or 10 to 40 mcg/day intranasally in divided doses every 8 to 24 hours. Alternative vasopressin agents include aqueous vasopressin (Pitressin), lysine vasopressin (Diapid), or vasopressin tannate. Be wary of adverse responses with administration of vasopressin agents, including abdominal cramps, HTN, and coronary insufficiency.
4. In patients with nephrogenic DI, thiazide diuretics may be used to deplete sodium and cause increased renal water reabsorption. Nephrogenic DI does not respond to hormonal replacement.
5. Carbamazepine, clofibrate, or chlorpropamide may be helpful to produce and release endogenous vasopressin in patients with insufficient amounts of circulating ADH.
6. Restrict salt and protein intake for patients with nephrogenic DI.
7. Encourage iced fluids when the patient is able to take oral fluids.

ENDO

8. Provide oral hygiene and meticulous skin care to preserve skin integrity. Vasopressin therapy may cause diarrhea, which is a risk factor for skin breakdown.
9. For hypernatremia, see p. 369.

DIABETIC KETOACIDOSIS (DKA)

Clinical Brief

DKA is an acute complication of type 1 diabetes mellitus that is characterized by hyperglycemia, uncontrolled lipolysis (decomposition of fat), ketogenesis (production of ketones), negative nitrogen balance, depletion of vascular volume, hyperkalemia and other electrolyte imbalances, and metabolic acidosis. As a result of a relative or absolute insulin deficiency, uptake of glucose by muscle cells is decreased, production of glucose by the liver is increased, and the metabolism of free fatty acids into ketones is increased. Despite hyperglycemia, cells are unable to use the glucose as their energy source, requiring the conversion of fatty acids and protein into ketone bodies for energy.

Osmotic diuresis occurs; leading to cellular dehydration, hypotension, electrolyte loss, and an anion gap metabolic acidosis. Intracellular potassium is exchanged for excessive extracellular hydrogen ions as an attempt to correct acidosis, resulting in hyperkalemia.

Most cases of DKA are precipitated by common infections, including influenza and urinary tract infections. These infections cause an increase in metabolic needs and increased insulin requirements. Other common causes of DKA include a failure to maintain prescribed insulin and/or dietary regimen and dehydration.

Presenting Signs and Symptoms

Neurologic response may range from alert to comatose. RR may be rapid, or respirations may be deep and rapid (Kussmaul) with a fruity acetone breath. The patient will be dehydrated and may complain of extreme thirst, polyuria, and weakness. Nausea, vomiting, severe abdominal pain, and bloating are often present and can be mistaken for manifestations of an acute condition of the abdomen. Headache, muscle twitching, or tremors may also be present.

Physical Examination

Vital signs:
  BP: orthostatic hypotension

ENDO

HR: tachycardia
RR: tachypnea to Kussmaul's breathing
Temperature: may be elevated (infection) or decreased
Skin:
    Dry, flushed
    Decreased turgor
    Dry buccal membranes
Pulmonary:
    Lungs clear
    Pleuritic pain, friction rubs (dehydration)
Abdominal:
    Vague pain, discomfort, bloating
Musculoskeletal:
    Weakness
    Decreased deep tendon reflexes

ENDO

Diagnostic Findings

Serum glucose >300 mg/dL but not >800 mg/dL
Urine ketones strongly positive
Serum ketones >3 mOsm/L
Blood pH <7.3
Serum bicarbonate <15 mEq/L
Serum osmolality increased but usually <330 mOsm/L
Anion gap >20 mmol/L
Serum potassium initially may be normal or high but will decrease to
    normal or low with successful treatment, as potassium shifts back
    into the intracellular compartment.

ACUTE CARE PATIENT MANAGEMENT

Goals of Treatment

Provide cellular nutrition.
    Insulin therapy
Restore fluid and electrolyte balance and correct acidosis.
    Crystalloids
    Colloids
    Electrolyte therapy
Determine and treat the cause.
    Appropriate treatment
Detect/prevent clinical sequelae (Table 5-42).

Table 5-42 CLINICAL SEQUELAE ASSOCIATED WITH DIABETIC KETOACIDOSIS

Complication	Signs and Symptoms
Circulatory collapse	SBP <90 mm Hg; HR >120 beats/min; change in mental status; cool, clammy skin; diminished pulses
Renal failure	Oliguria, increasing BUN and creatinine
Electrolyte imbalances	Life-threatening dysrhythmias, ileus
Cerebral edema	Lethargy, drowsiness, headache during successful therapy

BUN, Blood urea nitrogen; *HR,* heart rate; *SBP,* systolic blood pressure.

Priority Nursing Diagnoses and Potential Complications

Priority Nursing Diagnoses	PC: Potential Complications
Deficient fluid volume	Hypovolemia, decreased cardiac output, electrolyte imbalances
Risk for injury	Hyperglycemia, metabolic acidosis
Risk for imbalanced nutrition (see p. 53)	Negative nitrogen balance
Risk for interrupted family processes (see p. 45)	

ENDO

Nursing Diagnosis: DEFICIENT FLUID VOLUME related to osmotic diuresis secondary to hyperglycemia and lack of adequate oral intake

Outcome Criteria

CVP 2 to 6 mm Hg
PAS 15 to 30 mm Hg
PAD 5 to 15 mm Hg
SBP 90 to 120 mm Hg
MAP 70 to 105 mm Hg
HR 60 to 100 beats/min
RR 12 to 20 breaths/min
Urine output 30 mL/hr or 0.5 to 1 mL/kg/hr
Serum glucose 250 mg/dL during initial phase of treatment; eventual goal is to achieve normal serum glucose levels of 80 to 110 mg/dL
Serum osmolality 275 to 295 mOsm/kg
Serum sodium 135 to 145 mEq/L
Serum potassium 4 to 5 mEq/L
Elastic skin turgor
Moist buccal membranes

Patient Monitoring

1. Obtain PA pressures (if available), and CVP hourly or more frequently if the patient's condition is unstable or during fluid resuscitation. Both parameters reflect the capacity of the vascular system to accept volume and can be used to monitor fluid volume status. Increasing values suggest fluid overload; decreasing values suggest hypovolemia.

2. Monitor MAP; a MAP <60 mm Hg can adversely affect cerebral and renal perfusion.

3. Continuously monitor ECG to detect life-threatening dysrhythmias that may be caused by hyperkalemia or hypokalemia.

4. Monitor serum glucose levels with a glucometer every 1 to 2 hours during acute phase to evaluate the patient's response to therapy.

5. Accurately monitor fluid volume status: measure urine output hourly, determine fluid balance every 8 hours, and compare serial weights. Fluid deficit may be as high as 6 L.

6. Calculate serum osmolality and monitor trends.

Patient Assessment

1. Obtain VS: BP, MAP, HR, and RR, hourly or more frequently if the patient's condition is unstable or during fluid resuscitation to evaluate the patient's response to therapy. Kussmaul's breathing is associated with a pH <7.2.

2. Assess hydration status: note skin turgor on inner thigh or forehead, condition of buccal membranes, and development of edema or crackles after fluid resuscitation initiated.

3. Assess LOC carefully during fluid resuscitation because cerebral edema may result from overly aggressive volume replacement. Children with type 1 diabetes who presented with DKA at the time of diagnosis are particularly at risk for cerebral edema, which is often fatal.

4. Assess respiratory status to determine the rate and depth of respirations or adventitious breath sounds. Potassium imbalance can cause respiratory arrest; rapid fluid resuscitation may cause fluid overload.

5. Assess GI status: nausea, abdominal distention, and absence of bowel sounds may indicate ileus.

6. Assess the patient for clinical sequelae (see Table 5-42).

ENDO

Diagnostics Assessment

1. Review serial serum glucose levels (in addition to bedside monitoring) to evaluate the patient's response to insulin therapy.
2. Review serum electrolytes (e.g., sodium, potassium, and magnesium) because imbalances are associated with osmotic diuresis. Potassium in particular should be evaluated every 1 to 2 hours. Seizures may be associated with hyponatremia; ileus and dysrhythmias may result with potassium imbalances.
3. Review indicators of renal function: creatinine and BUN. Patients could be at risk for prerenal acute renal failure from profound vascular volume depletion.
4. Review ABGs to evaluate oxygenation status and resolution or worsening of metabolic acidosis.
5. Review culture reports to identify presence of infecting organism.

Patient Management

1. Administer crystalloids as ordered to correct dehydration. NS boluses of up to 1000 mL/hr may be required until urine output, VS, and clinical assessment reflect an adequate hydration state. Less aggressive fluid resuscitation may be necessary for patients with a history of cardiovascular disease, particularly HF. Half-strength saline rather than NS may be required in these patients. Anticipate addition of 5% dextrose to intravenous infusions when serum glucose is ≤250 mg/dL, to prevent rebound hypoglycemia.
2. Offer small, frequent sips of water or ice chips if the patient is permitted to take fluids by mouth.
3. Provide frequent oral hygiene because dehydration causes drying of the mucous membranes.
4. Provide intravenous insulin therapy as ordered. Typical regimen begins with a loading dose of 0.15 units of insulin/kg, followed by maintenance infusion of 0.1 units of insulin/kg/hr. Insulin drip may be discontinued and subQ insulin may be initiated when serum glucose is ≤250 mg/dL, acidosis is corrected, and the patient is able to tolerate oral intake.

ENDO

Nursing Diagnosis: RISK FOR INJURY related to altered mental status secondary to acidosis, electrolyte imbalances, and impaired glucose utilization secondary to lack of insulin

Outcome Criteria

Patient alert and oriented

Patient will not injure self

Serum glucose 250 mg/dL during initial phase of treatment; eventual goal is to achieve normal serum glucose levels of 80 to 110 mg/dL

pH 7.35 to 7.45

Absence of serum and urine ketones

Serum bicarbonate 22 to 26 mEq/L

Patient Monitoring

None specific

ENDO

Patient Assessment

1. Assess LOC, which may range from confusion to frank coma. Too rapid a reduction in serum glucose (>100 mg/dL/hr) also may impair cerebral function. If the patient experiences headache, lethargy, or drowsiness during successful therapy, suspect cerebral edema.
2. Assess the patient for clinical sequelae (see Table 5-42).

Diagnostics Assessment

1. Review serial serum glucose levels (in addition to bedside monitoring with glucometer) to evaluate the patient's response to insulin therapy.
2. Review ABGs to evaluate oxygenation status and resolution or worsening of metabolic acidosis.

Patient Management

1. Administer regular insulin as ordered, after serum potassium levels are obtained. Rarely, some patients have hypokalemic DKA; in these instances, administration of intravenous insulin before the potassium level is corrected could be lethal. Typical regimen begins with a loading dose of 0.15 units of insulin/kg, followed by maintenance infusion of 0.1 units of insulin/kg/hr. Glucose should drop 40 to 80 mg/dL/hr. Too

rapid a fall in serum glucose levels can cause cerebral edema. If the serum glucose level does not decrease in 2 hours, doubling the dose of insulin infusion may be necessary. If cerebral edema occurs, anticipate mannitol administration.

2. Anticipate addition of dextrose with half normal saline (0.45 NS) when the glucose level is ≤250 mg/dL to prevent hypoglycemia and cerebral edema.

3. Subcutaneous administration of insulin can be started when serum glucose is ≤250 mg/dL, pH is >7.2, or CO_2 is 15 to 18 mEq/L, and the patient is able to tolerate oral intake. Generally, an insulin infusion will be discontinued 1 to 2 hours after the patient receives subQ insulin.

4. Anticipate potassium supplementation (potassium chloride, potassium phosphate, and potassium acetate) to replace potassium loss as a result of urinary excretion, as a result of correction of metabolic acidosis, or secondary to cellular uptake with insulin therapy. Validate urine output before administering potassium. If hypokalemia is refractory to therapy, consider magnesium replacement.

5. Sodium bicarbonate is considered only if the serum pH is <7.

6. NG intubation may be required to reduce the risk of vomiting and aspiration in the patient with altered mentation. Keep the patient NPO until he or she is alert and vomiting has ceased.

7. Intubation and mechanical ventilation may be required if the patient is unable to protect the airway or to adequately ventilate and oxygenate. Position patient to decrease risk of aspiration and ventilator-acquired pneumonia.

8. Assist the conscious patient to C&DB to prevent pulmonary stasis and atelectasis. Reposition the unconscious patient every 1 to 2 hours and suction secretions as needed.

9. Provide meticulous skin care to prevent impaired skin integrity; inspect bony prominences. Maintain body alignment in the unconscious patient.

10. Frequently orient the patient to the surroundings. Keep the bed in low position and side rails up.

HYPERGLYCEMIC HYPEROSMOLAR NONKETOSIS (HHNK)

Clinical Brief

HHNK is a rare condition known interchangeably as nonketotic hyperosmolar syndrome (NKHS), nonketotic hyperglycemia (NKH), and hyperosmolar hyperglycemic nonketotic state (HHNS). As its multiple names or titles imply, it is a syndrome characterized by extreme hyperglycemia and intravascular volume depletion without ketonemia and with minimal or absent acidosis and ketonuria. It occurs most often in older patients with type 2 diabetes mellitus and is precipitated by another acute illness, such as influenza or bacterial pneumonia. Other factors associated with HHNK can include a change in diet or the introduction of new medications to the patient's daily regimen, including corticosteroids, thiazide diuretics, furosemide, interferon, potassium supplements, phenytoin sodium, and propranolol. The inciting physiologic stressor causes a disruption in the body's metabolism so that the body does not have sufficient insulin to prevent hyperglycemia yet has enough endogenous insulin to prevent lipolysis, and thus ketosis. The ensuing hyperglycemia, however, can be significant, resulting in an osmotic diuresis and increased serum osmolality. In the presence of serum glucose levels >1000 mg/dL, profound dehydration, and hyperosmolar plasma >330 mOsm/L, the patient typically exhibits clinical manifestations consistent with hypovolemic shock and a hypertonic encephalopathy or cerebral edema that results in coma. This serious consequence is called hyperglycemic hyperosmolar nonketotic coma (HHNC).

ENDO

Presenting Signs and Symptoms

Signs and symptoms include severe dehydration with mild or no N/V. HHNK resembles DKA in many ways (with the exception of the profound dehydration): polyuria, polyphagia, weakness, and confusion (Table 5-43). Neurologic signs are more predominant, and often increased lethargy is the chief complaint. Up to half of the patients present comatose (HHNC). Focal neurologic signs such as hemisensory deficits, hemiparesis, aphasia, and seizures may mimic a cerebrovascular accident.

Physical Examination

Vital signs:
    HR: tachycardia
    BP: low systolic, orthostatic hypotension
    RR: rapid and shallow (not Kussmaul), absence of fruity breath
    Temperature: normothermic or hyperthermic, depending on underlying process
Neurologic:
    Altered mental status
    Focal neurologic signs may be present
    +4 reflexes

Table 5-43   Comparison of Clinical Signs of Diabetic Ketoacidosis (DKA) and Hyperglycemic Hyperosmolar Nonketosis (HHNK)

Parameter	DKA	HHNK
Respirations	Kussmaul	Regular
Serum glucose	300-800 mg/dL	Typically >800 mg/dL
Serum osmolality	295-330 mOsm/L	320-350 mOsm/L
Serum bicarbonate	<15 mEq/L	22-26 mEq/L
Blood pH	<7.3	Normal to mild acidosis
Serum ketones	>3 mOsm/L	Absent
Urine ketones	Strongly positive	Negative or slight
Serum sodium	Mean 132 mEq/L	Mean 145 mEq/L
BUN	Mean 41 mg/dL	Mean 65 mg/dL

BUN, Blood urea nitrogen.

ENDO

Skin:

    Pale, dry, with decreased turgor

    Dry buccal membranes

    Tongue dry, furrowed

Cardiovascular:

    Pulse weak and thready

    Capillary refill >3 sec

Diagnostic Findings

Serum glucose >800 mg/dL, averaging 1200 mg/dL

Serum sodium >147 mEq/L

Serum potassium initially may be normal or high

pH normal to mild acidosis <7.3

Serum bicarbonate 22 to 26 mEq/L

Serum osmolality 320 to 350 mOsm/L

Urine acetone/ketones negative or trace amounts

Urine specific gravity >1.022

ACUTE CARE PATIENT MANAGEMENT

Goals of Treatment

Restore fluid and electrolyte balance.

    Crystalloids

    Electrolyte therapy

Improve glucose/insulin ratio.

Insulin therapy
Determine and treat the cause.
Appropriate therapy
Detect/prevent clinical sequelae (Table 5-44).

Table 5-44 CLINICAL SEQUELAE ASSOCIATED WITH HYPERGLYCEMIC
HYPEROSMOLAR NONKETOSIS (HHNK)

Complication	Signs and Symptoms
Neurologic deficits	Focal changes, generalized seizures, hemiparesis, sensory deficits, coma (HHNC)
Hypovolemic shock	SBP <90 mm Hg; HR >120 beats/min; weak, thready pulse; progressive deterioration in LOC; cool, clammy skin
Renal failure	Decreased urinary output, increasing BUN and creatinine
Venous thromboemboli (VTE)	Calf pain, SOB, neurologic deficits

BUN, Blood urea nitrogen; *HHNC,* hyperglycemic hyperosmolar nonketotic coma; *HR,* heart rate; *LOC,* level of consciousness; *SBP,* systolic blood pressure; *SOB,* shortness of breath.

Priority Nursing Diagnoses and Potential Complications

Priority Nursing Diagnoses	PC: Potential Complications
Deficient fluid volume	Hypovolemia, electrolyte imbalances
Risk for injury	Hyperglycemia, seizures
Risk for imbalanced nutrition: less than body requirements (see p. 53)	
Risk for ineffective protection (see p. 48)	
Risk for interrupted family processes (see p. 45)	

Nursing Diagnosis: DEFICIENT FLUID VOLUME related to osmotic diuresis, inability to take oral fluids, nausea, and vomiting

Outcome Criteria

CVP 2 to 6 mm Hg
PAS 15 to 30 mm Hg
PAD 5 to 15 mm Hg

ENDO

SBP 90 to 120 mm Hg
MAP 70 to 105 mm Hg
Absence of nausea and vomiting
Moist buccal membranes
Elastic skin turgor
Serum osmolality 275 to 295 mOsm/L
Serum potassium 3.5 to 5.5 mEq/L
Urine output 30 mL/hr or 0.5 to 1 mL/kg/hr

Patient Monitoring

1. Obtain CVP, PA pressures (if available), and BP readings every 15 minutes during fluid resuscitation and evaluate the patient's response to therapy. Monitor MAP; MAP <60 mm Hg adversely affects cerebral and renal perfusion.
2. Monitor fluid volume status: measure urine output hourly, determine fluid balance every 8 hours, and compare serial weights for rapid (0.5-1 kg/day) changes that suggest fluid imbalance.
3. Continuously monitor ECG because dysrhythmias may be precipitated by electrolyte imbalance associated with diuresis.

Patient Assessment

1. Monitor HR, RR, and BP every 15 minutes during fluid resuscitation and note the patient's response to therapy.
2. Assess the patient's hydration status: note skin turgor on inner thigh or forehead, condition of buccal membranes, and development of edema or crackles. Calculate osmolality.
3. Assess tissue perfusion: note LOC, peripheral pulses, and skin temperature and moisture. Hypovolemia may lead to shock.
4. Assess for pressure ulcer development secondary to hypoperfusion.
5. Assess for gastric distention and absent bowel sounds, which would suggest ileus.
6. Assess the patient for clinical sequelae (see Table 5-44).

Diagnostics Assessment

1. Review serial ABGs to evaluate hypoxemia and acidosis, which may be present with shock.
2. Review serial electrolyte levels (e.g., sodium, potassium, and magnesium) to evaluate the need for replacement or the patient's response to therapy.

3. Review serial serum osmolality and evaluate patient response to therapy.
4. Review serial Hgb and Hct levels; increased levels are associated with profound diuresis and increase blood viscosity.

Patient Management

1. Fluid resuscitation with NS ≤1 L/hr may be required if the patient is hypotensive and tachycardic. Fluid requirements may exceed 10 L; 0.45 NS may be used if hypernatremia is present or the patient manifests signs and symptoms of HF. D_5W is administered when serum glucose reaches between 250 and 300 mg/dL. May need to administer fluids with caution with patients with known or suspected history of cardiovascular disease.
2. Administer insulin as ordered, usually regular insulin 0.1 to 0.2 units/kg/hr.
3. Plasma expanders such as albumin may be required if isotonic solutions do not improve intravascular volume.
4. Administer potassium supplements as ordered to prevent adverse effects on the myocardium and GI and respiratory muscles; validate adequate urine output before potassium administration. If hypokalemia is refractory to therapy, consider magnesium replacement.
5. Keep the patient NPO while nauseated and vomiting; NG intubation may be required if ileus develops or the patient is at risk for aspiration.
6. Prophylactic low-dose heparin or LMWH therapy may be ordered to prevent clotting associated with increased blood viscosity secondary to profound diuresis.
7. Antibiotic therapy will be ordered if the patient has an underlying infection.
8. Initiate pressure ulcer prevention strategies. e.g., meticulous skin care, repositioning, relieving pressure points.
9. See information on electrolyte imbalances, pp. 348-375.

Nursing Diagnosis: RISK FOR INJURY related to altered level of consciousness secondary to insulin insufficiency, cerebral edema, or cellular dehydration

Outcome Criteria

Patient alert and oriented
Patient will not injure self
Absence of seizure activity

ENDO

Serum sodium 135 to 145 mEq/L
Serum glucose <250 mg/dL
Serum osmolality 275 to 295 mOsm/kg

Patient Monitoring

Monitor bedside serum glucose levels at least hourly.

Patient Assessment

1. Assess neurologic status every 15 to 30 minutes during fluid resuscitation when risk of cerebral edema is especially high. LOC will improve as osmolality decreases.
2. Assess the patient for clinical sequelae (see Table 5-44).

Diagnostics Assessment

1. Evaluate serum glucose and serum osmolality to determine effectiveness of therapy.
2. Carefully monitor hourly potassium levels; while hyperglycemia and deficient fluid volume are corrected, potassium will shift intracellularly, resulting in hypokalemia.

Patient Management

1. Administer insulin as ordered. Generally, a bolus of regular insulin 0.1 to 0.2 units/kg is given IV, followed by an insulin infusion at 0.1 to 0.2 units/kg/hr until the serum glucose reaches 250 mg/dL. Lowering serum glucose too rapidly (>100 mg/dL/hr) may result in hypoglycemia.
2. Institute seizure precautions: pad side rails, reduce environmental stimuli, place bed in low position, and have emergency equipment (oral airway, suction) available.
3. Keep HOB elevated if BP has stabilized and keep NG tube patent to decrease the risk of aspiration.

HYPOGLYCEMIA (HYPERINSULINISM, INSULIN SHOCK, INSULIN COMA)

Clinical Brief

Hypoglycemia is a condition characterized by a serum glucose level <50 mg/dL caused by glucose production inadequate to meet glucose demands. It is characterized either as postprandial or fasting. Postprandial primarily occurs after surgical modification of the upper GI tract. Fasting hypoglycemia is most commonly caused by excessive administration of insulin or oral hypoglycemics, too much exercise, or too little food. Ingestion of alcohol or salicylates, use of β-adrenergic blocking agents, and tapering of corticosteroids can be contributing factors. Iatrogenically induced hypoglycemia can result if serum glucose is rapidly reduced in the treatment of DKA or if the rate of a parenteral nutrition (PN) infusion abruptly drops or ceases. Onset is rapid and the symptoms are primarily neurologic. Repeated or prolonged periods of hypoglycemia can lead to permanent neurologic damage (especially in children) or to death. Older patients who have other disease conditions that cause them to be debilitated and patients with "hypoglycemia unawareness" (low blood sugar episodes without early-stage symptoms) are at risk for developing severe hypoglycemia.

Presenting Signs and Symptoms

Mild hypoglycemia is associated with adrenergic symptoms: pallor, diaphoresis, tachycardia, palpitations, hunger, widened pulse pressure, and shakiness. Patients who are taking β-adrenergic blocking agents may not exhibit these symptoms. Patients are totally alert during mild hypoglycemic episodes.

Moderate hypoglycemia is characterized by neuroglycopenic signs: headache, inability to concentrate, confusion, irrational behavior, slurred speech, blurred vision, paresthesias, fatigue, or somnolence. Severe hypoglycemia includes neuroglycopenic signs or loss of consciousness and seizures. Signs and symptoms are particularly prominent if the serum glucose falls rapidly.

Physical Examination

Vital signs:
    HR: tachycardia
    BP: hypertension (HTN) initially, progressing to shock; widened
        pulse pressure
    RR: shallow and rapid initially, progressing to bradypnea
    Temperature: normal
Neurologic:
    Visual disturbances
    Dilated pupils
    Numbness of tongue and lips
    Change in LOC
    Seizures
    Paresthesias or paralysis
Skin:
    Pallor

ENDO

Diaphoresis
Cool to touch

Diagnostic Findings

Serum glucose <50 mg/dL
Serum ketones negative

ACUTE CARE PATIENT MANAGEMENT

Goals of Treatment

Restore serum glucose level.
10% to 50% dextrose IV
Intravenous therapy with 5% to 10% glucose solution

Priority Nursing Diagnoses and Potential Complications	
Priority Nursing Diagnoses	**PC: Potential Complications**
Risk for injury	Hypoglycemia (and rebound hypoglycemia), seizures
Risk for ineffective protection (see p. 48)	
Risk for imbalanced nutrition: less than body requirements (see p. 53)	
Risk for interrupted family processes (see p. 45)	

Nursing Diagnosis: RISK FOR INJURY related to central nervous system (CNS) dysfunction secondary to lack of glucose energy source

Outcome Criteria

Patient will not injure self
Patient alert and oriented
Absence of seizures
Serum glucose between 80 and 110 mg/dL

Patient Monitoring

Bedside glucose monitoring with glucometer for quick evaluation of glucose level. May be performed hourly during initial treatment. Glucose should be raised to 100 mg/dL.

Patient Assessment

1. Observe for adrenergic symptoms: tachycardia and HTN. Note onset of palpitations, shakiness, pallor, or diaphoresis.

These symptoms may indicate recurrence of a hypoglycemic episode.

2. Assess for changes in LOC, speech, vision, and behavior, which may signal neuroglycopenia.

3. Be particularly attuned to acute onset of diaphoresis and tachycardia in patients receiving neuromuscular blockade. Patients may additionally evidence acute change in train-of-four twitches with peripheral nerve stimulator (PNS).

Diagnostics Assessment

1. Review serum glucose levels to monitor the patient's response to nutritional and glucose support.

2. If the patient remains unconscious with a serum glucose of 200 mg/dL, suspect neurologic residual.

Patient Management

1. If the patient is symptomatic but conscious, administer a rapidly absorbed, glucose-containing food or liquid (e.g., 120 mL of orange juice or apple juice, sugar cubes, honey, hard candy, or syrup). At least 10 g of carbohydrate is required to raise the blood sugar. Repeat every 5 to 10 minutes until symptoms begin to subside. Recheck glucose level in 20 to 30 minutes. Intravenous therapy of D_5W may be ordered for continued glucose support.

2. If the patient is unconscious, administer dextrose 10% to 50% solution IV as ordered. Intravenous therapy of D_5W or $D_{10}W$ may be ordered for continued glucose support. Supplement intravenous dextrose with oral carbohydrates when the patient awakens to prevent rebound hypoglycemia.

3. If long-acting oral antidiabetic agents (e.g., sulfonylureas) have been implicated as the cause of the hypoglycemic episode, the patient is at heightened risk for rebound hypoglycemia. Octreotide may be useful in preventing rebound.

4. Institute seizure precautions: pad side rails; place the bed in low position; and have emergency equipment available, such as oral airway and suction.

5. To prevent Wernicke-Korsakoff syndrome, patients with known or suspected alcoholism should receive thiamine 100 mg IV because it promotes carbohydrate metabolism.

6. Maintain a safe environment.

ENDO

MYXEDEMA COMA

Clinical Brief

Myxedema coma is a life-threatening condition in which patients with underlying thyroid dysfunction exhibit exaggerated manifestations of hypothyroidism. Precipitating factors may include (but are not limited to) infection, trauma, surgery, HF, stroke, or CNS depressants. Hypothyroidism depresses metabolic rate, thus seriously affecting all body systems. The clinical signs of myxedema coma and thyroid storm are compared in Table 5-45.

Table 5-45 COMPARISON OF CLINICAL SIGNS OF THYROID STORM AND MYXEDEMA COMA

	Thyroid Storm	Myxedema Coma
Blood pressure	Increased	Decreased
Heart rate	Tachycardia	Bradycardia
Respiratory rate	Tachypnea	Bradypnea
Temperature	>102.2° F (39° C)	<95° F (<35° C)
Fluid balance	Dehydrated	Overload
Serum glucose	Hyperglycemia	Hypoglycemia
Cardiac index	Increased	Decreased
SVRI	Decreased	Increased
Serum sodium	Hyponatremia or hypernatremia	Hyponatremia
TSH	<0.1 microU/mL	>20 microU/mL
Serum T_4	>12.5 mcg/dL	<5 mcg/dL
Serum T_3	>230 ng/100 mL	<110 ng/100 mL
Resin T_3 uptake	>35%	<25%

SVRI, Systemic vascular resistance index; *TSH,* thyroid-stimulating hormone.

Presenting Signs and Symptoms

The predominant features are hypothermia, hypoventilation, and decreased mental function. Profound fatigue, activity intolerance, and hyporeflexia may precede its onset. Signs and symptoms of cardiac or respiratory failure may also be present.

ENDO

Physical Examination

Vital signs:
   BP: hypotension or hypertension
   HR: bradycardia
   RR: bradypnea
   Temperature: hypothermic <95° F (35° C)
Skin: coarse and dry, possibly carotene color, periorbital and facial
   edema
Neurologic:
   Obtunded, coma or seizures
   Delayed reflexes
Gastrointestinal: decreased bowel sounds
Endocrine: thyroid may be nonpalpable, enlarged, or nodular

Diagnostic Findings

Diagnosis is based on a high index of suspicion. Thyroid studies
indicating primary hypothyroidism include the following:
Elevated thyroid-stimulating hormone (TSH) level (gold standard test) and low free thyroxine index (if TSH results not
   definitive).
Other: hyponatremia and hypoglycemia may be present; ECG
   demonstrates low-voltage, prolonged QT interval and flattened or
   inverted T wave.
Cortisol level also may be low.

ACUTE CARE PATIENT MANAGEMENT

Goals of Treatment

Increase thyroid hormone levels.
   Thyroid replacement
Improve ventilation/oxygenation.
   Supplemental oxygen
   Intubation/mechanical ventilation
Restore normothermia.
   Warming methods
Restore hemodynamic stability.
   Crystalloids
   Vasopressor agents
Detect/prevent clinical sequelae (Table 5-46).

Table 5-46   CLINICAL SEQUELAE ASSOCIATED WITH MYXEDEMA COMA

Complication	Signs and Symptoms
Respiratory failure	Pao_2 <50 mm Hg, $Paco_2$ >50 mm Hg, pH <7.35
Cardiac failure	PAWP >20 mm Hg, increased JVP, crackles, S_3, decreased heart sounds, murmur
Bowel obstruction	Distended abdomen, vomiting, hypoactive/absent bowel sounds
Acute adrenal insufficiency	Hyponatremia, decreased cortisol, hypoglycemia

JVP, Jugular venous pressure; *PAWP,* pulmonary artery wedge pressure.

ENDO

Priority Nursing Diagnoses and Potential Complications

Priority Nursing Diagnoses	PC: Potential Complications
Hypothermia	
Impaired gas exchange	Hypoxemia
Decreased cardiac output	Dysrhythmias
Risk for injury	Seizures, hyponatremia
Ineffective protection (see p. 48)	
Risk for interrupted family processes (see p. 45)	

Nursing Diagnosis: **HYPOTHERMIA** related to decreased metabolism secondary to hypothyroidism

Outcome Criterion

T 97.7° to 100° F (36.5°-37.8° C)

Patient Monitoring

1. Continuously monitor core temperature (if possible) to evaluate the patient's response to therapy.
2. Assess the patient for clinical sequelae (see Table 5-46).

Patient Assessment

Assess neurologic status: note LOC.

Diagnostics Assessment

None specific

Patient Management

1. Administer thyroid hormone as ordered and carefully monitor cardiac patients for myocardial ischemia, chest pain, and ECG changes using one of the two following typical regimens.

2. Levothyroxine: given at 50 to 100 mcg IV every 6 to 8 hours for 24 hours, followed by a daily dose of 50 to 100 mcg IV until oral agents can be tolerated.

   Or levothyroxine: loading dose of 300 to 500 mcg IV, followed by a daily dose of 50 to 100 mcg IV until oral agents can be tolerated. (This loading dose regimen may be associated with increased myocardial ischemic sequelae and is reserved for only the most profoundly ill patients with myxedema coma.)

3. Corticosteroids may also be administered; these are particularly indicated for patients who receive a loading dose bolus of levothyroxine.

4. Institute passive rewarming methods; a thermal blanket may be necessary to increase body temperature. Use cautiously; rewarming may cause vasodilation and hypotension. (See p. 605 for information about thermal regulation.)

ENDO

Nursing Diagnosis: IMPAIRED GAS EXCHANGE related to respiratory muscle weakness and blunted central respiratory response to hypoxemia and hypercapnia

Outcome Criteria

Patient alert and oriented
RR 12 to 20 breaths/min, eupnea
PaO_2 80 to 100 mm Hg
$PaCO_2$ 35 to 45 mm Hg
pH 7.35 to 7.45
O_2 sat ≥95%

Patient Monitoring

1. Continuously monitor oxygen saturation with pulse oximetry (SpO_2). Monitor patient activities and interventions that can adversely affect oxygen saturation.

2. Continuously monitor ECG for dysrhythmias that may be related to hypoxemia or acid-base imbalance.

Patient Assessment

1. Assess respiratory status: note RR, rhythm, and depth. Patients are generally intubated and their lungs are mechanically ventilated.
2. Assess the patient for clinical sequelae (see Table 5-46).

Diagnostics Assessment

Review serial ABGs to evaluate oxygenation and acid-base balance.

Patient Management

1. Administer supplemental oxygen as ordered (for patient management of ventilation therapies, see p. 506.)
2. Administer levothyroxine as prescribed.
3. Reposition the patient to improve oxygenation and mobilize secretions. Evaluate the patient's response to position changes with SpO_2 or ABGs to determine the best position for oxygenation.
4. As the patient stabilizes hemodynamically, provide pulmonary hygiene to prevent complications.
5. Avoid administering CNS depressants because they are slowly metabolized by the hypothyroid patient.

Nursing Diagnosis: DECREASED CARDIAC OUTPUT related to bradycardia and decreased stroke volume

Outcome Criteria

Patient alert and oriented
SBP 90 to 120 mm Hg
MAP 70 to 105 mm Hg
HR 60 to 100 beats/min
Urine output 30 mL/hr or 0.5 to 1 mL/kg/hr
Peripheral pulses palpable
PAS 15 to 30 mm Hg
PAD 5 to 15 mm Hg
CI 2.5 to 4 L/min/m^2

Patient Monitoring

1. Continuously monitor ECG for dysrhythmias or profound bradycardia that can adversely affect CO. A prolonged QT interval is associated with torsades de pointes. Monitor for ST-T changes suggestive of the untoward complication of

ENDO

    myocardial ischemia with introduction of levothyroxine therapy.

2. Continuously monitor PA pressures, CVP (if available), and BP. Obtain CI and PAWP to evaluate cardiac function and the patient's response to therapy. Monitor MAP; a MAP <60 mm Hg adversely affects cerebral and renal perfusion.

3. Monitor fluid volume status: measure urine output hourly and determine fluid balance every 8 hours; compare serial weights; a rapid (0.5-1 kg/day) change suggests fluid imbalance.

Patient Assessment

1. Assess cardiovascular status: note quality of peripheral pulses and capillary refill. Observe for increase in JVP and pulsus paradoxus, which may indicate pericardial effusion. Obtain HR and auscultate heart sounds, and breath sounds for development of HF. Observe for tachycardia and myocardial ischemia with thyroid hormone replacement therapy.

2. Assess the patient for clinical sequelae (see Table 5-46).

Diagnostics Assessment

Review thyroid studies as available. TSH levels should decline within 24 hours of therapy and should normalize after 7 days of therapy.

Patient Management

1. Administer intravenous fluids as ordered to maintain SBP >90 mm Hg; carefully monitor for fluid overload and development of HF.

2. Vasopressor agents may be used if hypotension is refractory to volume administration and if thyroid replacement has not had time to act. Carefully monitor the patient for lethal dysrhythmias.

Nursing Diagnoses: RISK FOR INJURY related to altered level of consciousness and deficient fluid volume secondary to impaired free water clearance

Outcome Criteria

Patient alert and oriented
Absence of seizures
Patient will not injure self
Intake approximates output
Serum sodium 135 to 145 mEq/L

ENDO

Serum osmolality 275 to 295 mOsm/L
Urine specific gravity 1.001 to 1.035

Patient Monitoring

1. Monitor fluid volume status: measure I&O hourly, determine fluid balance every 8 hours. Compare serial weights; a rapid (0.5-1 kg/day) change indicates fluid imbalance. Weight gain without edema may be observed.
2. Monitor LOC with Glasgow Coma Scale. Deterioration in LOC may be associated with water intoxication.

Patient Assessment

1. Assess for complaints of headache, fatigue, or weakness.
2. Assess hydration status: note skin turgor on inner thigh or forehead, observe buccal membranes, and assess thirst.
3. Assess the patient's lungs for adventitious sounds; assess heart sounds for development of S_3 (a hallmark of HF).
4. Assess the patient for clinical sequelae (see Table 5-46).

Diagnostics Assessment

Review serum sodium, serum osmolality, and urine specific gravity. Hyponatremia may be contributing to the obtunded state.

Patient Management

1. If the sodium level is <120 mEq/L, isotonic saline may be administered and free water restricted. (See p. 369 for management of hyponatremia.)
2. Carefully administer fluids and diuretics. Explain fluid restriction to patient.
3. Institute seizure precautions.
4. Hydrocortisone 50 to 100 mg IV every 6 to 8 hours may be ordered until adrenal function normalizes.
5. Maintain safe environment. Reorient the confused patient with each interaction. Institute fall precautions.

SYNDROME OF INAPPROPRIATE ANTIDIURETIC HORMONE (SIADH)

Clinical Brief

SIADH is a condition that results from failure in the negative feedback mechanisms that regulate inhibition and secretion of ADH. It produces excess ADH, resulting in hyponatremia and hypoosmolality of serum. The kidneys respond by reabsorbing water in the tubules and excreting sodium; thus the patient becomes severely water intoxicated. SIADH is most commonly caused by ectopic production of ADH by malignant tumors. It can be the result of CNS disorders, such as Guillain-Barré syndrome, meningitis, brain tumors, and head trauma. Pulmonary-related conditions, such as pneumonia, and positive pressure ventilation can cause SIADH. Pharmacologic agents such as general anesthetics, thiazide diuretics, oral hypoglycemics, chemotherapeutic agents, and analgesics are also associated with SIADH release.

Presenting Signs and Symptoms

Signs and symptoms depend on the degree and rate of onset of hyponatremia. The patient may complain of a headache, muscle cramps, and lethargy or have seizures or coma. If alert, the patient usually complains of nausea, vomiting, and anorexia with related muscle weakness and loss. Weight gain may result from increased water retention, although the patient does not appear edematous.

Physical Examination

    Vital signs:
        BP: ↑ or may be normal
        HR: tachycardia
        Temperature: ↓ or may be normal
    Neurologic:
        Alert to unresponsiveness
        Seizures
Cardiovascular: bounding pulses
Pulmonary: crackles may be present
Gastrointestinal:
    Cramps
    Decreased bowel sounds
    Vomiting
Musculoskeletal:
    Weakness
    Cramps
    Absent deep tendon reflexes

Diagnostic Findings

    A water load test confirms the diagnosis.
Serum sodium <120 mEq/L, normalizes with water restriction
Serum osmolality <250 mOsm/kg
Serum potassium <3.8 mEq/L

Serum calcium <8.5 mg/dL
Serum aldosterone level <5 ng/dL
Serum ADH >5 pg/mL
Urine osmolality >900 mOsm/kg, 50 to 150 mOsm/L
Urine sodium >200 mEq/24 hr, 20 mEq/L

ACUTE CARE PATIENT MANAGEMENT

Goals of Treatment

Restore fluid and electrolyte balance.
    Fluid restriction <1000 mL/day
    Diuretic therapy
    Potassium supplementation
Control ADH excretion.
    Lithium
    Demeclocycline
    Phenytoin
    Surgery
Prevent seizures.
    Hypertonic saline
    Phenytoin
Treat the cause.
    Appropriate therapy

Priority Nursing Diagnoses and Potential Complications	
Priority Nursing Diagnoses	**PC: Potential Complications**
Excess fluid volume	Electrolyte imbalances
Risk for injury	Seizures, hyponatremia
Risk for ineffective protection (see p. 48)	
Risk for imbalanced nutrition: less than body requirements (see p. 53)	
Risk for interrupted family processes (see p. 45)	

Nursing Diagnosis: **EXCESS FLUID VOLUME** related to excessive amounts of antidiuretic hormone secretion

Outcome Criteria

    Intake approximates output
    Serum potassium 3.5 to 5 mEq/L

Serum sodium 135 to 145 mEq/L
Serum chloride 95 to 105 mEq/L
Serum osmolality 275 to 295 mOsm/kg
Urine specific gravity 1.003 to 1.035
CVP 2 to 6 mm Hg
PAWP 4 to 12 mm Hg

Patient Monitoring

1. Monitor PA pressures and CVP hourly (if available) or more frequently to evaluate the patient's response to treatment. Both parameters reflect the capacity of the vascular system to accept volume and can be used to monitor fluid volume status.
2. Monitor hourly intake and urine output, and determine fluid balance every 8 hours. Compare serial weights and note rapid (0.5-1 kg/day) changes in weight, suggesting fluid imbalance.
3. Continuously monitor ECG for dysrhythmias resulting from electrolyte imbalance.

Patient Assessment

1. Obtain VS every hour or more frequently until the patient's condition is stable.
2. Evaluate hydration status every 4 hours. Note skin turgor on inner thigh or forehead, condition of buccal membranes, development of edema or crackles, and complaints of thirst.
3. Assess for pressure ulcer development secondary to edematous state

Diagnostics Assessment

Review serum sodium and potassium, serum osmolality, urine specific gravity, and urine osmolality to evaluate the patient's response to therapy.

Patient Management

1. Restrict fluid as ordered, generally <500 mL/day in severe cases and 800 to 1000 mL/day in moderate cases. Water intake should not exceed urine output and insensible loss until sodium is normal and the patient is asymptomatic. Encourage fluids high in sodium.
2. Administer potassium supplements as ordered; assess renal function and ensure adequate urine output before administering potassium.

ENDO

3. As adjuncts to water restriction, demeclocycline may be ordered to inhibit the renal response to ADH in patients with lung malignancies; lithium carbonate may be used to alter psychogenic behavior.

4. Avoid hypotonic enemas to treat constipation because water intoxication can be potentiated.

5. Institute pressure ulcer prevention strategies, e.g., meticulous skin care, repositioning, relieving pressure points.

Nursing Diagnosis: RISK FOR INJURY related to changes in mentation and seizures related to low serum sodium

Outcome Criteria

Patient alert and oriented
Patient will not injure self
Absence of seizures
Serum sodium 135 to 145 mEq/L

Patient Monitoring

Obtain PA pressures and CVP (if available) hourly or more frequently during hypertonic saline infusions to monitor for development of fluid overload.

Patient Assessment

Assess LOC hourly to evaluate effects of water intoxication. Patients may exhibit neurologic symptoms (e.g., confusion, seizures, coma) at sodium levels <125 mEq/L.

Diagnostics Assessment

Review serial serum sodium levels to evaluate the patient's response to therapy.

Patient Management

1. If the patient's sodium level is <105 mEq/L, hypertonic saline (3% NaCl) may be used to slowly raise serum sodium to 125 mEq/L (serum sodium should be increased no faster than 1-2 mEq/L/hr). Too rapid an increase in serum sodium may further impair neurologic function. Closely monitor for fluid overload and HF during hypertonic infusion: dyspnea, increased RR, crackles, moist cough, and bounding pulses. Furosemide or other diuretic agents may be administered with hypertonic saline infusions to increase urinary excretion of free water.

2. Maintain airway.
3. Institute seizure and fall precautions.
4. Reorient the confused patient to place, person, and time with each interaction.

THYROTOXICOSIS (THYROID STORM)

Clinical Brief

Thyroid storm is a life-threatening condition in which patients with underlying thyroid dysfunction exhibit exaggerated signs and symptoms of hyperthyroidism. Thyroid storm is precipitated by stressors such as infection, trauma, DKA, surgery, HF, or stroke. The condition can result from discontinuation of antithyroid medication or as a result of untreated or inadequate treatment of hyperthyroidism. The excess thyroid hormones increase metabolism and affect the sympathetic nervous system, thus increasing oxygen consumption and heat production and altering fluid and electrolyte levels. The clinical signs of thyroid storm and myxedema coma are compared in Table 5-45.

Presenting Signs and Symptoms

Signs and symptoms include sudden onset of fever ≤102.2° F (39° C), tremors, flushing, profuse palm sweating, tachydysrhythmias, and extreme restlessness. The patient may be unresponsive. GI symptoms may be present: nausea, vomiting, diarrhea, and weight loss. Fatigue and muscle weakness and atrophy are common. Older patients may manifest principally cardiac symptoms (e.g., HF, angina, dysrhythmias).

Physical Examination

Vital signs:
   BP: systolic HTN or hypotension (if shock)
   HR: tachycardia disproportionate to the degree of fever
   RR: >20 breaths/min
   Temperature: >102.2° F (39° C), can be up to 105.9° F (41° C)
Neurologic: agitated, tremulous, delirious to coma
Cardiovascular: bounding pulses, systolic murmur, widening pulse pressure; ↑ JVP, S_3, weak thready pulses (depending on the degree of CV compromise)
Pulmonary: tachypnea, crackles may be present
Gastrointestinal: ↑ bowel sounds
Endocrine: thyroid may be enlarged or nodular

ENDO

Diagnostic Findings

Diagnosis is based on a high index of suspicion (fever, tachycardia out of proportion to the fever, and CNS dysfunction). Studies indicating hyperthyroidism include the following:

Decreased TSH (gold standard diagnostic test)

Increased T_3 resin uptake and T_4 (useful if TSH results ambiguous)

ECG may show atrial fibrillation and SVT.

ACUTE CARE PATIENT MANAGEMENT

Goals of Treatment

Reduce oversecretion of thyroid hormone.
　　Antithyroid agents
　　β-Adrenergic blocking agents
　　Glucocorticoids
　　Surgery
　　Treatment of precipitating factor
Restore hemodynamic stability.
　　Supplemental oxygen
　　Crystalloids
　　Vasopressor agents
　　Inotropic agents
　　Diuretic agents
Restore normothermia.
　　Cooling methods
　　Acetaminophen
Support nutrition.
　　Supplemental feedings
　　Enteral nutrition
Detect/prevent clinical sequelae (Table 5-47).

ENDO

Table **5-47** CLINICAL SEQUELAE ASSOCIATED WITH THYROID STORM

Complication	Signs and Symptoms
Shock	SBP <90 mm Hg, HR >120 beats/min, altered mental state, cool clammy skin, ↓ urine output
Respiratory failure	Pao_2 <50 mm Hg, $Paco_2$ >50 mm Hg, paradoxical breathing, restlessness, RR >30 breaths/min
Cardiac failure/ pulmonary edema	Tachycardia, S_3, hypotension, ↑ JVP, crackles, tachypnea, dyspnea, frothy sputum

HR, Heart rate; *JVP,* jugular venous pressure; *RR,* respiratory rate; *SBP,* systolic blood pressure.

Priority Nursing Diagnoses and Potential Complications

Priority Nursing Diagnoses	PC: Potential Complications
Hyperthermia	
Decreased cardiac output	Dysrhythmias
Ineffective breathing pattern	Atelectasis, pneumonia, hypoxemia
Imbalanced nutrition: less than body requirements	Negative nitrogen balance
Ineffective protection (see p. 48)	
Risk for interrupted family processes (see p. 45)	

Nursing Diagnosis: HYPERTHERMIA related to increased metabolism

Outcome Criteria

T 97.7° to 100° F (36.5°-37.8° C)
SBP 90 to 120 mm Hg

Patient Monitoring

1. Continuously monitor core temperature (if possible) to evaluate the patient's response to therapy.
2. Continuously monitor BP because fever increases peripheral vasodilation, which can lead to hypotension.

Patient Assessment

1. Assess the patient for diaphoresis and shivering; shivering increases metabolic demand.
2. Assess the patient for clinical sequelae (see Table 5-47).

Diagnostics Assessment

Review culture reports for possible infection.

Patient Management

1. Administer acetaminophen as ordered and evaluate the patient's response.
2. Avoid aspirin administration because salicylates increase circulating thyroid hormones.
3. Administer antithyroid pharmacologic agents as prescribed:
    Propylthiouracil (PTU): blocks thyroid hormone synthesis and inhibits conversion of T_4 to T_3; administer doses of 300 mg every 6 hours.
    Iodide: inhibits the release of thyroid hormone and should be given at least 2 hours after the first dose of PTU has been

ENDO

administered, saturated solution of potassium iodide (SSKI) 1 to 2 gtt every 12 hours.

Dexamethasone: may be used to suppress conversion of T_4 and T_3 and to replace rapidly metabolized cortisol, 2 mg every 6 hours.

Colestipol: may be used in extreme cases, 10 g every 8 hours.

4. Institute cooling methods; a hypothermia blanket may be necessary to reduce body temperature (see p. 605).
5. Provide comfort measures, checking the patient for diaphoresis and changing patient's gown and bed linens as necessary.
6. Peritoneal dialysis and plasmapheresis have been reported to reduce thyroid hormone levels in extreme cases.

ENDO

Nursing Diagnoses: DECREASED CARDIAC OUTPUT related to increased cardiac work secondary to increased adrenergic activity; DEFICIENT FLUID VOLUME secondary to increased metabolism and diaphoresis

Outcome Criteria

Patient alert and oriented
Peripheral pulses palpable
Lungs clear to auscultation
Urine output 30 mL/hr or 0.5 to 1 mL/kg/hr
SBP 90 to 120 mm Hg
MAP 70 to 105 mm Hg
HR 60 to 100 beats/min
Absence of life-threatening dysrhythmias
PAS 15 to 30 mm Hg
PAD 5 to 15 mm Hg
PAWP 4 to 12 mm Hg
CI 2.5 to 4 L/min/m^2
SVRI 1700 to 2600 dynes/sec/cm^{-5}/m^2
LVSWI 45 to 60 g-m/m^2

Patient Monitoring

1. Continuously monitor ECG for dysrhythmias or HR ≥140 beats/min that can adversely affect CO and monitor for ST segment changes indicative of myocardial ischemia.
2. Continuously monitor oxygen saturation with pulse oximetry (SpO_2). Be alert for patient activities or interventions that adversely affect oxygen saturation.

3. Continuously monitor PA pressures, CVP (if available), and BP. Obtain CI and PAWP to evaluate cardiac function and the patient's response to therapy. Monitor MAP; a MAP <60 mm Hg adversely affects cerebral and renal perfusion.

4. Monitor fluid volume status: measure urine output hourly, and determine fluid balance every 8 hours. Compare serial weights; a rapid (0.5-1 kg/day) change suggests fluid imbalance.

Patient Assessment

1. Assess cardiovascular status: extra heart sounds (S_3 is a hallmark of HF), complaints of orthopnea or dyspnea on exertion (DOE), ↑ JVP, crackles, and prolonged capillary refill suggest HF, which can progress to pulmonary edema (increasing dyspnea, frothy sputum). Assess the patient for myocardial ischemic pain.

2. Assess hydration status (e.g., thirst, mucous membranes, skin turgor) because dehydration can further decrease circulating volume and compromise CO.

3. Assess for pressure ulcer development secondary to hypoperfusion.

4. Assess the patient for clinical sequelae (see Table 5-47).

Diagnostics Assessment

1. Review thyroid studies as available.

2. Review serial serum electrolytes, serum glucose, and serum calcium levels to evaluate the patient's response to therapy.

3. Review serial ABGs for hypoxemia and acid-base imbalance, which can adversely affect cardiac function.

4. Review serial chest radiographs for cardiac enlargement and pulmonary congestion.

Patient Management

1. Administer dextrose-containing intravenous fluids as ordered to correct fluid and glucose deficits. Carefully assess the patient for HF or pulmonary edema. Dopamine may be used to support BP.

2. Provide supplemental oxygen as ordered to help meet increased metabolic demands. Once the patient is hemodynamically stable, provide pulmonary hygiene to reduce pulmonary complications.

ENDO

3. Administer β-adrenergic blocking agents such as propranolol as ordered to control tachycardia and HTN (also inhibits conversion of T_4 to T_3). Monitor HR for bradycardia and PA pressures (if available) to evaluate left ventricular function. A short-acting β-adrenergic blocking agent such as esmolol may also be tried.

4. If the patient is in HF, typical pharmacologic agents for treatment of HF may also be indicated, including ACE inhibitors, diuretics, potassium supplements, β-blockers, and digoxin. (See discussion of heart failure, p. 237.)

5. Reduce oxygen demands: decrease anxiety, reduce fever, decrease pain, and limit visitors if necessary. Schedule uninterrupted rest periods. Approach the patient in a calm manner, explain procedures, or provide information to decrease misperceptions. Keep the room cool and dimly lit and reduce external stimuli as much as possible.

6. Anticipate aggressive treatment of precipitating factor.

7. Institute pressure ulcer prevention strategies, e.g., meticulous skin care, repositioning, relieving pressure points.

Nursing Diagnosis: INEFFECTIVE BREATHING PATTERN related to intercostal muscle weakness

Outcome Criteria

Patient alert and oriented
RR 12 to 20 breaths/min, eupnea
PaO_2 80 to 100 mm Hg
$PaCO_2$ 35 to 45 mm Hg
pH 7.35 to 7.45
O_2 sat ≥95%

Patient Monitoring

1. Continuously monitor oxygen saturation with pulse oximetry (SpO_2). Monitor patient activities and interventions that can adversely affect oxygen saturation.

2. Continuously monitor ECG for dysrhythmias that may be related to hypoxemia or acid-base imbalance.

Patient Assessment

1. Assess respiratory status: note RR, rhythm, and depth and use of accessory muscles. Observe for paradoxical breathing pat-

tern and increased restlessness, increased complaints of dyspnea, and changes in LOC. Cyanosis is a late sign of respiratory distress.

2. Assess the patient for clinical sequelae (see Table 5-47).

Diagnostics Assessment

1. Review serial ABGs to evaluate oxygenation and acid-base balance.
2. Review serial chest radiographs for pulmonary congestion.

Patient Management

1. Administer supplemental oxygen as ordered. (For patient management of ventilation therapies, see p. 506.)
2. Reposition the patient to improve oxygenation and mobilize secretions. Evaluate the patient's response to position changes with SpO_2 or ABGs to determine the best position for oxygenation.
3. As the patient's hemodynamics stabilize, provide pulmonary hygiene to prevent complications.
4. Decrease oxygen demands (e.g., reduce fever, alleviate anxiety, limit visitors if necessary, and schedule uninterrupted rest periods).
5. Administer antithyroid medications as prescribed.

Nursing Diagnosis: IMBALANCED NUTRITION: LESS THAN BODY REQUIREMENTS related to increased metabolism

Outcome Criteria

Stabilized weight
Positive nitrogen balance

Patient Monitoring

Monitor for changes in serial weights; rapid (0.5-1 kg/day) changes indicate fluid imbalance and not an imbalance between nutritional needs and intake.

Patient Assessment

1. Assess GI status: absent or hyperactive bowel sounds, vomiting, diarrhea, or abdominal pain may interfere with nutritional absorption.
2. Assess the patient for clinical sequelae (see Table 5-47).

ENDO

Diagnostics Assessment

1. Review serial serum glucose levels for hyperglycemia because excessive circulating thyroid hormones increase glycogenolysis and decrease insulin levels.
2. Review serum albumin levels; hypoalbuminemia may suggest muscle breakdown.
3. Review urine urea nitrogen (UUN) as indicated to estimate nitrogen balance.

Patient Management

1. Conduct calorie counts to provide information about the adequacy of intake required to meet metabolic needs. Consult with a nutritionist to maximize intake of calories and protein to reverse the negative nitrogen balance.
2. Assist the patient with small, frequent feedings if oral intake can be tolerated. Enteral feedings may be required. (See p. 561 for information on enteral nutrition.)
3. Sliding scale insulin therapy may be required to control hyperglycemia.
4. Avoid caffeine products, which may increase peristalsis.

ENDO

RENAL DISORDERS

ACUTE RENAL FAILURE

Clinical Brief

Acute renal failure (ARF) is a clinical syndrome characterized by a sudden, rapid deterioration in kidney function, which results in the retention of nitrogen waste (urea nitrogen and creatinine) and fluid, electrolyte, and acid-base imbalances. Risk factors for ARF include volume depletion, CHF, contrast exposure, aminoglycoside therapy, and septic shock. Causes of acute renal failure can be divided into three categories.

Prerenal: factors that decrease renal perfusion without cellular injury (e.g., intravascular volume depletion, CHF, cirrhosis, pharmacologic agents). Rapid intervention with volume replacement can reverse prerenal failure.

Intrarenal: factors that damage the renal parenchyma (e.g., nephrotoxic agents [antibiotics, contrast media, pesticides, myoglobin], inflammation, trauma, and any prerenal process that results in renal ischemia); acute tubular necrosis (ATN) is a type of intrarenal failure

Postrenal: factors that result from obstruction of urine flow from the kidneys to the external environment (e.g., prostatic hypertrophy, uric acid nephropathy, or bladder tumor)

ATN is the most common cause of acute renal failure in the critical care environment. Patients with acute renal failure and ATN often have oliguria (<700 mL of urine in 24 hours). Patients must receive continuous renal replacement therapy (CRRT) (e.g., hemodialysis) for at least the short term, in the face of persistent oliguria with increasing azotemia, hyperkalemia, vascular overload, or metabolic acidosis.

The phases of ARF are:

Oliguric—<0.5 mL/kg/hr (<450-500 mL/day); increase in serum electrolytes and metabolites as renal function deteriorates

Polyuric/diuretic—results when nephrons recover and new tubule cells grow; dilute urine is secondary to ineffective functioning of immature cells

RENAL

Postdiuretic—regeneration of tubules, renal function is restored

Presenting Signs and Symptoms

The acute onset of acute renal failure is often accompanied by oliguria (but may be nonoliguric) and azotemia (accumulation of nitrogen waste products), hyperkalemia, and metabolic acidosis.

Physical Examination

Vital signs:
  BP: increased or decreased
  HR: increased
  RR: increased
  Temperature: normal or increased
Neurologic: irritability, restlessness, change in LOC
Cardiovascular: S_3, S_4, JVD may be present
Pulmonary: deep and rapid respirations, crackles
Gastrointestinal: nausea, vomiting, anorexia

RENAL

Table 5-48 CATEGORIES OF ACUTE RENAL FAILURE AND RELATED LABORATORY VALUES

	Prerenal	Intrarenal (ATN)	Postrenal
URINE			
Volume	Low	Low or high	Low or high
Sodium	<20 mEq/L	>40 mEq/L	>40 mEq/L
Osmolality	>500 mOsm	<350 mOsm (fixed)	<350 mOsm (varies)
Specific gravity	>1.020	<1.010	1.008-1.012
Creatinine	~Normal	Low	Low
FEna	≤1%	>3%	>1%
Sediment	Normal	Normal	Cells, casts, protein
PLASMA			
Urea (BUN)	High	High	High
Creatinine	~Normal	High	High
BUN:creatinine	20:1 or more	<20:1	10:1

ATN, Acute tubular necrosis; *BUN,* blood urea nitrogen; *FEna,* fractional excretion of sodium.

Diagnostic Findings

Diagnostic findings vary with category (Table 5-48).

NOTE: Diuretic administration will affect urine analysis.

ACUTE CARE PATIENT MANAGEMENT

Goals of Treatment

Optimize hydration and volume status.

Maintain blood pressure.

    Correct suspected cause.

    Fluid challenge

    Diuretic agents

    Antihypertensive agents

    Vasodilator agents

    Avoidance of nephrotoxic agents

Normalize fluid status.

    Fluid challenge in prerenal patients

    Fluid restriction in oliguric patients

    Renal replacement therapy

Remove nitrogen waste products.

    Restriction of protein intake

    Increase in caloric intake

    Renal replacement therapy

Maintain electrolyte balance.

    Restriction of sodium

    Restriction of potassium

    Phosphate-binding pharmacologic agents

For hyperkalemia:

    Sodium polystyrene sulfonate (Kayexalate) (with sorbitol)

    Glucose with insulin

    Renal replacement therapy

Treat metabolic acidosis.

    Sodium bicarbonate

    Renal replacement therapy

Treat hypercatabolism.

    Renal replacement therapy

    Nutrition: high calorie, low protein, high essential amino acids

Treat anemia

    Erythropoietin

Detect/prevent clinical sequelae (Table 5-49).

RENAL

Table 5-49 CLINICAL SEQUELAE ASSOCIATED WITH ACUTE RENAL FAILURE

Complication	Signs and Symptoms
Hyperkalemia	Peaked T waves, prolonged PR interval, prolonged QRS duration, dysrhythmias; twitching, cramps, hyperactive reflexes
Pericarditis	Chest discomfort aggravated by supine position or deep inspiration, intermittent friction rub and/or fever may be present
Metabolic acidosis	pH <7.35 with ↓ HCO_3^- and normal or ↓ $Paco_2$; Kussmaul respirations (hyperventilation); headache, fatigue, altered mental status
Anemia	Decreasing hematocrit, active bleeding; pale, weak, tired; SOB
GI bleed	Occult or visible blood in stools or gastric contents, decreasing hematocrit
Infection	↑ Temperature (may be subtle); lungs, urinary tract, or wounds may be sources
Uremia	Lethargy progressing to coma, seizures, asterixis, heart failure, volume disturbances, pericarditis, N/V, anorexia, diarrhea, GI bleeding

GI, Gastrointestinal; *N/V,* nausea and vomiting; *SOB,* shortness of breath.

Priority Nursing Diagnoses and Potential Complications

Priority Nursing Diagnoses	PC: Potential Complications
Excess fluid volume	Renal insufficiency, metabolic acidosis, electrolyte imbalances (see pp. 348-376)
Deficient fluid volume	
Imbalanced nutrition: less than body requirements (see p. 53)	Negative nitrogen balance
Ineffective protection (see p. 48)	
Risk for interrupted family processes (see p. 45)	

Nursing Diagnosis: **EXCESS FLUID VOLUME** related to decreased renal excretion (oliguria) and excess sodium and water retention

Outcome Criteria

Patient at target body weight
Intake approximates output
MAP 70 to 105 mm Hg
SBP 90 to 140 mm Hg

Absence of edema
Lungs clear to auscultation
Patient alert and oriented
Absence of HF
CVP 2 to 6 mm Hg
Electrolytes WNL
Urine output 0.5 mL/kg/hr
Creatinine 0.6 to 1.2 mg/dL
BUN <100 mg/dL
Urine specific gravity 1.003 to 1.030
Skin intact

Patient Monitoring

1. Monitor fluid volume status: measure urine output hourly, determine fluid balance every 8 hours and include other bodily drainage. Compare serial weights for rapid changes; an increase of 0.5 to 1 kg/day indicates fluid retention (1 kg is approximately 1000 mL of fluid). The oliguric phase (urine output <400 mL/day) in ATN usually lasts 10 to 16 days and may be followed by a diuretic phase.

2. Obtain CVP, PA pressures (if available), and BP hourly or more frequently to evaluate the extent of excess fluid volume and the patient's response to therapy. Monitor MAP, an indicator of tissue perfusion; a decrease in MAP further insults the kidney.

3. Continuously monitor ECG for dysrhythmias secondary to electrolyte imbalance.

Patient Assessment

1. Assess fluid volume status: note any onset of S_3 and crackles; presence of edema, cough, or frothy sputum; increased work of breathing; decreased peripheral perfusion; and increased JVP to determine development of HF or pulmonary edema.

2. Assess for pressure ulcer development secondary to edema.

3. Assess the patient for clinical sequelae (see Table 5-49).

Diagnostics Assessment

1. Review BUN, creatinine, and BUN/creatinine ratio. Serum creatinine reflects glomerular filtration rate (GFR). Estimating GFR is not accurate in acute renal failure and is assumed to be <10 mL/min. Uremic symptoms may manifest if BUN is >70 mg/dL or GFR is <15 mL/min. A rise in BUN without a corresponding rise in creatinine is unlikely to be caused by a renal failure.

RENAL

2. Review urine sodium, urine osmolality, and urine specific gravity to evaluate renal function. Urine samples for laboratory analysis should be obtained prior to diuretic administration.
3. Review serial chest radiographs to evaluate pulmonary congestion.
4. Review serial ABGs to evaluate extent of acid-base imbalances.
5. Review serial electrolytes: hyperkalemia, hyponatremia, hypocalcemia, hyperphosphatemia, and hypermagnesemia are common in acute renal failure.

Patient Management

1. Anticipate sodium and fluid restriction in oliguric patients (e.g., approximately 600 mL/day plus insensible losses). Consult with dietitian for increased caloric intake and protein restriction. Restrict protein intake to limit nitrogen accumulation. Increase caloric intake to minimize protein catabolism.
2. Concentrate medications when possible to minimize fluid intake.
3. If diuretics (furosemide, bumetanide) are ordered, monitor for signs of hypovolemia, hypotension, hypokalemia, and hyponatremia.
4. If vasoactive drugs are ordered, carefully monitor BP and MAP every 15 minutes to every hour. Generally SBP should be >90 mm Hg and MAP 70 to 105 mm Hg.
5. Raise HOB if the patient is SOB without being hypotensive.
6. Institute pressure ulcer prevention strategies, e.g., meticulous skin care, repositioning, relieving pressure points.
7. Anticipate hemodialysis or CRRT to remove excess fluid and/or solutes. See p. 575 for information on renal replacement therapy.
8. Be alert for nephrotoxic agents, e.g., NSAIDs, ACE inhibitors, contrast media, amphotericin B, aminoglycosides.
9. Be prepared to administer preprocedure hydration if ordered.
10. Be prepared to administer erythropoietin if ordered.

Nursing Diagnosis: DEFICIENT FLUID VOLUME related to volume depletion (diuretic phase)

Outcome Criteria

MAP 70 to 105 mm Hg
Urine output 30 mL/hr or 0.5 to 1 mL/kg/hr

RENAL

Intake approximates output
Elastic skin turgor
Moist mucous membranes
HR 60 to 100 beats/min
Electrolytes WNL

Patient Monitoring

1. Monitor I&O hourly to assess the fluid balance trend, which is reflective of renal function. The diuretic phase (>400 mL/day) of ATN may last 2 to 3 days or up to 12 days.
2. Compare daily weights to assess fluid volume status.
3. Obtain CVP, PA pressures (if available), HR, and BP hourly or more frequently as the patient's condition dictates. Monitor MAP, an indicator of tissue perfusion; a MAP <70 mm Hg further insults the kidney. Be alert for tachycardia and postural hypotension, which may indicate volume depletion.

Patient Assessment

1. Assess hydration state: note skin turgor on inner thigh or forehead, and condition of buccal membranes. Flat neck veins, complaints of thirst, and decreased LOC may signal volume depletion.
2. Assess the patient for clinical sequelae (see Table 5-49).

Diagnostics Assessment

1. Review urine sodium, osmolality, and specific gravity to assess volume status.
2. Review serial electrolytes because severe imbalances can occur.

Patient Management

1. Administer aggressive fluid and electrolyte replacements as ordered to increase volume and maintain normal electrolyte and acid-base balance. Carefully monitor for increase in urine output and early signs of excess fluid volume when administering fluid challenges.
2. Avoid administration of nephrotoxic agents (e.g., NSAIDs, ACE inhibitors, contrast media, amphotericin B, aminoglycosides) or administer at reduced dose or frequency as ordered to prevent additional renal damage.

RENAL

3. Avoid rapidly placing the patient in an upright position because postural hypotension may result.
4. Provide meticulous skin care to prevent skin breakdown and oral care to soothe dry mucous membranes.
5. Check for occult blood in stools and NG aspirate because GI bleeding can occur in patients with renal failure, contributing to signs and symptoms of volume deficit.
6. Consult with dietitian to reduce protein and increase caloric intake. Restrict protein intake to reduce nitrogen waste product accumulation. Increase caloric intake to minimize protein catabolism.

ELECTROLYTE IMBALANCE: CALCIUM

Clinical Brief

Calcium imbalances occur as a result of changes in calcium ion concentrations in extracellular fluid (ECF). Because approximately half of the calcium is bound to albumin, evaluation of calcium levels must be done in conjunction with albumin levels. A falsely low total calcium level is seen in the presence of low albumin levels, although ionized calcium levels are not greatly affected. Changes in pH alter the amount of calcium bound to albumin, requiring that assessment of serum calcium levels ideally be done when the pH is normal.

Hypocalcemia often results from respiratory alkalosis associated with hyperventilation, receiving large amounts of stored blood, acute pancreatitis, decreased intake, or decreased absorption (from vitamin D deficiency, decreased parathyroid hormone release, hyperphosphatemia, chronic renal failure [CRF], or malabsorption). *Hypercalcemia* commonly occurs with malignancy (primarily cancer of the lung, breast, and hematologic tissues) and hyperparathyroidism. However, immobility and resumption of kidney function following renal transplantation also can cause hypercalcemia.

Presenting Signs and Symptoms

Signs and symptoms depend on the severity of the imbalance. (See following discussion of physical examination.)

RENAL

Physical Examination

	Hypocalcemia	Hypercalcemia
Appearance	Tired	Tired, lethargic, confused, bone pain
Cardiovascular	ECG: prolonged QT interval Palpitations Hypotension Dysrhythmias, torsades de pointes	ECG: shortened QT interval
Pulmonary	Stridor, bronchospasm, laryngospasm, respiratory arrest	
Neurologic	Cramping of hands and feet, hyperreflexia, tetany, carpal and pedal spasm, numbness and tingling around the mouth and extremities, twitching, seizures, altered mental status	Hyporeflexia, altered mental status, headache
Gastrointestinal	Abdominal cramps	Anorexia, thirst, nausea, vomiting, constipation

RENAL

Diagnostic Findings

Hypocalcemia is defined as an ionized serum calcium level of <4.5 mg/dL (total calcium of <9 mg/dL); hypercalcemia is an ionized calcium of >5.5 mg/dL (total calcium >11 mg/dL).

ACUTE CARE PATIENT MANAGEMENT

Goals of Treatment

Goal	Hypocalcemia	Hypercalcemia
Maintain normal serum calcium level	Correct underlying problem High-calcium diet Vitamin D supplements Oral calcium supplements Intravenous 10% calcium gluconate	Correct underlying problem Low-calcium diet Normal saline and diuretics Corticosteroids Calcitonin Plicamycin Pamidronate

Hypocalcemia

Priority Nursing Diagnosis and Potential Complications	
Priority Nursing Diagnosis	**PC: Potential Complications**
Risk for injury	Dysrhythmias, seizures, hypocalcemia

Nursing Diagnosis: RISK FOR INJURY related to altered mental status, seizures, and tetany secondary to calcium imbalance: hypocalcemia

Outcome Criteria

Serum calcium 4.5 to 5.5 mg/dL (total calcium 9-11 mg/dL)
Normal reflex activity
Normal peripheral sensation and movement
Patient alert and oriented
HR 60 to 100 beats/min
PR interval 0.12 to 0.20 second
QT interval <½ of R-R interval
Absence of life-threatening dysrhythmias
MAP 70 to 105 mm Hg
Absence of injury
Absence of seizure activity
RR 12 to 20 breaths/min
Nonlabored respirations
Absence of laryngeal stridor
Absence of Trousseau's sign
Absence of Chvostek's sign

Patient Monitoring

1. Continuously monitor ECG for dysrhythmias. Measure serial QT intervals; torsades de pointes is associated with prolonged QT intervals.
2. Monitor BP because decreased myocardial contractility and hypotension are cardiovascular manifestations associated with hypocalcemia.

Patient Assessment

1. Assess for presence of cramps in hands, feet, and legs and assess for circumoral paresthesia.
2. Assess RR and depth, work of breathing, and breath sounds at least every 4 hours. Airway obstruction and respiratory

RENAL

arrest can occur. Monitor for stridor, bronchospasm, and laryngospasm.

3. Assess for signs of tetany: numbness and tingling in the fingers, around the mouth, and over the face, which may be followed by spasms of the face and extremities.

4. Assess for Trousseau's sign by inflating a BP cuff above SBP for 2 to 5 minutes and assessing for carpopedal spasm of the hand. A positive test, which results when carpopedal spasm is present, is associated with hypocalcemia.

5. Assess for Chvostek's sign by tapping the facial nerve anterior to the ear and observing for lip and cheek spasms. Spasms indicate a positive test result and are associated with hypocalcemia.

6. Be alert for seizures because hypocalcemia causes CNS irritability.

7. Assess patients taking digitalis for signs of digitalis toxicity; increasing calcium may cause digitalis toxicity.

Diagnostics Assessment

1. Review albumin levels because hypoalbuminemia is the most common cause of hypocalcemia.

2. Review serial serum calcium levels in conjunction with pH and albumin levels because alkalosis and hypoalbuminemia decrease calcium ionization. To correct for calcium in the presence of hypoalbuminemia, the following formula can be used: Corrected Ca = total calcium + 0.8 (4 − albumin). In addition, drugs can cause hypocalcemia: aminoglycosides, aluminum-containing antacids, corticosteroids, and loop diuretics.

Patient Management

1. Initiate seizure precautions by padding side rails, minimizing stimulation, assisting the patient with all activities, and keeping airway management equipment available. If seizures do occur, protect the patient and be prepared to correct hypocalcemia and administer antiseizure medications if ordered.

2. Have a tracheostomy tray available; be prepared to administer humidified air or oxygen, administer bronchodilators, and/or assist with a tracheostomy if bronchospasm and laryngospasm occur.

3. If respiratory arrest occurs, institute emergency respiratory and cardiac support.

RENAL

4. Administer vitamin D and oral calcium supplements 1 hour after meals and at bedtime to maximize calcium absorption and utilization.

5. For symptomatic hypocalcemia, calcium gluconate or calcium chloride may be ordered. Intravenous administration can be diluted and given slowly over 30 minutes. Infusions can be administered over several hours until oral calcium takes over. Calcium gluconate contains 90 mg of elemental calcium in 10 mL of a 10% solution; calcium chloride contains 272 mg of elemental calcium in 10 mL of a 10% solution. Administer through a central line if one is available because calcium is very irritating to the veins and will cause tissue damage if it extravasates. Too rapid intravenous administration of calcium can lead to cardiac arrest. Monitor patients receiving digitalis closely for fatal dysrhythmias.

6. Evaluate the patient for hypomagnesemia because magnesium deficiency is often associated with hypocalcemia and impairs the restoration of normal calcium levels.

7. Encourage foods high in calcium (e.g., milk products, meats, and leafy green vegetables).

8. Assist with self-care activities because the patient may develop poor coordination.

Hypercalcemia

Priority Nursing Diagnosis and Potential Complications	
Priority Nursing Diagnosis	PC: Potential Complications
Risk for injury	Hypercalcemia, dysrhythmias

Nursing Diagnosis: RISK FOR INJURY related to mental lethargy, decreased muscle tone, and neuromuscular excitability secondary to calcium imbalance: hypercalcemia

Outcome Criteria

Serum calcium 4.5 to 5.5 mg/dL (total calcium 9-11 mg/dL)
Normal reflex activity
Normal peripheral sensation and movement
Patient alert and oriented
HR 60 to 100 beats/min
PR interval 0.12 to 0.20 second
QT interval <½ of R-R interval

RENAL

Absence of life-threatening dysrhythmias

MAP 70 to 105 mm Hg

Absence of injury

Patient Monitoring

1. Continuously monitor ECG for dysrhythmias. Measure the QT interval.
2. Monitor fluid volume status: measure I&O hourly; acute hypercalcemia may induce acute renal failure. Polyuria may also result. Volume restoration may result in fluid volume overload. Monitor CVP closely.

Patient Assessment

1. Assess mentation and observe for behavioral changes. Patients may be confused or develop psychotic behavior.
2. Assess patients receiving digitalis for signs of digitalis toxicity because the inotropic effect of digitalis is enhanced by calcium. Digitalis dose may need to be reduced.
3. Assess GI function: note abdominal distention and absent bowel sounds, anorexia, or N/V, which may suggest paralytic ileus.

Diagnostics Assessment

Review serial calcium levels to evaluate the patient's response to therapy.

Patient Management

1. Anticipate the administration of NS to expand ECF volume along with diuretics, such as IV furosemide, to increase urinary excretion of calcium. Monitor for signs of fluid volume imbalances. Thiazide diuretics are avoided because they inhibit calcium excretion.
2. Etidronate may be ordered IV for hypercalcemia associated with malignancy. Generally 7.5 mg/kg is given in 250 mL NS daily for 3 days. Pamidronate may be ordered for hypercalcemia associated with malignancy; a single infusion of 30 mg may be ordered.
3. Calcitonin may be ordered for patients who cannot tolerate sodium; 3 to 4 units/kg subQ every 12 to 24 hours may be ordered.
4. Corticosteroids may be initiated if hypercalcemia is associated with some types of granulomatous disorders.

RENAL

5. Plicamycin may be given in hypercalcemia associated with malignancy. Administer over 4 hours to reduce nausea. Dilute medication to minimize irritation to the veins. Be alert for thrombocytopenia, hepatotoxicity, and nephrotoxicity.

6. Phosphates administered IV may be given as a last resort to lower calcium; fatal hypotension and widespread metastatic calcification may occur.

7. If the patient develops heart block, check BP, HR, and pulse pressure; be prepared to administer atropine and calcium and to assist with pacemaker insertion. Be prepared to initiate immediate emergency measures for cardiac arrest.

8. Encourage a diet low in calcium and protein.

9. Encourage mobility as soon as possible because immobility results in the release of bone calcium; assist with ambulation because muscle weakness may be present.

10. To prevent the formation of kidney stones, encourage a high-fluid intake (avoiding milk products, which are high in calcium), to a level that maintains urine output of 3 to 4 L/day. Encourage prune or cranberry juice to maintain acidic urine because calcium solubility is increased in acidic urine.

ELECTROLYTE IMBALANCE: MAGNESIUM

Clinical Brief

Magnesium imbalances occur as a result of changes in magnesium ion concentrations in ECF. Hypomagnesemia occurs as a result of malabsorption, starvation, parenteral nutrition without magnesium, alcoholism, excessive diuretics, GI losses, pancreatitis, pregnancy toxemia, hypocalcemia, and hyperaldosteronism. Hypermagnesemia is associated with renal insufficiency, acidosis, adrenal insufficiency (AI), hyperparathyroidism, and increased magnesium intake.

Magnesium is essential for the production of energy (all cellular enzymatic reactions require adenosine triphosphate [ATP]) and the maintenance of normal intracellular electrolyte composition. Magnesium is critical for the activation of the sodium/potassium ATPase pump, which moves potassium into the cell and sodium out of the cell against the concentration gradient. Magnesium is also needed for protein synthesis within the cell and for neuromuscular transmission.

Abnormalities in magnesium are often mistaken for potassium imbalances. Magnesium deficiency often makes hypokalemia refractory to treatment. Most significantly, magnesium has a profound

RENAL

effect on cardiac activity, and magnesium deficiency may cause HTN and coronary artery vasospasm. Magnesium deficiency may contribute to sudden death from nonocclusive ischemic heart disease and increase the risk of MI.

Presenting Signs and Symptoms

See discussion of physical examination.

Physical Examination

	Hypomagnesemia	Hypermagnesemia
Appearance	Weak, dizzy, cramping	Lethargic, flushed
VS	↑HR, ↑BP	↓RR, ↓HR, ↓BP
Cardiovascular	ECG: peaking of T waves, prolonged PR or QT interval, dysrhythmias	ECG: wide QRS; prolonged PR and QT intervals, bradycardia, complete heart block, cardiac arrest
Pulmonary	Stridor, bronchospasm, laryngospasm	Shallow respirations, apnea
Neurologic	Confusion, altered mental status, tremors, tetany, hyperreflexia, seizures, positive Trousseau's and Chvostek's signs	Altered mental status, hyporeflexia, seizures, muscle paralysis, coma
Gastrointestinal	Anorexia, nausea	

Diagnostic Findings

Hypomagnesemia is defined as a serum magnesium level <1.5 mEq/L. Hypermagnesemia is a serum magnesium level >2.5 mEq/L. Reduced body stores of magnesium, referred to as magnesium deficiency, may be present with normal magnesium levels.

ACUTE CARE PATIENT MANAGEMENT

Goals of Treatment

	Hypomagnesemia	Hypermagnesemia
Normalize serum magnesium levels	High-magnesium diet	Low-magnesium diet
	Magnesium sulfate	Diuretics
		Calcium gluconate, calcium chloride

RENAL

Hypomagnesemia

Priority Nursing Diagnosis and Potential Complications	
Priority Nursing Diagnosis	PC: Potential Complications
Risk for injury	Hypomagnesemia, seizures, dysrhythmias

Priority Nursing Diagnosis: RISK FOR INJURY related to seizures and neuromuscular changes secondary to magnesium imbalance: hypomagnesemia

Outcome Criteria

Serum magnesium 1.5 to 2.5 mEq/L
Normal reflex activity
Normal peripheral sensation and movement
HR 60 to 100 beats/min
PR interval 0.12 to 0.20 second
QT interval ½ of R-R interval
T wave rounded
Absence of life-threatening dysrhythmias
MAP 70 to 105 mm Hg
RR 12 to 20 breaths/min
Nonlabored respirations
Absence of laryngeal stridor
Absence of injury
Absence of seizure activity

Patient Monitoring

Continuously monitor ECG for changes in rate and rhythm. Measure PR and QT intervals. Torsades de pointes is associated with prolonged QT intervals. Dysrhythmias may occur: premature ventricular contractions (PVCs), ventricular tachycardia (VT), and ventricular fibrillation (VF).

Patient Assessment

1. Assess mentation, changes in behavior, and ability to swallow.
2. Assess RR and depth, work of breathing, and breath sounds at least every 4 hours. Monitor for stridor, bronchospasm, and laryngospasm, which can occur during acute hypomagnesemia.
3. Assess for signs of hypocalcemia, which often accompanies hypomagnesemia: muscle weakness, muscle pain, numbness

RENAL

and tingling, positive Trousseau's sign, and positive Chvostek's sign.

4. Assess patients taking digitalis for signs of digitalis toxicity because hypomagnesemia predisposes the patient to toxicity. Digitalis dose may need to be adjusted.

5. Be alert for seizures.

Diagnostics Assessment

1. Review magnesium levels when available, although serum levels do not reflect total body magnesium stores and thus are poor indicators of magnesium deficiency. Urinary excretion of magnesium or a magnesium load test may be done to further assess magnesium levels.

2. Review potassium levels because magnesium imbalances are often mistaken for potassium imbalances.

3. Review calcium levels because hypocalcemia often accompanies hypomagnesemia.

Patient Management

1. Encourage foods high in magnesium, such as seafood, green vegetables, bananas, grapefruits, oranges, nuts, and legumes. Diet can correct mild hypomagnesemia.

2. For symptomatic hypomagnesemia, administer intravenous magnesium as ordered. A rapid infusion may result in cardiac or respiratory arrest; 10% magnesium sulfate (1 g/10 mL) should be administered no faster than 1.5 mL/min.

   a. Assess renal function before administering magnesium because magnesium is removed from the body through the kidneys.

   b. Obtain BP, HR, and respirations every 15 minutes during infusion of large doses of magnesium because vasodilation, bradycardia, and respiratory depression may occur.

   c. Before and during the administration of magnesium, monitor for hypermagnesemia by assessing the patellar (knee-jerk) reflex. If the reflex is absent, stop the magnesium infusion and notify the physician. Hyporeflexia will precede respiratory depression.

   d. If hypotension or respiratory depression occurs during magnesium infusion, stop the magnesium infusion, notify the physician, and be prepared to administer calcium and to support cardiac and respiratory functioning.

RENAL

3. Seizures may result from hypomagnesemia. Initiate seizure precautions by padding side rails, minimizing stimulation, assisting the patient with all activities, and keeping airway management equipment available. If seizures do occur, protect the patient and be prepared to correct hypomagnesemia and administer antiseizure medications if ordered.

4. Have tracheostomy tray available. Be prepared to administer humidified air or oxygen, administer bronchodilators, and/or assist with a tracheostomy if bronchospasm and laryngospasm occur.

5. If dysrhythmia occurs, be prepared to begin treatment to increase the serum magnesium level. Be aware that antidysrhythmic agents and defibrillation are often ineffective in the presence of hypomagnesemia.

6. If respiratory arrest occurs, institute emergency respiratory and cardiac support.

7. Correct the magnesium level before correcting the potassium level because hypokalemia is difficult to treat in the presence of hypomagnesemia.

8. Because patients with hypomagnesemia often experience muscle weakness, teach the patient methods for conserving energy; provide for rest periods, and assist with self-care activities and ambulation.

RENAL

Hypermagnesemia

Priority Nursing Diagnosis and Potential Complications	
Priority Nursing Diagnosis	**PC: Potential Complications**
Risk for injury	Hypermagnesemia, dysrhythmias

Priority Nursing Diagnosis: RISK FOR INJURY related to lethargy and muscle weakness secondary to magnesium imbalance: hypermagnesemia

Outcome Criteria

Serum magnesium 1.5 to 2.5 mEq/L
Normal reflex activity
Normal peripheral sensation and movement
HR 60 to 100 beats/min
PR interval 0.12 to 0.20 sec
QT interval ½ of R-R interval
T wave rounded

Absence of life-threatening dysrhythmias
MAP 70 to 105 mm Hg
RR 12 to 20 breaths/min
Nonlabored respirations
Absence of laryngeal stridor
Absence of injury

Patient Monitoring

1. Continuously monitor the ECG for bradycardia and heart block. Measure PR and QT intervals.
2. Monitor BP for hypotension.

Patient Assessment

1. Assess LOC and note lethargy or drowsiness.
2. Assess the RR and pattern; note shallow respirations or periods of apnea.
3. Monitor patellar (knee-jerk) reflex because absence of the reflex indicates severe hypermagnesemia that may proceed to respiratory or cardiac arrest.

Diagnostics Assessment

1. Review magnesium levels when available.
2. Review potassium levels because magnesium imbalances are often mistaken for potassium imbalances.
3. Review calcium levels because hypercalcemia often accompanies hypermagnesemia.

Patient Management

1. Restrict food high in magnesium, including seafood, green vegetables, bananas, grapefruits, oranges, nuts, and legumes.
2. Administer NS and diuretics as ordered to increase renal excretion of magnesium (if the patient has urine output). If the patient is anuric, dialysis may be used.
3. If the patient is symptomatic (e.g., hypotension, shallow respirations, and/or decreased LOC), administer calcium gluconate (5 to 10 mL of 10% solution) as ordered. Hemodialysis may be required.
4. If dysrhythmia occurs, be prepared to begin treatment to decrease the serum magnesium level and to administer antidysrhythmic agents as ordered.
5. If respiratory or cardiac arrest occurs, institute emergency respiratory and cardiac support.

RENAL

ELECTROLYTE IMBALANCE: PHOSPHORUS

Clinical Brief

Phosphorus imbalances occur as a result of changes in phosphorus ion concentrations in ECF. Phosphorus concentration in the ECF is in an inverse relationship with calcium concentration. Hypophosphatemia is associated with hyperparathyroidism, excessive diuresis, chronic alcohol abuse, carbohydrate load, parenteral nutrition without phosphorus supplementation, respiratory alkalosis secondary to mechanical ventilation, malabsorption syndromes, refeeding syndrome and chronic use of antacids. Hyperphosphatemia occurs with hypoparathyroidism, acute and chronic renal failure [CRF], rhabdomyolysis, cytotoxic agents, metabolic acidosis, and excessive phosphate intake.

Presenting Signs and Symptoms

See physical examination.

Physical Examination

	Hypophosphatemia	Hyperphosphatemia
Cardiovascular	Decreased myocardial contractility	
Respiratory	Respiratory failure from diaphragmatic weakness	
Neuromuscular	Malaise, muscle pain, muscle weakness, paresthesia, neuroirritability, confusion, tremors, seizures, coma	Fatigue, S/S of tetany, muscle cramping, hyperreflexia, seizures
Gastrointestinal	Anorexia	

Diagnostic Findings

Hypophosphatemia is defined as a serum phosphorus level <3 mg/dL or 1.8 mEq/L. *Hyperphosphatemia* is a serum phosphorus level >4.5 mg/dL or 2.6 mEq/L.

ACUTE CARE PATIENT MANAGEMENT

Goals of Treatment

	Hypophosphatemia	Hyperphosphatemia
Maintain normal serum phosphorus level	High-phosphorus diet	Low-phosphorus diet

RENAL

	Hypophosphatemia	Hyperphosphatemia
	Low-calcium diet	High-calcium diet
	Correct hypercalcemia	Correct hypocalcemia
	Phosphate replacement	Hydration and diuretic agents; dialysis if life threatening; phosphate-binding antacids (aluminum hydroxide, aluminum carbonate) or calcium carbonate; sevelamer hydrochloride (renal failure)

Hypophosphatemia

Priority Nursing Diagnosis and Potential Complications

Priority Nursing Diagnosis	PC: Potential Complications
Risk for injury	Hypophosphatemia, bleeding

RENAL

Priority Nursing Diagnosis: RISK FOR INJURY related to confusion, muscle weakness secondary to phosphorus imbalance: hypophosphatemia

Outcome Criteria

Serum phosphorus 3 to 4.5 mg/dL (1.8-2.6 mEq/L)
Serum calcium 4.5 to 5.5 mg/dL (total calcium 9-11 mg/dL)
Normal peripheral sensation and movement
Absence of injury
Hgb 12 to 16 g/dL (females); 13.5 to 17.5 g/dL (males)
Hct 37% to 47% (females); 40% to 54% (males)

Patient Monitoring

None specific

Patient Assessment

1. Assess peripheral sensation and strength. Muscle weakness, muscle pain, numbness, and tingling often occur in patients with hypophosphatemia.
2. Assess neurologic status for changes in mentation, confusion, or decreased LOC.
3. Be alert for development of decreased tissue perfusion. Profound hypophosphatemia can impair oxygen delivery to the tissues (decreased 2,3-DPG)

Diagnostics Assessment

Review serum phosphorus levels in conjunction with calcium levels because hypophosphatemia is usually associated with hypercalcemia.

Patient Management

1. Because patients with hypophosphatemia often experience muscle weakness, teach the patient methods for conserving energy and provide for rest periods.
2. Assist with self-care activities and ambulation.
3. Encourage a diet high in phosphorus by encouraging intake of hard cheeses, meats, fish, nuts, eggs, dried fruits and vegetables, and legumes.
4. When administering oral phosphorus supplements, mix them with ice water to increase palatability. Monitor for diarrhea.
5. Administer intravenous phosphate slowly to prevent rapidly decreasing calcium levels. The usual range is 0.08 to 0.32 mM/kg as a loading dose over 6 hours. Observe for signs and symptoms of hypocalcemia, including tetany, fatigue, palpitations, hypotension, numbness and tingling, positive Trousseau's and Chvostek's signs. Avoid IV phosphate in patients with hypercalcemia (metastatic calcification can result).

Hyperphosphatemia

Priority Nursing Diagnosis and Potential Complications	
Priority Nursing Diagnosis	**PC: Potential Complications**
Risk for injury	Hyperphosphatemia, hypocalcemia, seizures

Priority Nursing Diagnosis: RISK FOR INJURY related to tetany secondary to phosphorus imbalance: hyperphosphatemia

Outcome Criteria

Serum phosphorus 2.6 to 4.5 mg/dL (1.8-2.6 mEq/L)
Serum calcium 4.5 to 5.5 mg/dL (total calcium 9-11 mg/dL)
Normal peripheral sensation and movement
Absence of injury
Absence of seizure activity

Patient Monitoring

None specific

RENAL

Patient Assessment

1. Assess BP to detect hypotension resulting from the hypo-calcemia that often accompanies hyperphosphatemia.
2. Observe for signs and symptoms of hypocalcemia, including tetany, fatigue, palpitations, hypotension, numbness and tingling, and positive Trousseau's and Chvostek's signs because hypocalcemia often accompanies hyperphosphatemia.
3. Be alert for the development of tremors and seizures.

Diagnostics Assessment

Review serial serum phosphorus levels in conjunction with calcium levels because hyperphosphatemia is usually associated with hypocalcemia.

Patient Management

1. Administer IV fluids and diuretics as ordered. Anticipate dialysis for life-threatening hyperphosphatemia. Consult with dietitian regarding dietary phosphorus restriction, e.g., foods high in phosphorus such as hard cheeses, meats, fish, nuts, eggs, dried fruits and vegetables, and legumes.
2. Because seizures may result from hyperphosphatemia, initiate seizure precautions by padding side rails, minimizing stimulation, assisting the patient with all activities, and keeping airway management equipment available. If seizures do occur, protect the patient and be prepared to correct hyperphosphatemia and hypocalcemia and administer antiseizure medications if ordered.
3. If ordered, administer phosphate-binding antacids (aluminum hydroxide, aluminum carbonate) before meals to reduce absorption of phosphorus. This intervention is indicated for short-term use only because use of these agents is associated with aluminum toxicity. Alternative agents that may be administered include sucralfate, which also binds phosphorus, or calcium carbonate tablets, which lower the phosphorus levels by increasing calcium levels. Sevelamer is a calcium-free phosphate binder that does not produce hypercalcemia or aluminum toxicity.

ELECTROLYTE IMBALANCE: POTASSIUM

Clinical Brief

Potassium imbalances occur as a result of changes in the concentration of potassium ions in the ECF. Hypokalemia is most often caused

RENAL

by losses of GI secretions, diuretic usage, decreased potassium intake, alkalemia, and aldosterone excess and is often associated with magnesium deficiency. Hyperkalemia occurs with decreased urine output, trauma to cells, potassium-sparing diuretics, ACE inhibitors, increased catabolism, increased potassium intake, acidemia, and hypoaldosteronism.

Presenting Signs and Symptoms

Signs and symptoms depend on the severity of the imbalance. See discussion of physical examination.

Physical Examination

Appearance: Weak, tired

	Hypokalemia	Hyperkalemia
Cardiovascular	ECG: flat T waves, U waves, ST depression, prolonged QT interval, wide QRS, prolonged PR interval, ventricular dysrhythmias	ECG: tall, peaked T waves; prolonged PR interval; flat or absent P waves; prolonged QRS duration; dysrhythmias
Pulmonary	SOB may progress to respiratory arrest	SOB may progress to respiratory arrest
Neuromuscular	Hypoactive reflexes, numbness, cramps, weakness, paralysis	Hyperactive reflexes, numbness, tingling, weakness in arms and legs, paralysis
Gastrointestinal	GI irritability, distention, ileus	Nausea, cramps, diarrhea

Diagnostic Findings

Hypokalemia is defined as serum potassium <3.5 mEq/L; hyperkalemia is a serum potassium >5.5 mEq/L.

ACUTE CARE PATIENT MANAGEMENT

Goals of Treatment

	Hypokalemia	Hyperkalemia
Normalize serum potassium level to prevent cardiac and neuromuscular complications	Treat underlying cause	Treat underlying cause

RENAL

High-potassium diet	Low-potassium diet
Correct alkalosis	Sodium polystyrene sulfonate (Kayexalate) with sorbitol
Oral potassium supplements	Hypertonic glucose and insulin
	Inhaled β_2-adrenergic agonist (albuterol)
Intravenous potassium	Sodium bicarbonate (if not fluid overloaded and acidosis present)
	Calcium gluconate
	Correct hypomagnesemia

Hypokalemia

Priority Nursing Diagnosis and Potential Complications	
Priority Nursing Diagnosis	**PC: Potential Complications**
Risk for injury	Hypokalemia, dysrhythmias, paralytic ileus

Priority Nursing Diagnosis: RISK FOR INJURY related to muscle weakness secondary to hypokalemia

Outcome Criteria

Serum potassium level 3.5 to 5.5 mEq/L
Rounded P and T waves
PR interval 0.12 to 0.20 second
QRS duration 0.04 to 0.10 second
Absence of dysrhythmias
MAP 70 to 105 mm Hg
RR 12 to 20 breaths/min
Nonlabored respirations
Deep, symmetric chest expansion
Normal reflex activity
Normal peripheral sensation and movement
Active bowel sounds
Absence of injury

Patient Monitoring

1. Monitor ECG for changes in complex configuration, waveform, and duration. Flat or inverted T waves, U waves, ST

segment depression, prolonged QT interval, wide QRS, and prolonged PR interval may be present. Dysrhythmias such as PVCs, heart blocks, VT, VF, and torsades de pointes may occur.

2. Monitor changes in intake or output that might affect potassium balance. Hypokalemia may occur with diuretics, renal insufficiency, and GI losses.

Patient Assessment

1. Observe for signs of alkalosis (pH >7.45, decreased RR, tingling, dizziness) because alkalosis shifts potassium into the cells, resulting in hypokalemia.
2. Assess patients on digitalis for signs of digitalis toxicity because hypokalemia increases sensitivity to digitalis.
3. Assess muscle strength and monitor deep tendon reflex activity because hypokalemia is associated with muscle weakness and hyporeflexia that may progress to tetany and respiratory arrest.
4. Assess abdomen size, shape, and bowel sounds every 4 hours because hypokalemia is associated with paralytic ileus.

Diagnostics Assessment

1. Review serial potassium levels to evaluate response to therapy and before administering diuretics. Note: furosemide, dopamine, theophylline, β_2-agonists, catecholamines, and antibiotics such as carbenicillin and gentamicin can cause hypokalemia.
2. Review magnesium levels because abnormalities in magnesium are often mistaken for potassium imbalances. Hypokalemia that is refractory to treatment is often due to hypomagnesemia.

Patient Management

1. Ensure adequate urine output before administering potassium.
2. When administering oral potassium supplements, administer with food or immediately after meals to minimize GI irritation and diarrhea.
3. Ensure patency of the intravenous line before and during potassium administration because potassium is irritating and potentially damaging to tissues. Dilute intravenous potassium to minimize irritation to the veins. A central line is

RENAL

preferable for potassium infusion. Administer intravenous potassium at a rate not to exceed 20 mEq/100 mL/hr; continuous cardiac monitoring should be employed. Rapid potassium infusions can result in cardiac arrest; potassium should never be given undiluted. Check the potassium level and be alert for overcorrection of hypokalemia.

4. Evaluate for hypomagnesemia because magnesium deficiency is often associated with hypokalemia and impairs restoration of normal potassium levels.

5. Withhold oral intake and notify the physician if bowel sounds are severely diminished or absent. Otherwise, encourage foods rich in potassium such as apricots, bananas, cantaloupes, dates, raisins, avocados, beans, meats, potatoes, and orange juice.

6. If cardiac dysrhythmias or respiratory distress occurs, institute immediate treatment for hypokalemia while supporting cardiac and respiratory functioning.

Hyperkalemia

RENAL

Priority Nursing Diagnosis and Potential Complications

Priority Nursing Diagnosis	PC: Potential Complications
Risk for injury	Hyperkalemia, dysrhythmias

Priority Nursing Diagnosis: RISK FOR INJURY related to muscle weakness secondary to hyperkalemia

Outcome Criteria

Serum potassium level 3.5 to 5.5 mEq/L
Rounded P and T waves
PR interval 0.12 to 0.20 second
QRS duration 0.04 to 0.10 second
Absence of dysrhythmias
MAP 70 to 105 mm Hg
RR 12 to 20 breaths/min
Nonlabored respirations
Deep, symmetric chest expansion
Normal reflex activity
Normal peripheral sensation and movement
Active bowel sounds
Absence of injury

Patient Monitoring

1. Monitor ECG for changes in complex configuration, waveform, and duration; tall peaked T waves and a shortened QT interval occur with potassium >6.5 mEq/L; the PR interval increases and QRS widens with potassium >8 mEq/L. Cardiac and renal patients are especially at risk for lethal effects of increased potassium on the electrical conduction system of the heart. Dysrhythmias such as bradycardia, heart blocks, extrasystole, junctional rhythm, idioventricular rhythm, ventricular tachycardia or fibrillation, sine wave, and asystole can occur.
2. Note changes in I&O that might affect potassium balance. A decrease in renal function, such as occurs with acute renal failure, is a risk factor for hyperkalemia.

Patient Assessment

1. Observe for signs of acidosis (pH <7.35, increased RR and depth, confusion, drowsiness, headache) because acidosis shifts potassium out of the cells, resulting in hyperkalemia.
2. Assess muscle strength and monitor deep tendon reflex activity because hyperkalemia is associated with muscle weakness and hyperreflexia. Numbness, tingling, muscle flaccidity, or paralysis may develop. Respiratory arrest may also occur.

Diagnostics Assessment

1. Review serial potassium levels and note the patient's response to therapy. Potassium-sparing diuretics (spironolactone, triamterene, and amiloride), penicillin G, succinylcholine, ACE inhibitors, β-adrenergic blocking agents, and salt substitutes, as well as hemolyzed blood samples, can cause hyperkalemia.
2. Review magnesium levels because abnormalities in magnesium are often mistaken for potassium imbalances.
3. Review serial ABGs because metabolic acidosis is associated with hyperkalemia.

Patient Management

1. Administer sodium polystyrene sulfonate (Kayexalate) with sorbitol orally (15 g, one to four times per day) or as a retention enema (30-50 g) as ordered to treat mild hyperkalemia (potassium of 5.5-6.5 mEq/L). If administered rectally, encourage retention for 30 to 60 minutes for maximum effect. Sodium polystyrene sulfonate increases potassium

excretion in the GI tract and each gram will remove 1 mEq of potassium. If sodium polystyrene sulfonate is used for several days, monitor for hypocalcemia, hypomagnesemia, and fluid overload (as a result of hypernatremia).

2. Anticipate furosemide and NS infusion to rid the body of excess potassium.

3. Inhaled albuterol, 10 to 20 mg by inhaler over 10 minutes, can be administered in patients without IV access. This results in temporarily shifting potassium into the cells.

4. Hypertonic glucose (25 g of 50% dextrose) and regular insulin (10 units regular) may be ordered to temporarily shift potassium into the cells for potassium levels >6.5 mEq/L.

5. Sodium bicarbonate may be ordered to temporarily shift potassium into the cells in cases of acidosis. Carefully assess for signs of hypernatremia and fluid volume overload.

6. To antagonize the cardiac suppression associated with severe hyperkalemia (potassium of >7.5 mEq/L), calcium supplements may be indicated. Administer 10 mL of 10% calcium chloride IV. Alternatively, calcium gluconate may be ordered. Administer calcium gluconate slowly over 2 to 3 minutes while observing for ECG changes. Stop any calcium infusion if bradycardia occurs. Administer with particular caution with patients concomitantly taking digitalis glycosides.

7. While administering medications to treat hyperkalemia, monitor for correction of hyperkalemia and signs of hypokalemia that might result from overcorrection. Observe closely for returning signs of hyperkalemia 30 minutes after calcium administration and 2 to 3 hours after sodium bicarbonate or insulin with glucose treatment.

8. For rapid removal of potassium, dialysis may be ordered.

9. After emergency treatment of hyperkalemia, consult with the physician regarding follow-up treatment to stabilize potassium levels for the long term.

10. Restrict foods rich in potassium such as apricots, bananas, coffee, cocoa, tea, dried fruits, cantaloupes, avocados, beans, meats, potatoes, and orange juice.

ELECTROLYTE IMBALANCE: SODIUM

Clinical Brief

Sodium imbalances occur as a result of changes in sodium ion concentrations in ECF. Hyponatremia is a deficiency of sodium relative to water and can occur from (1) excess water, such as with excessive water intake or syndrome of inappropriate antidiuretic hormone (SIADH) release; (2) sodium depletion, such as with GI losses, diaphoresis, diuretics, renal excretion of sodium, and adrenal insufficiency (AI); and (3) combined water and sodium retention, such as with HF, cirrhosis, or nephrotic syndrome. Hypernatremia is an excess of sodium relative to water and can occur from water depletion, such as with diuretics, decreased intake, GI losses, hyperglycemia, and diabetes insipidus (DI); and from sodium excess, such as with a large sodium intake (rare).

Sodium concentration is largely responsible for determining plasma osmolality. Symptoms associated with sodium imbalances are largely determined by the patient's volume status.

Presenting Signs and Symptoms

Patients with hypernatremia usually have an ECF volume deficit (dehydration). The symptoms of hypernatremia are nonspecific. Abnormalities in the CNS are most common and are a result of water moving out of the brain cells, e.g., confusion, weakness and lethargy progressing to seizures, coma, and death. Patients with hyponatremia can have dehydration (circulatory insufficiency) or overhydration (fluid overload, pulmonary edema). Intracellular swelling in the CNS results in cerebral edema. Symptoms of acute hyponatremia include nausea, vomiting, lethargy and confusion progressing to seizures, coma, and herniation.

Physical Examination

Dehydration (Hyponatremia or Hypernatremia)

Appearance: fatigued, lethargic, loss of skin turgor, dry mucous membranes; with hypernatremia, flushed skin
Vital signs:
    HR: tachycardia
    BP: ↓ or orthostatic BP
    Temperature: elevated
Cardiovascular: weak peripheral pulses, flat neck veins
Neurologic: confused, decreased mentation; irritability, twitching, and seizures (associated with sodium imbalances)
Genitourinary: decreased urine output
Gastrointestinal: abdominal cramps and nausea (hyponatremia)

Overhydration (Hyponatremia or Hypernatremia)

Appearance: malaise, edema, flushed skin (hypernatremia)

Vital signs:
  BP: increased
Cardiovascular: ↑ CO—bounding pulses, hypertension (HTN) or ↓
  CO—weak pulses, S_3, JVD
Pulmonary: crackles, dyspnea
Neurologic: headache, confusion; irritability, twitching, and seizures
  (associated with sodium imbalances)
Gastrointestinal: abdominal cramps and nausea (hyponatremia)

Diagnostic Findings

Hyponatremia is defined as a serum sodium of <135 mEq/L; hypernatremia is a serum sodium of >145 mEq/L.

ACUTE CARE PATIENT MANAGEMENT

Goals of Treatment

	Hyponatremia	Hypernatremia
Maintain normal serum sodium and osmolality level.	Correct underlying problem	Correct underlying problem
	High sodium intake 3% saline 0.45 NS or 0.9 NS	Low sodium intake
Normalize fluid status and serum osmolality.	Correct underlying problem	Correct underlying problem
	If volume deficit: fluids	If volume deficit: fluids without salt
	If volume excess: restrict fluids	If volume excess: restrict fluids
	Diuretics	Diuretics

RENAL

Priority Nursing Diagnoses and Potential Complications

Priority Nursing Diagnoses	PC: Potential Complications
Deficient fluid volume	Hypovolemia, hypernatremia
Excess fluid volume	Hyponatremia
Risk for injury: neurologic dysfunction	Seizures

Nursing Diagnosis: DEFICIENT FLUID VOLUME related to hypernatremia (hypertonic dehydration) or hyponatremia (hypotonic dehydration) associated with decreased fluid intake, GI losses, diaphoresis, diuretics, diabetes insipidus, increased renal excretion of sodium

Outcome Criteria

Patient alert and oriented
Serum sodium 135 to 145 mEq/L
Serum osmolality 275 to 295 mOsm/L
MAP 70 to 105 mm Hg
SBP 90 to 120 mm Hg
Urine output 30 mL/hr or 0.5 to 1 mL/kg/hr
CVP 2 to 6 mm Hg

Patient Monitoring

1. Monitor fluid volume status: obtain hourly I&O; include gastric and diarrheal fluid and diaphoresis in output when calculating fluid balance. Compare serial weights; a rapid decrease in weight (0.5-1 kg/day) suggests fluid volume loss (1 kg is approximately 1000 mL of fluid).
2. Monitor BP, HR, and PA pressures (if available) to evaluate fluid volume status. An orthostatic BP suggests hypovolemia. Monitor MAP; a MAP <60 mm Hg adversely affects renal and cerebral perfusion.

Patient Assessment

1. Assess hydration status: note poor skin turgor on inner thigh or forehead, dry buccal membranes, flat neck veins, complaints of thirst, decreased LOC, decreased weight, and output greater than intake may signal volume depletion.
2. Assess for the development of hypovolemic shock: decreased mentation, SBP <90 mm Hg, urine output <0.5 mL/kg/hr, weak pulses, and cool and clammy skin

Diagnostics Assessment

Review serial serum sodium, serum osmolality, urine osmolality, and specific gravity to assess fluid volume status. Sodium value <135 mEq/L, specific gravity <1.01, and serum osmolality <285 mOsm/L suggest overhydration; sodium value >145 mEq/L, specific gravity >1.02, and serum osmolality >295 mOsm/L suggest dehydration.

RENAL

Patient Management

1. Administer fluids and electrolytes as ordered. Lactated Ringer's (LR) or 0.9 NS may be ordered for patients with hypovolemic hyponatremia. Patients should be carefully monitored for possible fluid overload while ECF volume is replaced. Adjust oral intake of sodium as indicated by the serum sodium level.

2. Keep the patient supine until volume has been replaced. Assist the patient with position changes or ambulation because orthostatic changes may occur while the patient is volume depleted.

3. For a patient with hyponatremia, encourage fluids high in sodium such as chicken or beef broth and canned tomato juice. For a patient with hypernatremia, encourage fluids low in sodium such as distilled water, coffee, tea, and orange juice. Assist the patient with hypernatremia to avoid foods high in sodium.

Nursing Diagnosis: EXCESS FLUID VOLUME related to hypernatremia or hyponatremia (excess fluid intake, heart failure, cirrhosis, or nephrotic syndrome)

RENAL

Outcome Criteria

Patient alert and oriented
Serum sodium 135 to 145 mEq/L
Serum osmolality 275 to 295 mOsm/L
MAP 70 to 105 mm Hg
SBP 90 to 140 mm Hg
Lungs clear to auscultation
CVP 2 to 6 mm Hg
Intake approximates output
Skin intact

Patient Monitoring

1. Monitor fluid volume status: obtain hourly I&O; calculate fluid balance every 8 hours. Compare serial weights; a rapid increase in weight (0.5-1 kg/day) suggests fluid volume retention.

2. Monitor BP, HR, and PA pressures (if available) to evaluate fluid volume status.

Patient Assessment

1. Assess fluid volume status; note the onset of S_3 and crackles; presence of edema, cough, or frothy sputum; increased

work of breathing; decreased peripheral perfusion; and increased JVP to determine development of HF or pulmonary edema.

2. Assess for headache, blurred vision, and altered mentation; and note pupil size and reaction, speech, motor strength, and tremors to determine development of cerebral edema. Neurologic dysfunction is a major concern with sodium imbalances.

3. Assess for pressure ulcer development secondary to edema/changes in perfusion.

Diagnostics Assessment

Review serial serum sodium, serum osmolality, urine osmolality, and specific gravity to assess fluid volume status. Sodium value <135 mEq/L, specific gravity <1.010, and serum osmolality <285 mOsm/L suggest overhydration; sodium value >145 mEq/L, specific gravity >1.020, and serum osmolality >295 mOsm/L suggest dehydration.

Patient Management

1. If the patient is hypervolemic with hyponatremia, administer treatment ordered to correct the primary problem, e.g., heart failure, nephritic syndrome. Anticipate sodium and fluid restrictions and diuretic therapy. Concentrate medications when possible to minimize fluid intake.

2. If the patient is hypervolemic with hypernatremia, anticipate hypotonic fluids and diuretics. In patients with hypovolemia and hypernatremia, anticipate isotonic saline administration during hemodynamic instability.

3. Institute pressure ulcer prevention strategies, e.g., meticulous skin care, repositioning, relieving pressure points.

Nursing Diagnosis: RISK FOR INJURY: NEUROLOGIC DYSFUNCTION related to hypernatremia or hyponatremia

Outcome Criteria

Patient alert and oriented
Absence of neurologic deficits
Serum sodium 135 to 145 mEq/L

Patient Monitoring

None specific

Patient Assessment

Assess neurologic status: note any change in mental status and presence of neuromuscular irritability, headache, blurred vision, focal neurologic deficits, or seizure activity. Note pupil size and reaction, speech, motor strength, and presence of tremors to determine development of cerebral edema. Neurologic dysfunction is a major concern with hypernatremia.

Diagnostics Assessment

Review serial serum sodium levels. Neurologic signs generally manifest at sodium levels <125 mEq/L and become more severe at levels <115 mEq/L.

Patient Management

1. If the patient is asymptomatic, aggressive therapy to correct serum sodium is not indicated. Treating the underlying cause of hyponatremia is indicated, e.g., DI, SIADH, or AI.
2. If patient is *symptomatic* from hyponatremia, anticipate correction of serum sodium. Generally, the target is an increase in sodium no more than 2 mEq/L/hr for acute symptomatic hyponatremia. In patients with *symptomatic* hyponatremia >48 hours, the target is an increase in sodium no more than 1.5 mEq/L/hr. Monitor serum sodium frequently; overcorrection or rapid normalization of serum sodium can result in central demyelination syndrome (assess for quadriparesis, quadriplegia, dysarthria, mutism, abnormal pupils or oculomotor function, and coma).
3. If the patient is *symptomatic* from hypernatremia, anticipate water repletion to gradually lower serum sodium. Rapid lowering of sodium can result in cerebral edema; carefully monitor neurologic status.

RENAL

MULTISYSTEM DISORDERS

ACQUIRED IMMUNODEFICIENCY SYNDROME (AIDS)

Clinical Brief

AIDS is caused by a retrovirus, human immunodeficiency virus type 1 (HIV-1), that infects and destroys T-helper lymphocytes (CD4 cells), resulting in impairment of the immune system. HIV infection is transmitted in three ways: sexually; through transfer of infected blood; and perinatally, either from mother to fetus or from mother to infant via breast milk. People infected with HIV may exhibit variable clinical manifestations that range from no symptoms to complications associated with profound immunosuppression (AIDS). Those infected with HIV are diagnosed with AIDS if they exhibit any of the following manifestations: low CD4 counts (<200 cells/mm³), any one of many characteristic opportunistic infections or malignancies, AIDS dementia complex (ADC), or wasting syndrome.

Presenting Signs and Symptoms

Signs and symptoms are highly variable, depending on the clinical manifestations of immunodeficiency.

Physical Examination

The patient may exhibit any or all of the following, dependent on the clinical manifestations of the disease:

Skin: purplish lesions (Kaposi's sarcoma); maculopapular rash along dermatomes (varicella-zoster virus [VZV])

Neurologic: irritability, personality changes (*Toxoplasma gondii* encephalitis), depression, ADC, weakness, nuchal rigidity, photophobia, seizures (cryptococcal meningitis), progressive multifocal leukoencephalopathy (from CJ virus)

Pulmonary: dyspnea; chills; fever; hypoxemia; dry, nonproductive cough (*Pneumocystis jiroveci* pneumonia [PCP]); hemoptysis, night sweats (*Mycobacterium tuberculosis* [TB] infection)

Gastrointestinal: watery diarrhea, weight loss

Oral: ulcerative lesions (herpes simplex virus 1 [HSV1]), hairy leukoplakia (*Candida albicans* infection) from Epstein-Barr virus (EBV)

Gynecologic: ulcerative lesions (HSV2 or HSV1), hairy leukoplakia (*C. albicans* infection), cervical neoplasia

Eye: visual changes (cytomegalovirus [CMV] retinopathy)

General: cachexia (wasting syndrome)

MULTI

Diagnostic Findings (to determine HIV infection)

Two positive results to ELISA or enzyme immunoassays (EIA), then
confirmed with positive result on the Western blot test; if results
are unclear or indeterminate, then positive result on polymerase
chain reaction (PCR)

ACUTE CARE PATIENT MANAGEMENT

Goals of Treatment

Minimize further immune system damage through preventing ram-
pant HIV replication.

Antiretroviral agents: nucleoside reverse transcriptase inhibitors
(NRTIs), protease inhibitors, nonnucleoside reverse transcriptase
inhibitors (NNRTIs)

Prevent opportunistic infections.

Maintain up-to-date vaccinations, including pneumococcal vaccine, hepatitis B vaccine (HBV), hepatitis A vaccine (HAV),
and influenza vaccine.

Preventive treatment may include the following for those at particular risk:

PCP prophylaxis: trimethoprim-sulfamethoxazole (TMP-SMX),
dapsone, or pentamidine aerosol

TB prophylaxis: isoniazid (INH) and pyridoxine or rifampin

VZV prophylaxis: varicella-zoster immune globulin (VZIG) or
acyclovir

Treat opportunistic infections and malignancies as they arise.

P. jiroveci

TMP-SMX and corticosteroids

Alternative therapy: pentamidine, trimetrexate, and corticosteroids

Kaposi's sarcoma

Interferon α-2A

Vinblastine, vincristine

Toxoplasmosis

Pyrimethamine, sulfadiazine, folinic acid

Herpes

Acyclovir, vidarabine, foscarnet

Cytomegalovirus (CMV)

Ganciclovir

Foscarnet

Cidofovir

Cryptococcus

MULTI

Amphotericin B
Flucytosine, fluconazole
Candida
Fluconazole
Itraconazole
M. tuberculosis
INH, rifampin, and pyrazinamide and ethambutol or rifampin
Detect/prevent clinical sequelae (Table 5-50).

***Table* 5-50** CLINICAL SEQUELAE ASSOCIATED WITH HUMAN IMMUNODEFICIENCY VIRUS

Complication	Signs and Symptoms
Respiratory failure	Restlessness, tachypnea, Pao_2 <50 mm Hg, $Paco_2$ >50 mm Hg, pH <7.35
Septic shock	SBP <90 mm Hg, HR >90 beats/min, RR >20 breaths/min or $Paco_2$ <32 mm Hg, Pao_2/Fio_2 <280, T >100.4° F or <96.7° F (>38° C or <36° C), WBCs >12,000/mm^3 or <4000/mm^3 or >10% neutrophils; altered mental status, urine output <0.5 mL/kg/hr, plasma lactate >2 mmol/L
DIC	Bleeding from any orifice and mucous membranes; cool, clammy skin; abnormal clotting studies, D-dimer >2; FDP 1:40
AIDS dementia complex	Forgetfulness, personality changes, clumsiness, ataxia, weak or paralyzed extremities, aphasia
Meningitis	Nuchal rigidity, headache, fever, lethargy, confusion, seizures
Lymphoma (CNS)	Symptoms depend on tumor site, paresthesias, visual loss, ataxia, paresis, seizures
CMV retinitis	Progressive visual loss
Peripheral nervous system disease	Ascending paralysis, burning pain in feet, absent Achilles' tendon reflex, hypersensitivity, decreased sensation, muscle weakness

AIDS, Acquired immunodeficiency syndrome; *CMV,* cytomegalovirus; *CNS,* central nervous system; *DIC,* disseminated intravascular coagulation; *FDP,* fibrin degradation products; *HR,* heart rate; *RR,* respiratory rate; *SBP,* systolic blood pressure; *T,* temperature; *WBC,* white blood cell.

Priority Nursing Diagnoses and Potential Complications	
Priority Nursing Diagnoses	**PC: Potential Complications**
Impaired gas exchange	Hypoxemia, pneumonia
Risk for infection, ineffective protection	Opportunistic infections, sepsis (see p. 405), seizures (see p. 136)
Deficient fluid volume	
Diarrhea	
Imbalanced nutrition: less than body requirements (see p. 53)	Negative nitrogen balance
Risk for interrupted family processes (see p. 45)	

Nursing Diagnosis: IMPAIRED GAS EXCHANGE related to infectious processes impairing oxygen diffusion and decreasing lung compliance

Outcome Criteria

Patient alert and oriented
PaO_2 80 to 100 mm Hg
pH 7.35 to 7.45
$PaCO_2$ 35 to 45 mm Hg
O_2 sat ≥95%
RR 12 to 20 breaths/min, eupnea
Lungs clear to auscultation
Minute ventilation <10 L/min
Vital capacity (VC) 15 mL/kg
Lung compliance 60 to 100 mL/cm H_2O

Patient Monitoring

1. Continuously monitor oxygenation status with pulse oximetry (SpO_2). Be alert for effects of interventions and patient activities, which may adversely affect oxygen saturation.
2. Monitor serial lung compliance values to assess progression of lung stiffness.
3. Monitor pulmonary function by assessing minute ventilation and VC measurements. A VC of >15 mL/kg is generally needed for spontaneous breathing.

Patient Assessment

1. Assess respiratory status: RR >30 breaths/min suggests respiratory distress. Note the use of accessory muscles and the respiratory pattern. Note the presence of breath sounds and

MULTI

adventitious sounds, suggesting worsening pulmonary congestion.

2. Assess for signs and symptoms of hypoxemia: increased restlessness, increased complaints of dyspnea, and changes in LOC. Cyanosis is a late sign.

3. Assess the patient for clinical sequelae (see Table 5-50).

Diagnostics Assessment

1. Review ABGs for decreasing trends in PaO_2 (hypoxemia) or pH (acidosis). O_2 sat should be ≥95%.

2. Review serial chest radiographs to evaluate patient progress or worsening lung condition.

3. Review culture reports for identification of the infecting organism. Review WBC counts and differential for evidence of bacterial infection or pneumonia.

Patient Management

1. Provide supplemental oxygen as ordered. If the patient develops respiratory distress, be prepared for intubation and mechanical ventilation. (See p. 503 for information on ventilation therapies.)

2. Promote pulmonary hygiene with chest physiotherapy and postural drainage if necessary. Assist the patient to C&DB and reposition at least every 2 hours. Encourage incentive spirometry to decrease risk of atelectasis. Suction secretions as needed and note the color and consistency of sputum. Position the patient for maximum chest excursion.

3. Minimize oxygen demand by decreasing anxiety, fever, and pain.

4. Administer chemotherapeutic agents as ordered. Be alert for further decreases in WBC, RBC, and platelets and fluid and electrolyte imbalances. Orthostatic hypotension can occur with parenteral pentamidine administration.

5. Corticosteroids may be administered to decrease the interstitial inflammatory response.

Nursing Diagnoses: RISK FOR INFECTION related to immune dysfunction, and INEFFECTIVE PROTECTION related to immune dysfunction, chemotherapeutic agents, and central nervous system involvement

Outcome Criteria

Absence of injury
Absence of aspiration

Absence of additional infections or neoplasms
T 97.7° to 100° F (36.5°-37.8° C)
Urine output 30 mL/hr or 0.5 to 1 mL/kg/hr
BUN 10 to 20 mg/dL
Creatinine 0.6 to 1.2 mg/dL
WBCs 5000 to 10,000/mm³
RBCs 4.2 to 6.2 million/mm³
Platelets >150,000/mm³

Patient Monitoring

1. Monitor urine output hourly and note a decreasing trend, which may suggest renal insufficiency.
2. Monitor temperature to evaluate the patient's condition and response to therapy.

Patient Assessment

1. Assess for fever, chills, and night sweats. Be alert to signs of sepsis and septic shock (see p. 405).
2. Assess neurologic status: a decreased sensorium decreases protective reflexes and increases the risk for aspiration. Changes in LOC, cognition, or personality or the onset of numbness or tingling, weakness of extremities, incoordination, paralysis, or visual loss may indicate CNS infection or side effects of chemotherapeutic agents. Nuchal rigidity may indicate meningitis.
3. Assess for signs and symptoms of infection: fever, redness, tenderness, drainage at intravenous sites, cloudy urine, purulent sputum, white patches on oral mucosa, and foul vaginal drainage.
4. Assess for bleeding: test urine and stool for blood; note gingival bleeding or oozing of blood from intravenous sites; note any petechiae.
5. Inspect for new lesions, rashes, or breaks in skin.
6. Assess the patient for clinical sequelae (see Table 5-50).

MULTI

Diagnostics Assessment

1. Review CD4 counts to evaluate immune status.
2. Review all culture reports for identification of infecting organism.
3. Review WBC counts and differential for evidence of bacterial infection.

4. Review serial Hgb, Hct, and platelet values to evaluate anemia and the extent of thrombocytopenia.
5. Review serial BUN and creatinine levels to evaluate renal function.

Patient Management

1. Provide oral hygiene before and after meals to treat stomatitis associated with chemotherapy. Apply lip balm to prevent cracks and crusting.
2. Provide meticulous body hygiene, especially after diarrheal episodes, to prevent spread of organisms from stool. Use of A&D ointment or zinc oxide may prevent skin excoriation around the anorectal area.
3. Turn and reposition the patient at least every 2 hours and provide range of motion (ROM) and skin care to improve circulation and prevent skin breakdown. A therapeutic bed may be required.
4. Encourage fluids to maintain hydration and minimize nephrotoxic drug effects.
5. Keep HOB elevated or the patient in a side-lying position to prevent aspiration if the LOC is decreased and/or the patient is receiving enteral feedings. Keep suction equipment available.
6. Ensure a safe environment: bed in low position, call bell in reach, and soft restraints if indicated.
7. Institute seizure precautions as necessary.
8. Institute bleeding precautions if the patient is thrombocytopenic.
9. Assist the patient with activities to prevent falls. Institute fall precautions.
10. Hematest body fluids for occult blood. Spontaneous bleeding (e.g., hemoptysis, hematuria) may indicate DIC.
11. Orient the patient as needed.
12. Administer vaccines and other pharmacologic agents as ordered to ensure prophylaxis of other opportunistic infections.

Nursing Diagnoses: DEFICIENT FLUID VOLUME related to severe diarrhea, vomiting, poor oral intake, and night sweats; and DIARRHEA related to intestinal malabsorption and/or intestinal *Mycobacterium avium* or *Salmonella* infections

Outcome Criteria

Moist mucous membranes
Elastic skin turgor

MULTI

T C 97.7° to 100° F (36.5° to 37.8° C)
Intake approximates output
Urine specific gravity 1.001 to 1.035
Serum osmolality 275 to 295 mOsm/kg
SBP 90 to 120 mm Hg
MAP 70 to 105 mm Hg

Patient Monitoring

1. Continuously monitor CVP and PA pressures (if available) to evaluate trends. Decreasing trends suggest hypovolemia.
2. Monitor MAP; a value <60 mm Hg adversely affects renal and cerebral perfusion.
3. Monitor fluid status: calculate hourly I&O to determine fluid balance. Compare daily weights; a loss of 0.25 to 0.5 kg/day reflects excess fluid loss. Include an accurate stool count because patients may exceed 10 L of fluid per day with watery diarrhea.
4. Measure urine specific gravity to evaluate hydration status. Increased values reflect dehydration or hypovolemia.

Patient Assessment

1. Obtain BP and HR every hour to evaluate the patient's fluid volume status: HR >120 and SBP <90 mm Hg suggest hypovolemia; orthostatic hypotension reflects hypovolemia.
2. Evaluate mucous membranes by checking the area where the cheek and gum meet; dry, sticky membranes are associated with hypovolemia. Test skin turgor on the sternum or the inner aspects of thighs for best assessment.
3. Assess the patient for clinical sequelae (see Table 5-50).

Diagnostics Assessment

1. Review stool cultures for identification of any infectious agent.
2. Review serial electrolytes because diarrhea and vomiting can result in a severe electrolyte imbalance.
3. Review serial serum osmolality to evaluate hydration status; increased values are associated with dehydration and hypovolemia.

Patient Management

1. Administer fluids as ordered, carefully monitoring for fluid overload.

MULTI

2. Administer antidiarrheal agents as ordered to help control diarrhea.

3. Administer antiemetic agents as ordered to help control vomiting and increase the patient's ability to take oral food and fluids. Anticipate administration of nutritional supplementation either parenterally or enterally. Consult with a nutritionist to assess the patient's needs.

4. Administer antipyretics as ordered to control temperature, and antibiotics as ordered to treat intestinal infections.

5. Provide small portions of food more frequently. Include high-calorie, high-protein snacks. Avoid spicy or greasy foods. Cold entrées may be more palatable.

6. Low-fiber or fiber-enriched, lactose-free, or pectin-containing formulas may help reduce diarrheal episodes.

ANAPHYLACTIC SHOCK

Clinical Brief

Drugs (particularly antibiotics, radiologic contrast dye, and muscle relaxants) and blood products can cause iatrogenic anaphylaxis. Insect stings and bites and many foods (e.g., peanuts) are common noniatrogenic causes of anaphylaxis. In these instances, a stimulus (allergen) triggers a release of biochemical mediators from mast cells and eosinophils, which disrupts vascular permeability, leading to rapid fluid extravasation into the interstitial spaces, a decreased circulating volume, and circulatory collapse that is clinically consistent with a state of shock. Increased bronchial reactivity produces bronchial edema and bronchoconstriction, causing alveolar hypoventilation, respiratory distress, and respiratory failure.

Presenting Signs and Symptoms

Signs and symptoms include itching, chest tightness, difficulty breathing, and a feeling of impending doom.

Physical Examination

Appearance: restless, anxious
Vital signs:
    BP: normal to hypotensive
    HR: >100 beats/min
    RR: tachypnea
Neurologic: anxious progressing to unresponsive
Cardiovascular: tachycardia with ectopic beats

Pulmonary: stridor, wheezes, crackles
Skin: erythema, urticaria, flushing, angioedema

Diagnostic Findings

Clinical manifestations are the basis for diagnosis.

ACUTE CARE PATIENT MANAGEMENT

Goals of Treatment

Remove cause if possible (e.g., stop antibiotic infusion, search for
   insect stinger).
Maintain airway.
   Oxygen, intubation/mechanical ventilation
   Epinephrine (first-line agent)
   Diphenhydramine
   Inhaled β_2-adrenergic agonists
   Histamine-2 (H_2) antagonists
Optimize oxygen delivery.
   Colloids (albumin)
   Epinephrine
   Vasopressors: dopamine, norepinephrine

Priority Nursing Diagnoses and Potential Complications	
Priority Nursing Diagnoses	**PC: Potential Complications**
Impaired gas exchange	Hypoxemia, tracheobronchial constriction
Ineffective tissue perfusion	Hypovolemia
Ineffective protection (see p. 48)	
Risk for interrupted family processes (see p. 45)	

MULTI

Nursing Diagnosis: IMPAIRED GAS EXCHANGE related to bronchoconstriction,
pulmonary edema, or obstructed airway

Outcome Criteria

Patient alert and oriented
PaO_2 80 to 100 mm Hg
pH 7.35 to 7.45
$PaCO_2$ 35 to 45 mm Hg
O_2 sat ≥95%
Lungs clear to auscultation, no wheezes, no stridor
RR 12 to 20 breaths/min, eupnea

Patient Monitoring

Continuously monitor oxygenation status via pulse oximetry (SpO_2).

Patient Assessment

1. Obtain VS every 5 to 15 minutes during the acute phase.
2. Assess for hoarseness, stridor, and upper airway obstruction. Late airway reaction may occur 6 to 12 hours after the initial event.
3. Assess lung sounds and RR and depth to evaluate the degree of respiratory distress. Decreased air movement indicates severe respiratory distress.
4. Assess for signs and symptoms of hypoxemia: increased restlessness, increased complaints of dyspnea, and changes in LOC. Cyanosis is a late sign.

Diagnostics Assessment

Review ABGs to evaluate hypoxemia and acid-base status. Hypoxemia and acidosis are risk factors for dysrhythmias. O_2 sat should be ≥95%.

Patient Management

1. Establish and maintain an airway and provide supplemental oxygen. Endotracheal intubation or tracheostomy may be required.
2. Racemic epinephrine may be prescribed via nebulizer (0.3 mL racemic epinephrine in 3 mL NS) for laryngeal edema.
3. Epinephrine 1 to 5 mL of 1:10,000 solution (0.1-0.5 mg) may be prescribed IV to reverse bronchoconstriction and hypotension. May be administered via ET tube if unable to establish IV access. Alternatively, may administer 1 to 3 mL of 1:000 solution IM into the thigh.
4. Corticosteroids may be administered to decrease or control edema and prevent late airway reaction.
5. Metaproterenol 0.2 to 0.3 mL (5% solution) in 2.5 mL NS may be administered via nebulizer, or ipratropium bromide (36 mcg inhaled) may be used for persistent bronchospasm.
6. Diphenhydramine (Benadryl) may be used to reduce the effects of histamine. Usual dose is 25 to 50 mg IV.
7. H_2 antagonists, such as cimetidine or ranitidine, may be ordered as adjuvant intravenous agents.
8. Position the patient for maximum chest excursion.
9. Administer CPR and follow the ACLS protocol should cardiopulmonary arrest occur.

MULTI

Nursing Diagnosis: INEFFECTIVE TISSUE PERFUSION related to decreased circulating volume associated with permeability changes and loss of vasomotor tone

Outcome Criteria

Patient alert and oriented
Skin warm and dry
Peripheral pulses strong
Urine output 30 mL/hr or 0.5 to 1 mL/kg/hr
Absence of edema
SBP 90 to 120 mm Hg
MAP 70 to 105 mm Hg
O_2 sat ≥95%

Patient Monitoring

1. Monitor BP continuously via arterial cannulation if possible. Monitor MAP, an indicator that accurately reflects tissue perfusion. MAP <60 mm Hg adversely affects cerebral and renal perfusion.
2. Continuously monitor ECG to detect life-threatening dysrhythmias or HR >140 beats/min, which can adversely affect SV.
3. Continuously monitor oxygenation status via pulse oximetry (SpO_2).
4. Monitor hourly urine output to evaluate renal perfusion.
5. Monitor PA pressures and CVP (if available) hourly or more frequently to evaluate the patient's response to treatment. Both parameters reflect the capacity of the vascular system to accept volume and can be used to monitor for fluid overload and pulmonary edema.

Patient Assessment

1. Obtain HR, RR, and BP every 15 minutes to evaluate the patient's response to therapy and to detect cardiopulmonary deterioration.
2. Assess mentation, skin temperature, and peripheral pulses to evaluate CO and state of vasoconstriction.
3. Assess periorbital area, lips, hands, feet, and genitalia to evaluate interstitial fluid accumulation.

Diagnostics Assessment

1. Review lactate levels, an indicator of anaerobic metabolism. Increased levels may signal decreasing oxygen delivery.

2. Review ABGs for hypoxemia and acidosis because these conditions can precipitate dysrhythmias and affect myocardial contractility.
3. Review BUN, creatinine, and electrolytes and note trends to evaluate renal function.

Patient Management

1. Administer colloids (albumin) or crystalloids (LR) as ordered to restore intravascular volume.
2. An infusion of epinephrine (2-4 mcg/min) or norepinephrine (4-8 mcg/min) may be required.
3. Dopamine may also be tried to improve BP.
4. Provide oxygen therapy as ordered. Anticipate intubation and mechanical ventilation if the oxygenation status deteriorates or cardiopulmonary arrest ensues. See p. 503 for information on ventilation therapies.

BURNS

Clinical Brief

Thermal, electrical, chemical, or radiation-contaminated media are common causes of burns. The severity of the burn is determined by the percentage of body surface area burned (or the extent or total body surface area [TBSA] of the burn wound) and the depth of the burn wound. In addition to burn depth and TBSA percentage, the patient's age, medical history, and cause and location of the burn are investigated. Burn depth is described as superficial (or first degree), partial thickness (or second degree), deep partial thickness (also described as second degree), or full thickness (or third degree). Thermal burns can also be classified into concentric zones of injury. Hyperemia is the outermost zone and is the least damaged; stasis is the middle zone in which tissue perfusion is compromised; the innermost zone is coagulation, where cellular death occurs. In full-thickness burns, the zone of coagulation involves the entire thickness of the dermis.

Presenting Signs and Symptoms

Superficial: skin is red, blanches, and is painful (e.g., sunburn)
Partial thickness: pink or red, blisters; wound is painful
Deep partial thickness: pale, mottled, pearly white; dry, painful, no blanching

MULTI

Full thickness: involves all layers of the skin and subcutaneous tissue; the wound varies from waxy white or charred to red or brown and leathery; the area is insensitive to pain, although surrounding areas are typically painful. Injury may involve muscles, tendons, or bones.

Inhalation injury: chest tightness, hoarseness, dyspnea, tachypnea. If severe, singed nares and black sputum

Carbon monoxide inhalation or poisoning: clinical manifestations of inhalation injury, plus:

Mild: headache, nausea

Moderate: dizziness, confusion, ataxia, visual changes, pallor

Severe: dysrhythmias, coma, cherry-red buccal membranes, cherry-red cast to skin

Electrical: variable manifestations. Patient may have obvious charring at entry and exit wounds. Most common manifestations of electrical burns include cardiac dysrhythmias, rhabdomyolysis, or spinal cord trauma.

Physical Examination

Skin: area of body burned (Figure 5-2, Table 5-51), depth of burn.

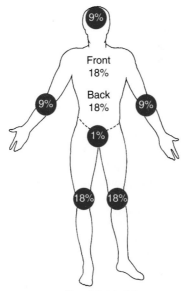

Figure 5-2 Rule of nines

Table 5-51 BERKOW FORMULA FOR CALCULATING % BODY SURFACE AREA (BSA) BURNS

Area	AGE IN YEARS					
	0-1	2-4	5-9	10-14	15	>15
Head	19	17	13	11	9	7
Neck	2	2	2	2	2	2
Ant. trunk	13	13	13	13	13	13
Post. trunk	13	13	13	13	13	13
R buttock	2.5	2.5	2.5	2.5	2.5	2.5
L buttock	2.5	2.5	2.5	2.5	2.5	2.5
Genitalia	1	1	1	1	1	1
R U arm	4	4	4	4	4	4
L U arm	4	4	4	4	4	4
R L arm	3	3	3	3	3	3
L L arm	3	3	3	3	3	3
R hand	2.5	2.5	2.5	2.5	2.5	2.5
L hand	2.5	2.5	2.5	2.5	2.5	2.5
R thigh	5.5	6.5	8	8.5	9	9.5
L thigh	5.5	6.5	8	8.5	9	9.5
R leg	5	5	5.5	6	6.5	7
L leg	5	5	5.5	6	6.5	7
R foot	3.5	3.5	3.5	3.5	3.5	3.5
L foot	3.5	3.5	3.5	3.5	3.5	3.5

L, Left; *LL*, left lower; *LU*, left upper; *R*, right; *RL*, right lower; *RU*, right upper.

MULTI

- Burns of head, neck, face, chest, mouth, nose, and pharynx correlate with inhalation injury.
- Hallmark of smoke inhalation: hypercapnia, hypoxemia, widened alveolar-arterial oxygen gradient, stridor, crackles, and carbonaceous sputum may be present. Charred eyebrows, eyelashes, nasal hair, and facial hair may also be present. Suspect carbon monoxide poisoning if history includes exposure in confined space and the patient appears delirious or comatose; note increased carboxyhemoglobin levels.

Diagnostic Findings

Other findings may include the following:
SBP <90 mm Hg and HR >120 beats/min if shock is present.

ACUTE CARE PATIENT MANAGEMENT

Goals of Treatment

Maintain airway and oxygenation.

>   Supplemental oxygen

>   Intubation/mechanical ventilation

Restore intravascular volume.

>   Crystalloids, colloids (after first 24 hours postinjury)

Control pain.

>   Opioid analgesics

Control anxiety.

>   Benzodiazepine antianxiety agents

Maximize wound closure.

>   Topical antimicrobials; wound management, including debridement, escharotomies, and grafts

Detect/prevent clinical sequelae (Table 5-52).

Table 5-52   CLINICAL SEQUELAE ASSOCIATED WITH BURNS

Complication	Signs and Symptoms
Burn shock (hypovolemic)	SBP <90 mm Hg, HR >100 beats/min, urine output <5 mL/kg/hr, cool, clammy skin
Renal failure	Urine output <5 mL/kg/hr, steady rise in BUN, creatinine
Respiratory distress	Carbon flecks in sputum, carbon monoxide levels >15%, RR >30 breaths/min, Pao_2 <60 mm Hg, stridor, noisy respirations, restlessness, change in LOC
Loss of limb	Pulselessness, pain, paresthesias, paralysis
Burn wound sepsis	Purulent exudate; focal black, gray, or dark brown discoloration; hemorrhagic discoloration and vascular thrombosis of underlying fat; erythema or edema of unburned skin at the wound margins; unexpected rapid eschar separation; greater than 100,000 organism per gram of tissue
Curling's ulcer	Blood in emesis, NG aspirate, or stool; decreasing trend in Hgb and Hct
Septic shock	SBP <90 mm Hg, HR >90 beats/min, RR >20 breaths/min or $Paco_2$ <32 mm Hg, Pao_2/Fio_2 <280, T >100.4° F or <96.7° F (>38° C or <36° C), WBCs >12,000/mm³ or <4000/mm³ or >10% neutrophils; altered mental status, urine output <0.5 mL/kg/hr, plasma lactate >2 mmol/L

BUN, Blood urea nitrogen; *Hct,* hematocrit; *Hgb,* hemoglobin; *HR,* heart rate; *LOC,* level of consciousness; *NG,* nasogastric; *RR,* respiratory rate; *SBP,* systolic blood pressure; *T,* temperature; *WBC,* white blood cell.

MULTI

Priority Nursing Diagnoses and Potential Complications

Priority Nursing Diagnoses	PC: Potential Complications
Impaired gas exchange	Hypoxemia, atelectasis, pneumonia, tracheobronchial constriction, ARDS, pulmonary edema
Deficient fluid volume	Hypovolemia, GI bleeding
Ineffective tissue perfusion	
Acute pain	
Risk for infection; Impaired skin integrity	Opportunistic infections
Imbalanced nutrition: less than body requirements (see p. 53)	Negative nitrogen balance, delayed wound healing
Ineffective protection (see p. 48)	
Risk for interrupted family processes (see p. 45)	

Nursing Diagnosis: IMPAIRED GAS EXCHANGE related to inhalation injury: carbon monoxide poisoning, chemical pneumonitis, and/or upper airway obstruction

Outcome Criteria

Patient alert and oriented
PaO_2 80 to 100 mm Hg
$PaCO_2$ 35 to 45 mm Hg
pH 7.35 to 7.45
O_2 sat ≥95% (with absent or normal carboxyhemoglobin)
Lungs clear to auscultation
RR 12 to 20 breaths/min, eupnea

Patient Monitoring

1. Continuously monitor oxygenation status with pulse oximetry (SpO_2) *if* carboxyhemoglobin levels are normal. Remember that hemoglobin has a much higher affinity for carbon monoxide than oxygen; therefore a high SpO_2 may be a toxic indication of hemoglobin saturation with carbon monoxide. Be alert for effects of interventions and patient activities that may adversely affect oxygen saturation.

2. Calculate $P(a/A)O_2$ ratio to estimate intrapulmonary shunting and evaluate the degree of lung dysfunction. The higher the ratio, the better the lung function.

Patient Assessment

1. Obtain BP, HR, and RR every 15 minutes during the acute phase. Patients with carbon monoxide poisoning are tachycardic and tachypneic.

MULTI

2. Assess for headache, confusion, N/V, and dyspnea. Note skin and mucous membranes—cherry-red color reflects severe carbon monoxide poisoning. As the carbon monoxide level increases, the patient will become more confused and eventually comatose.

3. Assess the rate and depth of respirations; note stridor or noisy respirations that may indicate respiratory distress. Laryngeal edema can develop over 72 hours after the burn event. In patients with burns of the chest, carefully assess chest excursion because burns to this area may result in hypoventilation and decreased compliance.

4. Note the presence of singed nasal hairs or carbonaceous sputum, indicators of inhalation injury.

5. Assess for signs and symptoms of hypoxia: increased restlessness, increased complaints of dyspnea, and changes in LOC.

6. Assess the patient for clinical sequelae (see Table 5-52).

Diagnostics Assessment

1. Review carboxyhemoglobin levels for carbon monoxide reflecting smoke inhalation (normal is <5% saturation of Hgb in nonsmokers, <10% in smokers).

2. Review ABGs for decreasing trends in PaO_2 (hypoxemia) or pH (acidosis). O_2 sat should be ≥95%.

3. Review serial chest radiographs to evaluate the patient's progress or a worsening lung condition.

4. Review Hgb and Hct levels and note trends. Decreased RBCs can adversely affect oxygen carrying capacity.

Patient Management

1. Maintain oral airway and administer supplemental oxygen as ordered. FIO_2 of 1 is used to treat carbon monoxide poisoning, initially. Anticipate hyperbaric oxygen treatment in moderate and severe cases of carbon monoxide poisoning. Anticipate intubation and mechanical ventilation with PEEP for respiratory failure. See p. 503 for information on ventilation therapies. Carbon monoxide poisoning may be treated with hyperbaric oxygenation.

2. Anticipate escharotomies to chest if full-thickness burns are present, to improve compliance and ventilation.

3. Promote pulmonary hygiene: position the patient for maximum chest excursion, assist the patient to C&DB to mobilize secretions, and encourage incentive spirometry to prevent atelectasis; chest physiotherapy and suction may be required.

MULTI

If mechanically ventilated, position patient to decrease risk of aspiration and ventilator-acquired pneumonia.

4. Bronchodilators may be used to treat bronchospasm.

Nursing Diagnosis: DEFICIENT FLUID VOLUME related to plasma loss, increased capillary permeability with interstitial fluid accumulation, and increased insensible water loss

Outcome Criteria

Patient alert and oriented
HR 60 to 100 beats/min
SBP 90 to 120 mm Hg
Urine output 30 to 50 mL/hr or 0.5 to 1 mL/kg/hr
Urine specific gravity 1.005 to 1.03
Lungs clear to auscultation
Serum sodium 135 to 145 mEq/L
Serum potassium 3.5 to 5.5 mEq/L

Patient Monitoring

1. Monitor fluid volume status: massive fluid shifts will occur within the first 72 hours of a burn event. Measure hourly I&O to determine fluid balance. Urine output reflects renal perfusion; ideally, urine output should be at least 1 mL/kg/hr. Compare daily weights (1 kg is approximately 1000 mL of fluid); a 15% to 20% weight gain within the first 72 hours can be anticipated and is indicative of fluid retention in the interstitium. The diuresis phase begins approximately 48 to 72 hours after the burn event.

2. Monitor MAP; a value <60 mm Hg adversely affects renal and cerebral perfusion.

3. If a PA catheter has been inserted, monitor PAWP to evaluate fluid status. CO/CI will be increased as a result of a hypermetabolic state.

4. If a CVP line is indicated, frequently monitor pressure during fluid resuscitation to evaluate the patient's response to therapy. CVP can be estimated; see p. 24.

5. Continuously monitor the ECG for dysrhythmias.

Patient Assessment

1. Obtain VS every 15 minutes during the acute phase to detect cardiopulmonary deterioration. Continuously monitor ECG for dysrhythmias in patients with electrical burns.

2. Assess fluid volume status: dry mucous membranes, decreased pulse pressure, tachycardia, furrowed tongue, absent JVD, and

complaints of thirst suggest hypovolemia. Bounding pulses, cough, dyspnea, and crackles suggest volume overload.

3. Assess the patient for clinical sequelae (see Table 5-52).

Diagnostics Assessment

1. Review serum electrolyte levels closely during the fluid resuscitation period; either hyperkalemia or hypokalemia can occur; hyponatremia is not uncommon. Electrolyte imbalances can occur as a result of loss of fluids via burns, shifts into interstitial spaces, drainage, fluid resuscitation, and tissue death.

2. Review serial Hgb, Hct, osmolality, and urine specific gravity and note trends. An increase in values may indicate hypovolemia.

Patient Management

1. Fluid administration is usually instituted for burns involving >20% of the TBSA. Administer LR as ordered. The American Burn Association (ABA) recommends 2 to 4 mL/kg/% BSA burned. Give the first half during the first 8 hours from the time of the burn injury and the second half during the next 16 hours. Colloids are contraindicated during the first 24 hours after the burn because the capillary membranes are unstable and colloids can seep into the interstitium. Colloids are administered during the second 24 hours after the burn, when the capillary membranes stabilize, to maintain intravascular volume. While diuresis occurs, infusion rates may be decreased. Dextrose in water solutions may be used to prevent hypernatremia in the second 24 hours. Hyperglycemia may occur with nonjudicious use of dextrose in water solutions.

2. Blood or blood products may be administered as needed. See p. 585 for information on blood transfusion.

3. Administer potassium as ordered to replace potassium loss.

Nursing Diagnosis: INEFFECTIVE TISSUE PERFUSION related to hypovolemia, circumferential burns of extremities, and presence of myoglobin

Outcome Criteria

Patient alert and oriented
Peripheral pulses strong
Bowel sounds present
Absence of GI bleeding
Gastric pH 5 to 7
Urine output 30 to 50 mL/hr or 0.5 to 1 mL/kg/hr

SBP 90 to 120 mm Hg
MAP 70 to 105 mm Hg
CVP 2 to 6 mm Hg

Patient Monitoring

1. Monitor MAP, an indicator of tissue perfusion. A MAP <60 mm Hg adversely affects cerebral and renal perfusion.
2. If a CVP line is indicated, continuously monitor pressure as an index of fluid volume status. CVP can be estimated (see p. 24).
3. Measure hourly I&O and urine specific gravity to evaluate adequacy of hydration; if urine output falls below 30 mL/hr, suspect renal ischemia secondary to hypovolemia or damage to tubules by myoglobin.
4. Monitor the color of the urine; if it is a port-wine color, suspect myoglobinuria.

Patient Assessment

1. Assess for systemic hypoperfusion: absent or decreased peripheral pulses; cool, pale skin; and capillary refill ≥3 seconds.
2. Assess neurovascular status every 15 to 30 minutes the first 24 to 48 hours: pulselessness, pallor, pain, paresthesia, and paralysis can signal nerve ischemia. Damaged sensory nerve fibers may be misinterpreted as improvement in neurovascular status, when in fact a loss of a limb may be the outcome. In burned extremities, monitor Doppler signal of palmar arch vessel in the arms and posterior tibial artery pulse in the legs. Maintain extremities free of restrictive clothing and jewelry.
3. Assess GI status: test gastric pH, auscultate bowel sounds, and test stool for occult blood. GI ischemia contributes to Curling's ulcer.
4. Assess the patient for clinical sequelae (see Table 5-52).

Diagnostics Assessment

1. Check the urinalysis for myoglobin level (myoglobin can cause tubular destruction and ATN).
2. Check urine specific gravity to determine hydration status and renal function.
3. Review serial BUN, creatinine, and potassium results for a steady rise in values, which may indicate renal failure.
4. Review Hgb and Hct levels for decreasing trends, which may suggest blood loss secondary to Curling's ulcer.
5. Review serum albumin, total protein, and glucose levels as indicators of stress hypermetabolism or catabolism. Review

MULTI

urine urea nitrogen (UUN) results to determine nitrogen balance. The basal metabolic rate is doubled in severe burn injuries, and profound catabolism occurs. Note that weight gain will reflect fluid retention, not gain of muscle mass.

Patient Management

1. Administer fluids as ordered to optimize oxygen delivery and tissue perfusion. Inotropic agents may be required.
2. Anticipate administration of mannitol, an osmotic diuretic, to flush kidneys and to maintain a urine output >100 mL/hr if the patient has myoglobinuria.
3. Anticipate NG intubation for abdominal distention secondary to paralytic ileus and/or for antacid administration.
4. Maintain gastric pH at 5 to 7 with proton pump inhibitors, antacids, cytoprotectives, and H_2-antagonists as ordered to help prevent Curling's ulcer.
5. Elevate edematous extremities to increase venous return and to decrease edema, which may adversely affect tissue perfusion. Be prepared for an escharotomy or fasciotomy to improve circulation if circumferential burns are present.
6. Maintain a warmer than normal room temperature and keep wounds covered to prevent hypothermia and vasoconstriction.

MULTI

Nursing Diagnosis: ACUTE PAIN related to burned tissues and wound debridement

Outcome Criterion

Patient will communicate pain relief.

Patient Monitoring

None specific

Patient Assessment

1. Assess pain using the patient's self-report whenever possible. See p. 35 for information about acute pain. An increase in intensity of pain may indicate ischemia. A decrease in pain may be misinterpreted as an improvement, when in fact sensory nerve fibers may be damaged. Note changes in HR, BP, and RR that may suggest SNS stimulation, which may signal pain. However, the absence of changes in HR, BP, and RR do not necessarily mean absence of pain.
2. Observe for cues such as grimacing, grunting, sobbing, irritability, withdrawal, or hostility, which may signal pain.

However, absence of these behaviors does not necessarily mean absence of pain.

<u>*Diagnostics Assessment*</u>

None specific

<u>*Patient Management*</u>

1. Administer an opioid analgesic as ordered (usually IV morphine sulfate or fentanyl) or self-administered oral transmucosal fentanyl before debridement and at frequent intervals for controlled pain management. Most patients should receive opioid analgesia around the clock, either via an intravenous drip or via a PCA pump with a set basal rate. Intramuscular and subcutaneous injections are not indicated during the acute burn phase because medications are poorly absorbed. Pain increases catecholamine release and the metabolic rate, which puts an added burden on an already hypermetabolic state.

2. Administer anxiolytic agents IV as needed and before debridements or escharotomies. Midazolam may induce retrograde amnesia, so that patients may not recall unpleasant debridements or other treatments.

3. Plan diversional activities appropriate for the patient's developmental level and the severity of burn incurred (e.g., music, television).

4. Promote relaxation through controlled breathing and guided imagery.

5. Reposition the patient frequently to promote comfort and avoid deformities.

6. Keep partial-thickness burn wounds covered because any stimulus to these wounds can cause pain.

7. See Acute Pain, p. 35.

Nursing Diagnoses: RISK FOR INFECTION secondary to impaired skin integrity related to severe burns

<u>*Outcome Criteria*</u>

T 97.7° to 100° F (36.5°-37.8° C)

Negative wound biopsy report

Healing by secondary intention or skin grafting without purulent drainage

Patient Monitoring

None specific

Patient Assessment

1. Obtain temperature every 4 hours to monitor inflammatory response.
2. Assess the wound daily and note color, drainage, odor, and the presence of epithelial buds. Rapid eschar separation, disappearance of well-defined burn margins, discoloration, and purulent exudates are indicative of infection. In skin grafts, bright red blood drainage and pooling of fluid will inhibit successful grafting. Check for adherence and closure of interstices. Check the donor site for infection development.
3. Assess the patient for clinical sequelae (see Table 5-52).

Diagnostics Assessment

1. Review wound biopsy reports for identification of the infecting organism (>100,000 organisms per gram of tissue = burn wound sepsis).
2. Review serial WBC counts; silver sulfadiazine may decrease WBCs; an increase may be associated with sepsis, although the leukocytosis may be caused by the inflammatory process.

Patient Management

1. Handwashing is the most effective weapon against transmission of infection.
2. Patients should be assigned their own equipment including stethoscopes and thermometers.
3. Avoid placing intravenous lines through burned skin. Remove invasive lines as early as possible.
4. Verify tetanus prophylaxis.
5. Regulate environmental temperature to 85° to 90° F (29°-32° C) to avoid excess heat loss when wounds are open.
6. Provide wound management per institutional protocol. General principles include premedicating the patient; daily wound cleansing and debridement using aseptic technique; and clipping hair around burn wounds to prevent infection. Wounds may be exposed (open treatment) or may be covered with a topical agent and dressing (closed treatment).
7. Document wound characteristics daily.

MULTI

8. Anticipate a wound excision and skin grafting to speed healing, prevent contractures, and shorten convalescence. Potential treatments may also include use of artificial skin products and vernix caseosa.

9. Administer antibiotics as ordered when an invasive burn wound infection has been identified.

10. Anticipate nutritional support that supplies adequate protein, carbohydrate, and fat calories; zinc; vitamins; and minerals to promote tissue healing. Energy requirements may be as high as 5000 kcal/day. High-nitrogen diets by the enteral route may offer immunologic benefits.

DISSEMINATED INTRAVASCULAR COAGULATION (DIC)

Clinical Brief

DIC is a coagulation disorder characterized by inappropriate concurrent thrombus formation and hemorrhage secondary to overstimulation of the clotting cascade. It is a secondary complication of many underlying conditions (e.g., shock, sepsis, crush injuries, obstetric complications, burns, malignancies, venom exposure, and ARDS).

Presenting Signs and Symptoms

Initial signs and symptoms include abdominal, back, or joint pain; mild bleeding from wounds and intravenous access sites; and a feeling of impending doom. As the disease progresses, the patient exhibits widespread, frank hemorrhage that results from excessive plasmin generation, widespread micro- and macrothrombosis from excessive thrombin generation, and shock.

Physical Examination

Depends on the underlying condition
Vital signs:
    HR: >100 beats/min
    BP: <90 mm Hg
    RR: >20 breaths/min
Neurologic: restless, anxious, altered LOC, seizures, unresponsive
Skin: mottled, cold fingers and toes; ecchymoses, petechiae, gingival bleeding
Cardiovascular: tachycardia
Pulmonary: dyspnea, tachypnea, hemoptysis

Gastrointestinal: hematemesis, melena, abdominal tenderness

Renal: urine output <0.5 mL/kg/hr, hematuria

Other: bleeding from any orifice

Diagnostic Findings

Clinical manifestations are the basis for diagnosis. Sudden onset of bleeding (petechia, purpura, ecchymosis, oozing from puncture sites) and thrombosis (gangrene, acral cyanosis, skin necrosis, deep vein thrombosis [DVT]). Other findings include the following:

D-dimer >2

Platelets <100,000/mm^3

PT >15 sec

PTT >40 sec

Fibrinogen <150 mg/dL

Fibrin split products >8 mcg/mL

Fibrin degradation products >1:40

Antithrombin III decreased

Blood smear shows schistocytes and burr cells

Positive protamine sulfate test results

ACUTE CARE PATIENT MANAGEMENT

MULTI

Goals of Treatment

Treat primary problem.

    Surgery, antibiotics

Optimize oxygen delivery.

    Crystalloids

    Supplemental oxygen/mechanical ventilation

    RBCs

    Positive inotropes: dopamine, dobutamine

Reverse clotting mechanism.

    Heparin (controversial)

    Hirudin (controversial)

    Protein C infusions (controversial)

Replace coagulation components.

    Platelets, FFP, cryoprecipitate

Correct hemostatic deficiency.

    Vitamin K

Detect/prevent clinical sequelae (Table 5-53).

Table 5-53 CLINICAL SEQUELAE ASSOCIATED WITH DISSEMINATED
INTRAVASCULAR COAGULATION (DIC)

Complication	Signs and Symptoms
ARDS	Dyspnea, hypoxemia refractory to increases in FIO_2, cyanosis, PaO_2/FIO_2 <175, PAWP <18 mm Hg
Intracerebral bleeding	Change in sensorium, headache, seizures, extremity weakness/paralysis
GI dysfunction	Absent bowel sounds, abdominal pain, diarrhea, upper and lower GI bleeding
Renal failure	Urine output <0.5 mL/kg/hr, steady rise in creatinine
Shock	SBP <90 mm Hg; HR >100 beats/min; patient anxious to unresponsive; cold, clammy skin; urine output <0.5 mL/kg/hr

ARDS, Acute respiratory distress syndrome; *GI,* gastrointestinal; *HR,* heart rate; *PAWP,* pulmonary artery wedge pressure; *SBP,* systolic blood pressure.

Priority Nursing Diagnoses and Potential Complications

Priority Nursing Diagnoses	PC: Potential Complications
Ineffective tissue perfusion	Venous thromboemboli, thrombocytopenia
Ineffective protection (see p. 48)	
Imbalanced nutrition: less than body requirements (see p. 53)	
Risk for interrupted family processes (see p. 45)	

MULTI

Nursing Diagnosis: INEFFECTIVE TISSUE PERFUSION (PERIPHERAL, RENAL, CEREBRAL, GI, AND PULMONARY) related to concurrent thrombus formation and bleeding

Outcome Criteria

Patient alert and oriented
Absence of neurologic deficits
Skin warm and dry
Peripheral pulses strong
Absence of acral cyanosis (mottled, cool toes and fingers)
Absence of chest pain
Absence of hemoptysis
RR 12 to 20 breaths/min, eupnea

Absence of hematemesis, melena

Active bowel sounds

Urine output 30 mL/hr or 0.5 to 1 mL/kg/hr

Absence of hematuria

Absence of pain, tenderness, redness, and venous distention in calves

Platelets >50,000/mL

Fibrinogen >100 mg/dL

SBP 90 to 120 mm Hg

MAP 70 to 105 mm Hg

CI 2.5 to 4 L/min/m^2

O_2 sat ≥5%

Svo_2 60% to 80%

Hct 37% to 47% (females); 40% to 54% (males)

Patient Monitoring

1. Monitor BP continuously via arterial cannulation because cuff pressures can cause further injury and bleeding. Monitor MAP, an indicator that accurately reflects tissue perfusion. MAP <60 mm Hg adversely affects cerebral and renal perfusion.

2. Monitor PA pressures and CVP hourly or more frequently to evaluate the patient's response to treatment. Both parameters reflect the capacity of the vascular system to accept volume and can be used to monitor for fluid overload and pulmonary edema.

3. Obtain CO/CI at least every 8 hours or more frequently to evaluate the patient's progress or deterioration.

4. Calculate $\dot{D}o_2I$ and $\dot{V}o_2I$ to evaluate oxygen transport; inadequate oxygen delivery and consumption produce tissue hypoxia.

5. Continuously monitor Svo_2 (if available). A decreasing trend may indicate decreased oxygen delivery and/or increased tissue oxygen extraction.

6. Continuously monitor oxygen status with pulse oximetry. Be alert for effects of interventions and patient activities, which may adversely affect oxygen saturation.

7. Continuously monitor ECG to detect life-threatening dysrhythmias and ST segment and T-wave changes.

8. Monitor fluid balance: record hourly I&O; include blood loss in determining fluid balance.

MULTI

Patient Assessment

1. Obtain HR, RR, and BP every 15 minutes to evaluate the patient's response to therapy and detect cardiopulmonary deterioration.
2. Assess peripheral pulses, capillary refill, and the color and temperature of the extremities to evaluate thrombotic-ischemic changes.
3. Assess skin, mucous membranes, and all orifices for bleeding. Test emesis; urine; stool; NG aspirate; and drainage from tubes and drains for blood. Assess invasive line sites for oozing blood.
4. Assess for the presence of headache or any change in LOC that might suggest impaired cerebral perfusion or intracranial bleeding; check extremities for strength and movement to identify neurologic involvement.
5. Assess the patient for clinical sequelae (see Table 5-53).

Diagnostics Assessment

1. Review coagulation studies: INR; PTT; D-dimer; fibrinogen level; platelet count; fibrin degradation products; and factors II, V, VII, and VIII to evaluate resolution or worsening of DIC.
2. Review Hgb and Hct levels and note trends. Decreased RBCs can adversely affect oxygen carrying capacity.
3. Review ABGs for hypoxemia and acidosis, which can signal pulmonary involvement and impaired gas exchange.

Patient Management

1. Administer blood and blood products as ordered to replace coagulation components. (See p. 585 for information on blood transfusion.)
2. Administer crystalloids (LR or NS) as ordered to optimize oxygen delivery. Monitor CVP and PAWP to evaluate response to fluid resuscitation.
3. Avoid dextran infusions for hypovolemia secondary to hemorrhage because coagulation problems can occur and enhance the bleeding problem.
4. Heparin may be ordered in select cases. Observe the patient for increased bleeding.
5. Dopamine or dobutamine may be used to enhance contractility; dopamine may be used to improve renal and splanchnic blood flow.
6. Provide oxygen therapy as ordered.

MULTI

7. Do not disturb established clots; use cold compresses or pressure to stop bleeding. Use an arterial line to minimize the number of peripheral sticks, thus minimizing thrombosis.

8. Avoid trauma and excessive manipulation of the patient to prevent further bleeding. Use gentle oral care, keep the patient's lips moist, avoid tape on the skin, use an electric razor, and use suction at the lowest pressure possible.

9. Avoid aspirin products, which could potentiate bleeding.

10. Administer pharmacologic agents, such as vitamin K, as ordered to correct hemostatic deficiency.

SYSTEMIC INFLAMMATORY RESPONSE SYNDROME (SIRS), SEPSIS, SEPTIC SHOCK, AND MULTIPLE ORGAN DYSFUNCTION SYNDROME (MODS)

Clinical Brief

SIRS is a massive systemic inflammatory response mounted against a variety of overwhelming insults.

Sepsis is a specific type of systemic inflammatory response to an infection. *Severe sepsis* is a disruption in homeostasis involving inflammation, coagulation and impaired fibrinolysis. This cascade of events leads to global tissue hypoxia.

Septic shock is defined as sepsis-induced hypotension that persists despite adequate fluid resuscitation along with hypoperfusion and abnormalities or organ dysfunction.

MODS refers to a profound disruption in organ function in critically ill patients that typically results from SIRS.

Presenting Signs and Symptoms

SIRS: manifested by two or more of the following:

T >100.4° or <96.8° F (>38° or <36° C)

HR >90 beats/min

RR >20 breaths/min or $PaCO_2$ <32 mm Hg

WBC >12,000/mm³ or <4000/mm³ or >10% immature neutrophils

Sepsis

SIRS + infection

Septic shock

Sepsis + hypotension (despite fluid resuscitation) and hypoperfusion

SBP <90 mm Hg

Lactic acidosis, oliguria, altered mental status, Pao_2/Fio_2 <280

MODS: presence of altered organ function, e.g.:
   ARDS
   Acute liver failure
   Coma
   Ischemic bowel injury
   GI bleeding
   Acute pancreatitis
   DIC
   Acute renal failure

Physical Examination

Neurologic: unresponsive, difficult to arouse
Cardiovascular: weak, thready pulses
Pulmonary: crackles, wheezes, respiratory distress
Skin:
   Cool, clammy skin
   Color pale
   Other: evidence of multiple organ failure

Diagnostic Findings

Clinical manifestations are the basis for diagnosis.

ACUTE CARE PATIENT MANAGEMENT

Goals of Treatment

Optimize oxygen delivery.
   Colloids, crystalloids
   Vasopressors: dopamine, norepinephrine, phenylephrine
   Inotropes: dobutamine
   Intubation/mechanical ventilation
   Blood products
Treat underlying problem.
   Antibiotics
   Surgery
Treat dysfunctional organs and organ systems when they show signs
   of failure. (See pertinent previous sections.)
Institute severe sepsis bundles (measure serum lactate, obtain blood
   cultures before antibiotic administration, ensure timely antibiotic
   administration, provide fluid resuscitation for hypotension or
   elevated lactate level, and initiate vasopressors as indicated; main-
   tain CVP >8 mm Hg and Svo_2 ≥65%)
Detect/prevent clinical sequelae (Table 5-54).

MULTI

Table 5-54 CLINICAL SEQUELAE ASSOCIATED WITH SEPTIC SHOCK

Complication	Signs and Symptoms
Cardiopulmonary arrest	Nonpalpable pulse, absent respirations
Multiple organ dysfunction syndrome (MODS)	
Acute respiratory distress syndrome (ARDS)	Hypoxemia refractory to increases in F_{IO_2}, decreased compliance, Pao_2/F_{IO_2} <175, PAWP <18 mm Hg
Renal dysfunction	Urine output <0.5 mL/kg/hr, steady rise in creatinine
GI bleed/dysfunction	Blood in NG aspirate, emesis, stool; absent bowel sounds, distention
Hepatic dysfunction	Jaundice, bilirubin >2 mg/dL, rise in LFTs, decreased albumin
Disseminated intravascular coagulation (DIC)	Bleeding from puncture sites and mucous membranes, hematuria, ecchymoses, prolonged PT and PTT; decreased fibrinogen, platelets, factors V, VIII, XIII, II; increased FSP; FDP 1:40; D-dimer >2

FDP, Fibrin degradation products; *FSP,* fibrin split products; *GI,* gastrointestinal; *LFT,* liver function test; *NG,* nasogastric; *PAWP,* pulmonary artery wedge pressure; *PT,* prothrombin time; *PTT,* partial thromboplastin time.

MULTI

Priority Nursing Diagnoses and Potential Complications

Priority Nursing Diagnoses	PC: Potential Complications
Ineffective tissue perfusion	Dysrhythmias, hypovolemia, acidosis (metabolic), renal insufficiency, paralytic ileus, hepatic dysfunction
Impaired gas exchange	Hypoxemia, atelectasis, pneumonia
Ineffective thermoregulation	
Ineffective protection (see p. 48)	
Imbalanced nutrition: less than body requirements (see p. 53)	
Risk for interrupted family processes (see p. 45)	

Nursing Diagnosis: INEFFECTIVE TISSUE PERFUSION related to inflammation, coagulation, and impaired fibrinolysis cascade

Outcome Criteria

Patient alert and oriented
Skin warm and dry
Peripheral pulses strong
Urine output 30 mL/hr or 0.5 to 1 mL/kg/hr
SBP 90 to 120 mm Hg
MAP 70 to 105 mm Hg
CVP >8 mm Hg
Lactate <4 mmol/L
CI ~4.5 L/min/m^2
O_2 sat ≥95%
Svo_2 60% to 80%
$\dot{D}o_2I$ >600 mL/min/m^2
$\dot{V}o_2I$ >165 mL/min/m^2
ERo_2 25%

Patient Monitoring

1. Monitor BP continuously via arterial cannulation because cuff pressures are less accurate in shock states. Monitor MAP, an indicator that accurately reflects tissue perfusion. MAP <60 mm Hg adversely affects cerebral and renal perfusion.

2. Monitor PA pressures and CVP hourly or more frequently to evaluate the patient's response to treatment. Both parameters reflect the capacity of the vascular system to accept volume and can be used to monitor for fluid overload and pulmonary edema.

3. Obtain CO/CI at least every 4 hours or more frequently to evaluate the patient's response to changes in therapy.

4. Calculate $\dot{D}o_2I$ and $\dot{V}o_2I$ to evaluate effectiveness of therapy. Calculate ERo_2; a value >25% suggests increased oxygen consumption, decreased oxygen delivery, or both.

5. Continuously monitor Svo_2. A decreasing trend may indicate decreased CO and increased tissue oxygen extraction (inadequate perfusion). Calculating $Ca\text{-}vo_2$ (arteriovenous oxygen content difference) also provides information regarding oxygen uptake at the tissue level.

6. Monitor hourly urine output to evaluate renal perfusion.

MULTI

Patient Assessment

1. Monitor HR, RR, and BP continuously; in particular note the patient's response to therapy and detect cardiopulmonary deterioration.
2. Assess mentation, skin temperature, and peripheral pulses and the presence of cardiac or abdominal pain to evaluate CO and the state of vasoconstriction.
3. Assess for evidence of frank or occult bleeding when drotrecogin alfa (activated) administered.
4. Assess the patient for clinical sequelae (see Table 5-54).

Diagnostics Assessment

1. Review ABGs for hypoxemia and acidosis because these conditions can precipitate dysrhythmias or affect myocardial contractility. Hypoxemia refractory to increasing FIO_2 may signal ARDS.
2. Review WBC counts for leukocytosis as the body attempts to fight infection or for leukopenia as the bone marrow becomes exhausted.
3. Review culture reports for identification of the infecting pathogen.
4. Review Hgb and Hct levels, and note trends. Decreased RBCs can adversely affect oxygen carrying capacity.
5. Review lactate levels, an indicator of anaerobic metabolism, which can identify tissue hypoperfusion in patients who may not be hypotensive. Increased levels signify that cells are not consuming the oxygen they need . However, lactate levels may be less useful in severe septic shock.
6. Review BUN, creatinine, and electrolytes and note trends to evaluate renal function.

Patient Management

1. Administer colloids (albumin) and crystalloids (LR or NS) to increase preload as ordered. Monitor CVP and PAWP to evaluate the patient's response to fluid resuscitation.
2. To increase oxygen transport, inotropes such as dobutamine may be required to increase myocardial contractility, SV, CO, and BP. Blood may also be given to increase Hgb level.
3. Administer antibiotics as ordered; obtain cultures before initiating antibiotics. Antibiotic therapy may not be effective in

MULTI

the first 48 to 72 hours; thus interventions to support BP and oxygenation are required.

4. Administer vasopressors such as dopamine or norepinephrine as ordered to oppose vasodilation.

5. Be prepared to administer insulin infusion to maintain glycemic control.

6. Be prepared to administer drotrecogin alfa (activated) (Xigris) for its immunomodulatory effects that include antiinflammatory, antithrombotic, and profibrinolytic properties. Administer intravenously in dedicated sole-use line at a dose of 24 mcg/kg/hr for 96 hours. Be alert for any signs of frank or occult bleeding, and discontinue the infusion if hemorrhage occurs.

7. Provide oxygen therapy as ordered. Anticipate intubation and mechanical ventilation before severe respiratory distress or cardiopulmonary arrest ensues.

8. Neuromuscular blockade with sedation and pain control may be instituted to reduce oxygen consumption and improve ventilation.

9. Treat dysrhythmias according to ACLS.

10. Prepare the patient for surgical intervention if required (e.g., abscess drainage).

MULTI

Nursing Diagnosis: IMPAIRED GAS EXCHANGE related to increased pulmonary vascular resistance, pulmonary interstitial edema, and pulmonary microthrombi

Outcome Criteria

Patient alert and oriented
pH 7.35 to 7.45
PaO_2 80 to 100 mm Hg
$PaCO_2$ 35 to 45 mm Hg
O_2 sat $\geq$95%
RR 12 to 20 breaths/min, eupnea
Lungs clear to auscultation

Patient Monitoring

1. Continuously monitor oxygenation status with pulse oximetry (SpO_2). Be alert for effects of interventions and patient activities, which may adversely affect oxygen saturation.

2. Continuously monitor PAS pressure (if available) because hypoxia can increase sympathetic tone and increase pulmonary vasoconstriction.

Patient Assessment

1. Monitor HR, RR, and BP continuously; in particular note the patient's response to therapy and detect cardiopulmonary deterioration.
2. Assess respiratory status: RR >30 breaths/min suggests respiratory distress. Note the use of accessory muscles and respiratory pattern. Note the presence of adventitious breath sounds, suggesting worsening pulmonary congestion.
3. Assess for signs and symptoms of hypoxemia: increased restlessness, increased complaints of dyspnea, and changes in LOC. Cyanosis is a late sign.
4. Assess the patient for clinical sequelae (see Table 5-54).

Diagnostics Assessment

1. Review ABGs for Pao_2 refractory to increases in Fio_2 that may suggest ARDS. O_2 sat should be ≥95%.
2. Review serial chest radiographs to evaluate the improvement or worsening of the patient's lung condition.
3. Review Hgb and Hct levels and note trends. Decreased RBCs can adversely affect oxygen carrying capacity.

Patient Management

1. Provide supplemental oxygen as ordered. Anticipate low tidal volumes and permissive hypercapnia in patients who are mechanically ventilated. Monitor plateau pressures (<30 cm H_2O is desirable).
2. When hemodynamically stable, promote pulmonary hygiene: assist the patient to C&DB and reposition the patient every 2 hours to mobilize secretions and to prevent atelectasis.
3. Minimize oxygen demand by decreasing anxiety, fever, shivering, and pain.
4. Position the patient for maximum chest excursion and comfort.

Nursing Diagnosis: INEFFECTIVE THERMOREGULATION related to infecting pathogen (in sepsis)

Outcome Criteria

T 97.7° to 100° F (36.5°-37.8° C)
Absence of shivering

Patient Monitoring

Continuously monitor core temperature for any changes.

Patient Assessment

1. Obtain HR and BP and evaluate trends to detect hemodynamic compromise.
2. Assess skin temperature and presence of diaphoresis. Note any chills or shivering, which increases oxygen demand.
3. Assess the patient for clinical sequelae (see Table 5-54).

Diagnostics Assessment

1. Review culture reports for identification of infecting pathogen.
2. Review WBC counts; an increase suggests that the body is attempting to fight the infection; a decrease suggests bone marrow exhaustion.

Patient Management

1. Regulate environmental temperature to help maintain the patient's temperature between 97.7° and 100.4° F (36.5°-38° C).
2. Apply extra bed linens, blankets, or thermal tent (e.g., BAIR hugger) during hypothermia and shivering episodes.
3. Remove extra linens during hyperthermia episodes.
4. Tepid sponge baths or a cooling blanket may be needed during hyperthermia episodes.
5. Administer antipyretics as ordered to reduce fever.
6. Administer antibiotics as ordered to eradicate infection.
7. See p. 605 for information on thermal regulation.

BIBLIOGRAPHY

NEUROLOGIC DISORDERS

Arbour M: Intracranial hypertension: monitoring and nursing assessment, *Crit Care Nurse* 24(5):19-32, 2004.

Bader MK: *AANN core curriculum for neuroscience nursing*, ed 4, Philadelphia, 2004, Saunders.

Bernard SA, Buist M: Induced hypothermia in critical care medicine: a review, *Crit Care Med* 31(7):2041-2051, 2003.

Brain Trauma Foundation, Inc. and American Association of Neurological Surgeons: Guidelines for the management of severe traumatic brain injury. Accessed January 8, 2005, from www.guidelines.gov/summary/aummary.aspx?doc_id=3794&nbr=3020&strin.

Chesnut RM: Management of brain and spine injuries, *Crit Care Clin* 20:25-55, 2004.

Clifton GL et al: Fluid thresholds and outcome from severe brain injury, *Crit Care Med* 30(4):924-935, 2002.

Demetriades D et al: Mortality prediction of head abbreviated injury score and Glasgow outcome coma scale: analysis of 7,764 head injuries, *J Am Coll Surg* 199(2):216-222, 2004.

Fahy BG, Sivaraman V: Current concepts in neurocritical care, *Anesthesiol Clin North Am* 20:441-462, 2002.

Fulgham JR et al: Management of acute ischemic stroke, *Mayo Clin Proc* 79(11):1459-1469, 2004.

Green GB et al: *The Washington manual of medical therapeutics*, ed 31, St Louis, 2004, University of Washington.

Greenberg MS: *Handbook of neurosurgery*, ed 5, New York, 2001, Thieme Medical Publishers.

Griffen MM, Frykberg ER, Kerwin HA: Clearance of blunt cervical spine injury: plain radiograph or computed tomography scan? *J Trauma* 55:222-227, 2003.

Hadley MM, Walters BC: Guidelines for the management of acute cervical spine and spinal cord injuries. Accessed January 9, 2003, 2005 from the World Wide Web, www.soineuniverse.com/displayarticle.php/article2081.html.

Hauser CJ, Visvikis G, Hinrichs C: Prospective validation of computed tomographic screening of the thoracolumbar spine in trauma, *J Trauma* 55:228-235, 2003.

Hickey JV: *The clinical practice of neurological and neurosurgical nursing*, ed 4, Philadelphia, 1997, Lippincott Williams & Wilkins.

Hickey JV: *Neurological and neurosurgical nursing*, ed 5, Philadelphia, 2003, Lippincott Williams & Wilkins.

Hoyt DB: What's new in general surgery: trauma and critical care, *J Am Coll Surg* 194(3):335-351, 2002.

Hunt W, Hess R: Surgical risk as related to time of intervention in the repair of intracranial aneurysms, *J Neurosurg* 28:14, 1968.

Jackson AB et al: A demographic profile of new traumatic spinal cord injuries: change and stability over 30 years, *Archives of PM&R* 85(11):1740-1748, 2004.

Kerr ME et al: Relationship between apoE4 allele and excitatory amino acid levels after traumatic brain injury, *Crit Care Med* 31:2371-2379, 2003.

Lee TL, Green BA: Advances in the management of acute spinal cord injury, *Orthop Clin North Am* 33:211-315, 2002.

Manly G, Knudson MM, Marabito D: Hypotension, hypoxia, and head injury: frequency, duration, and consequences, *Ann Em Med* 40(5):1118-1123, 2002.

Marik PE, Varon J: The management of status epilepticus, *Chest* 126(2):582-591, 2004.

Mitchell E, Moore K: Stroke: holistic care and management, *Nurs Stan* 18(31):43-52, 2004.

Okonkwo DO, Stone JR: Basic science of closed head injuries and spinal cord injuries, *Clin Sports Med* 22:467-481, 2003.

Plum F, Posner J: *The diagnosis of stupor and coma,* ed 3, Philadelphia, 1980, FA Davis.

Sinha PK, Neema PK, Rathod RC: Anesthesia and intracranial arteriovenous malformation, *Neurol India* 52(2):163-170, 2004.

Sirven JI, Waterhourse E: Management of status epilepticus, *AFP* 68(3):469-476, 2003.

Smythe PR, Samra SK: Monitors of cerebral oxygenation, *Anesthesiol Clin North Am* 20:293-313, 2002.

Sommargren CE: Electrocardiographic abnormalities in patients with subarachnoid hemorrhage, *Am J Crit Care* 37(supp):48-62, 2002.

Suarez JI: *Critical care neurology and neurosurgery,* Totowa, N.J., 2004, Humana Press.

PULMONARY DISORDERS

AHRQ:(2003). *Diagnosis and treatment of deep venous thrombosis and pulmonary embolism.* Retrieved November 5, 2004, from www.ahrq.gov/clinic/epcsums/dvtsum.htm.

Benditt JO: Surgical therapies for chronic obstructive pulmonary disease, *Respir Care* 49(1):53-61, 2004.

Collard HR, Saint S, Matthay MA: Prevention of ventilator-associated pneumonia: an evidence-based systematic review, *Ann Intern Med* 138(6):494-501, 2003.

Craig K: Prone positioning made easy, *Br J Perioper Nurs* 13(12):522-527, 2003.

El-Masri MM, Williamson KM, Fox-Wasylyshyn SM: Severe acute respiratory syndrome: another challenge for critical care nurses, *AACN Clin Issues* 15(1):150-159, 2004.

Grap MJ, Munro CL: Preventing ventilator-associated pneumonia: evidence-based care, *Crit Care Nurs Clin North Am* 16(3):349-358, 2004.

Happ MB: Communicating with mechanically ventilated patients: state of the science, *AACN Clin Issues* 12(2):247-258, 2001.

Haynes Hockman, R: Pharmacologic therapy for acute exacerbations of chronic obstructive pulmonary disease: a review, *Crit Care Nurs Clin North Am* 16(3):293-310, 2004.

Hubble MW, Hubble JP: *Principles of advanced trauma care,* Albany, N.Y., 2002, Delmar.

Keough V, Pudelek B: Blunt chest trauma: review of selected pulmonary injuries focusing on pulmonary contusion, *AACN Clin Issues* 12(2):270-281, 2001.

Kruse JA, Fink MP, Carlson RW: *Saunders manual of critical care,* Philadelphia, 2003, Saunders.

McAllister J: An overview of the current asthma disease management guidance, *Br J Nurs* 13(9):512-517, 2004.

Nava S, Ceriana P: Causes of failure of noninvasive mechanical ventilation, *Respir Care* 49(3):295-303, 2004.

Pierson DJ: Indications for mechanical ventilation in adults with acute respiratory failure, *Respir Care* 47(3):249-262, 2002.

Rowe C: Development of clinical guidelines for prone positioning in critically ill adults, *Nurs Crit Care* 9(2):50-57, 2004.

Suchyta MR, Orme JF Jr, Morris AH: The changing face of organ failure in ARDS, *Chest* 124(5):1871-1879, 2003.

Thompson JM et al: *Mosby's clinical nursing,* ed 5, St Louis, 2002, Mosby.

Vollman KM: Prone positioning in the patient who has acute respiratory distress syndrome: the art and the science, *Crit Care Nurs Clin North Am* 16(3):319-336, 2004.

Wilkins RW, Stoller JK, Scanlan CL: *Egan's fundamentals of respiratory care,* ed 8, St Louis, 2003, Mosby.

Winters AC: Management of severe acute asthma, *Crit Care Nurs Clin North Am* 16(3):285-291, 2004.

CARDIOVASCULAR DISORDERS

American Heart Association: *Heart disease and stroke statistic—2003 update,* Dallas, 2003, American Heart Association.

Bosin DM, Flemming M: Electrophysiology testing. *Dimens Crit Care Nurs* 22(1):10-19, 2003.

Braunwald E, Zipes D: *Braunwald's heart disease: a textbook of cardiovascular medicine,* Philadelphia, 2002, WB Saunders.

Braunwald E et al: ACC/AHA guidelines for the management of patients with unstable angina and non-ST-segment elevation myocardial infarction. A report of the American College of Cardiology/American Heart Association Task Force on Practice Guidelines, *Circulation* 102:1193-1209, 2000.

Gregoratos G et al: ACC/AHA/NASPE 2002 guideline update for implantation of cardiac pacemakers and antiarrhythmia devices. A report of the American College of Cardiology/American Heart Association Task Force on Practice Guidelines 2002, *J Cardiovasc Electrophysiol* 13(11):1183-1199, 2002.

Griffin BP, Topol EJ: *Manual of cardiovascular medicine,* ed 2, Philadelphia, 2004, Lipincott Williams & Wilkins.

Gura MT, Forman L: Cardiac resynchronization therapy for heart failure management, *AACN Clin Issues* 15(3):325-339, 2004.

Mancini M et al: The management of immunosuppression, *Crit Care Nurs Q* 27(1):61-64, 2003.

Martgaker MT, Keresztes PA: Evidence-based practice for the use of *N*-acetylcysteine, *Dimens Crit Care Nurse* 23(6):270-273, 2003.

Mohan SB et al: Idiopathic dilated cardiomyopathy: a common but mystifying cause of heart failure, *Cleveland Clin J Med* 69(6):481-487, 2002.

Neinaber C, Eagle K: Aortic dissection: new frontiers in diagnosis and management, part II therapeutic management and follow-up, *Circulation* 108(6):772-778, 2003.

Obias-Manno D, Wijetunga M: Risk stratification and primary prevention of sudden cardiac death, *AACN Clin Issues* 15(3):404-415, 2004.

Reiswig Timothy P, Rodeman BJ: Temporary pacemakers in critically ill patients: assessment and management strategies, *AACN Clin Issues* 15(3):305-325, 2004.

Smith AL, Brown CB: New advances and novel treatments in heart failure, *Crit Care Nurse* Feb (Suppl):11-18, 2003.

Stanik-Hutt JA: Drug-coated stents: preventing restenosis in coronary artery disease, *JCN* 19(6):404-408, 2004.

Wade CR et al: Postoperative nursing care of cardiac transplant recipient, *Crit Care Nurs Q* 27(1):17-28, 2003.

GASTROINTESTINAL DISORDERS

Bucher L, Melander S: *Critical care nursing,* Philadelphia, 1999, WB Saunders.

Conrad SA: Acute upper gastrointestinal bleeding in critically ill patients: causes and treatment options, *Crit Care Med* 30(6 Suppl):365S-368S, 2002.

DeFranchis R: Somatostatin, somotostatin analogues and other vasoactive drugs in the treatment of bleeding oesophageal varices, *Dig Liver Dis* 36(1 Suppl):93S-100S, 2004.

Higgins PD, Fontana RJ: Liver transplantation in acute liver failure, *Panminerva Med* 45(2):85-94, 2003.

Huang CD, Lichtenstein DR: Nonvariceal upper gastrointestinal bleeding, *Gastroenterol Clin North Am* 32(4):1053-1078, 2003.

Kessler CA: Hyperglycemic emergencies, *AACN Clin Issues* 3:350-360, 1992.

Lee WM: Acute liver failure in the United States, *Semin Liver Dis* 23(3):217-226, 2003.

Malangoni MA: Current concepts in peritonitis, *Curr Gastroenterol Rep* 5(4):295-301, 2003.

Marrero J, Martinez FJ, Hyzy R: Advances in critical care hepatology, *Am J Respir Crit Care Med* 168:1421-1426, 2003.

Mascarenhas R, Mcbarhan S: New support for branched-chain amino acid supplementation in advanced hepatic failure, *Nutr Rev* 62(1):33-38, 2004.

McCashland TM: Current use of transjugular intrahepatic portosystemic shunts, *Curr Gastroenterol Rep* 5(1):31-38, 2003.

Morgan D: Intravenous proton pump inhibitors in the critical care setting, *Crit Care Med* 30(6 Suppl):369S -372S, 2002.

Ranson JC: Risk factors in acute pancreatitis, *Hosp Pract* 20(4):69-73, 1985.

Spirt MJ: Stress-related mucosal disease: risk factors and prophylactic therapy, *Clin Ther* 26(3):197-213, 2004.

Steinberg KP: Stress-related mucosal disease in the critically ill patient: risk factors and strategies to prevent stress-related bleeding in the intensive care unit, *Crit Care Med* 30(6 Suppl):362S-364S, 2002.

Vaquera J et al: Pathogenesis of hepatic encephalopathy in acute liver failure, *Semin Liver Dis* 23(3):259-269, 2003.

Yadav D, Agarwal N, Pitchumoni SC: A critical evaluation of laboratory tests in acute pancreatitis, *Am J Gastroenterol* 97(6):1309-1318, 2002.

Yang YX, Lewis JD: Prevention and treatment of stress ulcers in critically ill patients, *Semin Gastrointest Dis* 14(1):11-9, 2003.

ENDOCRINE DISORDERS

Bhattacharyya A, MacDonald J, Lakhadar AA: Acute adrenal crisis: three different presentations, *Int J Clin Pract* 55(2):141-144, 2001.

Bhuvana G, Krishnaswamy G, Peiris A: The diagnosis and management of hypothyroidism, *South Med J* 95(5):475-480, 2002.

Boughey JC, Yost MJ, Bynoe RP: Diabetes insipidus in the head injured adult, *Am Surg* 70(6):500-503, 2004.

Carpenito-Moyet J: *Nursing diagnosis application to clinical practice,* ed 10, Philadelphia, 2004, Lippincott Williams & Wilkins.

Cooper DS: Combined T3 and T4 therapy—back to the drawing board, *JAMA* 290(22):3002-3004, 2003.

Coursin DB, Wood KE: Corticosteroid supplementation for adrenal insufficiency, *JAMA* 287:236-240, 2002.

Decaux G et al: Hyponatremia in the syndrome of inappropriate secretion of antidiuretic hormone. Rapid correction with urea, sodium chloride, and water restriction therapy, *J Am Soc Nephrol* 13:1433-1441, 1982.

Disckerson LM et al: Glycemic control in medical inpatients with type 2 diabetes mellitus receiving sliding scale insulin regimens versus routine diabetes medications: a multicenter randomized controlled trial, *Ann Fam Med* 1(1):29-35, 2003.

Farwell AP et al: Thyroidectomy for amiodarone-induced thyrotoxicosis, *JAMA* 263(11):1526-1528, 1990.

Finney SJ et al: Glucose control and mortality in critically ill patients, *JAMA* 290(15):2041-2047, 2003.

Giddons JF: Nursing management endocrine problems. In Lewis et al, editors: *Med Surg Nurs*, ed 6, St Louis, 2004, Mosby.

Goh KP: Management of hyponatremia, *AFP* 69(10):287-294, 2004.

Graber AL, McDonald T: Newly identified hyperglycemia among hospitalized patients. *South Med J* 93(11):1070-1072, 2001.

Huether S: Mechanisms of hormone regulation. In Huether SE, McCance KL, editors: *Understanding human pathophysiology*, ed 3, St Louis, 2004, Mosby.

Huether S: Alterations of hormone regulation. In Huether SE, McCance KL, editors: *Understanding human pathophysiology*, ed 3, St Louis, 2004, Mosby.

Kanda M et al: SIADH closely associated with non-functioning pituitary adenoma, *Endocr J* 51(4):435-438, 2004.

Kruse JA: Endocrine crisis. In Hall JB, Freid EB, editors: *SCCM ACCP 4th combined critical care course multidisciplinary review and board preparation*, 2002, 2003, American College of Chest Physicians and The Society of Critical Care Medicine, 469-481.

Lin L, Achermann JC: Inherited adrenal hypoplasias: not just for kids, *Clin Endocrinol* 60(5):529-537, 2004.

Liolios A: Intensive glucose control in the ICU: an expert interview with James S. Krinsley, MD, *Medscape Gen Med* 6(2):1-4, 2004.

Litwack K: The endocrine system. In Alspach JG, editor: *Core curriculum for critical care nursing*, Philadelphia, 1998, WB Saunders.

Loriaux DL: Glucocorticoid therapy in the intensive care unit, *NEJM* 350:1601-1602, 2004.

Medscape.com: Addison's disease: diagnosis can be more difficult than treatment, *Drug Ther Perspec* 17(8):12-15, 2001.

Mitchell DH, Owens B: Replacement therapy: arginine vasopressin, growth hormone, cortisol, thyroxine, testosterone and estrogen, *J Neuroscience Nurs* 28(3):140-154, 1996.

Montori VM, Bistrian BR, McMahon MM: Hyperglycemia in acutely ill patients, *JAMA* 288(17):2167-2169, 2002.

Preuss JM: Adrenal emergencies, *Top Emerg Med,* 23(4):1-12, 2001.

Rivers EP, Gaspari M, Saad GA: Adrenal insufficiency in high-risk surgical ICU patients, *Chest* 119:889-896, 2001.

Roberts SR, Hamedani B: Benefits and methods of achieving strict glycemic control in the ICU, *Crit Care Clin North Am* 16(4):537-546, 2004.

Schnell Z, Van Leeuwen AM, Kranpitz TR: *Davis's comprehensive handbook of laboratory and diagnostic tests with nursing implications*, Philadelphia, 2003, Davis.

Seute T et al: Neurologic disorders in 432 consecutive patients with small cell lung carcinoma, *Cancer* 100(4):801-804, 2004.

Shenkman L, Podrid P, Lowenstein J: Hyperthyroidism after propranolol withdrawal, *JAMA* 238(3):237-239, 1977.

Singer I, Oster JR, Fishman LM: The management of diabetes insipidus in adults, *Arch Intern Med* 157(12):1293-1301, 1997.

Singh KS et al: Standardization of intravenous insulin therapy improves efficiency and safety of blood glucose control in critically ill adults, *Intensive Care Med* 30(5):804-810, 2004.

Van den Berghe G et al: Intensive insulin therapy in critically ill patients, *N Engl J Med* 345(19):1359-1367, 2001.

RENAL DISORDERS

Berl T, Taylor J: Disorders of water balance. In Fink MP et al: *Textbook of critical care*, ed 5, Philadelphia, 2005, Saunders.

Bongard FS: Fluids, electrolytes and acid-base. In Bongard FS, Sue DY, editors: *Current critical care diagnosis and treatment*, New York, 2002, Lange Medical Books/McGraw-Hill.

Burger C: Hyperkalemia, *AJN* 104(10):66-70, 2004.

Cleaver N: Drugs used to promote diuresis: a treatment for fluid balance charts. *Nurs Crit Care* 9(2):80-85, 2004.

Kamel KS, Happerin ML: Disorders of plasma potassium concentration. In Fink MP et al, editors: *Textbook of critical care*, ed 5, Philadelphia, 2005, Saunders.

Poole BD, Schrier RW: Acute renal failure. In Fink MP et al, editors: *Textbook of critical care*, ed 5, Philadelphia, 2005, Saunders.

Popovtzer MM: Disorders of calcium and magnesium metabolism. In Fink MP et al, editors: *Textbook of critical care*, ed 5, Philadelphia, 2005, Saunders.

Rabinstein A, Wijdicks Eelco FM: Body water and electrolytes. In Layon AJ, Gabrielli A, Friedman W, editors: *Textbook of neurointensive care*, Philadelphia, 2004, Saunders.

Ruppel G: Solutions, body fluids and electrolytes. In Kruse J, Fink M, Carlson R, editors: *Saunders manual of critical care*, Philadelphia, 2003, Elsevier.

Womack KA: Fluids and electrolytes. In Newberry L, editor: *Sheehy's emergency nursing: principles and practice*, St Louis, 2003, Mosby.

MULTISYSTEM DISORDERS

ACCP/SCCM Consensus Conference Committee: Definitions for sepsis and organ failure and guidelines for the use of innovative therapies in sepsis, *Chest* 101:1644-1655, 1992. www.ihi.org/IHI/Topics/CriticalCare/Sepsis.

Ahrens T, Tuggle D: Surviving severe sepsis: early recognition and treatment, *Crit Care Nurse* 24 (Suppl):2-13, 2004.

Ahrens T, Vollman K: Severe sepsis management: are we doing enough? *Crit Care Nurse* 23(Suppl):2-15, 2003.

Bernard GR et al: Efficacy and safety of recombinant activated protein C for severe sepsis, *N Engl J Med* 344(10):699-709, 2001.

Bucher L, Melander S: *Critical care nursing*, Philadelphia, 1999, WB Saunders.

Hagstrom M et al: A review of emergency department fluid resuscitation of burn patients transferred to a regional, verified burn center, *Ann Plast Surg* 51(2):173-176, 2003.

Haubrich KA: Role of vernix caseosa in the neonate: potential application in the adult population, *AACN Clin Issues* 14(4):457-464, 2003.

Kemp SF, Lockey RF: Anaphylaxis: a review of causes and mechanisms, *J Allergy Clin Immunol* 110(3):341-348, 2002.

Kleinpell R: Advances in treating patients with severe sepsis: Role of drotrecogin alfa (activated), *Crit Care Nurse* 23(3):16-29, 2003.

Leiberman P: Anaphylactic reactions during surgical and medical procedures, *J Allergy Clin Immunol* 110(2 Suppl):964-969, 2002.

Rick RL: Disseminated intravascular coagulation: a review of etiology, pathophysiology, diagnosis, and management: guidelines for care, *Clin Appl Thromb Hemost* 8(1):1-31, 2002.

Sheridan RL: Burns, *Crit Care Med* 30(11 Suppl):500S-514S, 2002.

Sicherer SH: Advances in anaphylaxis and hypersensitivity reactions to foods, drugs, and insect venom, *J Allergy Clin Immunol* 111(3 Suppl):829S-834S, 2003.

Tang AW: A practical guide to anaphylaxis, *Am Family Physician* 68(7):1325-1332.

Taylor EB, Kinasewitz GT: The diagnosis and management of disseminated intravascular coagulation, *Curr Hematol Rep* 1(1):34-40, 2002.

Texas Tech University Managed Health Care Network Pharmacy & Therapeutics Committee: *HIV disease management,* National Guidelines Clearinghouse AHRQ, July 7, 2002, 1-13.

Wesley E, Kleinpell RM, Guyette RE: Advances in the understanding of clinical manifestations and therapy of severe sepsis: an update for critical care nurses, *Am J Crit Care* 12(2):120-133, 2003.

6

Monitoring the Critically Ill Patient

ARTERIAL BLOOD GAS (ABG) ANALYSIS

Clinical Brief

ABG analysis is done to assess the acid-base balance of the body, the adequacy of oxygenation and/or ventilation, and the adequacy of circulation and to detect metabolic abnormalities.

Indications

ABG analysis may be done in any of the following clinical situations: (1) serious respiratory problems or prolonged weaning from mechanical ventilation, (2) cardiac dysfunction associated with decreased cardiac output (CO), and (3) shock states.

Description

A sample of blood from an artery is analyzed and the partial pressures of oxygen (Pa_{O_2}) and carbon dioxide (Pa_{CO_2}), as well as the pH and bicarbonate ion levels and oxygen saturation, are determined.

The pH measures hydrogen ion concentration, which is an indication of acid-base balance. The body maintains a normal pH by keeping bicarbonate ion (a function of the kidneys) and Pa_{CO_2} (a function of the lungs) in a constant ratio of 20:1. When the acid-base balance is disturbed, there is compensation by the system (respiratory or renal) not primarily affected to return the pH to normal. If the disturbance is respiratory, the kidneys compensate by altering bicarbonate excretion to return the pH to normal; however, the kidneys are slow to respond to changes in pH, and compensation may take days. If the disturbance is metabolic, the respiratory system compensates by increasing or decreasing ventilation (Pa_{CO_2}) to return the pH to normal; the lungs respond to changes in pH within minutes.

The Paco$_2$ level is adjusted by the rate and depth of ventilation: hypoventilation results in high Paco$_2$ (Paco$_2$ >45 mm Hg) levels and respiratory acidosis, whereas hyperventilation results in low Paco$_2$ levels (Paco$_2$ <35 mm Hg) and respiratory alkalosis. If any abnormality in Paco$_2$ exists, the pH and HCO$_3$ parameters should be analyzed to determine if the alteration in Paco$_2$ is the result of a primary respiratory disturbance or a compensatory response to a metabolic acid-base abnormality.

The Pao$_2$ reflects the amount of oxygen dissolved in arterial blood. Pao$_2$ does not directly influence the acid-base balance, although hypoxemia with anaerobic metabolism can lead to lactic acidosis.

Oxygen saturation (Sao$_2$) reflects the amount of oxygen combined with hemoglobin (oxyhemoglobin) that is carried in the blood and is expressed as a percent. Hemoglobin has an affinity for oxygen that is directly related to the Pao$_2$. The oxygen-hemoglobin dissociation curve demonstrates the relationship between Po$_2$ and O$_2$ saturation. As tissues use the oxygen dissolved in arterial blood, oxygen dissociates from the hemoglobin, causing a decrease in saturation. Significant changes in oxygen saturation occur when the Pao$_2$ value is <60 mm Hg. The affinity of hemoglobin for oxygen progressively decreases. Thus small drops in Po$_2$ cause greater decreases in O$_2$ saturation. Various conditions can affect the oxygen-hemoglobin affinity and thus affect oxygen availability for tissues (Figure 6-1).

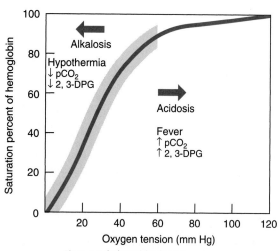

Figure 6-1 Oxyhemoglobin dissociation curve.

Base excess or deficit indicates the amount of blood buffer present. It reflects the tissue or renal presence or absence of acid. As the proportion of acid rises, the relative amount of base decreases (and vice versa). Abnormally high values (≥2) reflect alkalosis; low values (≤2) reflect acidosis.

The bicarbonate ion level represents the renal component of acid-base regulation. The kidneys adjust the level of bicarbonate ion by changes in its excretion rate. If the bicarbonate changes, acid changes in the opposite direction. To determine if the cause of the bicarbonate ion level change is either a primary problem or compensation, the relationship to pH must be evaluated because pH responds to the presence or absence of acid (Table 6-1).

VALUES

Normal

pH 7.35 to 7.45
$Paco_2$ 35 to 45 mm Hg
Pao_2 80 to 100 mm Hg
O_2 saturation 95% to 99%
Serum bicarbonate (HCO_3) 22 to 26 mEq/L

Table 6-1 DETERMINING THE IMBALANCE IN ARTERIAL BLOOD GASES (ABGS)

If	
pH ↑ and pCO_2 ↓ or pH ↓ and pCO_2 ↑	} Then respiratory disorder
If	
pH ↑ and HCO_3 ↑ or pH ↓ and HCO_3 ↓	} Then metabolic disorder
If	
pCO_2 ↑ and HCO_3 ↑ or pCO_2 ↓ and HCO_3 ↓	} Then compensation is occurring
If	
pCO_2 ↑ and HCO_3 ↓ or pCO_2 ↓ and HCO_3 ↑	} Then mixed imbalance

Significance of Abnormal Values

pH <7.35: acidosis, pH >7.45: alkalosis. It is impossible to determine the cause (respiratory or metabolic) of acidosis or alkalosis by looking at the pH alone.

$Paco_2$ <35 mm Hg: respiratory alkalosis, caused by hyperventilation (may be secondary to ventilatory support, central nervous system disease, fever, liver disease, heart failure, or pulmonary embolism)

$Paco_2$ >45 mm Hg: respiratory acidosis, caused by hypoventilation (may be secondary to impaired alveolar ventilation, respiratory depressants, or intracranial tumors)

Pao_2 <80 mm Hg: hypoxemia, with inadequate O_2 to meet tissue needs. If hypoxemia is left untreated, anaerobic metabolism and acidosis will result.

Pao_2 >100 mm Hg: hyperoxemia, usually a result of excessive concentration of oxygen. Fio_2 should be lowered to produce Pao_2 >60 to 70 mm Hg or O_2 saturation ≥95%.

O_2 saturation <95%: hypoxemia

HCO_3 <22 mEq/L: metabolic acidosis (may be secondary to renal failure, lactic acidosis, diabetic ketoacidosis, or diarrhea)

HCO_3 >26 mEq/L: metabolic alkalosis (may be secondary to vomiting, ingestion of diuretics, nasogastric suction, steroid therapy, hyperaldosteronism, or hyperadrenocorticism)

STEPS TO INTERPRET ARTERIAL BLOOD GASES (ABGS)

1. Check pH   ↑ = alkalosis; ↓ = acidosis
2. Check pCO_2 ↑ = CO_2 retention (hypoventilation); respiratory acidosis or compensating for metabolic alkalosis
          ↓ = CO_2 blown off (hyperventilation); respiratory alkalosis or compensating for metabolic acidosis
3. Check HCO_3 ↑ = Nonvolatile acid is lost; HCO_3 is gained (metabolic alkalosis or compensating for respiratory acidosis)
          ↓ = Nonvolatile acid is added; HCO_3 is lost (metabolic acidosis or compensating for respiratory alkalosis)
4. Determine imbalance.
5. Determine whether compensation exists. (See Table 6-1.)

ARTERIAL BLOOD GAS (ABG) MONITORING: POINT OF CARE (POC)

Description

POC ABG analysis is the testing or monitoring of ABGs at the point of patient care (bedside or near bedside) and is usually performed by nursing personnel. Various portable, handheld, or modular diagnostic equipment is used to obtain ABGs within 60 to 120 seconds. POC technology is preferable to traditional ABG analysis because it can be done without permanent blood loss, it decreases the cost of testing, and it reduces turnaround time for the availability of results.

Three types of POC systems commonly used are in vivo continuous systems, ex vivo intermittent systems, and portable in vitro systems.

An in vivo continuous system uses a flexible optical sensor, which relies on fiberoptic spectroscopy (similar to fiberoptic pulmonary artery [PA] or intracranial pressure [ICP] systems) using light to detect chemical changes in the body. The sensor can monitor PaO_2, $PaCO_2$, and pH for up to 96 hours. This system requires periodic recalibration to compensate for *drift* (erroneous readings) caused by the formation of fibrin or clot on the catheter.

Ex vivo intermittent systems use sensors that are located outside the vasculature. One system involves a volume-controlled syringe to draw blood into the sensor that is located in the fluid-filled tubing between the patient's arterial cannula and the monitor. ABG results are then displayed on the monitor within 60 seconds. Following the analysis, the blood is returned to the patient.

The third POC technology, in vitro testing, provides recent historical data and is usually used when intravascular access or equipment for the other types of POC testing is not available or contraindicated. The in vitro method involves placing two or three drops of blood into a test cartridge, which is inserted into a handheld analyzer or bedside monitor. The results are displayed within approximately 2 minutes.

Obtaining a Blood Sample

1. Observe Standard Precautions.
2. Follow unit policy and manufacturer's recommendations for specific system in use.
3. Ensure return of arterial waveform on monitor.

Removal of Arterial Catheter

1. Turn the stopcock off to the patient and disconnect the transducer from the monitor.

2. Remove the arterial line dressing from the site and remove any sutures.
3. Gently withdraw the catheter from the artery and apply direct, firm pressure above the puncture site with sterile gauze while continuously assessing the circulation of the distal extremity. Maintain pressure for a minimum of 5 minutes or until bleeding stops.
4. Apply a pressure dressing to the site.
5. Assess the site for signs of bleeding and the distal extremity for evidence of impaired circulation.
6. Remove the dressing 8 hours after the removal of the catheter.

ARTERIAL PRESSURE MONITORING

Clinical Brief

Direct arterial pressure monitoring provides a continuous display of the arterial blood pressure waveform and digital readings of the systolic, diastolic, and mean pressures. Mean arterial pressure (MAP) reflects the average pressure that pushes blood through the systemic circulation during the cardiac cycle; it is an important indicator of tissue perfusion. Because CO and systemic vascular resistance (SVR) determine MAP, an increase in either of these will cause an increase in MAP and a decrease in either value will decrease MAP.

MAP can be calculated using the following formula. However, when a pressure monitoring system is used, the bedside monitor displays the MAP and it does not have to be calculated.

$$MAP = \frac{\text{Systolic BP} + 2\,(\text{Diastolic BP})}{3}$$

An indwelling arterial line also provides continuous access to arterial blood for sampling, such as for blood gas analysis and/or for serum laboratory tests.

Complications include hemorrhage, clot formation, infection, vessel damage, air embolus, and electric shock.

Indications

Arterial pressure monitoring may be used for the following: to monitor patients with unstable blood pressure (BP), to measure trends and evaluate the efficacy of vasoactive drugs, to obtain frequent ABGs when weaning from mechanical ventilation, to obtain blood samples in the burn patient with limited vascular access through intact skin, or to monitor BP in shock states in which conventional cuff BP may be difficult to determine. In addition, direct arterial pressure monitoring allows easy determination of MAP, an indicator of tissue perfusion.

Description

An arterial catheter, usually a Teflon catheter over a needle, is inserted into an artery through a percutaneous or cutdown method. The radial artery is preferred because of its accessibility, although the axillary, femoral, brachial, or pedal arteries can be used. The catheter is then attached to a pressure transducer set-up with a continuous flush of heparinized saline (1 unit heparin per milliliter of saline or flush solution recommended by facility). When the pressure bag is inflated to 300 mm Hg, 3 mL/hr will be delivered through the line, thus promoting catheter patency. The pressure transducer is connected to the monitor, and a continuous waveform is displayed on the oscilloscope. Digital display of the pressure is also available.

VALUES

Normal

Systolic BP 90 to 120 mm Hg
Diastolic BP 60 to 80 mm Hg
MAP 70 to 105 mm Hg

Significance of Abnormal Values

Systolic BP values can be abnormal as a result of changes in stroke volume (e.g., hypervolemia, hypovolemia, or heart failure), changes in wall compliance (e.g., arteriosclerosis and hypertension), and changes in the rate of ejection of blood from the left ventricle (e.g., sympathetic nervous system stimulation and some vasoactive drugs) or when there is aortic insufficiency (elevated systolic BP) or aortic stenosis (lowered systolic BP).

Diastolic BP may be elevated as a result of increased stroke volume or SVR; it may be lowered as a result of hypovolemia, peripheral dilation of blood vessels, or aortic insufficiency.

PATIENT CARE MANAGEMENT

Preinsertion

Before insertion of a radial arterial line, an Allen test may be performed to assess adequacy of collateral circulation to the hand (Figure 6-2). The insertion of the arterial catheter is done under aseptic conditions.

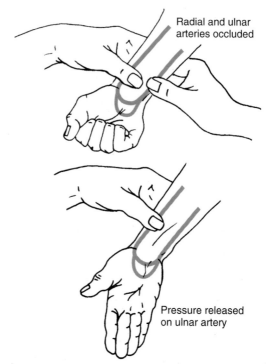

Radial and ulnar
arteries occluded

Pressure released
on ulnar artery

Figure 6-2   Allen test. Hold patient's hand up. Have patient clench and unclench hand while occluding the radial and ulnar arteries. The hand will become pale. Lower the hand and have the patient relax the hand. While continuing to hold the radial artery, release pressure on the ulnar artery. Brisk return of color (5-7 seconds) demonstrates adequate ulnar blood flow. If pallor persists for more than 15 seconds, ulnar flow is inadequate and radial artery cannulation should not be attempted. (From Stillwell S, Randall E: *Pocket guide to cardiovascular care,* ed 2, St Louis, 1994, Mosby.)

Postinsertion

Once the catheter is positioned and the waveform is immediately visible, perform a dynamic response test (Figure 6-3). Level and zero the transducer. The air reference port of the transducer should be at the level of the right atrium, e.g., at the phlebostatic axis (Figure 6-4), which is at the intersection of the fourth intercostal space and midchest. Mark the phlebostatic axis with ink or tape on the patient's skin and use this same point for taking readings; failure to do so will result in inaccurate readings.

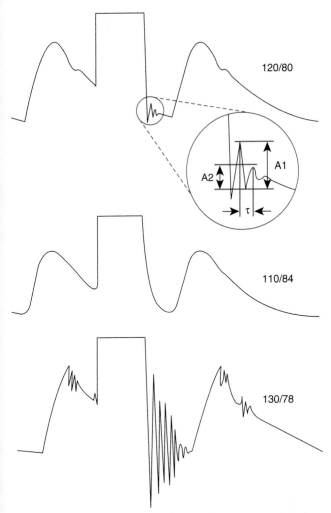

Figure 6-3 Pressure-time waveforms during fast-flush testing of dynamic response of arterial pressure monitoring systems. Top: optimal dynamic response showing true intraarterial blood pressure. Middle: overdamped system showing spuriously low systolic pressure. Bottom: hyperresonant, underdamped system showing spuriously elevated systolic pressure. Inset: method of determining amplitude ratio (A2/A1) and resonant waveform period (τ). A1 and A2 = successive amplitudes. (From Kruse JA, Fink MP, Carlson RW: *Saunders manual of critical care*, Philadelphia, 2003, Saunders.)

Alarm parameters should be set (usually 10-20 mm Hg higher and lower than the patient's baseline pressure) and activated. The alarms should remain on at all times so that a sudden change in pressure and/or disconnection of the line is immediately noted.

Be aware that BPs obtained by direct monitoring methods (e.g., arterial line) will not necessarily be the same as those derived by indirect methods (e.g., cuff) that are flow dependent. The routine practice of comparing cuff and arterial line pressure should be discouraged. More important is evaluation of each patient situation to determine the most appropriate method for assessing BP.

Obtaining Accurate Measurements

Relevel the transducer every time the patient or transducer is moved, including each time the bed height or head elevation is changed, as well as with any significant change in the patient's hemodynamic variables. Prevent kinks in the catheter by stabilizing it securely. Observe the line frequently for air, which may damp the waveform. Flush the line thoroughly each time blood is drawn. Peripheral arterial catheters are often positional, and the waveform may be damped if the extremity is flexed.

Waveform Interpretation

Systole is apparent on the waveform as a sharp rise in pressure; this is the anacrotic limb, and it signifies the rapid ejection of blood from

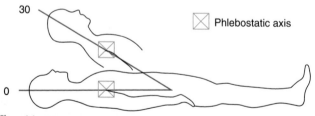

Figure 6-4 Phlebostatic axis. (From Stillwell S, Randall E: *Pocket guide to cardiovascular care*, ed 2, St Louis, 1994, Mosby.)

the ventricle through the open aortic valve. If there is a delay in this rapid rise, it could suggest a decrease in myocardial contractility, aortic stenosis, or damped pressure secondary to catheter position or clot formation. A steep rate of rise along with a high peak systolic pressure and a poorly defined dicrotic notch may be seen with aortic insufficiency.

Diastole follows closure of the aortic valve (seen as the dicrotic notch on the waveform) and continues until the next systole. The location of the dicrotic notch should be one third or greater of the height of the systolic peak; if it is not, suspect a decreased CO (Figure 6-5). Table 6-2 offers methods for troubleshooting invasive hemodynamic monitoring lines.

Critical Observations

Hemorrhage can occur if the arterial catheter inadvertently becomes disconnected from the transducer.

- The alarm system must be activated at all times, and Luer-Lok connections should be used at all connections in the pressure set-up. If the patient is restless or confused and is at risk for accidental dislodgment of the tubing or catheter, sedation or restraint should be considered.

Peripheral clot formation can occur at the insertion site or at the tip of the catheter. Patients with peripheral vascular disease or arteriosclerosis are particularly prone to clot formation and embolization. Use of the femoral artery is associated with a higher incidence of distal embolic complications than other sites.

- To prevent clot formation, a continuous infusion (3 mL/hr) of heparinized saline is connected to the arterial catheter. After the blood sample is obtained, the line must be flushed thoroughly

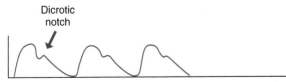

Figure 6-5 Arterial waveform. Dicrotic notch represents closure of the aortic valve.

Table 6-2   Troubleshooting Invasive Hemodynamic Monitoring Lines

Problem	Cause	Solution
Blood backup into tubing	Loose connections	Tighten connections
	Stopcock off to flush system	Open stopcock
	Inadequate pressure in bag	Inflate pressure bag to 300 mm Hg
Damped pressure tracing	Air bubbles in system	Purge air from system
	Clot formation	Aspirate blood from catheter and briefly flush system*
	Loose connections	Tighten connections
	Compliant tubing	Use stiff (high-pressure) tubing
	Change in patient condition	Assess and treat patient
	Inadequate pressure in bag	Inflate pressure bag to 300 mm Hg
No waveform	Transducer not open to catheter	Check system
	Transducer not connected to monitor	Connect transducer to monitor
	Incorrect scale selection	Select appropriate scale for physiologic pressure
	Kink in catheter	Reposition catheter; use armboard to prevent wrist flexion
Inaccurate readings	Change in transducer reference level	Keep transducer at phlebostatic axis
	Transducer above reference point results in false low readings	
	Transducer below reference point results in false high readings	
	Air or clotting within system	Check system: aspirate air or clots from system

Continued

Table 6-2 TROUBLESHOOTING INVASIVE HEMODYNAMIC MONITORING
            LINES—cont'd

Problem	Cause	Solution
Noise or fling in pressure waveform ("whip")	Excessive catheter movement: occurs when catheter in large vessel	Reposition catheter; use damping device to remove fling from waveform
	Excessive tubing length	Eliminate excessive tubing

*Do *not* flush intracranial pressure (ICP), left atrial pressure (LAP) systems.

to clear the catheter of blood. The tracing on the monitor must be observed frequently for loss of amplitude, which may be caused by clot formation. Assess capillary refill and color and temperature of the skin, as well as sensation and movement of the extremity distal to the cannulation site, at least every 2 hours. Signs of decreased circulation that result from embolization of a clot include pain, pallor, coolness, and cyanosis in the distal extremity.

Infection can occur with any invasive monitoring line; it can occur within the system set-up, at the cannulation site, or with the catheter. Flush solution containing glucose should be avoided to decrease the risk of bacterial growth.

- Strict aseptic technique is used during the system set-up and catheter insertion, as well as during blood sampling procedures and dressing changes. Sterile dead-end caps should be placed on all open ports of the stopcocks. A dry, sterile dressing should be maintained over the insertion site. The site should be inspected daily for redness, edema, tenderness to touch, or exudate. Gauze dressings should be changed every 48 hours and semipermeable dressings changed at least every 3 days (or per facility protocol) or sooner if the integrity is compromised. Flush solution should be changed every 24 hours. The hemodynamic tubing, stopcocks, and dead-end caps should be changed every 72 to 96 hours (or per facility protocol) and any time contamination is suspected.

Air embolus. Air that is trapped in the tubing can be inadvertently flushed into the artery and the systemic circulation.

- All air must be purged from the tubing during the set-up of the system. Also, the tubing should be frequently inspected for air, especially before fast-flushing the line. Observe the arterial waveform for decreased amplitude, which may indicate air in the line or in the transducer. Any detected air must be aspirated.

Vessel damage results from trauma to the vessel at the time of cannulation or from friction of the catheter in the vessel.

- The catheter should be handled gently at all times to minimize the friction on the wall of the vessel. If a clot is suspected, it should be aspirated instead of flushed into the artery. Vessel spasm can occur if too much force is used during blood sampling procedures; only minimal pressure should be used to draw blood into the syringe. If a radial catheter is used, support the patient's wrist on an armboard or other supportive device to prevent flexion and movement of the catheter.

Electric shock is a potential risk with any fluid-filled monitoring system. It can occur if current leaks from an electrical device to the fluid-filled catheter, which provides a low-resistance pathway directly to the heart.

- All electrical equipment used in patient rooms should be adequately grounded and have three-pronged plugs. Electrical devices used in the critical care unit should be checked by the biomedical department at regular intervals.

CAPNOMETRY

Clinical Brief

Capnometry is a continuous, noninvasive method for evaluating the adequacy of CO_2 exchange in the lungs.

Indications

Capnometry is useful in the mechanically ventilated patient who requires frequent blood gas sampling or who has an unstable respiratory status in which minute-to-minute assessment of gas exchange is necessary. Patient response to different modes of ventilation and tolerance to weaning can be assessed using capnometry. It is also recommended for use in confirming endotracheal tube placement.

Description

Capnometry is the measurement of exhaled CO_2 concentration. This concentration varies with the respiratory cycle; the inspired concentration is lowest, whereas the end-tidal ($P_{ET}CO_2$) concentration is highest and is assumed to represent alveolar gas. End-tidal CO_2 can be used to estimate the pressure of CO_2 in arterial blood (Pa_{CO_2}), thus allowing the clinician to evaluate adequacy of CO_2 exchange in the lung. CO_2 concentration can be displayed digitally or as a capnogram (a recorded tracing of the waveform).

VALUES

Normal

$P_{ET}CO_2$ is usually 1 to 5 mm Hg lower than the value of Pa_{CO_2} in normal individuals.

Significance of Abnormal Values

The gradient between Pa_{CO_2} and $P_{ET}CO_2$ is increased in patients with ventilation-perfusion mismatching and chronic obstructive pulmonary disease (COPD). Increased $P_{ET}CO_2$ suggests an increase in Pa_{CO_2}, perhaps as a result of hypoventilation, and decreased $P_{ET}CO_2$ suggests hyperventilation. Changes in $P_{ET}CO_2$ should prompt the nurse to assess the patient and to obtain ABGs when deterioration in respiratory status is suspected.

CENTRAL VENOUS PRESSURE (CVP) MONITORING

Clinical Brief

Intermittent or continuous CVP monitoring is used to evaluate right-sided heart function and to assess efficacy of fluid replacement therapy. *Complications* include hemorrhage, clot formation, infection, vessel damage, air embolus, electric shock, and catheter tip migration.

Indications

CVP monitoring may be used to assess (1) volume replacement therapy, (2) right-sided heart failure (acute left ventricular failure will eventually elevate the CVP but pulmonary edema is already well established), and (3) response to intravenous (IV) vasoactive drugs.

Description

The CVP catheter is inserted into a large vein by percutaneous or cutdown method. The catheter may be single lumen, or it may be a multilumen catheter that allows the infusion of several different or incompatible drugs or fluids simultaneously. The most common sites for insertion are the jugular (internal or external), subclavian, basilic, or femoral veins. Once the catheter is inserted, it is placed so that the tip is located in the superior vena cava, approximately 2 cm above the right atrium. The pressure waveform and digital value are displayed on the monitor.

VALUES

Normal

2 to 6 mm Hg

The waveform has systolic (positive) and diastolic (negative) variations, but the fluctuations are small (because the right atrium is a low-pressure chamber); thus the mean pressure is monitored.

Significance of Abnormal Values

Increased CVP may be caused by increased vascular volume, tricuspid or pulmonic valvular disease, ventricular septal defect with left-to-right shunting, constrictive pericarditis, right ventricular (RV) infarction, myocarditis, cardiac tamponade, COPD, pulmonary embolus, pulmonary hypertension, or chronic left ventricular failure.

Hypovolemia, excessive diuresis, or systemic venodilation secondary to sepsis, drugs, or neurogenic causes may cause a decrease in CVP.

PATIENT CARE MANAGEMENT

Preinsertion

The patient is placed in the Trendelenburg position if the subclavian or jugular approach is to be used; this will facilitate filling of the vessel and will diminish the risk of air embolism. In addition, the patient should be instructed to hold a breath at peak expiration at the moment of catheter insertion. This will increase the intrathoracic pressure and diminish the risk for an air embolism.

Postinsertion

Following the subclavian or jugular insertion of the catheter, both lung fields must be auscultated for symmetric breath sounds because pneumothorax or hemothorax can occur. A chest radiograph is obtained to verify catheter placement and to rule out pneumothorax. A hydrothorax can occur if large amounts of fluids are infused through the catheter before a radiograph rules out the possibility of a pneumothorax.

A sterile occlusive dressing is applied to the site. The dressing should be changed every 48 hours, and the site should be inspected for signs of infection or phlebitis. The flush solution should be changed every 24 hours; the tubing should be changed every 72 to 96 hours (or per facility protocol). During tubing changes, place the patient in the Trendelenburg position and instruct the patient to hold a breath to prevent air from entering the catheter.

The waveform should be monitored continuously or at regular intervals to ensure that the catheter tip has not migrated into the right ventricle; this would be apparent by a much taller waveform associated with higher pressures (25-30 mm Hg). In addition, the electrocardiogram (ECG) waveform must be monitored for ventricular dysrhythmias.

Alarm parameters should be set and remain on at all times.

Obtaining Accurate Measurements

Zero the transducer before obtaining the first reading. Level the transducer each time the patient or transducer is moved. The transducer should be kept at the level of the phlebostatic axis during readings (the phlebostatic axis should be marked with ink or tape on the patient's skin to ensure consistency). The waveform may fluctuate with respirations; readings should be taken at end-expiration to minimize the influence of intrathoracic pressure.

Waveform Interpretation

The CVP waveform (Figure 6-6) has positive waves and negative descents. The *a* wave indicates right atrial systole; it is followed by the *x* descent, which indicates the drop in pressure that occurs during right atrial (RA) relaxation. The *c* wave, which may not be distinguishable on the waveform, is caused by bulging of the closed tricuspid valve into the atrium during RV systole; the *x'* descent follows the *c* wave. The *v* wave indicates RA diastole, when blood is filling the atrium; it is followed by the *y* descent, which indicates passive RA emptying of blood into the right ventricle through the open tricuspid valve.

Various changes in the CVP waveform can indicate pathophysiologic changes in the heart and pulmonary vasculature. An elevated *a* wave is seen with tricuspid stenosis, RV hypertrophy secondary to pulmonic valve stenosis or pulmonary hypertension, constrictive pericarditis, and cardiac tamponade, all of which impede RA emptying. Tricuspid insufficiency with backflow of blood into the right atrium during ventricular systole will cause increased pressure and an

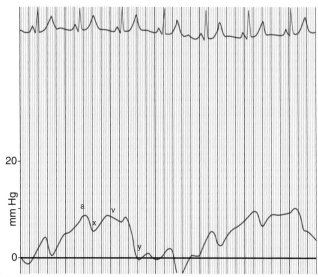

Figure 6-6 Central venous pressure (CVP) waveform. (From Daily EK, Schroeder JS: *Techniques in bedside hemodynamic monitoring*, ed 5, St Louis, 1994, Mosby.)

elevated *v* wave on the RA waveform. Tricuspid insufficiency can also cause an absence of the *c* wave on the waveform because the valve is incompetent and will not bulge back into the right atrium during ventricular systole.

Cannon waves (combined *a* and *c* waves) occur whenever the atrium contracts against a closed valve; for example, when junctional or ventricular beats occur, or with atrioventricular (AV) dissociation seen in complete heart block and ventricular tachycardia.

Troubleshooting

Table 6-2 offers troubleshooting suggestions for invasive hemodynamic monitoring lines.

Removal of Central Venous Pressure (CVP) Catheter

1. Place the patient flat or in Trendelenburg position to prevent air embolism during the catheter removal from the jugular or subclavian vein.
2. Turn the stopcock off to the patient and disconnect the transducer from the monitor.
3. Remove the dressing and remove the sutures.

4. Instruct the patient to hold a breath at full inspiration; remove the catheter slowly and inspect the tip to ensure the catheter is intact.
5. Apply pressure to the site until the bleeding has stopped, being careful not to compress any arteries (e.g., carotid) and impair blood flow.
6. Apply a sterile occlusive dressing to the site and leave in place for 24 hours.
7. Observe the site frequently for bleeding or hematoma.

Critical Observations

Catheter migration. The tip of the catheter may move forward to the right ventricle and irritate the endocardium, causing ventricular dysrhythmias. If the tip migrates far enough that the heart wall is perforated, cardiac tamponade can result because of bleeding into the pericardial sac.

• Monitor for cardiac dysrhythmias

Also see Critical Observations for Arterial Pressure Monitoring.

ELECTROCARDIOGRAM (ECG) MONITORING

CHOOSING A LEAD

Three-Lead System

1. Lead II (Figure 6-7): this is a common lead used in cardiac monitoring. An advantage of this lead is that it allows observation of QRS axis changes associated with left anterior hemiblock.
2. Modified chest lead (MCL_1) (Figure 6-8): this lead is a preferred monitoring lead for identifying type of bundle branch block (BBB) and differentiating ventricular ectopy from aberrant ventricular conduction.
3. Lewis lead: this lead is especially useful for identification of P waves. Positive electrode is at fourth intercostal space, right of sternum; negative electrode is at second intercostal space, right of sternum.
4. MCL_6 lead: the use of this lead enables the clinician to switch from viewing MCL_1 to MCL_6 (V_6) by moving only the positive electrode. It is a useful lead in those patients with a median sternotomy.

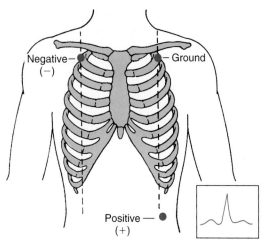

Figure 6-7 Lead II. Positive electrode—left leg; negative electrode—right arm. (From Stillwell S, Randall E: *Pocket guide to cardiovascular care*, ed 2, St Louis, 1994, Mosby.)

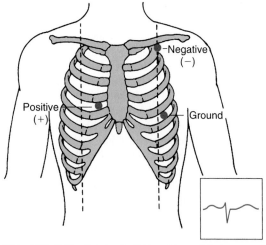

Figure 6-8 Lead MCL$_1$. Positive electrode—fourth intercostal space, right sternum; negative electrode—beneath left midclavicle. (From Stillwell S, Randall E: *Pocket guide to cardiovascular care*, ed 2, St Louis, 1994, Mosby.)

Five-Lead System

The five-lead system is shown in Figure 6-9 and allows the clinician to place the chest lead on select sites on the chest for ECG monitoring. More complete information can be obtained from the 12-lead ECG, which includes the six limb leads and six precordial leads (Figure 6-10).

RHYTHM STRIP ANALYSIS

Heart Rate (HR) Determination

Standard ECG paper is made up of a series of 1-mm squares, with each millimeter equal to 0.04 second. Each group of five small squares is marked by a darker line, so that one large square (5 mm) equals 0.20 second (Figure 6-11).

Figures 6-12 and 6-13 illustrate how to determine HR.

Rhythm Determination

To determine whether the rhythm is regular, measure the R-R or P-P intervals and determine whether the length of the intervals is constant.

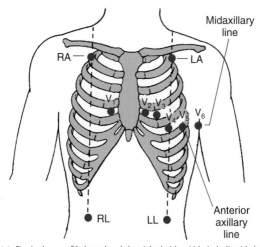

Figure 6-9 Five-lead system. RA electrode—below right clavicle, midclavicular line. LA electrode—below left clavicle, midclavicular line. RL electrode—right abdomen, midclavicular line. LL electrode—left abdomen, midclavicular line. (From Stillwell S, Randall E: *Pocket guide to cardiovascular care,* ed 2, St Louis, 1994, Mosby.)

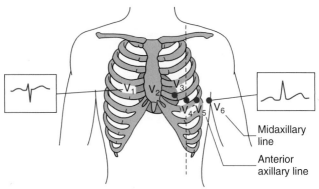

Figure 6-10 Precordial leads. V lead (positive) chest lead can be placed at identified locations to record V_1, V_2, V_3, V_4, V_5, and V_6. (From Stillwell S, Randall E: *Pocket guide to cardiovascular care,* ed 2, St Louis, 1994, Mosby.)

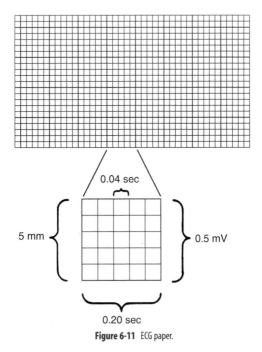

Figure 6-11 ECG paper.

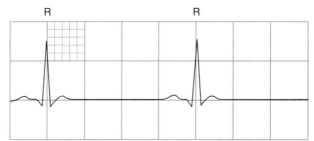

Figure 6-12 Heart rate determination with regular rhythm. Rate can be determined by dividing 300 by the number of large squares between cardiac cycles (300/4) or by dividing the number of small squares between cardiac cycles into 1500 (1500/20 = 75 beats/min). (From Stillwell S, Randall E: *Pocket guide to cardiovascular care,* ed 2, St Louis, 1994, Mosby.)

The rhythm is regular if the length of the shortest and longest interval varies by ≤0.12 second. If the rhythm is irregular, it should be determined whether there is any kind of pattern to the irregularity or if it is totally erratic.

In addition to the rate and regularity of the rhythm, the PR and QRS intervals must be determined, as well as the relationship of atrial activity (P waves) to ventricular activity (QRS complex). Normal PR interval is 0.12 to 0.20 second and normal QRS interval is up to 0.10 second. QT interval is usually less than half the preceding R-R interval (Table 6-3).

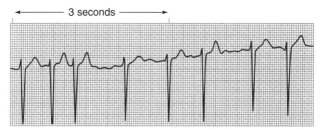

Figure 6-13 Heart rate determination with irregular rhythm. Heart rate can be approximated by multiplying the number of cardiac cycles in a 6-second period by 10; the heart rate in this example is approximately 80 beats/min. (From Stillwell S, Randall E: *Pocket guide to cardiovascular care,* ed 2, St Louis, 1994, Mosby.)

Table 6-3 Components of Normal Electrocardiogram (ECG)

Component	Criteria	Comment
Rhythm	Atrial and ventricular are same; R-R and P-P intervals vary ≤0.12 sec	
Rate	Atrial and ventricular rates are equal; 60-100 cycles/min	
P wave	Present; only one P for each QRS	
Direction	Upright in I, II, aV_F, and V_4 to V_6; inverted in aV_R; biphasic, flat or inverted in III, V_1, and V_2	
Shape	Rounded, symmetric, without notches, peaks	Upright and notched in I, II, V_4 to V_6 suggests left atrial abnormality; tall and peaked in II, III, aV_F suggests right atrial abnormality
Amplitude	<3 mm	
Width	1.5-2.5 mm (0.06-0.10 sec)	
Axis	0 to + 90 degrees	
PR interval	0.12-0.20 sec	>0.20 sec = AVB
QRS interval	0.06-0.10 sec	≥0.12 sec = BBB $V_1 V_2$ are best to measure QRS
QT interval	Less than half the preceding R-R interval in normal rates $$QTc = \frac{Qt \text{ (measured)}}{\sqrt{R\text{-}R \text{ interval(s)}}}$$ Normal ≤0.39 sec (men); ≤0.44 sec (women)	Prolonged QT interval associated with torsades de pointes
QRS complex	Follows each P	Uppercase and lowercase letters indicate the relative sizes of the QRS components

Continued

Table 6-3 COMPONENTS OF NORMAL ELECTROCARDIOGRAM (ECG)—cont'd

Component	Criteria	Comment
Configuration		

qRs   Rs   qR   rSR'   QS

Component	Criteria	Comment
Q wave	Width: <0.039 sec	Significant if 0.04 sec wide or 25% of the height of the R wave
	Depth 1-2 mm in I, aV_L, aV_F, V_5, and V_6; deep QS or Qr in aV_R and possibly in III, V_1, and V_2	
Amplitude	>5 mm and <25 mm in limb leads; 5-30 mm in V_1 and V_6; 7 to 30 mm in V_2 and V_5; 9 to 30 mm in V_3 and V_4	
R progression	Progressive increase in R wave amplitude from V_1 to V_6	
Axis	−30 to +110 degrees	
Transition	V_3 or V_4	
Intrinsicoid deflection	≤0.02 sec V_1; ≤0.04 sec in V_6	Delayed in BBB and chamber enlargement

V_6

Component	Criteria	Comment
ST segment	Isoelectric, but may be elevated ≤1 mm in limb leads and ≤2 mm in some precordial leads Not depressed more than 0.05 mm Curves gently into proximal limb of T wave	Elevation associated with vasospasm or acute injury; depression suggests ischemia

Continued

Table 6-3 Components of Normal Electrocardiogram (ECG)—cont'd

Component	Criteria	Comment
T wave		
Direction	Upright in I, II, and V_3 to V_6; inverted in aV_R; and varies in III, aV_L, aV_F, V_1, and V_2	Tall T wave associated with hyperkalemia, ischemia
Shape	Slightly rounded and asymmetric	
Height	≤5 mm in limb leads; ≤10 mm in precordial leads	
Axis	Left and inferior	
U wave		Increases in amplitude in hypokalemia
Direction	Upright	
Amplitude	0.33 mm in precordial leads (average); 2.5 mm (maximum)	
Width	≤0.24 sec	

AVB, Atrioventricular block; *BBB,* bundle branch block.
Adapted from Kinney M, et al: *AACN's clinical reference for critical-care nursing,* ed 4, New York, 1998, Mosby.

DYSRHYTHMIAS

Sinus Bradycardia (Figure 6-14)

1. Determinants
   Rhythm: regular
   Rate: <60
   P waves: present; same morphology
   PR interval: 0.12 to 0.20 second
   QRS: ≤0.10 second; same morphology
2. Treatment: if the patient is asymptomatic, none. If symptomatic, atropine, pacemaker, epinephrine, dopamine.

Sinus Tachycardia (Figure 6-15)

1. Determinants
   Rhythm: regular
   Rate: >100
   P waves: present; same morphology
   PR interval: 0.12 to 0.20 second
   QRS: ≤0.10 second; same morphology
2. Treatment: treat the cause (e.g., stress/anxiety, fever, heart failure, pain, hypoxia, hyperthyroidism)

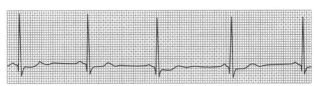

Figure 6-14 Sinus bradycardia. (From Conover MB: *Pocket guide to electrocardiography,* ed 5, St Louis, 2004, Mosby.)

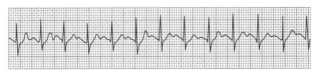

Figure 6-15 Sinus tachycardia. (From Conover MB: *Pocket guide to electrocardiography,* ed 5, St Louis, 2004, Mosby.)

Sinus Arrhythmia (Figure 6-16)

1. Determinants
   Rhythm: irregular; varies by >0.12 second
   Rate: variable; increases with inspiration, decreases with expiration
   P waves: present; same morphology
   PR interval: 0.12 to 0.20 second
   QRS: ≤0.10 second; same morphology
2. Treatment: none

Premature Atrial Complex (Figure 6-17)

1. Determinants
   Rhythm: irregular because of ectopic beats
   Rate: that of underlying rhythm
   P waves: present; same morphology except for ectopic beat
   PR interval: 0.12 to 0.20 second (PR interval of the ectopic beat may vary from the others)
   QRS: ≤0.10 second; same morphology
2. Treatment: usually none

Atrial Tachycardia (Figure 6-18)

1. Determinants
   Rhythm: regular
   Rate: atrial rate 130 to 250; ventricular rate may be less than atrial rate as a result of lack of conduction through the AV node
   P waves: present; same morphology

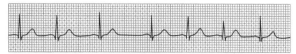

Figure 6-16 Sinus arrhythmia. (From Conover MB: *Pocket guide to electrocardiography,* ed 5, St Louis, 2004, Mosby.)

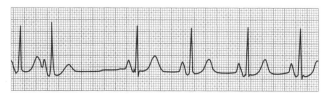

Figure 6-17 Premature atrial complex. (From Conover MB: *Pocket guide to electrocardiography,* ed 5, St Louis, 2004, Mosby.)

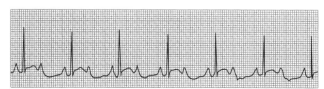

Figure 6-18 Atrial tachycardia. (From Conover MB: *Pocket guide to electrocardiography,* ed 5, St Louis, 2004, Mosby.)

PR interval: 0.12 to 0.20 second
QRS: ≤0.10 second, same morphology

2. Treatment: identify and treat the cause (e.g., if caused by digitalis toxicity, discontinue digoxin)

Atrial Flutter (Figure 6-19)

1. Determinants
   Rhythm: atrial rhythm is regular; ventricular rhythm regular or irregular, depending on the AV conduction pattern
   Rate: atrial rate 230 to 350; ventricular rate usually <150 (depends on AV conduction)
   P waves: absent; replaced by flutter waves, which have a saw-tooth appearance
   PR interval: none
   QRS: ≤0.10 second; same morphology

2. Treatment: if hemodynamically unstable, cardioversion

II

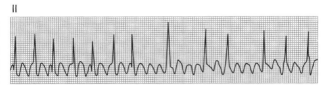

Figure 6-19 Atrial flutter. (From Conover MB: *Pocket guide to electrocardiography,* ed 5, St Louis, 2004, Mosby.)

Atrial Fibrillation (Figure 6-20)

1. Determinants
   Rhythm: irregular
   Rate: atrial rate >350; ventricular rate is variable
   P waves: none; fibrillatory waves create a wavy, undulating baseline
   PR interval: none
   QRS: ≤0.10 second; normal morphology
2. Treatment: if hemodynamically unstable, cardioversion

Paroxysmal Supraventricular Tachycardia (Figure 6-21)

1. Determinants
   Rhythm: regular; repeated episodes of tachycardia with an abrupt onset lasting from a few seconds to many hours
   Rate: 150 to 250
   P waves: cannot be clearly identified; may distort the preceding T wave
   PR interval: none measurable
   QRS: ≤0.10 second; same morphology
   Ratio: unable to determine
2. Treatment: treat underlying cause; if hemodynamically unstable, cardioversion

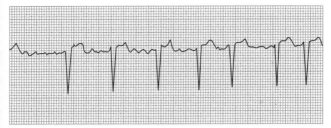

Figure 6-20 Atrial fibrillation. (From Conover MB: *Pocket guide to electrocardiography,* ed 5, St Louis, 2004, Mosby.)

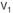

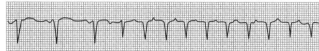

Figure 6-21 Paroxysmal supraventricular tachycardia. (From Conover MB: *Pocket guide to electrocardiography,* ed 5, St Louis, 2004, Mosby.)

Junctional Rhythm (Figure 6-22)

1. Determinants
   Rhythm: regular
   Rate: escape 40 to 60
   accelerated 62 to 99
   tachycardia 100 to 140
   P waves: absent, negative in II, III, aV$_F$; may be dissociated from QRS
   PR: not applicable (NA)
   QRS: ≤0.10 second; same morphology
2. Treatment: if asymptomatic, none. If symptomatic because of decreased HR, atropine or pacemaker may be indicated.

Premature Ventricular Complex (PVC) (Figure 6-23)

1. Determinants
   Rhythm: irregular because of the PVC
   Rate: varies with the underlying rhythm
   P waves: no P wave with the PVC
   QRS: PVC is wide and bizarre morphology
2. Treatment: none if benign

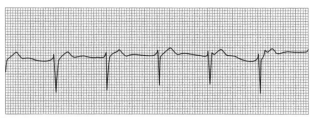

Figure 6-22 Accelerated idiojunctional rhythm. (From Conover MB: *Pocket guide to electrocardiography,* ed 5, St Louis, 2004, Mosby.)

V₁

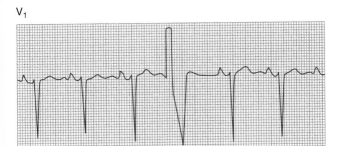

Figure 6-23 Premature ventricular complex. (From Conover MB: *Pocket guide to electrocardiography*, ed 5, St Louis, 2004, Mosby.)

Accelerated Idioventricular Rhythm (Figure 6-24)

1. Determinants
   Rhythm: regular
   Rate: 40 to 100 beats/min
   P waves: absent
   PR interval: none
   QRS: wide (>0.12 second); bizarre appearance with same morphology
2. Treatment: none unless hemodynamically unstable, then treat as with other bradydysrhythmias (atropine and/or pacemaker)

Ventricular Tachycardia (Figure 6-25)

1. Determinants
   Rhythm: regular or slightly irregular
   Rate: 100 to 250
   P waves: usually not seen; if present, will be dissociated from ventricular rhythm

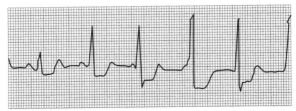

Figure 6-24 Accelerated idioventricular rhythm. (From Conover MB: *Pocket guide to electrocardiography*, ed 5, St Louis, 2004, Mosby.)

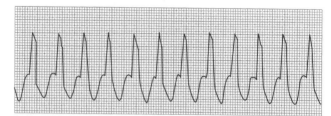

Figure 6-25 Ventricular tachycardia. (From Conover MB: *Pocket guide to electrocardiography*, ed 5, St Louis, 2004, Mosby.)

     PR interval: none measurable

     QRS: wide (>0.12 second) and bizarre morphology

  2. Treatment: defibrillation, CPR, vasopressor (i.e., vasopressin), epinephrine, amiodarone, lidocaine

Ventricular Fibrillation (Figure 6-26)

  1. Determinants

     Rhythm: irregular, chaotic baseline

     Rate: unable to measure

     P waves: none

     PR interval: none

     QRS: none

  2. Treatment: defibrillation, CPR, vasopressor (i.e., vasopressin), epinephrine, amiodarone, lidocaine

Torsades de Pointes (Figure 6-27)

  1. Determinants

     Rhythm: regular or slightly irregular

     Rate: 200 to 250

     P waves: usually not seen; if present, will be dissociated from ventricular rhythm

     PR interval: none measurable

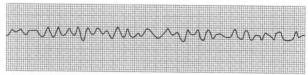

Figure 6-26 Ventricular fibrillation. (From Conover MB: *Pocket guide to electrocardiography*, ed 5, St Louis, 2004, Mosby.)

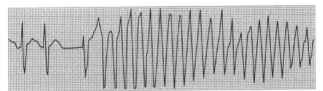

Figure 6-27   Torsades de pointes. (From Conover MB: *Pocket guide to electrocardiography,* ed 5, St Louis, 2004, Mosby.)

   QRS: wide (>0.12 second) and bizarre morphology; QRS complexes appear to be constantly changing and twist in a spiral pattern around the baseline

2. Treatment: if hemodynamically unstable, electrical therapy, magnesium, or overdrive pacing

First-Degree Atrioventricular (AV) Block (Figure 6-28)

   1. Determinants
      Rhythm: regular
      Rate: 60 to 100
      P waves: normal; same morphology
      PR interval: >0.20 second
      QRS: ≤0.10 second; same morphology
   2. Treatment: usually none unless associated with symptomatic bradycardia

Second-Degree Atrioventricular (AV) Block (Type I, Wenckebach) (Figure 6-29)

   1. Determinants
      Rhythm: irregular

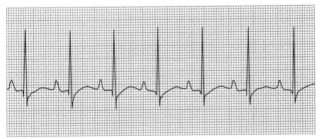

Figure 6-28   First-degree atrioventricular (AV) block. (From Conover MB: *Pocket guide to electrocardiography,* ed 5, St Louis, 2004, Mosby.)

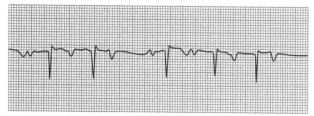

Figure 6-29 Second-degree atrioventricular (AV) block, type I. (From Conover MB: *Pocket guide to electrocardiography*, ed 5, St Louis, 2004, Mosby.)

Rate: atrial rate 60 to 100; ventricular rate is slower as a result of dropped beats

P waves: normal, same morphology

PR interval: progressive lengthening with each beat until a QRS is dropped; the PR interval is reset to normal with the dropped beat and the cycle of PR lengthening begins again

QRS: ≤0.10 second; same morphology

2. Treatment: usually none

Second-Degree Atrioventricular (AV) Block (Type II) (Figure 6-30)

1. Determinants

Rhythm: irregular

Rate: atrial 60 to 100; ventricular rate is slower as a result of dropped beats

P waves: normal; same morphology

PR interval: 0.12 to 0.20 second and fixed, except where beat is dropped

QRS: wide; same morphology

2. Treatment: pacemaker; there is a high tendency to progress to complete heart block

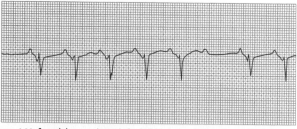

Figure 6-30 Second-degree atrioventricular (AV) block, type II. (From Conover MB: *Pocket guide to electrocardiography*, ed 5, St Louis, 2004, Mosby.)

Third-Degree Heart Block (Complete Heart Block) (Figure 6-31)

1. Determinants

   Rhythm: regular

   Rate: atrial 60 to 100; ventricular depends on site of escape rhythm, usually 20 to 60

   P waves: normal; same morphology

   PR interval: not measurable; no association between atrial rhythm and ventricular rhythm

   QRS: normal ($\leq$0.10 second) if from AV junction; widened (>0.12 second) if from below the bundle of His

2. Treatment: usually pacing is required

ELECTROCARDIOGRAPHY: TWELVE-LEAD

Clinical Brief

Twelve-lead ECG is used as a diagnostic tool in determining overall electrical functioning of the heart and can aid in identifying pathologic conditions. Normal and abnormal activity, as evidenced by examining individual waves, deflections, intervals, and segments, can be evaluated.

Twelve Leads

The 12 leads are either bipolar or unipolar. The precordial leads (V_1-V_6) are unipolar and provide information about anterior, posterior, right, and left electrical forces. The bipolar limb leads (I, II, III) consist of a positive and a negative electrode and compose Einthoven's triangle. Leads aV_R, aV_L, and aV_F are unipolar limb leads representing augmented vector right, left, and foot. The limb leads provide information about vertical electrical forces, as well as left and right forces.

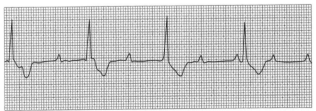

Figure 6-31 Third-degree atrioventricular (AV) block (complete heart block). (From Conover MB: *Pocket guide to electrocardiography,* ed 5, St Louis, 2004, Mosby.)

Deflections

Deflections signify individual cardiac cycle events and their electrical direction in relation to a positive electrode. When the electrical current moves in the general direction of a positive electrode, an upward or positive deflection is recorded. Conversely, a downward or negative deflection signifies movement away from the positive electrode. Major deflections are referred to as the P, Q, R, S, T, and U waves.

Waves, Intervals, and Segments

See Table 6-3 for components of a normal ECG.

Electrical Axis

An imaginary line drawn between two electrodes is called the axis of the lead. A vector signifies a quantity of electrical force that has both a given magnitude and direction. When the cardiac vector is parallel to the axis of the lead recording it, the ECG deflection is either the most upright or the most negative (Figure 6-32). When the direction of the electrical activity is perpendicular to the axis of the lead recording it, an equiphasic deflection will be recorded.

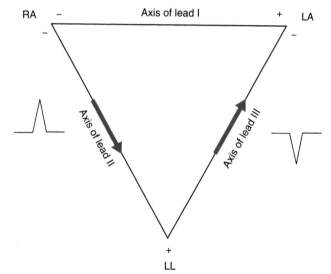

Figure 6-32 Axis. When a mean vector is parallel to the axis of a lead, the tallest (electrical current flowing toward the positive lead) or the deepest (electrical current flowing away from the positive lead) complex will result in that lead.

Hexaxial Reference System

The mean vector, or axis of the heart, can be measured in degrees using the hexaxial reference system. A normal QRS vector should lie between −30 and +110. Left axis deviation can be caused by left anterior hemiblock, left bundle branch block (LBBB), left ventricular hypertrophy, obesity, or inferior myocardial infarction (MI). Right axis deviation can be caused by left posterior hemiblock, RV hypertrophy, limb lead reversal, dextrocardia, or lateral MI.

Quick Method to Axis Determination

Figure 6-33 illustrates a quick method to determine axis.

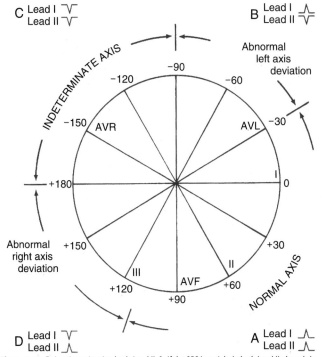

Figure 6-33 Estimating axis using leads I and II. **A,** If the QRS is upright in both I and II, the axis is normal. **B,** If the QRS is upright in I and down in II, left axis deviation is present. **C,** If the QRS is down in both I and II, indeterminate axis is present. **D,** If the QRS is down in I and upright in II, right axis deviation is present.

Electrocardiogram (ECG) Pattern Associated with Ischemia

Reduced blood supply is characterized by inverted T waves, transient ST depression during anginal episodes because of a fixed lesion, and transient ST elevation during anginal episodes that are due to vasospasm (Figure 6-34).

Electrocardiogram (ECG) Pattern Associated with Injury

Acuteness of an infarction is represented by ST segment elevation. ST segment elevation is one of the earliest changes characteristic of infarction. ST segment depression is characteristic of non–Q-wave infarction.

Electrocardiogram (ECG) Pattern Associated with Q-Wave Infarction

Indicative changes, significant Q waves, ST elevation, and T-wave inversion can be found in leads over infarcted myocardium.
Anterior MI—leads V_1-V_4
Lateral MI—leads I, aV_L, and V_5 and V_6
Inferior MI—leads, II, III, and aV_F
Posterior MI—reciprocal changes in anterior leads (e.g., tall R wave, ST depression, and tall symmetric T wave in V_1-V_4)
RV infarction is represented by lead V_{4R} and will exhibit ST elevation >1 mm.

Wellen's Syndrome—Critical Stenosis of Proximal Left Anterior Descending (LAD) Artery

Signs on ECG during pain-free period in patients with unstable angina indicating critical stenosis of the proximal LAD artery and impending infarction. These include little or no ST elevation in V_2 and V_3, ST segment turning down into a deeply inverted and symmetric T wave in V_2 and V_3, and no significant Q waves in precordial leads (Figure 6-35).

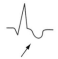

Ischemia
Symmetrically
inverted T waves

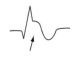

Injury
ST elevation
(indicates acuteness)

Infarction
Diagnosed by large
Q wave—0.04 sec wide
or 25% the height
of the R wave

Figure 6-34 ECG changes with infarction.

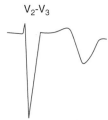

Figure 6-35 ECG changes associated with Wellen's syndrome. (From Conover MB: *Pocket guide to electrocardiography,* ed 5, St Louis, 2004, Mosby.)

Differentiating Bundle Branch Block (BBB)

LBBB characteristics include a mainly negative QRS in V_1 and an R wave with no Q or S wave in leads I, aV_L, and V_6. Right bundle branch block (RBBB) characteristics include an upright QRS in V_1; intrinsicoid deflection 0.07 second or later in V_1; and small Q wave and broad S wave in leads I, aV_L, and V_6. Figure 6-36 illustrates a quick identification of BBB.

Chamber Enlargement

Table 6-4 outlines changes on ECG indicative of chamber enlargement.

Ventricular Ectopy versus Aberrant Ventricular Conduction

Wide QRS complexes with bizarre morphology generally signify either ventricular ectopy or aberrant ventricular conduction. Ventricular ectopy has its origin in the ventricle and indicates increased ventricular

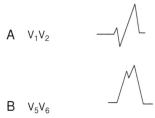

Figure 6-36 Right bundle branch block (RBBB) and left bundle branch block (LBBB). **A,** Check right precordial leads (V_1, V_2) for RR′, suggesting RBBB. **B,** Check left precordial leads (V_5, V_6) for RR′, suggesting LBBB.

Table 6-4 CHAMBER ENLARGEMENT

Chamber	Changes
Right atrium (RA)	Tall peaked P wave (>2.5 mm) in II, III, aV$_F$; low or isoelectric P wave in I; P waves in V$_1$, V$_2$ may be upright with increased amplitude
Left atrium (LA)	P-wave duration >0.12 sec, P wave notched and upright in I, II, V$_4$-V$_6$; wide, deep, negative component to P wave in V$_1$
Right ventricle (RV)	Right axis deviation, R/S ratio >1 in V$_1$; ST segment depression and T-wave inversion in V$_1$ or V$_2$
Left ventricle (LV)*	Increased voltage; R or S wave in limb leads >20 mm or S wave in V$_1$ or V$_2$ >30 mm or R wave in V$_5$ or V$_6$ >30 mm, 3 points
	ST changes; with digitalis, 1 point; without digitalis, 2 points
	LA enlargement, 3 points
	Left axis deviation (−30 or more), 2 points
	QRS duration ≥0.09 sec, 1 point
	Intrinsicoid deflection in V$_5$ or V$_6$ ≥0.05 sec, 1 point

*4 points, left ventricular hypertrophy (LVH) likely; 5 points, LVH present.

irritability. Aberrant ventricle conduction is caused by a supraventricular impulse (e.g., premature atrial contraction [PAC]) arriving at the ventricle too early; the ventricles are not totally repolarized so the impulse is conducted abnormally or aberrantly.

Both ventricular ectopy and aberrant conduction present as a wide QRS. Differential diagnosis is important because treatment is different.

Characteristics favoring aberrancy include QRS 0.12 to 0.14 second, and P waves (if identifiable) are associated with the QRS. Characteristics favoring ectopy include QRS >0.14 second and P waves (if identifiable) independent of the QRS. Additional diagnostic clues are seen in Figure 6-37.

Wolff-Parkinson-White Syndrome (WPW)

WPW is a form of ventricular preexcitation characterized by a short PR and a prolonged QRS and a delta wave (initial slurring of the QRS). An anomalous or accessory pathway between the atrium and ventricle allows the atrial impulse to bypass the AV node and therefore

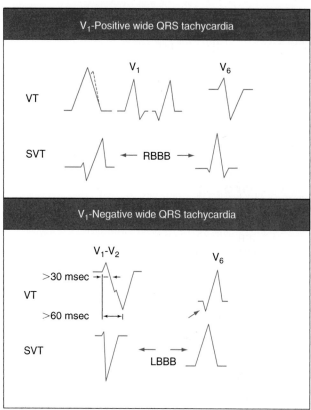

Figure 6-37 Differential diagnosis in wide QRS tachycardia. (From Conover MB: *Pocket guide to electrocardiography,* ed 5, St Louis, 2004, Mosby.)

reach the ventricle earlier than normal. The patient with WPW is predisposed to paroxysmal supraventricular ventricular tachycardia (PSVT) and atrial fibrillation. The tachydysrhythmias usually have a narrow QRS (orthodromic); however, a wide QRS tachycardia (antidromic) may occur and be confused with ventricular tachycardia (VT).

SYSTEMATIC APPROACH TO TWELVE-LEAD ELECTROCARDIOGRAM (ECG)

Review all 12 leads to determine (1) underlying rhythm; (2) patterns of ischemia, injury, or infarction; (3) chamber enlargement; and (4) ventricular axis.

1. Determine rate.

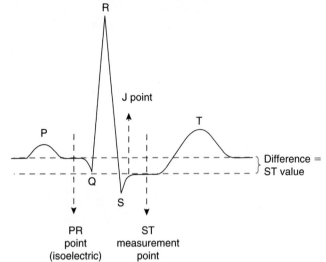

Figure 6-38 ST measurement points: PR point, J point, and ST point. The PR segment is used to identify the isoelectric line. The ST segment begins at the J point, which is the end of the QRS complex. The ST segment measurement point can be measured at 60 or 80 ms past the J point. (From Mims et al: *Critical care skills: a clinical handbook,* ed 2, St Louis, 2004, Saunders.)

2. Examine P-P and R-R intervals for regularity in rhythm.
3. Analyze P waves in each lead.
4. Measure PR, QRS, and QT intervals.
5. Analyze QRS complex.
6. Identify leads having significant Q waves.
7. Determine presence of R-wave progression and identify lead associated with transition.
8. Measure intrinsicoid deflection.
9. Determine axis.
10. Identify leads displaying ST segment elevation or depression (Figure 6-38).
11. Analyze T wave for increased amplitude.
12. Identify presence of U wave.

INTRACRANIAL PRESSURE (ICP) MONITORING

Clinical Brief

ICP monitoring is used to measure the pressure within the brain and to evaluate cerebral compliance so that changes can be detected early and effects of various medical and nursing interventions can be evaluated.

The traditional clinical signs of increased ICP (decreasing level of consciousness, increased systolic BP and widening pulse pressure, bradycardia, and slow irregular respirations) do not actually reflect early increases in ICP and in fact may occur too late for intervention and treatment to be effective.

ICP monitoring also provides the necessary data to calculate cerebral perfusion pressure (CPP); this is measured by subtracting mean ICP from the mean arterial blood pressure. Adequate cerebral circulation is ensured if the CPP remains approximately 70 to 90 mm Hg.

A pressure transducer set-up is connected, using sterile normal saline (without preservative) to provide a fluid column between the cerebrospinal fluid (CSF) within the ventricles and the transducer. The pressure is transmitted to a monitor, and the pressure waveform and digital readings are displayed. A continuous flush device is not used on any ICP monitoring system because it may contribute to further increased ICP.

Complications include CNS infection.

Indications

The Monroe-Kellie hypothesis states that the volume of the intracranium is equal to the volume of the brain plus the volume of the blood within the brain plus the volume of the CSF within the brain. Therefore any condition that results in an increase in the volume of one or more of these will increase the ICP, unless there is a concomitant decrease in one or more of the components.

Description

The intraventricular catheter is placed via a burr hole into the lateral ventricle of the nondominant hemisphere. When ICP is severely elevated, CSF can be drained using this type of system. This is the most invasive method of monitoring ICP, yet it is also the most accurate because the catheter is placed directly into the ventricle.

The subarachnoid screw or bolt is inserted into the subarachnoid space. This system is unreliable in patients with elevated ICP because the device becomes obstructed by brain tissue.

The epidural sensor is a transducer placed between the skull and dura. It is less invasive than the intraventricular catheter and the subarachnoid screw, so it may be less accurate. Once it is placed, recalibration is not necessary. Drainage of CSF cannot be performed with this system.

The fiberoptic transducer-tipped catheter can be placed in the ventricle, subarachnoid or subdural spaces, or parenchyma (Figure 6-39).

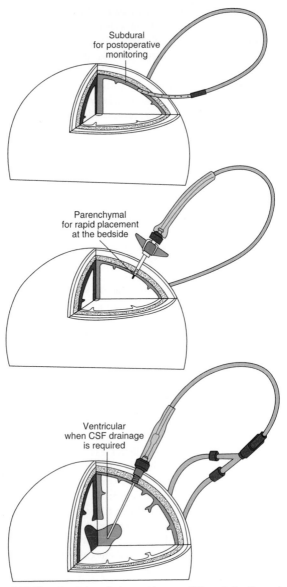

Figure 6-39 Fiberoptic techniques for intracranial pressure (ICP) monitoring. (Courtesy Integra Neurosciences, Camino, San Diego.)

With ventricular placement, CSF can be drained. Once it is placed, it cannot be recalibrated.

VALUES

Normal

0 to 15 mm Hg

Significance of Abnormal Values

Consistently elevated ICP suggests that the compensatory mechanisms of cerebral autoregulation (arterial constriction and dilation) have failed. Patients usually become symptomatic with an ICP of 20 to 25 mm Hg, and a sustained ICP >60 mm Hg is usually fatal. Factors that increase ICP include the following:

Hypercapnia ($Paco_2$ >42 mm Hg)

Hypoxia (Pao_2 <50 mm Hg)

Excessive fluid intake

Head, neck, and extreme hip flexion

Head rotation of 90 degrees to either side

Valsalva maneuver (straining, coughing)

Continuous activity without adequate rest

In addition, arousal from sleep, rapid eye movement (REM) sleep, emotional upset, and noxious stimuli such as suctioning are known to increase ICP.

PATIENT CARE MANAGEMENT

Preinsertion

For insertion, the patient is placed in a supine position with the head of the bed elevated 30 to 45 degrees. A twist drill is used to insert the device. Strict aseptic technique is essential, as is a sterile environment, during the procedure.

Postinsertion

The ICP waveform should be continuously displayed on the monitor, and alarms should be set to coincide with the patient's clinical status. The ICP should be monitored and recorded as ordered, and the mean arterial blood pressure should be monitored to determine CPP.

It is imperative that strict aseptic technique be maintained during the care of the insertion site and pressure line and during dressing changes. Assess for signs of infection, drainage, swelling, or irritation.

The site must be kept clean and dry and should be covered with an occlusive dressing at all times.

The patient should be positioned with the head of the bed elevated 15 to 30 degrees (unless contraindicated) and maintained in a neutral position with minimal hip and knee flexion to facilitate venous drainage from the brain and prevent further increases in ICP.

Additional measures to prevent sustained intracranial hypertension should be taken: prevent hypothermia and hyperthermia, keep $PaCO_2$ at 28 to 30 mm Hg, instruct the patient to avoid a Valsalva maneuver, and restrict fluids as ordered.

Obtaining Accurate Measurements

1. Zero the transducer by opening the transducer to air and adjusting the monitor to read zero; this eliminates the pressure contributions from the atmosphere, and only pressures within the chamber being monitored will be measured. Check with the manufacturer's recommendations for routine zeroing. Epidural sensors and fiberoptic devices are zeroed only before insertion.

2. Level the air reference port of the transducer to the level of the foramen of Monro (Figure 6-40) with each position change or a change in waveform and after any manipulation of the system. Epidural and fiberoptic devices do not require leveling after insertion.

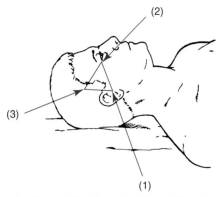

(2)

(3)

(1)

Figure 6-40 Location of foramen of Monro for transducer placement. Map an imaginary equilateral triangle from the external auditory meatus *(1)* to the outer canthus of the eye *(2)* to behind the hairline *(3)*. Point 3 is the location of the foramen of Monro.

3. Check the fluid-filled systems frequently for air because this will alter readings.
4. Obtain ICP readings at end-expiration to avoid the effects of thoracic pressures on the cerebral venous system.

Waveform Interpretation

The ICP waveform (Figure 6-41) is very similar in appearance to that of the CVP. Because the ventricles of the brain are relatively low-pressure chambers, the waveform has small systolic and diastolic fluctuations and thus the mean is monitored. The waveform consists of at least three peaks (Figure 6-41), although additional peaks may be present in some individuals. An increase in ICP will cause an increase in all waveform components initially; as ICP progresses, there is an elevation of P_2.

A P_2 equal to or higher than P_1 suggests decreased compliance, which may precede an actual increase in ICP. This signifies that compensatory mechanisms are failing and that a small increase in the volume can increase ICP significantly.

The intraventricular catheter and subarachnoid screw may develop a damped waveform as a result of tissue, blood, or debris blocking the transmission of the pressure. The line is irrigated only when ordered by a physician (Table 6-5). Air bubbles may cause a damped waveform in fluid-coupled systems.

Removal

The ICP monitoring device is removed by a physician. A wrench is required for the bolt. Sterile technique is used to prevent contamination of the insertion site. A sterile dressing is applied to the site for at least 24 hours; after this, the site is left open to air. If there is evidence of a CSF leak, additional sutures may be required.

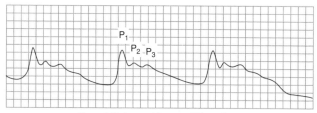

Figure 6-41 Intracranial pressure (ICP) waveform.

Table 6-5 Troubleshooting Intracranial Pressure (ICP) Monitoring
　　　　　Lines

Problem	Cause	Solution
ICP waveform damped or absent	Air in transducer system	Eliminate air
	Loose connections	Tighten connections
	Occlusion of monitoring device	Flush device only as directed by physician
False high-pressure reading	Transducer too low	Place transducer at level of foramen of Monro and zero balance
	Air in transducer system	Eliminate air
False low-pressure reading	Transducer too high	Place transducer at level of foramen of Monro and zero balance
	Air in transducer system	Eliminate air

Critical Observations

CNS infection. Risk factors that influence infection rate include the insertion environment and technique, type of device used, duration of monitoring, and patient factors such as age and state of immunosuppression.

- The entire pressure transducer set-up must remain a closed system to prevent contamination. Strict aseptic technique must be followed during insertion of the device and while manipulating the pressure line and changing dressings.

LEFT ATRIAL PRESSURE (LAP) MONITORING

Clinical Brief

LAP is monitored to evaluate left-sided heart pressures (left ventricular end diastolic pressure [LVEDP]) following open-heart surgery. *Complications* include hemorrhage, clot formation, infection, vessel damage, air embolus, electric shock, and catheter tip migration.

Indications

LAP monitoring can be used for the perioperative and postoperative assessment of left ventricular function and cardiovascular status and to assess the hemodynamic response to vasoactive drugs and fluids.

Description

The left atrium (LA) catheter is inserted into the left atrium during cardiac surgery; it is threaded through the superior pulmonary vein into the left atrium and the external end is brought out through a small incision at the inferior end of the mediastinal incision. The catheter is connected to a pressure transducer set-up, and the waveform is monitored continuously.

VALUES

Normal

4 to 12 mm Hg

Significance of Abnormal Values

Because the catheter is positioned in the left atrium, it indirectly reflects the LVEDP. Therefore the same factors that cause an increase or decrease in pulmonary artery diastolic (PAD) pressure and pulmonary artery wedge pressure (PAWP) will cause abnormal LAP values. (See Significance of Abnormal Values under Pulmonary Artery (PA) Pressure Monitoring significance of abnormal values, p. 474.)

PATIENT CARE MANAGEMENT

Preinsertion

The LA catheter is inserted during open-heart surgery, and the line will be in place when the patient arrives in the critical care unit.

Postinsertion

The LA line should never be irrigated or flushed. The remainder of the postinsertion care is the same as that described with the CVP and PA lines (see p. 476).

Obtaining Accurate Measurements

The air port of the pressure transducer must be leveled with the phlebostatic axis during pressure readings. Readings should be taken at end-expiration and obtained from a calibrated strip chart recording if respiratory variation is present. The transducer should be leveled each time the patient or transducer has been moved. The patient should not be removed from the ventilator or positive end-expiratory pressure (PEEP) during readings.

Waveform Interpretation

The LAP waveform closely resembles that of the PAWP, and the mean pressure is monitored (Figure 6-42). The waveform has *a* and *v* waves, as well as *x* and *y* descents; these correlate to the same mechanical events of the cardiac cycle as the waves and descents of the PAWP waveform (see p. 479).

If large *a* and *v* waves appear on the waveform, it may be the result of catheter migration to the left ventricle; if this occurs, notify the physician at once and monitor the patient for ventricular dysrhythmias.

Troubleshooting

Basic troubleshooting of the LA line is similar to that of other hemodynamic lines (see Table 6-2 on troubleshooting invasive hemodynamic monitoring lines) except that the LA catheter is never flushed. If damping of the waveform occurs and clot formation is suspected

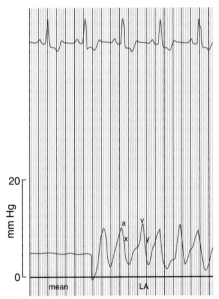

Figure 6-42 Left atrial pressure (LAP) waveform. (From Daily EK, Schroeder JS: *Techniques in bedside hemodynamic monitoring,* ed 5, St Louis, 1994, Mosby.)

as the cause, attempt to aspirate the clot. If the line cannot be aspirated or if the line remains damped, then the catheter must be discontinued.

Removal

The LA catheter is removed by a physician or nurse, depending on the institutional protocol. It is usually removed after 24 to 48 hours because of the increased risk for air embolus. Bleeding and pericardial tamponade can also occur following removal of the LA catheter. Mediastinal tubes should be left in place for at least 2 hours after the removal of the LA line so that blood does not collect in the mediastinum. The procedure for removal is the same as that for a CVP catheter (see p. 438). The site is covered with sterile occlusive dressing and must be observed frequently for bleeding. Following removal of the LA catheter, the patient must be monitored closely for signs of pericardial tamponade (jugular vein distention; cyanosis; elevation of CVP, PAD, and PAWP; pulsus paradoxus; decreased systolic BP).

Critical Observations

The potential risks of LAP monitoring are the same as those listed for CVP monitoring: *air embolus, clot formation, infection, cardiac tamponade, and electrical hazards* because the LA line provides direct access to the systemic circulation, the risk of air embolus is more threatening than with the CVP or PA lines.

- To decrease this risk, an inline air filter should be used, and the line should never be irrigated or flushed.

(See Critical Observations under CVP Pressure Monitoring, p. 439).

PULMONARY ARTERY (PA) PRESSURE MONITORING

Clinical Brief

The PA catheter is used to continuously monitor right intracardiac and PA pressures. The PA end-diastolic pressure can reflect left-sided heart pressures; LVEDP can be estimated and the hemodynamic response to fluid or drug therapy can be assessed. The PA catheter also allows for the sampling of mixed-venous blood from the PA to measure oxygen saturation. (See discussion under Sv_{O_2} monitoring, p. 482.) Finally, the PA catheter enables the measurement of CO and the calculation of the cardiac index (CI).

Complications include hemorrhage, clot formation, infection, vessel damage, air embolus, electric shock, catheter tip migration, perforation of the pulmonary artery by the catheter, pulmonary artery infarction, hemorrhage or embolism, ventricular dysrhythmias, bundle branch block, and balloon rupture.

Indications

The PA catheter may be used in the following clinical situations: (1) left-sided heart failure, (2) valvular disease, (3) titration of vasoactive drugs or fluids, (4) severe respiratory failure, and (5) perioperative and postoperative monitoring of surgical patients with cardiovascular or pulmonary dysfunction.

Description

The PA catheter is available in a wide variety of configurations depending on the type of patient condition being monitored. It has four main ports: (1) the proximal lumen ends in the right atrium and is used for infusion of fluids or monitoring of RA pressure and for the injection of a bolus of fluid to measure CO; (2) the distal lumen ends in the PA, allowing measurement of PA pressures and left-sided heart pressures reflected across the pulmonary vasculature; (3) the balloon port leads to an inflatable balloon at the tip of the catheter; when the balloon is inflated it blocks pressures behind it (the right side of the heart) and senses pressures through the pulmonary vasculature from the left side of the heart; and (4) the thermodilution port terminates 4 to 6 cm proximal to the tip of the catheter and senses temperature changes during CO measurement. Some PA catheters have additional ports for the infusion of fluids or for insertion of a temporary pacing wire; some have a sensor to continuously measure venous oxygen saturation. Other features include measurement of right-ventricular volumes and ejection fractions and continuous measurement of CO.

The catheter is inserted into a large vein (the same sites as those used for CVP catheters) via percutaneous or cutdown method. On entry into the right atrium, the balloon is inflated and the catheter is flow-directed into position in the PA. Continuous pressure monitoring of the waveform during insertion shows the anatomic location of the tip of the catheter, based on the characteristic waveforms of the right atrium, the right ventricle, and the PA (Figure 6-43). Once the PA has been reached, the balloon tip wedges into a small branch of the PA.

VALUES

Normal

RA: 2 to 6 mm Hg. The waveform has systolic (positive) and diastolic (negative) variations, but the fluctuations are small (because the right atrium is a low-pressure chamber); thus the mean pressure is monitored.

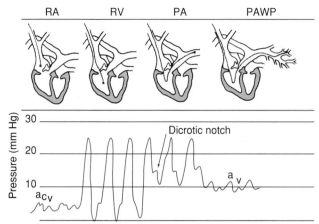

Figure 6-43 Pressure waveforms during pulmonary artery (PA) catheter insertion.

RV: 15 to 28/0 to 8 mm Hg. RV pressure is measured during catheter insertion only; this value provides information about the function of the right ventricle, as well as the tricuspid and pulmonic valves.

Pulmonary artery systolic (PAS): 15 to 30 mm Hg. The PAS pressure indicates the pressure in the PA during RV contraction, when the pulmonic valve is open.

PAD: 5 to 15 mm Hg. PAD pressure reflects the resistance to flow by the pulmonary vasculature. It indirectly measures the LVEDP because the pulmonic valve is closed during diastole (thereby eliminating right heart pressure influences) and the mitral valve is open, so that the catheter "sees" the pressure in the left atrium and the left ventricle. PAD can be used in place of the PAWP to estimate LVEDP when there is no pulmonary vascular obstruction, thereby decreasing the number of balloon inflations and potential patient risk. The PAD is normally 1 to 4 mm Hg higher than the PAWP because of the slight resistance to forward blood flow from the pulmonary vasculature; when the catheter is wedged there is no forward flow distal to the catheter tip and the effects of pulmonary vascular resistance do not affect the PAWP reading. The PAD/PAWP gradient is greater any time there is increased pulmonary vascular resistance (pulmonary embolus, hypoxia, chronic lung disease). Neither PAD nor PAWP accurately reflects LVEDP in the presence of mitral valve disease because the pressure is increased by the altered blood flow between the atrium and the ventricle.

PAWP: 4 to 12 mm Hg. PAWP, also known as *pulmonary artery occlusive pressure (PAOP)*, reflects the LVEDP most accurately because the pressures from the right side of the heart are blocked by the inflated balloon so that the tip of the catheter (distal to the balloon) senses pressures only forward of the catheter (Figure 6-44). The PAWP waveform has small fluctuations similar to the CVP waveform; thus the mean pressure is monitored.

Significance of Abnormal Values

RA: Increased RA pressure may be caused by increased vascular volume, tricuspid or pulmonic valvular disease, ventricular septal defect with left-to-right shunting, constrictive pericarditis, right ventricular (RV) infarction, myocarditis, cardiac tamponade, COPD, pulmonary embolus, pulmonary hypertension, or chronic left ventricular failure.

Hypovolemia, excessive diuresis, or systemic venodilation secondary to sepsis, drugs, or neurogenic causes may cause a decrease in RA pressure

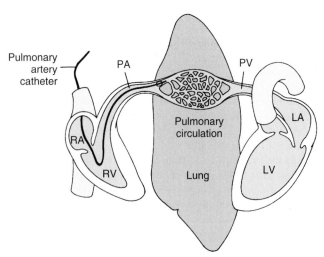

Figure 6-44 Pulmonary artery catheter in the wedged position. Balloon inflation allows for recording of pressures in the left heart as it "sees" the left atrium. *LA,* Left atrium; *LV,* left ventricle; *PA,* pulmonary artery; *PV,* pulmonary vein; *RA,* right atrium; *RV,* right ventricle.

RV: RV systolic pressures may be elevated as a result of pulmonic stenosis, pulmonary hypertension, pulmonary vascular volume overload, ventricular septal defect with left-to-right shunting, chronic lung disease, pulmonary embolism, hypoxemia, or acute respiratory distress syndrome (ARDS). Decreased RV systolic pressures may be the result of RV failure secondary to infarction or ischemia, as a result of myopathy, or secondary to hypovolemia.

RV diastolic pressure may be elevated because of pulmonic valve insufficiency, RV failure, pulmonary hypertension, cardiac tamponade, constrictive pericarditis, or intravascular volume overload. Decreased RV diastolic pressure occurs with hypovolemia.

PAS: PAS pressure may be elevated as a result of increased pulmonary blood volume or increased pulmonary vascular resistance secondary to pulmonary embolism, hypoxemia, lung disease, or ARDS. Decreased PAS pressure occurs with hypovolemia or vasodilation.

PAD: PAD pressure is elevated in the same circumstances as the PAS pressure, as well as in left heart dysfunction (from any cause), mitral stenosis and insufficiency, cardiac tamponade, or increased intravascular volume. Hypovolemia or vasodilation causes a decrease in pulmonary diastolic pressure.

PAWP: PAWP is increased in any situation in which there is left ventricular dysfunction: mitral stenosis/insufficiency, left ventricular failure, decreased left ventricular compliance, increased SVR, cardiac tamponade, or fluid volume overload. Decreased PAWP is seen with hypovolemia or vasodilation with resulting decreased afterload.

PATIENT CARE MANAGEMENT

Preinsertion

The patient is prepared in the same manner as for CVP insertion. Before insertion, the inflated balloon is tested for integrity by submerging it in saline and checking for air leaks. The transducer must be zeroed before catheter insertion, thereby ensuring accurate waveforms and pressure readings during catheter placement (see Figure 6-43). The pressures of the RA, RV, and PA are documented during insertion. It is important to monitor for ventricular dysrhythmias during insertion, especially during passage through the RV.

Postinsertion

A chest radiograph must be obtained to rule out pneumothorax and to verify correct placement. Fluids should not be infused directly into the distal lumen of the PA catheter.

　　Alarm parameters should be set and maintained at all times.

Obtaining Accurate Measurements

Zero the transducer before obtaining the first reading. Level the transducer with the phlebostatic axis every time the patient or transducer is moved. The head of the bed can be elevated up to 45 degrees for readings, but the patient should be supine.

　　Because the heart is subject to the same intrathoracic pressures as the lungs, there may be respiratory variation in the hemodynamic waveforms. When respiratory variation is present, there will be a decrease in the waveform during spontaneous inspiration and a rise in the waveform during expiration. The opposite occurs with positive-pressure ventilation—the waveform rises with inspiration and falls with expiration. When the patient is receiving intermittent mandatory ventilation, the waveform will peak and trough at different times during the respiratory cycle, depending on whether the breath is spontaneous or mechanically induced. Pressure readings should be taken at end-expiration because at this point the intrathoracic pressure is constant and the pressure waveform is most stable. The digital display is often inaccurate when respiratory variation is present, so the reading should be taken from a calibrated strip chart recording at end-expiration.

　　In patients receiving positive pressure ventilation or PEEP, the pressure reading should be taken without removing the ventilator so that the effects of positive pressure on the patient's hemodynamic status can be realized. In patients with normal lung compliance, the following equation can be used to estimate the effects of PEEP on PAWP.

$$PAWP \text{ (corrected)} = Measured\ PAWP - 0.5\ (PEEP)$$

　　In patients with ARDS or other conditions that decrease lung compliance, the following equation can be used to estimate the effects of PEEP on PAWP.

$$PAWP \text{ (corrected)} = Measured\ PAWP - 0.5\ (PEEP - 10)$$

　　The balloon should be inflated slowly when PAWP readings are taken, and inflation should cease as soon as the PAWP waveform is displayed. When obtaining a PAWP reading, do not leave the balloon inflated for more than 15 seconds; inflation longer than this can result in ischemia of the lung segment distal to the catheter. Never use more than the balloon capacity indicated by the manufacturer on the shaft of the catheter. Be sure that the PA waveform returns following passive deflation of the balloon.

PAD can be used to estimate LVEDP if the difference between PAD and PAWP is <5 mm Hg, there is no pulmonary vascular obstruction, and the HR is <130 beats/min.

Many different methods exist for measuring CO, providing invasive or noninvasive and intermittent or continuous assessments. The most commonly used procedure to determine intermittent CO at the bedside is the thermodilution method. This method uses room-temperature or iced injectate. For most patients, room-temperature injectate is preferred. Indications for iced injectate include a CO >10 L/min; dilated cardiomyopathy; patients receiving mechanical ventilation; and patients with erratic respiratory patterns, such as Cheyne-Stokes. A variety of injectate delivery systems are available, and it is important to use the correct computation constant (provided in the catheter package insert). If the wrong computation constant is inadvertently used, the following equation can be used to correct the obtained reading.

$$\text{Correct CO} = \frac{\text{Wrong CO} \times \text{Correct computaton constant}}{\text{Wrong computaton constant}}$$

To obtain a CO, iced or room-temperature solution (usually 10 mL) is injected via the proximal port of the PA catheter; generally three consecutive measurements are obtained and averaged to determine CO. Injection should be smooth, take <4 seconds, and produce a CO curve on the monitor that has a smooth and even upstroke (Figure 6-45).

Because CO, defined as the amount of blood that is pumped from the left ventricle into the aorta per minute, varies considerably in accordance to body size, the CI is used to achieve an accurate estimate of blood flow in proportion to the body surface area. Once CO has been determined, most bedside monitors have the ability to calculate parameters such as CI, stroke index (SI), systemic vascular resistance index (SVRI), pulmonary vascular resistance index (PVRI), left ventricular stroke work index (LVSWI), and right ventricular stroke work index (RVSWI). Formulas for hand calculating these values are found in Appendix D.

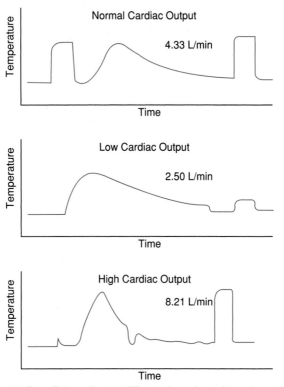

Figure 6-45 Thermodilution cardiac output (CO) curves. A normal curve shows a sharp upstroke from rapid injection of injectate, followed by a slightly prolonged downslope back to the baseline. When the cardiac output is low, more time is required for the temperature to return to baseline, producing a larger area under the curve. When the cardiac output is high, the injectate is carried through quickly and the temperature returns to baseline faster, producing a smaller area under the curve. (From Mims et al: *Critical care skills: a clinical handbook*, ed 2, St Louis, 2004, Saunders.)

Other methods for determining CO and calculated parameters do exist. Continuous CO catheters apply the same principles as the intermittent method but measure CO without use of manual boluses of injectate. Continuous CO catheters are modified with a thermal filament that gently warms the blood. A thermistor senses increased temperature (instead of the decreased temperature caused by an intermittent injectate bolus). The special CO computer, using an energy signal instead of the injectate, is capable of measuring CO every 30 to 60 seconds with average values continuously displayed. Various other methods of CO measurement include transesophageal, echocardiography, and noninvasive methods such as thoracic electrical bioimpedance (TEB) and Doppler echocardiography.

Waveform Interpretation

The PA waveform looks similar to that seen with arterial pressure monitoring. The systolic pressure is seen as a steep rise as blood is ejected from the right ventricle. The diastolic component of the waveform occurs after the closure of the pulmonic valve, seen as the dicrotic notch.

The PAWP waveform is similar in appearance to the CVP waveform. The *a* wave on the PAWP tracing indicates LA contraction; it is followed by the *x* descent, which indicates LA relaxation. The *c* wave is rarely seen in the PAWP tracing. The *v* wave represents LA filling, and the *y* descent following it represents the decrease in atrial pressure when the mitral valve opens.

Elevated *a* waves on the PAWP tracing can be indicative of mitral stenosis or left ventricular failure. Elevated *v* waves, on the other hand, indicate mitral insufficiency. Elevation of both *a* and *v* waves simultaneously indicates severe left ventricular failure.

Troubleshooting

Table 6-2 offers suggestions for troubleshooting invasive hemodynamic lines.

Additional problems that may be encountered with the PA catheter are spontaneous wedging of the balloon, migration of the catheter tip to the right ventricle, and RBBB.

If the catheter does not wedge and balloon rupture is not the cause, then the catheter may need to be advanced by the physician or designee. The chest radiograph should be used as a guide in determining correct placement.

Obtaining Mixed-Venous Blood Gases

The procedure for drawing mixed-venous blood gases is similar to that of drawing ABGs. However, mixed-venous gases are drawn from the distal lumen of the PA catheter. It is important to be sure the balloon is deflated during the aspiration of the sample; otherwise, only highly oxygen-saturated blood from downstream of the catheter tip will be drawn, causing erroneous results. Similarly, it is important to draw the sample slowly (not faster than 1 mL/20 sec), or arterial blood from the pulmonary capillaries that is highly oxygenated will be drawn into the syringe and cause erroneously high readings. Following completion of the procedure, ensure the return of the PA waveform.

Removal

Before removing the PA catheter, actively deflate the balloon. The procedure is similar to that of CVP catheter removal (see Removal of Central Venous Pressure [CVP] Catheter p. 478), except that the catheter should be rapidly pulled back to decrease the risk of ventricular dysrhythmias. If at any time resistance is felt, do not continue pulling, and notify the physician immediately. The site should be covered with a sterile, occlusive dressing. If the introducer with side port is left in place for central venous access, cap the introducer or insert an obturator.

Critical Observations

PA pressure monitoring is associated with the risk of developing the same complications as those seen with arterial and CVP monitoring (*air embolus, clot formation, hemorrhage, electrical shock, infection, and catheter tip migration* [see Critical Observations under Arterial Pressure Monitoring p. 431]). Additional complications may occur with PA pressure monitoring.

Perforation of the PA can occur during catheter positioning.
- The balloon should be inflated any time the tip is repositioned because the balloon provides some protection to the wall of the vessel.

PA infarction or *hemorrhage* can occur if the balloon is inadvertently left inflated or if the catheter spontaneously wedges, blocking blood flow to that branch of the vessel.
- The PA waveform must be monitored continuously so that inadvertent wedging of the catheter can be recognized immediately. If the PA waveform spontaneously develops a wedge appearance, the catheter has likely migrated forward into a smaller branch of the PA. To regain a PA waveform, the line should be aspirated, then flushed; if the problem continues, have the patient cough and/or turn to the side because this may help the catheter move back into a larger branch of the PA. The catheter may have to be pulled back slightly if these measures do not correct the problem. Pulmonary embolism can occur if a clot breaks off the tip of the catheter.

Ventricular dysrhythmias, secondary to irritation of the ventricular wall by the catheter tip, can occur during insertion of the catheter or if the catheter falls back into the right ventricle after placement in the PA.

- If this occurs, the catheter should be floated into the PA by a physician or designee or it should be removed. Additionally, RBBB may occur during manipulation of the catheter in the right ventricle. Generally this is not a problem unless the patient also has LBBB, in which case complete heart block could result.

Air embolus. The balloon of the catheter can rupture and cause an air embolus.

- The balloon should never be overinflated, and deflation should be passive (pulling back the air may damage the balloon). If balloon rupture is suspected (no resistance is felt during injection of air, failure to obtain wedge waveform, bleeding back into balloon port), the balloon port should no longer be used and should be labeled appropriately.

PULSE OXIMETRY

Clinical Brief

Pulse oximetry (SpO$_2$) is a noninvasive method of monitoring arterial oxygen saturation. It provides an early and immediate warning of impending hypoxemia.

Indications

Pulse oximetry may be used in any of the following clinical situations: (1) recovery from anesthesia, (2) assessment of adequacy of oxygen therapy or ventilatory management, and (3) in any patients who are at risk for hypoventilation or respiratory arrest (such as those receiving epidural anesthesia, neurologically damaged patients, or those who are receiving high doses of central nervous system depressants).

Description

The pulse oximeter is a noninvasive optical method of measuring oxygen saturation of functional hemoglobin. The amount of arterial hemoglobin that is saturated with oxygen is determined by beams of light passing through the tissue. The sensor with the light source is placed on the finger, earlobe, forehead, or the bridge of the nose; the saturation is displayed on the monitor, and visual and audible alarms can be set to alert the clinician of changes in oxygenation.

VALUES

Normal

SpO_2 ≥95%

Significance of Abnormal Values

When the arterial saturation is lower than 95%, it could be the result of a variety of causes. It may signify that the respiratory effort or oxygen delivery system is inadequate to meet the tissue needs or that CO is impaired, resulting in tissue hypoxia. If arterial flow to the sensor is impaired for any reason, it could result in an erroneously low reading while tissue oxygenation is adequate; therefore, it is important to correlate the reading with other assessment parameters.

PATIENT CARE MANAGEMENT

Obtaining Accurate Measurements

Place the sensor on clean, dry skin (finger, earlobe, forehead, or bridge of nose). If the HR displayed on the pulse oximeter and the patient's HR are within 5 beats/min, the reading is accurate. If readings are consistently inaccurate, change the sensor or the site. The sensor should not be on the same extremity that has an automatic BP cuff because this reduces arterial blood flow distally and will alter readings. The patient and extremity should be kept as still as possible to reduce artifact and interference with the signal. If severe peripheral vasoconstriction interferes with measurements from a finger, earlobe, or forehead site, the sensor should be placed more centrally (e.g., the bridge of the nose).

SVO_2 MONITORING

Clinical Brief

Continuous monitoring of mixed-venous oxygen saturation (SvO_2) provides ongoing information about the balance between oxygen supply and demand. The blood in the PA is a mixture of blood returned from the superior and inferior venae cavae, as well as the coronary sinus; the oxygen saturation of this blood returning from all perfused body parts indirectly reflects the amount of oxygen extracted systemically. The balance between oxygen supply and demand is affected by CO, arterial oxygen saturation, amount of hemoglobin available to carry oxygen, and tissue oxygen consumption.

When provided with an immediate warning that an imbalance exists, the clinician may be able to determine the cause of the imbalance and intervene appropriately.

Indications

Svo_2 monitoring may be used in any of the following clinical situations: cardiogenic shock, following open-heart surgery, acute MI, concomitant with intraaortic balloon pump (IABP) therapy, ARDS, cardiac tamponade, vasoactive drug therapy, and heart failure. In addition, Svo_2 monitoring is useful for early recognition of hemodynamic compromise because a decrease in Svo_2 often occurs before changes in other parameters. Patients with an unstable hemodynamic or respiratory status may require fewer CO or ABG measurements with the use of the Svo_2 monitor. Finally, the Svo_2 monitor is useful in assessing patient response to routine nursing interventions such as suctioning and repositioning.

Description

A thermodilution PA catheter with a fiberoptic light is used. Reflection spectrophotometry is the technique by which oxygen saturation of venous blood is measured. The light reflected by the blood is transmitted to a photodetector, where it is converted to electrical signals and the oxygen saturation is computed and displayed. The Svo_2 is updated every second and is displayed on the digital screen, as well as on a strip chart recording. The catheter has all other capabilities of the conventional PA catheter: RA, PA, and pulmonary wedge pressure monitoring; thermodilution CO; and infusion of IV fluids. Alarms can be set so that if the Svo_2 is outside the high and low limits, the clinician is immediately alerted.

VALUES

Normal

60% to 80%

Significance of Abnormal Values

A decreased (<60%) Svo_2 can be caused by (1) an increase in oxygen consumption secondary to shivering, seizures, pain, activity, hyperthermia, or anxiety or (2) a decrease in oxygen delivery secondary to decreased CO, dysrhythmias, hypoxemia, or anemia. An increased (80%-95%) Svo_2 can be caused by (1) a decrease in oxygen consumption by the tissues secondary to hypothermia, anesthesia, sepsis, or alkalosis or (2) an increase in oxygen delivery secondary to hyperoxia and left-to-right shunting.

PATIENT CARE MANAGEMENT

Preinsertion

See pulmonary artery (PA) pressure monitoring: preinsertion, p. 475.

Postinsertion

See pulmonary artery pressure (PA) monitoring: postinsertion, p. 476.

Obtaining Accurate Measurements

To maintain accuracy of the system, the oximeter should be calibrated daily to an in vivo measurement of mixed-venous blood. The connection between the optical module and the catheter must remain intact; if for any reason the system becomes disconnected, an in vivo calibration should be performed. If fibrin develops on the tip of the catheter, it will interfere with the light intensity and accuracy of the readings; therefore, it is important to maintain patency of the catheter and to flush the line if there is a damped waveform or poor signal from the processor.

Changes of $\geq 10\%$ in the Svo_2 reading or decreases in Svo_2 value to <60% are significant and should be followed by examination of other variables (CO, ABGs, hemoglobin level) to determine the cause of the change.

Critical Observations

There are no complications associated with fiberoptic monitoring of mixed-venous oxygen saturation. However, the same complications that are associated with the PA catheter pertain to the use of the Svo_2 catheter. (See Critical Observations under Pulmonary Artery [PA] Pressure Monitoring, p. 480.)

BIBLIOGRAPHY

Adams AB, Lim S: Monitoring and management of the patient in the intensive care unit. In Wilkins RL, Stoller JK, Scanlan CL, editors: *Egan's fundamentals of respiratory care*, ed 8, St Louis, 2003, Mosby.

Aherns T, Sona C: Capnography and application in acute and critical care, *AACN Clinical Issues* 14:123-132, 2003.

Baird MS: Dysrhythmias and conduction disturbances. In Baird MS, Keen JH, Swearingen PL, editors: *Manual of critical care nursing*, ed 5, St Louis, 2005, Mosby.

Baird MS, Keen JH, Swearingen PL: *Manual of critical care nursing*, ed 5, St Louis, 2005, Mosby.

Conover MB: *Pocket guide to electrocardiography*, ed 5, St Louis, 2004, Mosby.

Czekaj LA: Acid base balance. In Kinney MR et al, editors: *AACN's clinical reference for critical care nursing*, ed 4, St Louis, 1998, Mosby.

Daily EK, Schroeder JS: *Techniques in bedside hemodynamic monitoring*, ed 5, St Louis, 1994, Mosby.

Darovic GO: *Handbook of hemodynamic monitoring*, ed 2, Philadelphia, 2004, WB Saunders.

Dossey BM, Keegan L, Guzzetta CL: *Holistic nursing: a handbook for practice*, ed 3, Gaithersburg, Md, 2000, Aspen.

Fan JY: Effect of backrest position on intracranial pressure and cerebral perfusion pressure in individuals with brain injury: a systematic review, *J Neur Nurs*, 36(5):278-287, 2004.

Grap MJ: Protocols for practice: applying research at the bedside: pulse oximetry, *Crit Care Nurse* 18(1):94-99, 1998.

Hankins J et al: *Infusion therapy in clinical practice*, ed 2, St Louis, 2001, WB Saunders.

Kinney M et al: *AACN's clinical reference for critical-care nursing*, ed 4, New York, 1998, Mosby.

Kruse JA, Fink MP, Carlson RW: *Saunders manual of critical care*, Philadelphia, 2003, Saunders.

Layon AJ, Gabrielli A: Elevated intracranial pressure. In Layon AJ, Gabrielli A, Friedman WA, editors: *Textbook of neurointensive care*, Philadelphia, 2004, WB Saunders.

Lessig ML, Lessig PM: The cardiovascular system. In Alspach JG, editor: *Core curriculum for critical care nursing*, ed 5, Philadelphia, 1998, WB Saunders.

Lynn-McHale DJ, Carlson KK: *AACN procedure manual for critical care*, ed 4, Philadelphia, 2001, WB Saunders.

Mims BC, et al: *Critical care skills: a clinical handbook*, ed 2, St Louis, 2004, Mosby.

Nikas DL: The neurological system. In Alspach JG, editor: *Core curriculum for critical care nursing*, ed 5, Philadelphia, 1998, WB Saunders.

Otto SE: *Mosby's pocket guide to infusion therapy*, ed 5, St Louis, 2005, Mosby.

Smith RN: Concepts of monitoring and surveillance. In Kinney MR et al, editors: *AACN's clinical reference for critical care nursing*, ed 4, St Louis, 1998, Mosby.

Stillwell SB: *Mosby's nursing PDQ for critical care*, St Louis, 2005, Mosby.

Stillwell S, Randall E: *Pocket guide to cardiovascular care,* ed 2, St Louis, 1994, Mosby.

St. John R: The pulmonary system. In Alspach JG, editor: *Core curriculum for critical care nursing,* ed 5, Philadelphia, 1998, WB Saunders.

Urban N: Integrating the hemodynamic profile with clinical assessment, *AACN Clin Issues Crit Care Nurs* 4(1):161-179, 1993.

Urden LD et al: *Thelan's critical care nursing,* ed 4, St Louis, 2002, Mosby.

Urden LD, Stacy KM, Lough ME: *Priorities in critical care nursing,* ed 4, St Louis, 2004, Mosby.

US Department of Health and Human Services, Public Health Service, Centers for Disease Control and Prevention: Guideline for prevention of intravascular device-related infections, *Am J Infect Control* 24:262, 1996.

Williams LD: Hemodynamic monitoring. In Baird MS, Keen JH, Swearingen PL, editors: *Manual of critical care nursing,* ed 5, St Louis, 2005, Mosby.

7

Therapeutic Modalities

NEUROLOGIC MODALITIES

BARBITURATE COMA

Clinical Brief

Refractory increased intracranial pressure (ICP) is defined as ICP >25 mm Hg for 30 minutes, 30 mm Hg for 15 minutes or 40 mm Hg for 1 minute.[1] Sustained intracranial hypertension (ICH) can cause brain injury and patient death. Most commonly associated with severe traumatic brain injury, it also can occur in patients with intractable seizures; sagittal sinus thrombosis; Reye's syndrome; severe, refractory vasospasm; and ischemic stroke. Barbiturate coma is a second-tier treatment for refractory ICH. In patients whose ICP has not responded well to cerebrospinal fluid (CSF) drainage, hyperventilation, or osmotic therapy and in whom there is no surgical lesion, barbiturate coma may be instituted. Because the clinical examination is not reliable during the drug-induced coma, a surgical lesion must be removed before barbiturate coma is instituted.

The mechanism of barbiturate action is not fully understood, but it is believed to play a role in the reduction of cerebral blood flow, oxygen demand, and cerebral metabolism, thereby reducing ICP. The use of barbiturates also may reduce swelling and promote resolution of cerebral edema. Serial electroencephalogram (EEG) recordings guide induction of the coma and adjustments in dose maintenance of barbiturate infusion.[2]

Contraindications to barbiturate therapy include those patients whose ICP is normal or those patients who respond promptly to CSF drainage, hyperventilation, and/or osmotic therapy. Patients who suffer from cardiac disease, especially heart failure, are not candidates

NEURO

for barbiturate coma because of the myocardial depressive effects of barbiturates.

Complications

- Hypotension due to vasodilation from barbiturate
- Dysrhythmias, especially bradycardia, from barbiturate myocardial depressive effects
- Hypoxemia due to impaired gas exchange and risk for aspiration related to immobility and decreased consciousness
- Deep vein thrombosis and pulmonary emboli related to limited mobility
- Ileus and constipation from the parasympathetic effects of barbiturate administration

PATIENT CARE MANAGEMENT GUIDELINES

Patient Assessment

1. Continuously monitor arterial blood pressure (BP) and mean arterial pressure (MAP); assess the patient for hypotension and dysrhythmias.
2. Obtain ICP readings and calculate cerebral perfusion pressure (CPP).
3. Continuously monitor arterial and, if available, jugular or mixed-venous oxygen saturation as well as end-tidal CO_2 with capnometry. Review arterial and venous blood gases (ABGs) to evaluate oxygenation and acid-base status.
4. Obtain pulmonary artery (PA) and wedge pressures, as well as cardiac output/cardiac index (CO/CI), to evaluate the hemodynamic response to barbiturate coma.
5. Assess neurologic status to evaluate degree of coma.

Patient Management

1. Intubation and mechanical ventilation are required. Anticipate nasogastric (NG) tube placement to maintain gastric decompression and prevent the risk of aspiration.
2. Portable EEG monitoring or compressed spectral analysis (CSA) will be necessary to monitor the patient's response to the loading dose and to adjust maintenance dosing. Obtaining hourly EEG printouts is recommended.[3]
3. A loading dose of pentobarbital is 5 to 10 mg/kg intravenously (IV) at a rate no faster than 50 mg/min. Designate one intravenous line for pentobarbital infusion only. Have

phenylephrine 50 mg in 250 mL 5% dextrose in water (D_5W) available in case the patient becomes hypotensive; dopamine may also be prepared and ready to infuse during the loading dose of pentobarbital. Maintain systolic blood pressure (SBP) >90 mm Hg and cerebral perfusion pressure >70 mm Hg.

4. The maintenance dosage is usually 1 to 3 mg/kg/hr and may be given hourly as a bolus or as a constant infusion. Titrate to achieve either a 3-second burst suppression of EEG electrical activity or serum levels of 3 to 4 mg/mL. Check serum levels within 4 to 6 hours of initiating therapy, again at 12 hours and 24 hours, then daily. Correlate drug levels with EEG burst suppression.

5. During the first several hours of pentobarbital infusion, assess neurologic function. The patient will become unresponsive and flaccid; corneal, cough, gag, swallow, and/or pupillary reflexes will decrease or become absent; and spontaneous respirations will cease.

6. Osmotic therapy and CSF drainage may continue as needed (PRN) for intermittent ICP control during barbiturate coma.

7. Once the ICP has been lowered and remains stable for more than 48 hours, a slow taper (i.e., over 3-4 days) of barbiturates may begin. Osmotic diuretics and CSF drainage may continue PRN. If refractory ICH recurs, barbiturate therapy may be resumed.

Critical Observations

Consult physician for the following:

1. ICP unresponsive to barbiturate administration
2. CPP <70 mm Hg
3. Hypotension, especially SBP <70 mm Hg
4. O_2 saturation <95%
5. Suspected aspiration
6. Unilateral change in pupil size
7. Inadequate burst suppression or undesirable serum levels of pentobarbital

CAROTID ENDARTERECTOMY

Clinical Brief

Carotid surgery can be performed to repair traumatic injuries to the artery or to improve cerebral circulation in patients with occlusive vascular disease, reducing the risk of stroke.

Carotid endarterectomies are usually performed to remove atherosclerotic plaques that have significantly reduced the lumen of the artery or have become ulcerative and are the source of emboli. The symptoms in carotid disease are caused by a significant reduction in cerebral blood flow resulting from an area of tight stenosis or by transient ischemic attacks (TIAs) resulting from embolization of plaque fragments, platelet clumps, or small blood clots from the ulcer in the atheroma. The objective of endarterectomy is to remove the embolism source and to improve cerebral circulation.

Complications

- Stroke—due to embolization of plaque or thrombotic material
- Intracerebral hemorrhage—occurs within a few days of surgery, is usually associated with systemic hypertension, and is possibly due to altered cerebral blood flow autoregulation resulting in cerebral hyperperfusion
- Myocardial infarction—increased risk with hypertension, hypervolemia, and tachycardia
- Congestive heart failure—increased risk with valve insufficiency
- Airway obstruction—if hematoma forms at surgical site
- Cranial nerve injuries—common but usually transient

PATIENT CARE MANAGEMENT GUIDELINES

Patient Assessment

1. Assess the patient's pain using a self-report rating scale, such as the 0-to-10 numerical pain rating scale, to assess pain intensity.
2. Assess neurologic status hourly and compare findings with baseline assessment. Note the integrity of the cough and gag reflexes, visual fields, and motor and sensory integrity. Monitor speech for comprehension, hoarseness, and quality. Ask the patient to report signs and symptoms of TIAs.
3. Assess the patency of the carotid artery by palpating the superficial temporal artery and note the presence, quality, strength, and symmetry of pulses.
4. Assess vital signs (VS) hourly and carefully note BP: hypotension can occur secondary to carotid sinus manipulation during surgery; hypertension can occur secondary to surgical denervation of the carotid sinus.
5. Assess respiratory status: note rate and depth of respirations; observe respiratory pattern and note presence of stridor. Assess the patient's ability to handle secretions (gag, cough,

swallowing reflexes). Continuously monitor oxygen saturation via pulse oximetry (SpO_2).

6. Continuously monitor electrocardiogram (ECG) for dysrhythmias secondary to intraoperative manipulation of carotid sinus. Monitor closely for signs and symptoms of myocardial ischemia.

7. Examine the surgical dressing for bloody drainage. Assess for hematoma or swelling at the operative site, which may adversely affect airway patency; note the presence of any tracheal deviation.

Patient Management

1. Keep head of bed (HOB) at 30 degrees unless hypotensive events occur, then lower HOB to enhance cerebral blood flow.

2. Maintain a dry, occlusive dressing at the incision site for 48 hours. Keep firm pressure over the dressing if bleeding occurs.

3. Administer analgesics as ordered and evaluate the effectiveness of medication.

4. Administer vasopressors and/or antihypertensive agents as necessary to maintain BP within set parameters.

5. Turn and position the patient to prevent airway obstruction and aspiration. Provide incentive spirometry and assist the patient with cough and deep breathing (C&DB). Patient should have nothing by mouth (NPO) until the gag and swallow reflexes return to normal.

6. Resume antiplatelet agent such as aspirin 2 to 72 hours postoperatively as ordered.

Critical Observations

Consult physician for the following:

1. Symptoms reported by the patient that suggest TIAs
2. Hemiparesis/hemiplegia, pupillary irregularity, aphasia
3. Difficulty breathing, stridor, tracheal deviation
4. Excessive bleeding at incision site
5. Dysrhythmias, hypotension, or hypertension

CRANIOTOMY

Clinical Brief

A craniotomy provides a "bone window" through which to evacuate hematomas, clip or ligate aneurysms or feeding vessels of an arteriovenous malformation (AVM), resect tumors, or perform a biopsy of the brain. Craniotomies are also used in the surgical

NEURO

treatment of epilepsy (i.e., intraoperative EEG and resection of the cortex areas responsible for seizure activity). Pituitary tumors may be approached either transcranially through a craniotomy (especially when the tumor has a large suprasellar component) or by the transnasal transsphenoidal route.

Complications

Complications depend on the reason the surgery was performed, the location of the pathologic condition, and underlying medical conditions.

- Intracranial hemorrhage—can occur in subdural, epidural, intracerebral, or intraventricular space, resulting in a variety of signs and symptoms. Can be life threatening.
- Cerebral edema—can occur or if already present, increases due to surgical trauma
- Increased ICP—can occur due to other complications such as cerebral edema (most common), hemorrhage, meningitis, and surgery-related trauma
- Pneumocephalus—trapped air that is usually reabsorbed, but may require evacuation if of large volume and acts as a space-occupying lesion
- Hydrocephalus—occurs with edema or when there is bleeding into subarachnoid space
- Seizure—may occur as a result of surgical manipulation of brain or edema
- CSF leak—generally occurs at operative site and is spontaneously healed or occasionally requires surgical repair
- Infection—meningitis or infection of surgical wound may occur
- Fluid imbalance—diabetes insipidus (DI) or syndrome of inappropriate antidiuretic hormone (SIADH) may occur

---

PATIENT CARE MANAGEMENT GUIDELINES

Patient Assessment

1. Assess pupil size, reactivity, and visual fields; level of consciousness (LOC); quality and comprehension of speech; and sensorimotor function. Test gag, swallow, and corneal reflexes.
2. Observe for signs and symptoms of meningitis: lethargy, severe headache, photophobia, nuchal rigidity, positive Kernig sign.
3. Assess trends in ICP; initial readings may be required every 15 to 30 minutes. Calculate and record CPP readings (normal is 60-100 mm Hg) every hour. Note effects of patient and nursing activities on CPP, and plan care accordingly.

4. Obtain BP and MAP; CPP depends on adequate BP. Obtain central venous pressure (CVP) and PA pressures (if available) to determine imbalances in volume status that can adversely affect CPP.

5. Measure intake and output (I&O) hourly and determine fluid balance every 8 hours. Measure specific gravity at least every 8 hours and review serum electrolyte and osmolality levels. If urine output is <30 mL/hr or >200 mL/hr for 2 consecutive hours, suspect SIADH or DI.

6. Assess for CSF leaks. For transsphenoidal surgical approaches, question the patient about a feeling of a postnasal drip down the back of the throat. Note excess swallowing. Apply mustache dressing to check for CSF leaks from either nostril (transsphenoidal approach). Note amount and color of drainage and number of times dressing is changed.

7. Assess respiratory function. Monitor airway patency, oxygen saturation via pulse oximeter, and the patient's ability to handle secretions (i.e., gag and swallow reflexes). Note rate, depth, and pattern of respirations, and assess the lungs for adventitious sounds.

8. Examine the surgical dressing for bloody drainage or possible CSF drainage (CSF drainage will test positive for glucose).

Patient Management

1. Administer analgesics as ordered and evaluate the effectiveness of medication. Maintain a quiet environment and provide uninterrupted rest periods.

2. Administer oxygen as ordered and monitor ABGs; hypoxia and hypercarbia are disturbances that can cause an increase in ICP. Promote pulmonary hygiene to prevent atelectasis and pneumonia.

3. Fluid management depends on the type of surgery and potential complications. Generally hypotonic solutions are avoided because they may cause an increase in ICP.

4. Keep HOB at 30 to 45 degrees or as ordered to promote cerebral venous drainage. Maintain the patient's head and neck in proper alignment; teach the patient to avoid the Valsalva maneuver; hyperoxygenate the patient's lungs before and after suctioning secretions; and limit suctioning to 15 seconds.

5. Pharmacologic agents such as chlorpromazine may be needed to reduce shivering, and anticonvulsants may be needed to control seizures.

6. Vasoactive agents may be required to control BP because CPP depends on an adequate BP. For hypotension, a dopamine or phenylephrine infusion may be titrated to the desired BP. For hypertension, labetalol or hydralazine HCl may be ordered.

7. If a ventriculostomy is being used, drain CSF according to established parameters (generally to maintain ICP <20 mm Hg). Keep the CSF drainage system at the level ordered to prevent inadvertent collapse of the ventricles.

8. If a shunt was placed, avoid pressure on the shunt mechanism; keep head in neutral alignment to prevent kinking or twisting of shunt catheter.

9. Histamine-2 (H_2) blocking agents may be ordered to decrease gastric acid secretion. If an NG tube is in place, sucralfate may be ordered to reduce the risk of ulcer formation.

10. Nutritional needs may be met when the patient is alert and awake. If the patient is comatose or unable to take food or fluids orally, a feeding tube may be required or parenteral nutrition (PN) may be indicated.

11. Patients who have undergone transsphenoidal surgery may develop episodes of DI in the first 72 hours. Maintenance intravenous fluids plus replacement fluid and/or administration of aqueous vasopressin may be ordered. Carefully measure urine output hourly; specific gravity measurements may be required every 2 hours.

12. Patients who have developed subarachnoid hemorrhage from a ruptured aneurysm preoperatively are continued on calcium channel blocking agents postoperatively. If the patient develops neurologic deficits secondary to vasospasm, hypervolemic hemodilution therapy may be initiated. To increase intravascular volume and decrease hematocrit (Hct) levels, crystalloid infusions may be used to maintain a PA diastolic pressure at 14 to 16 mm Hg or CVP at 10 to 12 mm Hg. Hypertensive therapy (e.g., dopamine, phenylephrine) may be employed to raise SBP 25% to 40% in an effort to enhance cerebral blood flow during vasospasm.

13. See pp. 328 and 302 for information on SIADH and DI.

Critical Observations

Consult physician for the following:

1. Change in LOC, pupillary inequality, hemiparesis or hemiplegia, visual changes, onset or worsening of aphasia, or any deterioration in neurologic functioning

2. A loss of gag or swallow reflex
3. ICP >20 mm Hg and unresponsive to ordered therapy
4. Suspected CSF leak
5. Urine output >200 mL/hr for 2 hours (without diuretic) or urine output <30 mL/hr
6. Hypernatremia or hyponatremia
7. Sudden bloody drainage from ventriculostomy
8. Signs of meningitis: altered mental status, nuchal rigidity, Brudzinski sign, Kernig sign

HYPERVENTILATION THERAPY

Clinical Brief

Cerebral edema resulting from head injury, brain tumors, or cerebrovascular accidents raises ICP. The use of mild, chronic hyperventilation therapy to lower $Paco_2$ can be a useful adjunct in the treatment of increased ICP. The patient may be chemically sedated, paralyzed, and placed on a mechanical ventilator to maintain a $Paco_2$ of 30 to 35 mm Hg by controlling the rate of respirations. If unsuccessful in reducing ICP, $Paco_2$ levels of 27 to 30 mm Hg are sometimes used with extreme caution and very close monitoring for signs of cerebral ischemia. Effects on ICP, CPP, and ABG readings and side effects of therapy will determine the need for adjustment.

Hypercarbia produces cerebral vasodilation and consequently increases ICP. Hypocarbia, induced by hyperventilation, produces vasoconstriction of the cerebral arterioles, reducing ICP. If $Paco_2$ falls to <28 mm Hg, there may be compromised cerebral blood flow, contributing to secondary brain injury. Because of this and other potential adverse outcomes, hyperventilation therapy remains controversial, and prophylactic use is not recommended. It is also not recommended for use in the first 24 hours, and if possible the first 5 days, after head injury. Instead, mild hypocarbia is prescribed in the presence of increased ICP that does not respond to other interventions and is without contraindication.

Complications

- Cerebral ischemia—result of severe vasoconstriction, hypotension, and/or decreased cerebral perfusion
- Barotrauma—occurs with high-pressure ventilation
- Increased mean airway pressure—may ultimately lead to further increase in ICP
- Decreased cardiac filling pressures—may result from positive end-expiratory pressure (PEEP)

NEURO

- Acid-base imbalance—respiratory alkalosis can occur as a result of hyperventilation therapy. Hypoxemia (Pao_2 <50 mm Hg) can lead to cerebral vasodilation.

PATIENT CARE MANAGEMENT GUIDELINES

Patient Assessment

1. Obtain ICP readings to assess the patient's response to hyperventilation therapy. Calculate CPP (normal is 60-100 mm Hg). The inability to reduce ICP with hyperventilation is a poor prognostic indicator. See p. 462 for information on ICP monitoring.
2. Monitor $Petco_2$ with capnometry to evaluate the patient's response to hyperventilation therapy. Generally $Paco_2$ levels are maintained at 30 to 35 mm Hg. If $Paco_2$ drops to <25 mm Hg, there is significant risk for cerebral hypoxia due to severe vasoconstriction.
3. Review ABGs to assess oxygenation and acid-base balance.
4. Monitor body temperature. Hypothermia can shift the oxyhemoglobin dissociation curve to the left. This causes hemoglobin (Hgb) and oxygen to be more tightly bound and reduces oxygen availability to the tissues.
5. Continuously monitor BP and MAP; monitor CVP and PA pressures (if available).
6. Monitor fluid volume status: measure I&O hourly; determine fluid balance every 8 hours.

Patient Management

1. Sedatives and paralytics may be used to reduce ICP caused by agitation. Monitor LOC carefully.
2. Ensure airway patency; suction secretions only when necessary.
3. Inotropic or vasoactive agents may be ordered to maintain a MAP that results in a CPP of at least 60 mm Hg.
4. When ICP is stable, wean hyperventilation therapy slowly as ordered by physician.

Critical Observations

Consult physician for the following:
1. ICP unresponsive to maximum hyperventilation
2. CPP <60 mm Hg
3. O_2 sat <95%
4. SBP <90 mm Hg
5. pH consistently >7.45

PULMONARY MODALITIES

CHEST DRAINAGE

Clinical Brief

Chest tubes (CTs) drain blood, fluid, or air that has accumulated in the thorax to restore negative intrapleural pressure and allow reexpansion of a compressed lung. A pleural CT is inserted for a pneumothorax, hemothorax, hemopneumothorax, empyema, or pleural effusion. After cardiothoracic surgery, mediastinal tubes may be placed to prevent the accumulation of fluid around the heart, which could lead to cardiac tamponade.

A CT drainage system must have two components—a collection container and a seal to prevent air from entering the chest on inspiration. A three-bottle system contains a drainage bottle, a water seal bottle, and a third bottle that is attached to suction and serves as a pressure regulator. Suction is used to increase airflow from the pleural space. Disposable systems are available in either the one-bottle or three-bottle systems and as fluid-filled or waterless systems.

A flutter (Heimlich) valve may be used in place of a drainage system to prevent air from entering the chest on inspiration. This valve opens on expiration, allowing air to escape from the chest, and collapses on inspiration to prevent air from entering the thorax (Figure 7-1). The Heimlich valve is useful during patient transport and for increasing patient mobility. However, inadvertent closure of the valve can result in pneumothorax. The Heimlich valve is not recommended for patients with excessive pleural fluid or secretions and for patients who are confused or disoriented.

Complications

- Pain at the chest tube site
- Tube occlusion
- Infection

PATIENT CARE MANAGEMENT GUIDELINES

Patient Assessment

1. Obtain VS and assess oxygen saturation. Assess respiratory status: note rate, rhythm, and ease of respiration and palpate for subcutaneous emphysema around the area of the tube; conduct ongoing auscultation of breath sounds. An obstruction or kinked tube can cause a tension pneumothorax; a

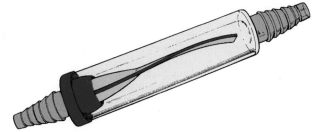

Figure 7-1 Heimlich valve.

defect in the system can cause recurrence of hemothorax or pneumothorax.

2. Assess CT drainage (pleural and mediastinal) after insertion of the CT and document the type, color, and amount of drainage. A sudden change in the amount of drainage or a CT output of 200 mL/hr may indicate the need for surgical intervention. Sudden drainage cessation may indicate tube obstruction. Check with a physician regarding the expected drainage for the condition or procedure.

3. Assess the dressing and note any drainage or odor.

Patient Management

1. The nurse should read the chest drainage system manufacturer's instructions carefully. Determine whether the system requires water to maintain a water seal, or if the device has a dry seal system.

2. If suction is being used, verify that suction is at the prescribed amount. If a wet system, refill the suction control chamber with sterile water as needed. The water level determines the level of suction. Gentle bubbling in the pressure-regulating chamber is normal; turbulent bubbling may indicate that the negative pressure in the chest drain may be too high. If a dry system, watch for changes in the negative pressure and suction indicators.

3. Ensure the patency of the drainage system. Keep tubing free of drainage, kinks, and dependent loops. Check that all connections are taped securely. Keep the drainage device below the level of the patient's chest. For wet systems, the water level should rise on inspiration and fall during spontaneous exhalation

(tidaling). The opposite water level movement occurs with mechanical ventilation. If tidaling stops, the lung may have fully expanded or there is an obstruction in the system. If an obstruction is suspected, check the tubing and have the patient deep breathe and cough or change positions; reassess tidaling.

4. Monitor for air leaks by observing for bubbling in the water seal chamber. If there is air in the pleural cavity, intermittent bubbling during expiration is normal. Prolonged air leaks are common after lung resection procedures. No bubbling should be observed in the water seal chamber when mediastinal CTs are used.

5. If an air leak is suspected, check for any loose connections or cracks in the chest drainage system that could be the cause of an external air leak. Leaks can be located by clamping the tube at different intervals along the tubing. If the bubbling continues when the CT is clamped close to the patient's chest, the source is external. Caution must be taken because a tension pneumothorax can quickly develop when bubbling CTs are clamped. CTs should be unclamped as soon as possible. Postthoracotomy CTs should not be clamped because of the potential for the development of pneumothorax and hemodynamic compromise. Do not clamp CTs for patients with known tracheobronchial leaks.

6. Milking or stripping CTs is not recommended as a routine practice because it creates excessively negative pressures in the thorax. Milking a CT should include only an area of visible clot in the tubing. If large amounts of drainage or clots continue, the physician may prescribe periodic stripping or milking to prevent an obstruction.

7. Should the CT accidentally be pulled out, apply a petrolatum gauze dressing to the site to prevent air from entering the chest. Monitor the patient for the development of a tension pneumothorax. Use a three-sided taping technique for the dressing so that air under pressure can escape on exhalation.

8. If the patient is transported away from the suction device, do not clamp the tubing. The drainage system continues to collect air or chest drainage even when the suction is not connected.

Chest Tube (CT) Removal

CTs can be removed when drainage and air leaks have ceased. Trial clamping of the CT may be done before CT removal; closely monitor the patient for respiratory distress. Chest radiographs are reviewed to ensure that the lung is reexpanded. Necessary equipment includes a suture set, plain or petrolatum gauze, sterile 4×4 gauze dressings, and adhesive tape. Premedicate the patient before removing the CT. The tube is removed quickly, in a continuous motion, while the patient is performing the Valsalva maneuver. After CT removal, monitor the patient's respiratory status closely and encourage the patient to take a few deep breaths.

Critical Observations

Consult physician for the following:
1. Respiratory rate (RR) >28 breaths/min
2. Absent or unequal breath sounds
3. Hypotension, shock
4. PaO_2 <60 mm Hg
5. Signs of hypoxia: restlessness, ↑ heart rate (HR), dyspnea
6. Bleeding or large amount of drainage on dressing
7. Subcutaneous emphysema that is increasing or travels to the neck and face
8. CT drainage ≥200 mL/hr
9. New bubbling in underwater seal chamber not related to loose connections
10. Dislodged or obstructed CT
11. Deviated trachea

LUNG TRANSPLANT

Clinical Brief

Lung transplantation is performed for patients with end-stage restrictive (e.g., idiopathic pulmonary fibrosis, sarcoidosis) or obstructive (e.g., chronic obstructive pulmonary disease [COPD], cystic fibrosis) lung disease and vascular disease (e.g., primary pulmonary hypertension). Evaluation and criteria for lung transplantation differ among centers. Double lung transplants are recommended for patients with cystic fibrosis or septic pulmonary diseases because the native, diseased lung would contaminate a single transplanted lung. Heart-lung transplantation is reserved for irreversible pulmonary or cardiac diseases associated with pulmonary hypertension. Single-lung transplantation is performed through a lateral thoracotomy incision and uses single-lung ventilation. Double-lung transplantation technique incorporates bilateral thoracotomy incisions with a transverse sternotomy. In the heart-lung transplant, the donor heart and lungs are implanted together en bloc through a median sternotomy incision using cardiopulmonary bypass (CPB).

PULM

Complications

- Pulmonary reimplantation response—characterized by alveolar and interstitial infiltrates, a decrease in compliance, and abnormal gas exchange
- Hemorrhage
- Organ rejection
- Infection
- Adverse effects of immunosuppressant medications
- General risks of thoracic surgery (see p. 510)

PATIENT CARE MANAGEMENT GUIDELINES

See thoracic surgery, p. 510, for guidelines for the general thoracic surgery patient.

Patient Assessment

1. Continuously monitor SpO_2 and SvO_2 (if available) and review serial ABGs. Single-lung transplant recipients may have different compliance and vascular resistance in each lung and experience altered ventilation-perfusion.
2. Conduct ongoing auscultation of lungs for presence of secretions. Be aware of the potential for pulmonary edema development. Monitor airway pressures and tidal volumes when mechanically ventilated.
3. Assess tissue perfusion; note level of mentation, skin color and temperature, peripheral pulses, and capillary refill.
4. Assess for dysrhythmia development that may result from electrolyte imbalance, hypoxemia, and/or hemorrhage. Atrial dysrhythmias are more common postoperatively.
5. Assess hemodynamic and fluid status: monitor CVP, PA pressures, CO/CI, HR, BP, and MAP. Note trends and patient response to therapy. Monitor pulmonary vascular resistance index (PVRI) and systemic vascular resistance index (SVRI) and note trends and patient response to therapy. Calculate left ventricular stroke work index (LVSWI) and right ventricular stroke work index (RVSWI) to evaluate contractility in the heart-lung transplant. Monitor I&O and daily weights.
6. Assess for bleeding: CT drainage >200 mL/hr; decrease in Hgb and Hct levels; abnormal coagulation studies.
7. Assess temperature. Patients may be hypothermic on returning from surgery. Monitor for signs of infection; consider intravenous sites, wound sites, the urinary tract, lungs, and

mucous membranes as potential sites of infection. Monitor sputum cultures, white blood cell (WBC) count, and titers for presence of infection.

8. Monitor pulmonary function tests to evaluate lung function.

9. Assess gastrointestinal (GI) status for paralytic ileus or diaphragmatic hernia (after omental wrap).

10. Assess for dehiscence of the airway anastomosis (e.g., hemoptysis, fever, secretion retention, pneumothorax, mediastinitis, pneumomediastinum, signs of lung collapse).

11. Assess the patient for side effects of immunosuppression therapy: nephrotoxicity, GI toxicity, musculoskeletal toxicity, central nervous system (CNS) toxicity, hematologic toxicity, endocrine toxicity, dermal toxicity, and psychiatric toxicity.

12. Use a self-report pain rating scale, such as a 0-to-10 scale, to assess pain intensity in patients who are awake and oriented. See Acute Pain in Chapter 2.

Patient Management

1. Patient may be sedated and pharmacologically paralyzed. See Neuromuscular Blockade in the Critically Ill, p. 595.

2. Monitor ventilatory modes and parameters as ordered. See Ventilation Therapies, p. 503.

3. Manage pain. See Chapter 2.

4. Anticipate diuretics, and albumin administration during reimplantation response. Low-dose pressor support and concentrating intravenous infusions may be required to maintain circulatory volume and reduce fluid overload.

5. High pulmonary systolic pressures may be seen in patients who are transplanted for pulmonary hypertension. Prostaglandin E_1 infusion or nitric oxide inhalation may be ordered.

6. Because the patient is immunosuppressed with medications to prevent organ rejection, reverse isolation protocol may be instituted. All dressing changes should be completed with strict aseptic technique. Intravenous access sites and dressings should be changed according to institutional protocol. Anticipate removal of invasive lines and devices as soon as the patient is stable.

7. To promote optimal inflation and reduce edema in the new lung, patients with single-lung transplant should be positioned in the lateral decubitus position with the transplanted lung up and the native lung down. If acute rejection is suspected (perfusion to transplanted lung is diminished) the native lung should be positioned up. Double-lung transplant

patients are generally maintained in a supine position for 6 to 8 hours or until hemodynamically stable before position changes are instituted. Patients can be positioned on a continuous lateral rotation bed to promote drainage of pulmonary secretions and gas exchange. Monitor hemodynamics and oxygen saturation closely during position changes.

8. Suction patients with a premeasured suction catheter according to measurement from operating room to avoid penetrating suture lines. Use an Ambu bag with airway pressure manometer attached to regulate airway pressures during preoxygenation and postoxygenation. Bronchoscopy may be needed to assess and remove pulmonary secretions.

9. Defer vigorous aggressive chest physiotherapy (CPT) during the intubated and unstable course of recovery. CPT, incentive spirometry, and postural drainage are critical after extubation. Patients need to be coached to cough because the cough reflex in the denervated lung is absent.

10. Passive range-of-motion exercises should be initiated postoperatively and an individualized plan for activity followed.

11. Medicate the patient for pain before physiotherapy and other activities and procedures (e.g., CT removal).

12. Cardiac function may be decreased postoperatively. Hemodynamic instability may be treated with vasoactive and inotropic agents. Titrate the infusion to achieve the desired hemodynamic response.

13. Anticipate enteral feeding when bowel sounds are auscultated. See nutrition, p. 561.

Critical Observations

Consult physician for the following:

1. Signs and symptoms of impaired oxygenation
2. Signs and symptoms of organ rejection
3. Signs and symptoms of hemodynamic instability
4. Signs and symptoms of infection
5. Signs and symptoms of adverse effects of immunosuppression
6. Signs of acute renal failure

VENTILATION THERAPIES

Clinical Brief

Invasive and noninvasive ventilation can improve alveolar ventilation and arterial oxygenation while reducing the work of breathing for the critically ill patient with overwhelming metabolic needs.

PULM

Noninvasive ventilation does not require an endotracheal airway. Noninvasive positive pressure ventilation (NPPV) is provided via a full oral/nasal mask, a nasal-only mask, or nasal "pillow" inserts. NPPV may take the place of short-term intubation in acute respiratory failure for patients able to protect their own airways. Noninvasive negative pressure ventilation equipment such as the chest cuirass, iron lung, or poncho wrap is rarely used.

Invasive positive-pressure ventilation requires endotracheal intubation or tracheostomy, and carries additional risks related to the tube placement and maintenance. Indications for intubation with positive pressure ventilation include general anesthesia, apnea, respiratory failure, hypoxemia, and respiratory muscle fatigue. Positive pressure ventilators, that is, volume-controlled or pressure-controlled ventilators, are most commonly used in critical care and operating room settings.

Complications

- Ventilator-associated pneumonia (VAP)
- Decreased cardiac output
- Fluid volume overload
- Gastrointestinal bleeding
- Increased ICP
- Oxygen toxicity
- Volutrauma and barotrauma

Lung-Protective Ventilation Strategies

The following lung-protective ventilation strategies minimize the oxygen and gas pressure–related complications of mechanical ventilation.

Fio_2: the concentration of oxygen delivered to the patient. The Fio_2 is adjusted to maintain a Pao_2 of at least 60 mm Hg and an Sao_2 ≥90% with an upper level limited to Fio_2 of 0.5 to 0.65. Initial setting may be set >0.6 until results of ABG are obtained.

PEEP: the pressure maintained by a mechanical ventilator at end of expiration. PEEP restores functional residual capacity (FRC), improves compliance, and decreases shunt in patients with restrictive disease. Addition of PEEP may promote adequate oxygenation at a lower Fio_2 than would be required without PEEP. PEEP levels are generally set at 5 to 20 cm of water.

Plateau pressure: the estimate of alveolar pressure at end inspiration. The target plateau pressure is 30 to 35 cm of water.

Limiting tidal volume is usually required to attain this plateau pressure, which is the pressure required to inflate the lungs to total lung capacity.

Tidal volume: the amount of gas delivered with each breath. Tidal volumes as small as 5 mL/kg are used in permissive hypercapnia therapy. Permissive hypercapnia is contraindicated in increased ICP.

High-frequency ventilation: an investigational ventilation mode that uses small tidal volumes at rates between 60 and 3600 cycles/min

Extracorporeal carbon dioxide removal: blood is diverted from the body to an extracorporeal filter, where carbon dioxide is removed and oxygen is infused in the blood and returned to the body.

Other lung-protective ventilation strategies include interventions that decrease the oxygen/ventilation demand and promote oxygen supply (e.g., control pain, reduce fever, relieve anxiety and agitation, administer blood transfusions, increase CO, and position patient).

Modes of mechanical ventilation are described in Table 7-1.

PULM

Table 7-1 MODES OF VENTILATORY SUPPORT

Type	Description
Assist-control (A/C)	Full assisted tidal volume delivered when triggered by patient or preset rate.
Continuous positive airway pressure (CPAP)	Positive pressure applied during spontaneous breathing and maintained throughout the entire respiratory cycle
Continuous mandatory ventilation (CMV)	Ventilator delivers the breaths at a preset rate and volume or pressure
Intermittent mandatory ventilation (IMV)	Ventilator delivers breaths at a set rate and volume or pressure. Patient is able to breathe spontaneously between machine breaths.
Mandatory minute ventilation (MMV)	Patient breathes spontaneously; ventilator adds breaths to ensure a preset minimum level of minute ventilation

Continued

Table 7-1 MODES OF VENTILATORY SUPPORT—**cont'd**

Type	Description
Pressure-controlled/ inverse-ratio ventilation (PC/IRV)	Provides inspiratory time greater than expiratory time, improves distribution of ventilation and prevents collapse of stiffer alveolar units (auto-PEEP). Patient is unable to initiate an inspiration.
Positive end-expiratory pressure (PEEP)	Positive pressure applied during machine breathing and maintained at end-expiration
Pressure support ventilation (PSV)	Patient's inspiratory effort triggers a preset amount of positive pressure assistance. PSV decreases work of breathing. PSV is often combined with SIMV to support patient's spontaneous breaths between machine breaths.
Synchronized IMV (SIMV)	Intermittent ventilator breaths synchronized with spontaneous breaths to reduce competition between ventilator and patient. If no inspiratory effort is sensed, the ventilator delivers the breath at a preset rate and volume.

PATIENT CARE MANAGEMENT GUIDELINES

Patient Assessment

1. Assess placement of the endotracheal tube (ETT): auscultate breath sounds immediately after intubation, then reassess every few hours for type and equality. Unilateral breath sounds may indicate that the ETT is too far into a mainstem bronchus, most often on the right side. Gurgling auscultated over the epigastric region may indicate esophageal intubation. Gurgling auscultated over the neck or the patient's ability to speak aloud may indicate a cuff leak or esophageal intubation. If the patient coughs repeatedly, the ETT might be resting near the carina. A chest radiograph should be obtained and reviewed to confirm proper placement of the ETT (see Figure 1-12). Once placement is confirmed, document tube placement each shift by using the ETT markings.

The placement depth varies with body size and structure. Examples: 25 cm at the teeth or 23 cm at the nares.

2. Assess oxygenation status: auscultate breath sounds and note the rate and depth of respirations. Monitor for signs that may indicate hypoxemia: a change in LOC, tachypnea, tachycardia, or dysrhythmias. Cyanosis is a late sign. Observe for patient-ventilator asynchrony: dyspnea, diaphoresis, hypertension, tachycardia, tachypnea.

3. Assess CO: HR, BP, skin temperature, urine output, and LOC.

PULM

Patient Management

1. Check ventilator settings (e.g., mode, FIO_2, tidal volume, respiratory rate (RR), PEEP, and plateau pressure). Verify the inspiratory/expiratory (I:E) ratio. An increase in peak inspiratory pressure and increased plateau pressure suggests a change in lung compliance. An increase in peak pressure without a change in plateau pressure suggests an increase in airway resistance (e.g., bronchospasm, secretion, kinking of ETT). Monitor static compliance in patients with acute respiratory distress syndrome (ARDS) daily to assess improvement in lung status.

2. Continuously monitor oxygen saturation with pulse oximetry (SpO_2). Measure PaO_2/FIO_2 ratio daily to assess improvement in patient's lung status.

3. Monitor ventilation with capnography (if available). The $PETCO_2$ is 1 to 4 mm Hg lower than $PaCO_2$.

4. Monitor airway cuff pressure to prevent tracheal pressure injury. ETTs have a pilot balloon and port to measure the pressure. A cuff manometer is used to determine that the pressure of the cuff is less than the tracheal capillary pressure; cuff pressure should not exceed 20 mm Hg. A cuff pressure <15 mm Hg increases the risk of aspiration, although a properly inflated cuff does not prevent aspiration.

5. Maintain secure placement of tube with tape or commercial tube device. Prevent pressure ulcers to the lip, tongue, or naris by alternating tube taping area daily. Avoid displacing the tube by having a second person hold the tube during retaping. Provide oral care and lip care to reduce risk of ulceration.

6. Talk with and reassure the patient. If necessary, sedate the patient when anxious and fighting the ventilator. Provide the patient with a communication board to make needs known or establish a communication system with the patient.

7. Ensure that the ventilator alarms are on and functional. Table 7-2 lists possible causes for ventilator alarming. Manually ventilate the patient's lungs with 100% oxygen if the cause of ventilator malfunction cannot be identified or be corrected quickly.

8. Review ABGs to ensure that the ventilator settings are supporting oxygenation and ventilation appropriately. Allow 20 to 30 minutes after ventilator changes before drawing ABGs to ensure equilibration between alveolar ventilation and arterial blood. Arterial oxygenation goals are based on the individual. Generally Sao_2 ≥90% is clinically acceptable using the lowest possible Fio_2. Permissive hypercapnia may be used to limit lung distention and injury.

9. Assess fluid balance every 8 hours, note the condition of skin and mucous membranes, and compare serial weights. Ventilated patients are at risk for excess fluid volume because of increased secretion of antidiuretic hormone (ADH), which may reduce urine production.

10. If PEEP or continuous positive airway pressure (CPAP) is used, do not remove the patient from the ventilator to obtain hemodynamic pressure readings or to suction the ETT; patients may desaturate rapidly when the ventilator is disconnected.

11. Suctioning can lead to airway trauma and infection. To decrease the likelihood of complications, use sterile technique and suction only when rhonchi are present. Ensure that the

Table 7-2 SUMMARY OF VENTILATOR ALARMS

Alarm	Possible Causes
High pressure	Secretion buildup, kinked airway tubing, bronchospasm, coughing, fighting the ventilator, decreased lung compliance, biting on endotracheal tubing, condensation in the tubing
Low exhaled volume	Disconnection from ventilator, loose connection, leaking airway cuff
Low inspiratory pressure	Disconnection from the ventilator, loose connection, patient increasing spontaneous respiratory effort
High respiratory rate	Hypoxia, anxiety, pain, fever
Apnea alarm	No spontaneous breath within preset time interval

suction device is not set higher than 120 mm Hg and that suction is applied only when the catheter is being withdrawn. Use closed tracheal suction devices in patients with PEEP or CPAP.

12. Administer H_2 antagonists, antacids, or cytoprotective agents as ordered to raise gastric pH and reduce risk of gastric ulceration. Monitor bowel function; assess bowel sounds, and test stool for occult blood.

13. Promote adequate oxygenation and decrease oxygen demand: reposition the patient frequently. Prone positioning improves oxygenation in patients with ARDS. Control pain, anxiety, and agitation. Reduce fever.

14. For neuromuscular blockade, see p. 595.

Weaning and Extubation

Box 7-1 lists weaning criteria. There are no criteria that guarantee successful weaning from mechanical ventilation. Many factors can affect the weaning outcome, including the original cause of the respiratory failure, cognitive/psychologic state, cardiovascular function, malnutrition, and electrolyte deficiencies. Nurses can promote successful weaning by clear communication, effective teaching, and timely emotional support. Patients may be anxious about the sensation of ventilation changes and fear that they will not be able to breathe without the ventilator.

Postextubation

Close observation of the patient is essential. Observe for signs of respiratory distress and increased patient effort: diaphoresis; restlessness; RR >30 breaths/min or <8 breaths/min or increase of 10 respirations from starting RR; increase or decrease in HR by 20 beats/min or <60 beats/min; increase or decrease in BP by 20 mm Hg; pulmonary artery wedge pressure (PAWP) >20 mm Hg; nasal flaring, retraction of suprasternal and intercostal spaces, and paradoxical motion of ribcage and abdomen; tidal volume

Box 7-1 Weaning Criteria

Vital capacity ≥10 mL/kg body weight
Spontaneous tidal volume ≥5 mL/kg
Minute ventilation ≤10 L/min
Negative inspiratory pressure > −20 cm H_2O
Positive expiratory pressure ≥ +30 cm H_2O

<250 to 300 mL; minute ventilation increase of 5 L/min; and Sao_2 ≤90%, Pao_2 <60 mm Hg, and increase in $Paco_2$ with a fall in pH <7.35.

Terminal Weaning

When mechanical ventilation is ordered withdrawn in the case of a terminal illness, the goal of ensuring patient comfort assumes a higher priority than maintaining gas exchange. Symptoms experienced during terminal weaning may include dyspnea, anxiety, and excessive secretions. Pharmacologic agents used to treat dyspnea include morphine sulfate, bronchodilators, and diuretics. To relieve anxiety, benzodiazepines (e.g., lorazepam) may be administered. The administration of both lorazepam and morphine sulfate may allow for reduced doses of both drugs; however, some patients may continue to require large doses for comfort (see p. 623 in Chapter 8).

Critical Observations

Consult physician for the following:
1. Unequal or absent breath sounds
2. Respiratory distress or increased patient effort
3. Sao_2 ≤90%, Pao_2 <60 mm Hg, $Paco_2$ >45 mm Hg with pH <7.35
4. Excessive coughing
5. Persistent cuff leak
6. High peak airway pressures
7. SBP <90 mm Hg
8. Fluid imbalance
9. GI bleeding
10. Signs and symptoms of infection

THORACIC SURGERY

Clinical Brief

Various procedures are performed to repair or to explore abnormalities of the thorax (Table 7-3). Indications include congenital or acquired deformities, traumatic injuries, lesions, and drainage of infections. Traditionally, the open incisional approach has been used for these procedures. However, biopsies and procedures such as pleurodesis, thoracic sympathectomy, empyema evacuation, and wedge resection can be performed via a closed approach (e.g., thoracoscopy).

Various pulmonary function tests can be performed as part of the preoperative assessment. The forced expiratory volume in 1 second

PULM

Table 7-3 THORACIC PROCEDURES

Procedure	Description	Indications
Segmental resection, wedge resection, lobectomy, or pneumonectomy	Removal of lung segment, lung peripheral wedge section, lobe(s) of lung, or an entire lung	Lung abscess, infection such as tuberculosis; congenital cyst or bleb; benign or malignant tumor
Lung reduction	Open chest or thoracoscopic; heavily diseased lung areas trimmed to allow expansion of relatively healthier lung tissues for better gas exchange	Severe emphysema
Tracheal resection	Partial resection and end-to-end reanastomosis of trachea	Tumors; significant tracheal stenosis, usually related to mechanical pressure of cuffed tracheal tube
Repair after thoracic trauma	Drainage of pleural cavity, control of hemorrhage, structural repair	Hemorrhage produced by injury to thoracic vessels causes massive blood loss as well as compression of lungs and mediastinum, resulting in cardiopulmonary compromise
Open thoracostomy	Partial resection of selected rib or ribs, with insertion of chest tube into infected material to provide for continuous drainage	Drainage of empyemas from pocketed pleural spaces
Decortication of lung	Removal of fibrinous, reactive membrane covering visceral and parietal pleura	Restrictive fibrinous membrane

Continued

Table 7-3 THORACIC PROCEDURES—cont'd

Procedure	Description	Indications
Closed thoracostomy	Insertion of chest tube through intercostal space into pleural space; chest tube is attached to water seal system, with or without suction	Provision of continuous aspiration of air, blood, or other fluid or from pleural cavity
Pleurodesis	Insertion of chemical through thoracostomy tube to cause adhesion of visceral and parietal pleura	Recurrent pleural effusion caused by malignancy or chronic disease, recurrent pneumothorax
Thoracoplasty	Surgical collapse of portion of chest wall by multiple rib resections to intentionally decrease volume in hemithorax	Closure of chronic cavitary lesions, empyema spaces, recurrent air leaks, reduction of open thoracic "dead space" after large resection
Correction of pectus excavatum ("funnel chest")	Depression of sternum and costal cartilage corrected by moving sternum outward and realigning cartilage-sternal junction	Prevention/relief of cardiopulmonary compromise caused by chronic restriction of ventilation
Open thoracotomy for cardiac surgery	Coronary artery bypass grafting, valve repair or replacement (see p. 315)	Coronary artery disease, valve disorder
Excision of mediastinal masses, thymectomy	Removal of masses/cysts in upper anterior/posterior mediastinum, removal of thymus gland	Mediastinal tumors (benign or malignant), cysts, abscesses, thymectomy for primary thymic neoplasm, myasthenia gravis
Esophagogastrectomy	Resection of esophagus and stomach with primary anastomosis of proximal esophagus to remaining stomach	Carcinoma of esophagus anywhere from neck to esophagogastric junction, chemical burns of esophagus, uncontrolled esophageal or gastric hemorrhage

(FEV_1) is most widely used to help determine any underlying obstructive disease, predict potential problems with extubation, or identify operative risk.

Complications

- Acute pain
- Hemorrhage
- Hypoxia
- Infection
- Pulmonary edema (in remaining lung after pneumonectomy)

PATIENT CARE MANAGEMENT GUIDELINES

Patient Assessment

1. Assess hemodynamic status: obtain BP and HR every 15 minutes until stable, hourly for the first 4 hours, then every 2 hours. Institutional protocols may vary. Assess capillary refill (normal <3 sec) and quality of peripheral pulses. Calculate MAP; a MAP <60 mm Hg adversely affects cerebral and renal perfusion.

2. Assess respiratory/oxygenation status: continuously monitor SpO_2. Assess respiratory rate and depth, presence of dyspnea, use of accessory muscles, and chest wall movement; auscultate breath sounds and the ability to cough and deep breathe. Review serial ABGs to evaluate oxygenation and acid-base status. Monitor PA systolic pressure (if available) because hypoxia can increase sympathetic tone and increase pulmonary vasoconstriction.

3. Assess pain: perform systematic initial and ongoing pain assessment (intensity, location, quality, aggravating and relieving factors). Use a self-report pain rating scale, such as 0-to-10 scale, to assess pain intensity in patients who are awake and oriented (see Chapter 2).

4. Monitor fluid volume status: record chest drainage, urinary output, and fluid intake hourly; determine fluid balance every 8 hours.

5. Continuously monitor ECG to detect dysrhythmias. Hypoxia, acidosis, and electrolyte imbalance are risk factors.

6. Monitor for air leak and drainage from CTs. See Chest Drainage, p. 497.

7. Assess surgical site for bleeding.

8. Assess temperature, sputum, and WBC count for potential infection.

Patient Management

1. Manage pain. Thoracic surgery can cause severe pain, which can result in hypoventilation, atelectasis, and pneumonia. (See Chapter 2; see also Intraspinal Analgesia, p. 590.)

2. Encourage incentive spirometry and deep breathing and coughing at least every hour. Reposition patient at least every 2 hours. Mobilize patient (e.g., dangle, chair, ambulate). More aggressive techniques and procedures may improve respiratory status (e.g., chest physiotherapy [CPT] and nebulizer treatments, suctioning, and bronchoscopy). Administer supplemental oxygen as ordered.

3. Monitor tube patency. Milking CTs may be necessary to maintain patency (see Chest Drainage, p. 497). Postthoracotomy CTs should not be clamped. Once air leak and drainage are minimal, the CT(s) may be changed to water seal.

4. Fluid management may include fluid restriction and diuretics, strict I&O, and daily weights.

5. To prevent venous stasis and the development of deep vein thrombosis (DVT), pneumatic compression boots may be ordered.

6. If the patient is intubated and mechanically ventilated, see Ventilation Therapies, p. 503.

Critical Observations

Consult physician for the following:

1. Tracheal deviation
2. Dysrhythmias
3. SBP <90 mm Hg
4. CT drainage ≥200 mL/hr
5. Urine output ≤20 mL/hr for 2 hours
6. O_2 sat <90%
7. Pao_2 <60 mm Hg
8. Svo_2 <60% or >80%
9. Potassium level <3.5 mEq/L
10. Decreasing trend in Hgb and Hct levels
11. Development of air leak: bubbling in water seal chamber or subcutaneous emphysema
12. Respiratory distress: restlessness, shortness of breath (SOB), increased RR, change in LOC, agitation
13. Hemodynamic instability, bleeding at surgical site
14. Elevated temperature >101° F (38.3° C)

CARDIOVASCULAR (CV) MODALITIES

CARDIAC SURGERY

Clinical Brief

The purpose of cardiac surgery is to optimize cardiac function, preserve myocardial tissue, and/or improve quality of life. Cardiac surgeries are performed under general anesthesia, on or off cardiopulmonary bypass (CPB), by using a sternotomy (most common) or thoracic approach. During CPB, a cannula is placed in the superior vena cava or right atrium for drawing blood out of the body into a CPB machine, where it becomes oxygenated. The oxygenated blood is then returned to the patient through a cannula placed in the aorta (distal to the cross-clamp), thereby effectively bypassing the heart. To preserve myocardial tissue and stop the heart, potassium-rich cardioplegia mixed with blood is infused into the coronary artery vasculature. Once the surgical procedure is completed, the patient is weaned off CPB. Epicardial wires and CTs may be placed before closing the chest.

The purpose, indications, and description of the various cardiac surgeries are detailed in Box 7-2. Contraindications for cardiac surgery include inability to tolerate general anesthesia and terminal illness.

Box 7-2 Cardiovascular Surgeries

Type: coronary artery bypass graft surgery (CABG)

Purpose: to restore adequate blood flow to the myocardium to meet metabolic demands distal to the coronary artery stenosis

Indications: myocardial ischemia refractory to medical management, extensive coronary disease, left main with stenosis >50% occlusion, three-vessel disease with ejection fraction of <50% or vessel(s) with large area of myocardium in jeopardy

Description: either vessels are harvested from the saphenous veins of the lower extremities or radial artery from arms, or internal mammary artery (IMA) is stripped down from the anterior chest wall. The saphenous vein and radial artery grafts are anastomosed to the aortic root at one end, and the other end of the graft is anastomosed to the coronary artery distal to the stenosis. If the IMA is used, only the distal end is anastomosed to the coronary artery distal to the stenosis. Another graft option not used very often is the gastroepiploic artery.

Type: valvular repair/replacement

Purpose: to restore normal or near-normal function to a valve that is stenotic or incompetent

Indications: critical tricuspid, pulmonic, mitral, or aortic stenosis or symptomatic incompetence

Continued

Box 7-2 Cardiovascular Surgeries—cont'd

Description: access is gained by an atrial incision or aortic/pulmonary artery root incision. Valves can be repaired by valvuloplasty, splitting fused commissures, shortening or lengthening chordae tendineae, or reattaching papillary muscle. Leaflets may be sewn to repair tears or stretching. During valve replacement (VR) the dysfunctional valve is removed and replaced with mechanical or bioprosthetic (tissue) valve.

Type: atrial/ventricular septal defect repair

Purpose: to repair left-to-right shunts that are a result of congenital defects or septal perforation related to acute myocardial infarctions

Indications: congenital septal defect or acute septal perforation related to myocardial infarctions. Surgical repair is reserved for hemodynamic instability or neurologic sequelae secondary to defect.

Description: an incision is made in the atrium or ventricle. The defect is patched with a synthetic graft or closed with sutures.

Type: ventricular aneurysm repair

Purpose: to improve symptoms and pump function or reduce chance of clot formation

Indications: surgical repair is performed when scar tissue causes life-threatening dysrhythmias, false aneurysm, or clot formation inside akinetic/dyskinetic ventricle wall or possibility of thin ventricular wall rupture

Description: incision is made through the aneurysm in the ventricular wall, the aneurysm is removed and healthy tissue is closed with sutures and/or felt strips

Type: myotomy/myomectomy

Purpose: to restore adequate flow through valves in the ventricle

Indications: symptomatic obstruction causing hypertrophic cardiomyopathy

Description: access to the left ventricle is gained via the aortic valve orifice or a ventricular incision. Excess myocardium is removed to create an adequate outflow tract. The aortic or mitral valves may need to be replaced.

Type: cardiomyoplasty

Purpose: to improve ventricular function as a bridge to transplantation and/or long-term alternative to transplantation

Indications: refractory end-stage heart failure

Description: the Bastista procedure is the resection of a large segment of the left ventricle and the closure of the ventricle in two layers, sometimes with replacement/repair of the mitral valve

Type: Maze procedure (Cox-Maze)

Purpose: to eradicate atrial fibrillation rhythm

Indications: refractory atrial fibrillation

Description: precise incisions/ablation are made in the right and left atria to interrupt the conduction of abnormal impulses and to direct normal sinus impulses to travel to the atrioventricular node (AV node)

Complications

- Excess bleeding
- Cardiac tamponade
- Perioperative myocardial infarction
- Decreased preload/hypotension
- Respiratory failure
- Dysrhythmias
- Increased afterload/hypertension
- Neurologic changes
- Fluid and electrolyte imbalance
- Acid-base imbalance
- Renal failure
- Cerebrovascular accident

PATIENT CARE MANAGEMENT GUIDELINES

Patient Assessment

1. A thorough head-to-toe assessment should be completed on arrival to the recovery area. The patient should be monitored continuously for instability, which is often present in the early postoperative period.
2. The CV system should be assessed every 15 minutes until stable and then per unit protocol, including VS, CVP, PA pressures, cardiac rhythm, incision or dressing appearance, hourly CT drainage, quality of peripheral pulses, and hourly urinary output. Heart sounds should be assessed for changes in quality and intensity of murmurs and muffled tones.
3. A complete cardiac profile including CO, CI, SVRI, and LVSWI should be done on admission, every 8 hours, and with any significant changes in hemodynamic status or pharmacologic therapies.
4. Respiratory system assessment should include lung sounds, O_2 saturation or Svo_2 (if available), airway pressures, tidal volume, and RR per protocol.
5. Assessment of neurologic status should include LOC, movement and strength of extremities, and the ability to follow commands.

Patient Management

1. Most patients regain consciousness within the first few hours postoperatively. Restlessness can occur as the patient is waking up from anesthesia and can be associated with hypertension,

pain, and hemodynamic instability. Restlessness may require the use of sedatives such as intravenous midazolam (Versed), or propofol (Diprivan). Pain can be managed with intravenous morphine sulfate or fentanyl (Sublimaze) as ordered.

2. It is recommended to keep SBP between 100 and 120 mm Hg to prevent damage to the anastomoses or the fresh suture lines in patients who have had CABG surgery and aortic root repair. Furthermore, a MAP of >70 mm Hg is desirable in these patients to prevent the acute collapse of the grafts.

3. Increased afterload, which may cause hypertension and reduced CO, may occur postoperatively and is usually managed with vasodilators such as sodium nitroprusside and/or nitroglycerin. Sodium nitroprusside may be administered by intravenous infusion to maintain SBP at 100 mm Hg or as ordered. Dose may range from 0.5 to 10 mcg/kg/min. Monitor patient for signs and symptoms of cyanide toxicity: tinnitus, blurred vision, delirium, and muscle spasm. Adding sodium thiosulfate to the nitroprusside infusion will reduce cyanide poisoning. Refer to facility policy or procedure regarding the administration of nitroprusside and sodium thiosulfate. Intravenous nitroglycerin may be administered to gain desired response: start with an infusion of 5 mcg/min; titrate to desired response or to maintain SBP >90 mm Hg. Increase dose every 5 to 10 minutes by 5 to 10 mcg/min. If hypotension or reflex tachycardia occurs, raise the patient's legs and reduce dose as needed to maintain SBP >90 mm Hg. Nitroglycerin infusion also prevents arterial vasospasm when internal mammary artery is used.

4. Decreased preload occurs as a result of hypovolemia or vasodilation. This may result from CPB, diuretics administered while weaning from CPB, postoperative bleeding, or postoperative warming of the patient. Blood products and colloids are usually the most effective in correcting hypovolemia. Reducing doses of vasodilator agents and achieving normothermia can resolve vasodilation.

5. ST segment and T-wave changes may indicate myocardial ischemia and/or infarction, resulting in potential decreased CO with subsequent hypotension and increased dysrhythmias. Ensure adequate myocardial oxygenation; nitroglycerin may be ordered to prevent ischemia and coronary vasospasm. Serial ECGs will reveal effectiveness of interventions. Decreased CO/CI can be treated with inotropic agents such

as dobutamine or milrinone administered per protocol. Dobutamine can be administered at 2.5 to 10 mcg/kg/min. Milrinone is administered as a 50-mcg/kg bolus over 10 minutes, followed by an infusion of 0.375 to 0.75 mcg/kg/min. Use lower doses with renal impairment.

6. CT drainage >100 mL in two hours may indicate an intrathoracic bleed, presence of coagulopathy, incomplete reversal of heparin, or bleeding from the graft site. Serum coagulation profiles, (e.g., activated clotting time [ACT], prothrombin time [PT], activated partial thromboplastin time [aPTT], platelet count, fibrinogen, thromboelastography [TEG]) may reveal deficits requiring replacement with fresh frozen plasma (FFP), platelets, cryoprecipitates, clotting factors, or protamine (25-50 mg IV) as ordered. Hypothermia can also affect the clotting cascade and the patient should be warmed to 98.6° F (37° C). PEEP can increase intrathoracic pressure to tamponade some of the bleeding in the chest. Antifibrinolytic drugs such as aprotinin and epsilon-aminocaproic acid may be ordered. Anemia associated with excess bleeding can lead to relative hypoxemia and myocardial ischemia requiring replacement with packed red blood cells (PRBCs).

7. To maintain adequate oxygenation, PEEP may be used to facilitate gas exchange, leading to improved PaO_2. As PEEP is increased, venous return may decrease, adversely affecting BP and CO/CI.

8. Shivering increases O_2 demands and can be controlled with warm blankets, meperidine 25 to 50 mg IV, or vecuronium (Norcuron) 40 to 80 mcg/kg over 5 to 10 minutes.

9. Dysrhythmias such as atrial fibrillation, supraventricular tachycardia (SVT), ventricular tachycardia (VT), bradycardias, junctional rhythms, heart blocks, and asystole are possible. Dysrhythmia management should follow the advanced cardiac life support (ACLS) guidelines or by pacing with the epicardial wires that are placed during surgery. Hypokalemia and hypomagnesemia should be managed promptly with frequent assessment of serum levels.

10. Cardiac tamponade usually occurs as a result of excessive intrathoracic bleeding and/or ineffective draining of CTs. Signs of cardiac tamponade include narrowing pulse pressure, increasing and equalization of CVP and pulmonary artery diastolic (PAD)/PAWP pressures, increasing cardiac silhouette on chest radiograph, and muffled heart sounds. Treatment

includes inotropic agents and increased intravascular volume replacement until thoracic reexploration can be performed.

Critical Observations

Consult physician for the following:

1. Acute drop in or trend of decreasing CO/CI
2. Inability to control BP (sustained hypotension or hypertension)
3. Sudden cessation of CT drainage
4. Excessive CT drainage
5. New onset of ST segment and T-wave changes
6. Muffling of heart sounds and equalizing PA and CVP pressures
7. Lethal dysrhythmias

CARDIAC TRANSPLANT

Clinical Brief

Cardiac transplantation is reserved for patients with end-stage cardiac disease with significant functional impairment who are unresponsive to medical or interventional therapy. The surgical procedure involves a sternotomy incision, hypothermia induction, and initiation of CPB. The recipient's heart is removed, leaving the posterior walls of the atria intact; the vena cava and pulmonary veins are left intact. The donor's atria are anastomosed to the recipient's atrial walls, and PA and aorta are then anastomosed. Temporary epicardial pacing wires and CTs are inserted and then the chest is closed. As a result of this procedure the heart is denervated and does not respond to autonomic nervous system (ANS) stimulation (HR changes in response to stressors).

Complications

See Cardiac Surgery, p. 515, for other complications.

- Organ rejection
- Adverse effects of immunosuppressive therapy
- Infection

PATIENT CARE MANAGEMENT GUIDELINES

Patient Assessment

1. Monitor CVP, PA pressures, CO/CI, HR, BP, MAP, PVRI, and SVRI. Note trends and patient response to therapy. Monitor LVSWI and RVSWI to evaluate contractility.
2. Assess tissue perfusion: note level of mentation, skin color and temperature, peripheral pulses, and capillary refill.

3. Continuously monitor ECG for dysrhythmias that may result from electrolyte imbalance, hypoxemia, and/or hemorrhage.

4. Assess for bleeding: CT drainage >200 mL/hr, development of cardiac tamponade, decrease in Hgb and Hct levels, or abnormal coagulation studies. A donor heart may be smaller than the native heart, which can result in a larger pericardial space and potential reservoir for bleeding and tamponade.

5. Monitor HR and cardiac rhythm. The denervated heart has no increase in HR in response to decreased CO. The donor sinus node stimulates electrical conduction; however, the recipient P waves may also be seen on ECG. Monitor for junctional rhythm with atrioventricular block.

6. Continuously monitor SpO_2 and SvO_2 (if available); review serial ABGs and auscultate lungs every 1 to 2 hours. Note any adventitious lung sounds and increased work of breathing. Assess cough and secretions.

7. Assess temperature. Patients may be hypothermic on returning from surgery. Also monitor for signs of infection. Consider intravenous sites, wound sites, the urinary tract, lungs, and mucous membranes as potential sites of infection.

8. Monitor serum immunosuppressive drug levels for therapeutic range.

9. Assess patient for side effects of immunosuppression therapy: hypertension, hyperkalemia, gingival hyperplasia, leukopenia, and hyperglycemia.

10. Monitor sputum cultures, WBC count, and titers for presence of infection.

11. Monitor renal function: blood urea nitrogen (BUN) and creatinine levels and urine output. Obtain daily weight. Monitor I&O each shift.

12. Assess neurologic status. Potential side effects of cyclosporine include confusion, cortical blindness, seizures, encephalopathy, quadriplegia, and coma.

Patient Management

1. Hemodynamic instability may be treated with fluids, amrinone, milrinone, prostaglandins, dobutamine, and dopamine. Prostaglandins may be used to decrease elevated pulmonary vascular resistance (PVR). Dobutamine or milrinone may be used to increase myocardial contractility. Dopamine or nesiritide is often used to enhance renal output. Titrate the infusions

to achieve desired hemodynamic response. Diuretics may be prescribed for heart failure symptoms.

2. Be prepared to pace the patient for bradycardia or heart block. Note: atropine has no effect on the denervated heart.

3. Isolation protocols should be followed. Dressings should be completed with aseptic technique. Intravenous sites should be changed according to institutional protocol. Catheters and other invasive equipment should be removed as soon as possible. The patient should be weaned from the ventilator as soon as possible. Vigorous pulmonary toilet and incentive spirometry should be initiated.

4. Administer H_2 blockers as prescribed to prevent stress ulcers. Test all stools and emesis for evidence of occult blood.

5. Administer cytomegalovirus (CMV)-negative blood products as prescribed.

6. Administer immunosuppressive therapy (e.g., azathioprine, cyclosporine, corticosteroids, OKT3, FK506) as prescribed to prevent and/or treat acute rejection.

7. See Cardiac Surgery, p. 515, for other patient management guidelines.

Critical Observations

Consult physician for the following:

1. Bleeding: CT drainage >200 mL/hr, cardiac tamponade, abnormal coagulation studies

2. Signs and symptoms of myocardial dysfunction: decreased CO/CI, heart failure, dysrhythmias, hemodynamic instability

3. Adverse effects of immunosuppression: GI bleeding, hyperglycemia, hyperkalemia

4. Signs of renal failure: rising BUN and creatinine levels, decreased urine output

5. Signs of infection: elevated temperature, abnormal WBC count, incisional drainage, purulent sputum

IMPLANTABLE CARDIOVERTER DEFIBRILLATOR (ICD) OR AUTOMATED IMPLANTABLE CARDIOVERTER DEFIBRILLATOR (AICD)

Clinical Brief

The ICD is an effective treatment option for patients with recurrent ventricular dysrhythmias at risk for sudden death. ICD is a multiprogrammable electronic device. ICD components include (1) a pulse generator (generally placed subcutaneously or in a submuscular pocket in the pectoral region), which contains the battery and capacitors, and (2) leads or electrodes that monitor heart activity and deliver electrical therapy. The ICD is implanted subcutaneously and offers programmable features including bradycardic backup pacing, antitachycardia pacing, low-energy cardioversion, and high-energy defibrillation therapy. Predicted battery life is 5 years. An ICD malfunction can result in inappropriate shock or failure to shock.

Complications

- Hemothorax or pneumothorax
- Vascular or cardiac perforation
- ICD malfunction
- Tamponade
- Infection
- Thromboembolism

PATIENT CARE MANAGEMENT GUIDELINES

Patient Assessment

1. Monitor heart rhythm and patient response before, during, and after ICD therapy. As long as the ICD continues to respond and the patient is stable, no intervention is necessary.
2. Assess the patient's risk factors for a lethal event (e.g., hypoxemia, electrolyte imbalances).

Patient Management

1. Be aware of the specific device implanted and how it is programmed (e.g., is the device on or off? what are the settings? tachycardia detection rate?). Place a sign with this information at the head of the bed and/or in the patient record.
2. Emergency care of the patient with an ICD should follow ACLS protocol.
3. When the ICD discharges, individuals touching the patient can receive up to a 2-joule shock. Wearing gloves will reduce the shock to caregiver. If VT/ventricular fibrillation (VF) continues, initiate cardiopulmonary resuscitation (CPR) and countershock. (An external defibrillator does not damage ICD.)
4. Inappropriate discharge of the ICD may occur infrequently (patient shocked while in normal sinus rhythm [NSR]). Be alert to this complication. Inactivate the ICD (depending on institutional policy, nurses may or may not use a magnet to inactivate

the ICD). It is likely that the ICD vendor representative will be consulted to check the function of the ICD with a physician.

5. Monitor for signs of infection after implantation of the ICD. Monitor temperature every 4 hours. Note any drainage, redness, and increased tenderness at the surgical site.

6. Continue antiarrhythmic medication for identified dysrhythmias.

7. Patient and family teaching must be done to prepare them to live with an ICD. The patient should be instructed to avoid electromagnetic interference because it may temporarily or permanently render the defibrillator nonfunctional. Magnetic resonance imaging and electrocautery are contraindicated.

Critical Observations

Consult physician for the following:

1. Inappropriate discharge of ICD
2. Failure (of ICD) to discharge
3. Evidence of wound infection: temperature >101° F (38.3° C), redness, drainage

INTRAAORTIC BALLOON PUMP (IABP) COUNTERPULSATION

Clinical Brief

The purpose of the IABP is to increase coronary artery perfusion and decrease myocardial oxygen consumption. Counterpulsation increases aortic pressure during diastole (balloon inflation), augmenting coronary and peripheral perfusion and oxygen supply. Counterpulsation decreases aortic pressure during systole (balloon deflation), decreasing afterload and myocardial oxygen consumption (Figure 7-2). Consequently, counterpulsation produces the following effects:

Increased Supply	Decreased Demand
↑ MAP/stroke index (SI)/CI	↓ Left ventricular end-diastolic pressure (LVEDP)/PAWP (preload)
↑ Renal perfusion	↓SVRI (afterload)
↑ Cerebral perfusion	↓ MVO$_2$
↑ Coronary artery perfusion	↓ HR

Indications for IABP include cardiogenic shock related to acute myocardial infarction (MI), following cardiac surgery, noncardiogenic shock, ventricular septal defect, papillary muscle dysfunction,

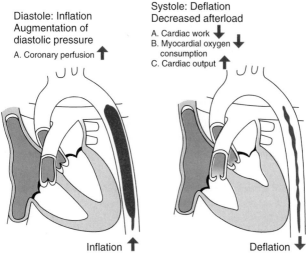

Diastole: Inflation
Augmentation of
diastolic pressure

A. Coronary perfusion ↑

Systole: Deflation
Decreased afterload

A. Cardiac work ↓ ↓
B. Myocardial oxygen ↓
   consumption
C. Cardiac output ↑

Inflation ↑   Deflation ↓

Figure 7-2 Intraaortic balloon inflation and deflation. (From Datascope Corp., Fairfield, NJ.)

unstable angina, and prophylactically for high-risk cardiovascular (CV) patients undergoing coronary interventions.

Contraindications include irreversible brain damage, end-stage cardiac disease, aortic regurgitation, dissecting aortic aneurysm, and significant peripheral vascular disease.

Description

The IABP device consists of a balloon-tipped catheter and power console that permits inflation and deflation of the balloon during diastole and systole, respectively. The catheter is inserted in the femoral artery via a percutaneous approach and advanced through the aorta. Chest radiograph and/or fluoroscopy can confirm correct placement in the descending aorta distal to the left subclavian artery (second to third intercostal space [ICS]) and proximal to the renal arteries (monitor urine output [UOP]). Inflation and deflation of the intraaortic balloon is most often triggered from the ECG, although pressure scales can be used. Timing is fine-tuned from the arterial waveform (Figure 7-3). The balloon inflation, at onset of diastole (dicrotic notch), causes an increase in diastolic aortic pressure and coronary artery pressure, thus improving coronary and cerebral artery blood flow. This period is called diastolic augmentation. Rapid

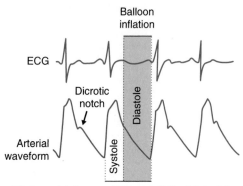

Figure 7-3 Intraaortic balloon pump (IABP) period of balloon inflation. Balloon inflation occurs during diastole and should begin at aortic valve closure (dicrotic notch); balloon deflation should occur just before the aortic valve opens. (From Stillwell S, Randall E: *Pocket guide to cardiovascular care,* ed 2, St. Louis, 1994, Mosby.)

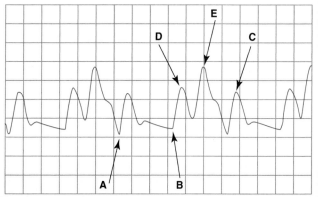

Figure 7-4 Intraaortic balloon pump (IABP) timing 1:2 assist mode. **A,** Balloon-assisted end-diastolic pressure. **B,** Patient aortic end-diastolic pressure. **C,** Balloon-assisted systole. **D,** Patient systole. **E,** Peak diastolic augmented pressure.

deflation of the balloon is timed to occur just before the onset of systole. Proper deflation of the balloon decreases the aortic pressure dramatically and allows the ventricle to empty more completely against less pressure. Initially, the IABP is usually set to augment every cardiac cycle or every other cycle (Figure 7-4). Timing must be monitored frequently to detect problems with early or late balloon inflation (Figure 7-5).

Early Inflation

Inflation of the IAB before aortic valve closure

Waveform Characteristics:

- Inflation of IAB prior to dicrotic notch
- Diastolic augmentation encroaches onto systole (may be unable to distinguish)

Physiologic Effects:

- Potential premature closure of aortic valve
- Potential increase in LVEDV and LVEDP or PCWP
- Increased left ventricular wall stress or afterload
- Aortic regurgitation
- Increased MVO_2 demand

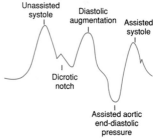

Late Inflation

Inflation of the IAB markedly after closure of the aortic valve

Waveform Characteristics:

- Inflation of the IAB after the dicrotic notch
- Absense of sharp V
- Suboptimal diastolic augmentation

Physiologic Effects:

- Suboptimal coronary artery perfusion

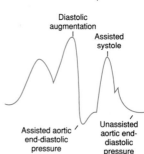

Early Deflation

Premature deflation of the IAB during the diastolic phase

Waveform Characteristics:

- Deflation of the IAB is seen as a sharp drop following diastolic augmentation
- Suboptimal diastolic augmentation
- Assisted aortic end-diastolic pressure may be equal to or less than the unassisted aortic end-diastolic pressure
- Assisted systolic pressure may rise

Physiologic Effects:

- Suboptimal coronary perfusion
- Potential for retrograde coronary and carotid blood flow
- Angina may occur as a result of retrograde coronary blood flow
- Suboptimal afterload reduction
- Increased MVO_2 demand

Figure 7-5 Problems with intraaortic balloon pump (IABP) timing. (Datascope Corp, Fairfield, NJ.)

Continued

CV

Late Deflation

Waveform Characteristics:

- Assisted aortic end-diastolic pressure may be equal to the unassisted aortic end diastolic pressure
- Rate of rise of assisted systole is prolonged
- Diastolic augmentation may appear widened

Physiologic Effects:

- Afterload reduction is essentially absent
- Increased MVO_2 consumption due to the left ventricle ejecting against a greater resistance and a prolonged isovolumetric contraction phase
- IAB may impede left ventricular ejection and increase the afterload

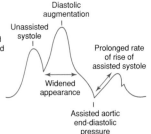

Figure 7-5, cont'd Problems with intraaortic balloon pump (IABP) timing. (Datascope Corp, Fairfield, NJ.)

Complications

Poor IABP augmentation
- Balloon leak
- Incorrect timing
- ↑ HR
- ↓ MAP/SI/SVRI
- Incorrect balloon size
- Incorrect balloon position
- Any condition that ↓ SV

Balloon migration
- Subclavian/carotid artery obstruction
- Renal artery obstruction

Embolization

Infection

Aortic dissection

Atelectasis secondary to immobility

Loss of peripheral pulses related to thrombus formation at access site

Hematoma formation at percutaneous access site

Bleeding
- Thrombocytopenia
- Related to anticoagulation

PATIENT CARE MANAGEMENT GUIDELINES

Patient Assessment

1. The CV system should be assessed every 15 to 30 minutes until stable after IABP insertion and then per unit protocol, include VS and cardiac rhythm; urine output should be monitored hourly. Assess for chest pain.

2. Assess pulmonary artery pressures (PA) and CVP hourly (if available). Complete hemodynamic profile, including CO/CI, SVRI, and LVSWI should be done on admission, every 8 hours, and with any significant changes in hemodynamics.

3. Assess peripheral pulses (both pedal and posttibial pulses) for strength and equality every 15 minutes for 1 hour and then every hour. Left arm radial and brachial pulses also should be assessed to check for possible catheter migration, which would result in a diminished or absent pulse. Verify that the skin remains pink and warm to the touch and that capillary refill is equally brisk bilaterally. If a change in quality of pulses is noted, a Doppler device should be employed to attempt to identify pulses.

4. Assess the percutaneous insertion site for oozing, ecchymosis, or hematoma formation every 15 minutes for 1 hour, then every hour after IABP insertion. Assess coagulation status, including platelets, via ordered laboratory tests.

5. Augmentation of IABP should be assessed hourly and as needed. Balloon-assisted systolic pressure should be lower than the patient's unassisted systolic pressure. Assisted aortic end-diastolic pressure should be less than the unassisted aortic end-diastolic pressure. Balloon migration should be ruled out with the development of poor IABP augmentation, changes in LOC (possible subclavian artery occlusion), a diminished radial pulse in the left arm, or a decrease in urinary output (possible renal artery occlusion). A STAT chest radiograph is crucial to verify placement. The radiopaque catheter tip should be just distal to the aortic arch in the second to third ICS.

6. Assess for discomfort at insertion site or secondary to immobility. Rule out bleeding.

7. Assess neurologic functioning every 1 to 4 hours as indicator of adequate cerebral perfusion.

Patient Management

1. Maintain proper functioning of the balloon pump according to the manufacturer's guidelines. Maintain airtight seals on all connections between the pump and the patient.

2. The inflation of the balloon should be timed to occur at the dicrotic notch and to deflate just before the next systole (see Figure 7-4). Instruct the patient to keep the affected leg immobilized and do not elevate the HOB more than 30 degrees.

3. Inflation and deflation timing are usually adjusted via slide bars. The goal of the adjustment is to achieve maximum diastolic augmentation and minimum aortic end-diastolic pressure. Avoid early or late inflation or deflation (see Figure 7-5).

4. Red or brownish discolorations inside the balloon connecting tubing indicates balloon leak. The IABP should be placed on standby and the physician called immediately to remove the balloon. The balloon should not be immobile for >30 minutes because of risk of thrombus formation and balloon entrapment.

5. When the balloon catheter is removed, direct pressure is applied per unit protocol, and then a pressure dressing and/or a sandbag may be applied at the insertion site per unit protocol. A large amount of blood may exsanguinate into the groin and upper thigh without any obvious evidence; therefore, close monitoring is warranted. Watch for hematoma formation at the access site. Mark the site carefully with a skin-marking pen and assess hourly for the first 4 hours and at least every 4 hours thereafter to determine the magnitude of the hematoma.

6. Provide and encourage pulmonary hygiene: coughing and deep breathing, incentive spirometry, and repositioning.

7. Administer analgesics as ordered and reposition patient to avoid discomfort and skin breakdown.

Critical Observations

Consult physician for the following:

1. Inability to maintain adequate augmentation
2. Accidental dislodgment or removal of catheter
3. Migration of balloon tip: decrease in urine output, changes in LOC, decrease or loss of pulse in an extremity
4. Excessive bleeding at access site (apply direct pressure)
5. Balloon leak

PERCUTANEOUS CORONARY INTERVENTIONS (PCI)

Clinical Brief

Numerous catheter-based cardiac interventions can be performed in the cardiac catheterization lab. These procedures are percutaneous transluminal coronary angioplasty (PTCA), stenting, atherectomy, and Rotablator. The purpose of these interventions is to restore blood flow to the myocardium by increasing lumen diameter of a coronary artery. Indications for these interventions are for asymptomatic to severely symptomatic patients with intraluminal narrowing (>60%). PCI is fast becoming a desirable option for managing acute coronary syndromes (ACS), that is, unstable angina, non–ST segment elevation MI, and ST segment elevation MI.

These different procedures are usually done after coronary angiography or intravascular ultrasound has identified the occluded vessel(s). Once percutaneous arterial access is established, the appropriate catheter is advanced over the guidewire to the lesion (or through the lesion). The patient will require anticoagulation with heparin or bivalirudin (Angiomax) at the beginning of the procedure. A summary of the various procedures follows:

PTCA: A wire is placed through the lesion and a specially equipped catheter with a balloon tip is passed over the wire. The balloon is then inflated to compress the atherosclerotic plaque, thereby increasing lumen diameter. The patient may experience angina during balloon inflation, as blood flow distal to the balloon is impaired. The balloon may need to be inflated several times to achieve optimal luminal opening. Note: intracoronary nitroglycerin may be administered to prevent or treat vasospasm during the procedure. Intracoronary thrombolytics may be administered to treat acute thrombus formation.

Bare metal stent: This is a stainless steal slotted wire device designed to mechanically support the coronary artery and prevent acute restenosis following PTCA and dissection. A delivery system positions the stent through the lesion site, where it is released. The stent expands by a balloon, which improves the vessel intraluminal diameter. Acute closure secondary to thrombus formation may occur; therefore, these patients receive anticoagulation with heparin, bivalirudin, clopidogrel (Plavix), and a glycoprotein IIb IIIa inhibitor (e.g., abciximab, tirofiban, eptifibatide).

Drug-eluting stent: These were developed to reduce in-stent restenosis due to cell proliferation. These stents are impregnated with antiproliferative agents—rapamycin and paclitaxel. The drug-eluting stents are placed with the same technique as a bare metal stent. These patients are medicated with aspirin (ASA) and clopidogrel for 3 to 6 months to prevent endothelialization of the stent surfaces.

Excimer laser therapy: This breaks up the plaque of a total occluded artery into subcellular debris and gases so that balloon angioplasty can be employed or the laser can be used to thermally seal the artery following angioplasty. Arterial perforation, embolization, and spasm are laser-related complications.

Rotablator atherectomy: A diamond-studded burr is advanced over the guidewire to the calcified lesion. It is rotated at very high speeds, which crumbles the lesion into microparticulates. These patients may be susceptible to emboli or coronary dissection as a result of the nature of the procedure.

Transluminal cutting balloon atherectomy: This device is positioned at the lesion and shaves away the plaque. A balloon is inflated to stabilize the catheter, and the excised plaque is collected in a housing compartment beyond the occlusion and removed. Restenosis of the artery can occur following the atherectomy.

Patient Selection

In general, patients who are candidates for PTCA or other PCI include individuals with discrete lesions, preferably involving one or two vessels, and not at large vessel bifurcations. These patients also should be a candidate for CABG surgery. Contraindications include <50% occluded lesion, nonviable myocardium distal to the stenotic lesion, diffuse disease with distal vessels suitable for bypass grafting, left main disease, and tortuous vessels.

Complications

- Acute occlusion/restenosis
- Reperfusion dysrhythmias
- Reaction to contrast agent
- Bleeding related to anticoagulation
- Vasovagal reaction
- Loss of peripheral pulses
- Hematoma formation at percutaneous access site
- Stroke or MI

PATIENT CARE MANAGEMENT GUIDELINES

Patient Assessment

1. Assess VS every 15 minutes four times, every 30 minutes four times, every hour four times, then per routine, if stable.
2. Assess cardiac rhythm continuously via bedside monitor. Note rate, rhythm, and/or ST segment and T-wave changes.
3. Assess access site for oozing, ecchymosis, or hematoma formation with VS check. If a hematoma develops at the groin access site, consider applying direct pressure. The size of the hematoma should be monitored by outlining the borders with a skin-marking pen. A large amount of blood may exsanguinate into the retroperitoneum, groin, and upper thigh without necessarily seeing an early drop in SBP or an increase in HR; therefore, close observation of the access site is warranted.
4. Assess patient comfort level every 1 to 2 hours for 12 hours. If pain develops at the groin access site, assess for local hematoma formation and/or back pain. Assist with repositioning but keep affected leg immobile.
5. Assess peripheral pulses (pedal and posttibial pulses) for strength and equality with VS check. A Doppler device may be helpful in identifying peripheral pulses.
6. Monitor coagulation studies (aPTT, ACT, platelets). The normal value for PTT is 30 to 45 seconds and for ACT is <150 seconds. Glycoprotein IIb IIIa inhibitors may reduce platelet levels especially abciximab (ReoPro). Monitor for drop in platelet counts.

Patient Management

1. The patient should be instructed to promptly report any chest pain, SOB, and moisture or warmth at the groin site (may indicate bleeding). Instruct the patient to not lift head off bed and to apply pressure to dressing when coughing or laughing.
2. Low-flow oxygen therapy should be administered as per protocol to keep SaO_2 >92%.
3. The HOB should not be elevated greater than 30 degrees and the affected extremity should be kept straight to prevent bleeding and/or dislodgment of the groin sheath. Educate the patient about activity restrictions.
4. Encourage PO fluids (if not contraindicated) to offset the effects of the hypertonic contrast. Intravenous fluids or

acetylcysteine (Mucomyst) may be ordered to preserve kidney function.

5. Maintain hypercoagulated state or platelet inhibition if ordered.

6. If the patient was sedated during the procedure and remains sedated, institute aspiration and fall precautions until the patient is fully alert. Consider pulse oximetry.

7. If the patient reports chest pain, intravenous or sublingual nitroglycerin may be ordered to relieve discomfort: sublingual, 1 tablet (0.4 mg) every 5 minutes × 3; IV, start with an infusion of 5 mcg/min and titrate to desired response or to maintain SBP >90 mm Hg. Increase dose every 5 to 10 minutes by 5 to 10 mcg/min. If hypotension or reflex tachycardia occurs, raise unaffected leg and reduce the dose and notify the physician.

8. If the patient becomes hypotensive, a fluid challenge may be ordered. If the patient is bradycardic, administer atropine per ACLS protocol.

9. If pain develops at the groin access site or in lower back, assess groin site for hematoma and bleeding, administer analgesics per protocol, and obtain hematocrit and hemoglobin (H&H) if ordered.

10. If a hematoma forms at the access site, direct pressure should be applied per unit protocol followed by a pressure dressing.

11. If nausea and/or vomiting occurs, administer antiemetics per protocol.

12. Promote and assist with pulmonary hygiene: reposition the patient, encourage coughing, deep breathing, and use of incentive spirometer.

Sheath Removal

1. Once the physician has ordered the sheath(s) removed, the patient should be informed of the forthcoming procedure.

2. The access site should be prepared as per protocol (local anesthesia, antimicrobial prep, suture removal).

3. The sheath(s) should be removed and direct pressure applied until hemostasis is achieved. For an arterial sheath, apply pressure 1 inch above the puncture site; for a venous sheath, apply pressure 1 inch below the puncture site. Apply enough pressure to obtain hemostasis but not occlude the distal pulse. A mechanical device may be employed to establish hemostasis. If so, follow the manufacturer's directions.

Continuous monitoring of site, ECG, HR, and intermittent assessment of peripheral pulses and blood pressure should be performed throughout procedure.

4. Once hemostasis is achieved, a pressure dressing should be applied and the site and peripheral pulses should be monitored frequently per protocol.

5. Educate the patient about activity restrictions. The patient should be instructed to promptly report any chest pain, SOB, or moisture or warmth at the groin site (may indicate bleeding). Instruct the patient to apply pressure to dressing when coughing or laughing.

Critical Observations

Consult physician for the following:

1. Increase or onset of chest pain or angina symptoms
2. Hypotension or bradycardia
3. Significant oozing, bleeding, or hematoma formation
4. A change in quality or loss of peripheral pulses
5. Increased times in coagulation studies
6. The onset of dysrhythmias or ST and T-wave changes

PERCUTANEOUS VALVULOPLASTY (PV)

Clinical Brief

The purpose of PV is to restore normal blood flow through a previously stenotic cardiac valve. The procedure is similar to a cardiac catheterization. Percutaneous access is established and the patient receives anticoagulation therapy. For tricuspid, pulmonic, or mitral PV, venous approach is used. Mitral PV requires an atrial transseptal approach and creates an increased risk for complications. For aortic PV, the most common form, arterial approach is used. Regardless of which valve is involved, a specially equipped balloon-tip catheter is used. Once the valve is crossed with the catheter, the balloon is inflated and the commissures are split or the calcium nodules are fractured. Indications for PV include a documented (via an echocardiogram or a ventriculogram) critical flow gradient across a valve in high–surgical risk patients. Contraindications include heavy calcification associated with the stenosis.

Complications

- Leaflet tearing, annulus disruption
- Fragmentation of leaflets

- Loss of peripheral pulses related to thrombus formation at access site
- Embolization to brain
- Hematoma formation at percutaneous access site
- Cardiac tamponade
- Bleeding related to anticoagulation therapy
- Dysrhythmias secondary to local edema resulting from balloon manipulation
- Vasovagal reaction
- Left to right shunt related to transseptal approach
- Reaction to contrast agent

PATIENT CARE MANAGEMENT GUIDELINES

Patient Assessment

1. Assess VS every 15 minutes for four times, every 30 minutes for four times, every hour for two times, then per routine, if stable. Assess cardiac rhythm continuously via bedside monitor. Note rate/rhythm and/or ST segment, T-wave changes. The patient will most likely have CVP and PA catheters in place, and these readings should be included in the CV assessment. Changes in CVP readings, PAP readings, and/or heart sounds may indicate acute valvular failure, cardiac tamponade, or exacerbation of left to right shunt resulting from the transseptal approach, requiring emergency surgery. Heart sounds should be auscultated and murmurs noted. Diastolic murmurs may develop because the procedure corrects the stenotic valve. The patient also should be monitored for dysrhythmias.

2. Assess access site for oozing, ecchymosis, or hematoma with VS check. If a hematoma develops at the groin access site, apply direct pressure. The size of hematoma should be monitored; outline the borders with a skin-marking pen. A large amount of blood may exsanguinate into the retroperitoneum, groin, and upper thigh without seeing an early drop in SBP or an increase in HR; close observation of the access site is warranted.

3. Assess the patient comfort level every 1 to 2 hours for 12 to 24 hours. If pain develops at the groin access site, assess for local hematoma formation. Assess the patient for back discomfort.

4. Assess peripheral pulses (pedal and posttibial pulses) for strength and equality with VS check. A Doppler device may be helpful in identifying peripheral pulses, especially if the patient is cool.

5. Monitor coagulation studies as ordered.

Patient Management

1. Low-flow oxygen therapy should be administered.
2. The HOB should be elevated 30 degrees or less and the affected extremity should be kept straight to prevent dislodgment of the groin access sheath. Educate the patient on activity restrictions.
3. Maintain the hypercoagulated state per protocol.
4. If the patient was sedated during the procedure and remains sedated, institute aspiration and fall precautions until the patient is fully alert. Consider pulse oximetry.
5. If the patient becomes hypotensive, place the patient flat and administer fluid challenges as ordered. If the patient is brady-cardic, administer atropine per ACLS protocols.
6. If pain occurs at the groin access site, administer analgesics per protocol after bleeding has been ruled out. Reposition and medicate for back pain as ordered.
7. If a hematoma forms at the access site, apply direct pressure per unit protocol followed by a pressure dressing.
8. If nausea and/or vomiting occurs, administer antiemetics per protocol.

Sheath Removal

See PCI, p. 531.

Critical Observations

Consult physician for the following:

1. Significant changes in BP, CVP, and PA pressure readings
2. Muffling of heart sounds or development or changes in the quality of a murmur
3. Significant oozing, bleeding, or hematoma formation at the groin site
4. A change in quality or loss of peripheral pulses

PERIPHERAL ANGIOPLASTY OR LASER THERAPY

Clinical Brief

The purpose of angioplasty or laser therapy is to restore blood flow distal to the lesion. This is accomplished in the same manner as with PTCA or coronary artery laser therapy.

Complications

- Ischemia to organ system with reduced blood supply
- See PCI and sheath removal complications, p. 531.

PATIENT CARE MANAGEMENT GUIDELINES

Patient Assessment

Assessment is similar to patients undergoing PCI (see p. 531).

Monitor affected organ system for return of functioning or acute loss of function.

Patient Management

Management is similar to patients undergoing PCI (see p. 531).

Critical Observations

Critical observations are similar to patients undergoing PCI (see p. 531).

PERIPHERAL VASCULAR SURGERY (PVS)

Clinical Brief

Peripheral arterial occlusive disease applies to any disease involving the aorta, its major branches, and the arteries. The cause of occlusive arterial disease may be (1) vasospastic, as in Raynaud's phenomenon; (2) inflammatory, as in thromboangiitis obliterans (Buerger's disease); (3) atherosclerosis (arteriosclerosis obliterans), in which an atheroma obstructs part or all of the lumen of the vessel, or (4) trauma. These conditions cause ischemia of the distal peripheral tissues, resulting in pain and/or ultimately necrosis or gangrene, necessitating amputation.

Abdominal aortic aneurysms occur when there is a weakening in the wall or intimal tear of the aorta, resulting in increased aortic wall tension. Rupture of the aorta can lead to death. Aneurysms may be either fusiform, in which the entire circumference of the diseased segment has expanded, or saccular, in which there is an outpouching at the site of the diseased segment. Risk factors associated with aortic aneurysms are atherosclerosis, coronary artery disease (CAD) risks, cigarette smoking, uncontrolled hypertension, hyperlipidemia, Marfan's disease, syphilis, autoimmune disease, and trauma.

The purpose of PVS is to bypass and/or remove the occlusion and to restore blood flow distal to the lesion. Common surgical procedures (see Box 7-2) include thoracic aortic aneurysm repair, abdominal aortic aneurysm repair, aortofemoral bypass, iliofemoral bypass, or femoropopliteal bypass.

Complications

- Increased afterload (relative)
- Respiratory insufficiency/failure

- Acute graft occlusion
- GI ileus
- Graft leakage

PATIENT CARE MANAGEMENT GUIDELINES

See cardiac surgery, p. 515, for procedures requiring CPB.

Patient Assessment

1. A head-to-toe assessment should be completed on patient's arrival to the recovery area. The patient frequently should be assessed because instability often presents in the early postoperative period.
2. The CV system should be assessed every 15 minutes until stable and then per unit protocol. The assessment should include VS, CVP, PA pressures; cardiac rhythm; and incisional dressing. CT drainage (if present) and urine output should be monitored hourly. Hourly monitoring of peripheral pulses for presence and quality, along with an assessment of sensation and capillary refill is necessary to detect early onset of graft occlusion. Adjunctive devices such as Doppler are useful in detecting faint pulses. Mark pulse sites with a skin-marking pen. Warming the extremity with thermal blankets may increase peripheral pulse amplitude.
3. A cardiac profile including CO, CI, and SVRI should be done on admission, every 8 hours, and with any significant changes in hemodynamics and intervention.
4. Compare serial complete blood counts (CBCs) to detect significant blood loss requiring replacement with PRBCs.
5. Assess the patient's ability to take a deep breath. Auscultate lung sounds every 2 to 4 hours and as clinically indicated for adventitious sounds that may indicate atelectasis or pneumonia.
6. Assess for return of bowel sounds postoperatively and check abdominal girth daily to monitor for distention. Mark the sites of measurement with a skin-marking pen for consistency in assessments. Ileus is a common complication of PVS that includes a major abdominal incision.
7. Assess comfort level via pain scale, monitoring facial expression, and ability to take a deep breath.

Patient Management

1. Nitroprusside may be ordered to maintain SBP <120 mm Hg, diastolic blood pressure (DBP) <70 mm Hg, and SVRI in the

CV

normal range (1700-2600) to prevent leaking or rupture of anastomoses. Monitor MAP—a MAP of 70 mm Hg is critical in preventing acute graft occlusion. Titrate intravenous infusion to maintain SBP at 100 mm Hg or as ordered. Dose may range from 0.5 to 10 mcg/kg/min. Monitor patient for signs and symptoms of cyanide toxicity: tinnitus, blurred vision, delirium, and muscle spasm. Refer to facility policy and procedure for the administration of nitroprusside.

2. Pain management (see Chapter 2) is crucial in BP control and in the patient's ability to C&DB. Intravenous morphine sulfate, patient-controlled analgesia (PCA), or intraspinal analgesia (see p. 590) is usually ordered in the immediate postoperative period. If managing pain with intravenous morphine sulfate, give intravenous push (IVP) in 2-mg increments every 5 minutes to relieve symptoms.

3. Encourage the patient to use incentive spirometry and C&DB. Instruct the patient how to splint an abdominal or thoracic incision with a pillow to decrease pain while coughing or moving.

4. Leave the NG tube in place until bowel sounds return to prevent vomiting and to reduce the risk of aspiration. Early postoperative mobility may be the most important intervention in preventing an ileus. Metoclopramide (Reglan) may be used to stimulate return of gastric mobility. Administer 10 mg IV over 1 to 2 minutes as ordered.

Critical Observations

Consult physician for the following:
1. Inability to control hypertension
2. Changes in intensity or quality of peripheral pulses
3. Signs of bleeding

RADIOFREQUENCY CATHETER ABLATION

Clinical Brief

Radiofrequency catheter ablation is a nonsurgical treatment used primarily for treatment of supraventricular tachycardias associated with Wolff-Parkinson-White syndrome (WPW) and atrioventricular nodal reentry. It also has been used in the treatment of ventricular tachycardia. The procedure is done in a cardiac catheterization laboratory.

Radiofrequency current (delivered by a catheter positioned in the heart) is used to destroy or ablate accessory pathway(s) or arrhythmogenic area(s). Heart block may occur if the area ablated is in proximity to the atrioventricular node.

Complications

- AV block
- Arterial occlusion
- Infection
- Thromboembolism
- Hemorrhage/pseudoaneurysm at catheter site
- See PCI and sheath removal complications, p. 531.

PATIENT CARE MANAGEMENT GUIDELINES

Patient Assessment

1. Assess VS every 15 minutes for four times; every 30 minutes for two times; every hour until stable. Assess tissue perfusion (peripheral, cerebral, renal, GI, cardiopulmonary) with VS checks.
2. Assess cardiac rhythm continuously for dysrhythmias and ST segment changes via bedside monitor.
3. Assess for pulsatile groin mass, bruit, and/or report of acute tearing sensation or flank pain.
4. Check groin site and dressing with VS checks; if bleeding occurs, apply pressure to the site.

Patient Management

1. Keep patient on bed rest for 6 to 12 hours (or as ordered).
2. Prevent flexion of affected extremity.
3. Encourage fluids if not contraindicated.

Critical Observations

Consult physician for the following:

1. Vascular insufficiency: cold, pale, mottled extremity; absent or diminished pulse; or sudden pain
2. Renal insufficiency: decreased urine output, increased BUN and creatinine levels
3. Hemorrhage: uncontrolled bleeding at puncture site
4. Dysrhythmias compromising CO/CI
5. Cerebral ischemia: change in neurologic status or worsening neurologic deficits
6. Cardiac tamponade: hypotension, tachycardia, pallor or cyanosis, JVD, decrease in pulse pressure, decrease in heart sounds, tachypnea

7. Myocardial ischemia: chest discomfort, ST segment changes
8. Heart failure: S_3, crackles, increased HR, decreased urine output

TEMPORARY PACEMAKERS

Clinical Brief

The purpose of a temporary pacemaker is to provide an artificial stimulus to the myocardium when the heart is unable to initiate an impulse or when the conduction system is defective. Types of pacemakers include temporary (external or internal) or permanent. Pacing modes can be asynchronous (impulse generated at a fixed rate despite the rhythm of the patient) or synchronous (impulse generated on demand or as needed according to the patient's intrinsic rhythm).

Indications for pacing include symptomatic or asymptomatic second-degree heart block type II (Mobitz II); complete heart block; sick sinus syndrome; symptomatic bradycardia; tachydysrhythmias such as SVT, atrial fibrillation, or atrial flutter with rapid ventricular response; and intermittent VT unresponsive to drug therapy.

The external temporary pacemaker (transcutaneous pacemaker) is used to emergently treat symptomatic bradydysrhythmias unresponsive to medications until more definitive treatment can be employed. The external pacemaker includes a pulse generator, pacing cable attached to large external electrodes, and an ECG cable for the demand mode. Place the pacing electrodes per the manufacturer's instructions. Usually one electrode is placed at V_3 or V_4 anteriorly and the other is placed in the left subscapular area. The milliampere setting necessary to achieve consistent capture will vary. A setting up to 200 mA occasionally may be necessary, although 40 to 80 mA is often sufficient.

Temporary internal pacing can be accomplished via epicardial or transvenous electrodes. Some PA catheters are designed to accommodate transvenous pacing electrodes. Epicardial electrodes are placed on the epicardium during cardiac surgery and exit through the chest wall. Transvenous electrodes are threaded into the right atrium or right ventricle using a venous approach. These electrodes are attached to a pulse generator. The milliampere setting necessary to achieve consistent capture with internal electrodes is much less than with external electrodes; often a setting of 5 to 20 mA will be adequate.

Complications

- Muscle twitching
- Failure to capture

- Failure to pace
- Failure to sense

PATIENT CARE MANAGEMENT GUIDELINES

Patient Assessment

1. Monitor ECG for proper pacemaker functioning (e.g., evidence of capture: pacer spike immediately followed by a P wave or wide QRS).
2. Assess for palpable pulses with each QRS complex.
3. Assess mentation, capillary refill, urine output, HR, BP, skin color, and temperature.

Patient Management

1. Muscle twitching or chest wall discomfort occurs often with the use of external pacemakers. Sedation or analgesia is a standard of care.
2. Failure to pace:
   a. Check the power supply (i.e., battery) and all connections between generator and patient.
   b. If the external pacemaker is in use, check the electrodes for adequate surface contact: excessive hair at the electrode placement should be trimmed; however, shaving may cause nicks and increase chest impedance. If the patient rolls onto the side, poor chest wall contact may result. Secure electrodes as necessary. Change electrode pads every 8 hours when pacing, and every 24 hours when on standby.
   c. With transvenous or epicardial pacing, lead displacement or fracture may cause failure to pace. If the situation cannot be quickly remedied, prepare to externally pace the patient until more definitive treatment can be rendered.
3. Failure to capture (Figure 7-6):
   a. The problem may arise from any of the problems mentioned in the previous section; the same interventions are warranted.
   b. The problem may also be due to low output (milliampere) and may be corrected by increasing the milliamperes.
   c. Transvenous pacing: repositioning the patient to the left side may also correct the problem. This may promote electrode to contact myocardium.

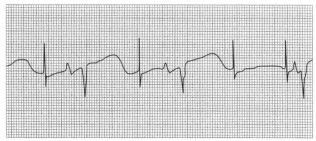

CV

Figure 7-6 Failure to capture. (From Stillwell S, Randall E: *Pocket guide to cardiovascular care,* St Louis, 1990, Mosby.)

      d. Always rule out physiologic conditions that may decrease the myocardial response to stimulation (e.g., hyperkalemia, acidosis, severe hypoxemia).

  4. Symptomatic hypotension may be a result of too slow a rate and may be corrected by merely increasing the rate.

  5. If defibrillation is required, defibrillate per unit protocol and then check pacer function.

  6. Failure to sense (Figure 7-7):

      a. Failure to sense may be a result of catheter tip migration, sensitivity setting too low (millivolts set too high), asynchronous mode selection, or battery failure.

      b. Turn the patient to the left side, change the power source (battery), or increase the sensitivity of the generator (by decreasing millivolts).

      c. For transvenous or epicardial pacing: if failure to sense is creating pacer spikes that are dangerously close to the pre-

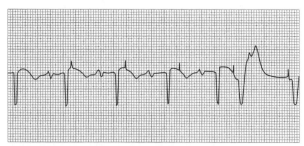

Figure 7-7 Failure to sense. (From Stillwell S, Randall E: *Pocket guide to cardiovascular care,* St Louis, 1990, Mosby.)

ceding T wave, change battery and consider turning off
the pacer and externally pacing the patient.
   d. Sustained dysrhythmias should be treated per ACLS protocol.

Critical Observations

Consult physician for the following:
   1. Failure to capture despite nursing interventions
   2. Failure to pace despite nursing interventions
   3. Failure to sense despite nursing interventions

THROMBOLYTIC THERAPY

Clinical Brief

The purpose of thrombolytic therapy is to lyse acutely formed
thrombi in the coronary artery and restore blood flow to the
myocardium. Thrombolytics also may be used to treat pulmonary
embolism, acute occlusion in peripheral vascular disease, and cerebral artery occlusion. Thrombolytic agents activate the conversion of
plasminogen to plasmin. Plasmin dissolves fibrin, thereby lysing the
clot. Current available thrombolytic agents are streptokinase,
alteplase, reteplase, anistreplase, and tenecteplase (Table 7-4).

   Traditional inclusion criteria for thrombolytic therapy include
chest pain or discomfort of ischemic nature lasting greater than

Table 7-4 THROMBOLYTICS

Name	Dose	Half-life
Alteplase (rt-PA), (t-PA)	15-mg bolus intravenously 0.75-mg/kg infusion over 30 min (≤50 mg) 0.50-mg/kg infusion over 60 min (≤35 mg)	4-5 min
Anistreplase (APSAC)	30 units IV over 5 min	90 min
Reteplase (r-PA)	10 units IV bolus, repeat in 30 min	13-16 min
Streptokinase (SK)	1.5 million units IV infusion over 1 hr	23 min
Tenecteplase (TNK)	Total dose ≤50 mg, based on weight (see package insert) given over 5-10 sec	20-24 min

IV, Intravenous.

30 minutes but less than 6 hours, chest pain unrelieved by nitroglycerin and ST segment elevation in two contiguous leads with or without Q waves. Current trend is to administer thrombolytics when PCI is not readily available or is contraindicated.

There are absolute and relative contraindications for the administration of thrombolytics. The absolute contraindications include previous hemorrhagic stroke, any other stroke within the past year, known intracranial neoplasm, active internal bleeding, and suspected aortic dissection. Relative contraindications include uncontrolled hypertension (>180/110 mm Hg), known bleeding disorder, major surgery or trauma within 2 weeks, noncompressible vascular punctures, pregnancy, active peptic ulcer, chronic severe hypertension, or previous allergic reaction.

Complications

- Acute reocclusion
- Reperfusion dysrhythmias
- Bleeding
- Allergic response (streptokinase, anistreplase)

PATIENT CARE MANAGEMENT GUIDELINES

Note: refer to policy and procedure and pharmacy protocol.

Patient Assessment

1. The CV system should be assessed on patient's arrival to the unit and every 15 minutes until the patient's condition is stable. This assessment should include pulse (P), RR, and BP and cardiac rhythm strip assessment. Carefully observe for and document rate, rhythm, ST segment, and T-wave changes. Monitor ECG lead with most significant ST elevation. Urinary output should be monitored hourly.
2. Obtain a baseline ECG and monitor serial ECGs as ordered to determine the efficacy of therapy as evidenced by normalization of ST segments and T waves. Although the patient may continue to experience minimal residual discomfort, notify physician of any change in the quality of pain.
3. Assess baseline neurologic status and monitor for change in LOC or other functions that may indicate intracranial bleeding.
4. Assess the patient for signs of bleeding. All recent puncture sites should be monitored for oozing or hematoma formation. Test all stools and emesis and dipstick urine for occult blood.
5. Monitor aPTT and CBC for acute changes. The aPTT is usually kept 2½ times normal during heparin therapy to prevent

thrombus formation. (Note: check ranges for aPTT based on reagent used.) Current standards include *lower*-dosed weight-adjusted heparin with thrombolytic therapy.

6. Monitor patient for allergic response: hives, fever, and rash.

Patient Management

1. Before the initiation of thrombolytic therapy, establish three IV access sites. If feasible, use double-lumen peripheral IV catheters. Avoid intramuscular (IM) injections and unnecessary trauma (e.g., continuous-use automatic BP cuffs). Insertion of a Foley catheter after therapy is initiated should be avoided.

2. Evaluate response to thrombolytic therapy by monitoring for pain relief, normalization of ST segments, and reperfusion dysrhythmias.

3. Nitroglycerin and/or morphine sulfate should be administered to treat angina. Recurrence of angina with documented ECG changes represents possible reocclusion, and the patient should be prepared for possible emergent cardiac catheterization, PTCA, or CABG surgery.

4. A wide variety of dysrhythmias occur with thrombolytic therapy, including nonsustained VT, bradydysrhythmias, junctional escape rhythms, and idioventricular rhythms. If the rhythm is self-limiting and the patient is asymptomatic, no treatment is needed. Symptomatic dysrhythmias are treated per ACLS protocol.

5. All puncture sites should be compressed until hemostasis is ensured.

6. Prophylactic antiulcer medication, such as intravenous H_2 blockers and/or PO antacids, may be ordered.

7. Educate the patient on bleeding precautions. Post a sign in the patient's room alerting other personnel of thrombolytic administration and bleeding precautions.

Critical Observations

Consult physician for the following:

1. Inability to achieve ordered PTT range
2. Signs of bleeding
3. Significant hematoma formation
4. New onset of chest pain
5. New changes in ECG after initial improvement
6. No change in ECG or pain level despite thrombolytic therapy
7. Neurologic changes

VENTRICULAR ASSIST DEVICES (VADS)

Clinical Brief

The purpose of a VAD is to maintain systemic circulation and improve tissue perfusion in patients with severe ventricular dysfunction while allowing the ventricle(s) to recover. Examples of VADs include resuscitative devices (CPB, extracorporeal membrane oxygenation systems), external nonpulsatile devices (Bio-Medicus, Sarns), external pulsatile assist devices (Thoratec VAD, Abiomed BVS 5000), and implantable left ventricular assist systems (Novacor LVAD, HeartMate LVAD). Both right and left VADs can be used if needed to support ventricular function. Improvement is generally observed within 48 hours.

Indications for a VAD include profound cardiogenic shock refractory to medications and counterpulsation and inability to wean from CPB. A VAD can also be used while the patient awaits cardiac transplantation. Contraindications include irreversible disease processes from which recovery is unlikely, although currently the VAD is being considered as a treatment option for end-stage heart failure.

Complications

See Complications Following Cardiac Surgery, p. 515.
- Significant postoperative bleeding
- Air embolus and thrombus
- Ventricular failure of unassisted ventricle
- Mechanical failure
- Sepsis

PATIENT CARE MANAGEMENT GUIDELINES

Note: follow the guidelines detailed under Cardiac Surgery (p. 515), as appropriate, in addition to the following:

Patient Assessment

1. A thorough assessment should be completed on the patient on arrival to the recovery area. The patient frequently should be assessed because of the instability present in the early postoperative period. Careful assessment of patient, tubing, VAD, and blood flow should be performed every 15 minutes until stable and then every hour.
2. Assess VS, CVP, PA pressures, cardiac rhythm, incision and dressing appearance, CT drainage, quality of the peripheral pulses, and urine output every 15 minutes until stable and then every hour.

3. A complete cardiac profile including CO/CI, and SVRI should be done on admission and every 1 to 2 hours. Note: thermodilution CO/CI is accurate only with LVADs, not RVADs.
4. Monitor serial Hgb and Hct levels and coagulation profiles as ordered for evidence of bleeding and/or coagulopathy.
5. Monitor temperature every 2 hours.

Patient Management

1. Once VS are stable, turn the patient every 2 hours unless contraindicated. Perform range of motion twice daily. Monitor for skin breakdown.
2. Avoid tension in the tubes; eliminating kinks in tubing will assist in preventing emboli or thrombi formation. The use of heparin via a continuous IV infusion may be necessary, especially with continuous flow devices. Use covers for tubing to prevent heat loss and hypothermia.
3. Monitor PA pressures and hemodynamics to maintain filling pressures. Maintain MAP >70 mm Hg.
4. RV failure may occur after initiation of LVAD use and may necessitate RVAD. Monitor for ↑ JVD, peripheral edema, ↑ BP, ↑ HR, fatigue, and weakness.
5. CT drainage in excess of 150 to 200 mL/hr for 2 hours may indicate increased bleeding and may require emergent thoracic reexploration. Excess bleeding may also be a result of coagulopathy. Serum coagulation profiles (e.g., PT, PTT, platelet count, fibrinogen) may reveal deficits requiring replacement with FFP, platelets, cryoprecipitate, and clotting factors. Anemia associated with excess bleeding can lead to relative hypoxemia and requires prompt replacement with PRBCs.
6. Prophylactic antibiotic therapy may be ordered.
7. If cardiac arrest occurs, internal cardiac massage and internal defibrillation should be substituted in the ACLS protocol.

Critical Observations

Consult physician for the following:

1. Dislodgment of cannulas
2. Tubing obstruction
3. Inability to maintain MAP
4. Evidence of infection
5. Bleeding
6. Neurologic changes
7. Decreased urine output

GASTROINTESTINAL (GI) MODALITIES

GASTROINTESTINAL (GI) INTUBATION

Clinical Brief

GI tubes are used to evacuate gastric contents, to decompress the stomach, to instill irrigants and/or medications, to tamponade (e.g., compress) the stomach and esophagus to temporarily control bleeding, and to provide enteral nutrition. Tubes used to evacuate and decompress the stomach are typically nasogastric, although these tubes may be placed orally in those patients with known or suspected basilar skull fractures or with recent transsphenoidal brain surgery. Nasointestinal tubes are rarely used for intestinal decompression in critical care units.

Enteral feedings may be delivered to the stomach. However, most critically ill patients have gastric atony, resulting in impaired motility and absorption of stomach feedings. Therefore, the preferred route for delivery of enteral feedings is at a site that is distal to the pylorus of the stomach (e.g., postpylorically), into either the duodenum or the jejunum. This may be accomplished by using weighted nasoduodenal feeding tubes, or via percutaneous insertion of jejunostomy tubes. In those patients who may anticipate long-term enteral feeding (e.g., >6 weeks), a percutaneous endoscopic gastrostomy tube (PEG) may be placed when the critical illness resolves and gastric peristalsis returns (refer to Nutrition: Enteral Feedings, p. 561).

Complications

General complications of NG suctioning of gastric contents:
- Hypovolemia
- Electrolyte imbalances (particularly loss of potassium)
- Disruption of acid/base balance, and aspiration of stomach contents
- Skin breakdown and pressure ulcer formation at insertion site

Less common complications may include:
- Esophageal ulceration or rupture
- Otitis media, sinusitis, and parotitis

GENERAL PATIENT CARE MANAGEMENT GUIDELINES (NG TUBE)

Patient Assessment

1. Before insertion, assess for history of nasal surgery, nasal fractures, or deviated septum. Notify physician if history is positive.

2. Assess LOC; patients with altered mentation may inadvertently remove the NG tube.

3. Examine the nares daily for redness or skin breakdown.

4. Be alert for complications related to nasoenteric intubation.

Patient Management

1. Once proper tube placement is confirmed, secure the tube per facility policy. Prevent movement at the nares to avoid skin irritation.

2. Attach to appropriate amount and type of suction as prescribed by the physician. If tube has an air vent, leave the port open to air.

3. Provide meticulous mouth care: teeth brushing, mouthwash, lozenges if permitted. Mucous membranes should be kept moist; apply lip balm as needed.

4. Provide care to nares daily: clean perinasal area and replace tape that anchors tube, taking care not to either advance or withdraw tubing. Reassess for tube placement as needed.

5. Keep HOB elevated to prevent the possibility of aspiration.

6. Irrigate the tube as ordered to ensure patency. Validate tube irrigation with physician if the patient has undergone gastric surgery.

7. Check placement of the tube before administering anything down the tube. Flush before and after instillation of medications. Clamp tube for 30 to 45 minutes after the instillation of medications.

8. To obtain a gastric pH reading, have the patient lie on the left side; stop NG suction and withdraw 10 to 15 mL; discard fluid and use a second syringe to withdraw a sample for testing. Use pH paper with appropriate pH range. Do not use the syringe used for antacid administration to obtain the gastric sample. Generally gastric pH should be kept >3.5 to decrease the chance for stress ulcers. An inability to raise pH >4 may indicate sepsis.

9. Record color, consistency, and amount of drainage.

Nasogastric (NG) Tube Patient Care Management

1. Check placement of tube in the stomach by aspirating with a syringe and testing pH of aspirate. Instill 10 to 30 mL of air into the tube and auscultate the gastric area: air rushing or gurgling will be heard if the tube is in the proper position.

2. See p. 561 for information on enteral feedings.

Nasoduodenal Feeding Tube Patient Care Management

1. If inserting a feeding tube that requires a stylet to facilitate placement, never reinsert the stylet into the tube after it is placed in the patient.

2. Tip of most feeding tubes should be postpyloric. Placing the patient in a right side–lying position may enhance tube advancement. Premedicating the patient with metoclopramide 10 mg IV may facilitate intubation, particularly if the patient is not receiving concurrent opioid agents, but its overall efficacy is unclear. Insufflating the stomach with 350 to 500 mL of air is advocated by some experts to help facilitate tube transit to the duodenum, but its overall efficacy is likewise unclear. Some patients may require fluoroscopic or endoscopic guidance if intubation of the duodenum is not achieved after several attempts.

3. Feeding tubes require radiographic verification of position before feedings can begin.

4. See information on p. 561 for enteral feedings.

Sengstaken-Blakemore and Minnesota Tube Patient Care Management

1. Intubation is recommended before insertion of a Sengstaken-Blakemore (Figure 7-8) or Minnesota tube to protect the airway from aspiration.

2. Tube placement is verified by air injection into the stomach or aspiration of gastric contents. A radiograph confirms the position of the gastric balloon against the cardia of the stomach.

3. After radiographic verification, the gastric balloon is inflated with 200 to 500 mL of air. Many institutions require a football helmet to be placed on the patient's head to secure the tractioned tube to the helmet. Be sure the helmet is a proper fit. A Salem sump is inserted into the esophagus to remove secretions if a Sengstaken-Blakemore tube is used because the patient will not be able to swallow. A gastric aspirate port and Salem sump (or esophageal aspirate port) are connected to low suction.

4. The esophageal balloon is inflated only after radiographic confirmation of the position of the gastric balloon and if bleeding continues. Pressure in the esophageal balloon (usually 2-25 mm Hg) should be checked every 2 hours to be sure it does not exceed 40 mm Hg. Esophageal balloon deflation should be done every 4 hours for 10 minutes by physician's order only. The gastric balloon is never deflated while the

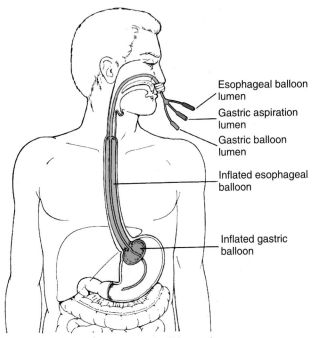

Figure 7-8 Sengstaken-Blakemore tube.

esophageal balloon is inflated. Generally the tube is not left inflated for more than 48 hours.

5. Scissors should be kept at the bedside to cut the balloon ports in case of airway obstruction from upward migration of the tube.

6. All ports of the tube should be clearly labeled. Never inject fluids in the esophageal port. Normal saline (NS) irrigation may be needed to keep the gastric aspirate port patent.

7. If bleeding appears to have stopped, the esophageal balloon is slowly deflated. Traction is relaxed on the gastric balloon and gastric aspirate is monitored for recurrence of bleeding. All air from the esophageal and gastric balloon is aspirated before the tube is removed.

8. Hgb and Hct levels are usually monitored every 2 to 4 hours. A drop in Hct by 3% indicates one unit of blood lost.

9. An acute onset of abdominal or back pain may indicate esophageal rupture.

Critical Observations

Consult physician for the following:

1. Fluid, electrolyte, or acid-base imbalance from prolonged gastric suctioning
2. Possible esophageal or gastric rupture and patient showing signs of shock
3. Respiratory distress from tube displacement or aspiration
4. Reports of ear or neck pain associated with otitis media or parotitis
5. Increasing abdominal distention
6. Obstructed tube that will not irrigate
7. Inability to remove the tube
8. Gastric pH <3.5 or value specified by physician

GASTROINTESTINAL (GI) SURGERY

Clinical Brief

Surgical intervention may be required to control gastric bleeding or relieve an intestinal obstruction if conservative medical therapy fails. The primary aim of surgery in either of these cases is to control the inciting source that can lead to shock, the systemic inflammatory response syndrome (SIRS), and multiple organ dysfunction syndrome (MODS). A secondary aim of GI surgical intervention is to prevent recurrence. Common surgical procedures to treat gastric ulcers may include laparoscopic vagotomy, pyloroplasty, and antrectomy accompanied by gastroduodenostomy with or without vagotomy. Common surgical procedures to treat duodenal ulcers may include vagotomy with antrectomy and either a gastroduodenostomy (Billroth I) or gastrojejunostomy (Billroth II). These procedures partially neutralize gastric acid and remove stimuli for acid secretion.

Surgical intervention to relieve a GI obstruction may be indicated for GI intussusception, perforation, rupture, or immovable masses. The nature of the surgery indicated is highly variable and depends on the site and extent of the obstruction, the surgical risk status of the patient, and the presence of other concomitant illnesses. In general, surgical intervention for GI obstruction occurs less commonly than in years past because of the advent of effective nonsurgical interventions other than gastrointestinal tubes. Pharmacologic agents that enhance GI motility that may be indicated include metoclopramide and octreotide. Instilling air via colonoscopy may be a useful nonsurgical intervention to relieve intussusception. When surgery is required, it often involves end-to-end anastomosis and may involve placement of a permanent or temporary colostomy.

Esophageal varices can be corrected with ligation or banding via endoscopy, sclerotherapy via endoscopy, or with a radiologically guided insertion of a transjugular intrahepatic portosystemic shunt (TIPS). Other surgically inserted shunts less commonly used include portacaval and distal splenorenal. Shunts decrease venous blood flow through the portal system and consequently reduce portal hypertension.

Complications

- Hemorrhage
- Infection (e.g., peritonitis, wound infection)
- Paralytic ileus
- Atelectasis
- Pneumonia
- Dumping syndrome
- Wound dehiscence

PATIENT CARE MANAGEMENT GUIDELINES

Patient Assessment

1. Assess hemodynamic status: a HR >100 beats/min, SBP <90 mm Hg, CVP <2 mm Hg, and a PAWP <4 mm Hg are signs of hypovolemia. A MAP <60 mm Hg reflects inadequate tissue perfusion. Assess the surgical dressing for excessive bleeding or drainage, or bleeding or drainage that is not diminishing over time. Review serial Hgb and Hct levels. Measure I&O hourly, including drainage from all tubes and drains. Urine output should be >30 mL/hr; 50 mL/hr is more desirable. Determine fluid balance every 8 hours: output should approximate intake. Compare serial weights to evaluate rapid changes (0.5-1 kg/day indicates fluid imbalance; 1 kg equals approximately 1000 mL fluid). Note skin turgor on the inner thigh or forehead, the condition of buccal membranes, and development of edema or crackles. Gastric surgery: NG drainage may be bright red postoperatively but should become dark red or brown within 12 hours after surgery; drainage should normalize to green-yellow within 24 to 36 hours postoperatively.
2. Continuously monitor ECG for lethal dysrhythmias that may result from electrolyte imbalance, hypoxemia, and hemorrhage.
3. Assess respiratory status: note depth, rate, and skin color every 15 minutes postoperatively until stable, then every 1 to 2

hours. Patients with abdominal surgery tend to take shallow breaths secondary to incisional pain.

4. Assess GI function: epigastric pain, tachycardia, and hypotension may signal gastric dilation; distention, rebound tenderness, or rigidity may signal internal bleeding. Note any hiccups or complaints of fullness or gagging and auscultate abdomen for return of bowel sounds.

5. Assess pain using patient's self-report whenever possible. See p. 35, acute pain. Note that opioid analgesic agents can cause diminished peristalsis.

6. Record temperature and monitor for development of infection: assess incision, intravenous sites, and drain sites. Consider the urinary tract and lungs as potential sites of infection. Review serial WBC counts and culture reports (if available).

7. Assess neurologic status, development of GI bleeding, and onset of ascites at intervals per orders or institutional protocols in patients after placement of portacaval shunts.

Patient Management

1. Provide supplemental oxygen as ordered (see p. 503 for information on ventilation therapies).

2. Administer intravenous fluids and/or blood products as ordered to correct intravascular volume and replace blood loss.

3. Monitor serum electrolyte levels and replace as ordered.

4. Use sterile procedure when manipulating GI tubes, surgical dressings, and indwelling lines. Protect the integrity of the skin during frequent dressing changes by using skin protectant products. Consult with wound/skin clinical nurse specialist as needed. Use an abdominal binder to protect against wound dehiscence as needed for patients with extensive surgical wounds and at risk for poor wound healing (e.g., patients who are older, who have diabetes, who concomitantly take corticosteroid agents, or who are hypoalbuminemic).

5. Maintain patency of the NG tube to prevent undue pressure on suture line. Do not irrigate or reposition tubes without the physician's order. Provide good care of the nares and mouth. Test gastric secretions for blood and pH. Generally gastric pH is maintained between 3.5 and 5 to prevent further development of stress ulcers. Proton pump inhibitors, H_2-receptor antagonists, and/or antacids may be prescribed.

6. Administer antiemetics to prevent vomiting and preserve the integrity of the suture line.

7. Administer nutritional supplements or support as ordered. Vitamin B_{12} will be ordered for patients undergoing a total gastrectomy to prevent pernicious anemia. Oral feedings may not be instituted until bowel sounds have returned.

8. Administer analgesics as indicated because abdominal pain may interfere with adequate ventilation; note RR before and after medication administration. Preemptively medicate patients for pain with opioid analgesia by administering via a PCA pump, with a set basal rate. Evaluate effectiveness of pain medication (see Chapter 2).

9. Assist patient with turning, coughing, and deep breathing at least every 2 hours to maintain oxygenation and prevent atelectasis.

Critical Observations

Consult physician for the following:

1. Signs of hypovolemia: increasing trend in HR; decreasing trend in urine output, CVP, PA pressures, and BP
2. Respiratory distress, new onset of crackles or cough
3. Temperature elevation or signs of infection
4. A sudden change in the color of or sudden increase in surgical or NG drainage
5. Increasing abdominal distention
6. Absence of drainage from the NG tube
7. Urine output <30 mL/hr or <0.5 mL/kg/hr
8. Wound dehiscence
9. Abnormal laboratory data
10. Uncontrolled pain

LIVER TRANSPLANTATION

Clinical Brief

Liver transplantation may be considered in patients with end-stage liver disease that is irreversible despite optimal medical management. The majority of liver transplants are performed on patients with chronic hepatocellular disease that may be a consequence of hepatitis B or C, alcohol-induced disease, or autoimmune hepatitis. End-stage liver disease may also be a consequence of chronic cholestatic diseases, including primary sclerosing cholangitis, primary biliary cirrhosis, or biliary atresia or metabolic liver disease, including Wilson's disease or hemochromatosis.

In general, contraindications for liver transplant include a known active extrahepatic malignancy or infection, severe cardiac or pulmonary disease, multisystem disease, active abuse of hepatotoxic drugs including alcohol, human immunodeficiency virus (HIV) antibody–positive status, and perceived inability to adhere to immunosuppressive regimen. One-year survival rates after transplant have improved to 84%; 5-year survival is >70%, with best results in patients with cholestatic liver disease and poorest results in patients with hepatitis C and hepatobiliary malignancy. The most important determinant of survival is the patient's clinical condition at the time of transplant.

Complications

- Hyperacute rejection
- Acute rejection
- Infection
- Hemorrhage
- Acute liver failure (encephalopathy, ascites, coagulopathy)
- Paralytic ileus
- Acute renal failure
- Hemorrhage
- Atelectasis
- Pneumonia

PATIENT CARE MANAGEMENT GUIDELINES

Patient Assessment

1. Assess hemodynamic status: CVP, PA pressures, CI, HR, and BP. Patients in liver failure often have an increased CI and decreased SVRI before surgery; this may continue into the early postoperative period. Fluid shifts often occur, affecting circulating volume. Hemorrhage may also occur, and Hgb and Hct level should be monitored. Hypertension is often seen postoperatively.

2. Assess fluid status: measure I&O hourly, including drainage from all tubes and drains. Urine output should be >30 mL/hr; 50 mL/hr is more desirable. Determine fluid balance every 8 hours. Compare serial weights to evaluate rapid changes (0.5-1 kg/day indicates fluid imbalance). Note skin turgor on inner thigh or forehead, condition of buccal membranes, and development of edema or crackles.

3. Assess tissue perfusion: note level of mentation, skin color and temperature, peripheral pulses, and capillary refill.

4. Continuously monitor ECG for dysrhythmias that may result from electrolyte imbalance, hypoxemia, and/or hemorrhage.

5. Assess temperature. Patients may be hypothermic on returning from surgery. Monitor for signs of infection: incision lines, T-tube site, drain tubes. Consider the urinary tract, lungs, and mucous membranes as potential sites of infection, especially because of immunosuppression. Review serial WBC counts and culture reports (if available).

6. Assess respiratory status: note depth, rate, and skin color every 15 minutes postoperatively until stable, then every 1 to 2 hours. Monitor pulse oximetry continuously and ABGs as ordered. Patients with abdominal surgery tend to take shallow breaths secondary to incisional pain.

7. Assess GI function: reaccumulation of ascites, bowel sounds. Abdominal tenderness, nausea and vomiting (N/V), or abdominal distention may indicate ileus or a more significant event (e.g., bowel infarction, hemorrhage). Measure abdominal girth every shift.

8. Monitor for clinical manifestations of acute rejection, which may include fever, headaches, nausea, vomiting, chills, general malaise, increasing weight, and an increasing bilirubin level. Assess bile production: quality and quantity. Bile should be thick and viscous and range from dark gold to brown. Variation from these findings may indicate a primary nonfunctioning graft.

9. Assess pain using the patient's self-report whenever possible (see Chapter 2).

10. Assess liver function: monitor coagulation times, potassium and glucose levels, and liver function tests closely. Normal coagulation times, decreased potassium levels, increased glucose levels, and decreased liver function tests indicate a functioning liver. Decreased coagulation times, increased potassium levels, decreased glucose levels, and continued elevation of liver function tests are indicative of a nonfunctioning liver.

11. Monitor acid-base balance. Patients are often in a metabolic alkalosis in the first 24 to 48 hours because of the large citrate load, decreased potassium level, diuretics, and large amounts of FFP.

12. Monitor neurologic status. Patients receiving tacrolimus may experience neurologic adverse effects that may include tremors, confusion, encephalopathy, and seizures.

GI

13. Assess renal function: monitor BUN and creatinine levels daily. Patients receiving tacrolimus or mycophenolate mofetil are at risk for renal failure.

Patient Management

1. Provide supplemental oxygen as ordered (see p. 503 for information on ventilation therapies).
2. Administer intravenous fluids and/or blood products as ordered to correct intravascular volume and to replace blood loss and coagulation factors.
3. Monitor serum electrolyte levels, and replace as ordered.
4. Use sterile procedure when manipulating GI tubes, surgical dressings, and indwelling lines. Protect the integrity of the skin by using skin protectants and consulting with wound/skin clinical nurse specialist.
5. Maintain patency of the NG tube to prevent undue pressure on suture line. Do not irrigate or reposition tubes without physician's order. Provide good care of the nares and mouth.
6. Administer corticosteroids, azathioprine, tacrolimus, mycophenolate mofetil, and/or OKT3 as ordered. Monitor for side effects.
7. Administer pain medication as ordered and evaluate its effectiveness and safety. (Use a sedation scale to monitor sedation level and prevent opioid-induced respiratory depression; see Sedation Scale, p. 41.)
8. Assist patient with turning, coughing, and deep breathing at least every 2 hours once extubated to maximize oxygenation and prevent atelectasis.
9. Administer prophylactic antibiotics as ordered.
10. Administer meticulous skin and mouth care, using nystatin for oral care.
11. When the patient is able to eat, ensure a high-calorie, high-protein diet because protein synthesis is decreased by liver damage and steroids have a catabolic effect.

Critical Observations

Consult physician for the following:

1. Signs of hypovolemia: increasing trend in HR; decreasing trend in urine output, CVP, PA pressures, and BP
2. Signs of respiratory distress; onset of crackles or cough
3. Temperature elevation or signs of infection
4. Change in bile production or drainage; increase in serum bilirubin

5. Increasing abdominal distention and tenderness, particularly at site of wound or T-tube

6. Increased potassium levels, decreased glucose levels, abnormal coagulation times, and increased liver function tests

7. Urine output <30 mL/hr, increasing BUN and creatinine levels

8. Uncontrolled pain

NUTRITION: ENTERAL FEEDINGS

Clinical Brief

The stress of critical illness causes an acceleration of patients' metabolic rates, referred to as *stress hypermetabolism*. A necessary consequence of stress hypermetabolism is catabolism or muscle breakdown. The critically ill experience varying rates of hypermetabolism and catabolism, based partly on the type and magnitude of the critical illness. Delivering enteral nutrients to patients early during the course of a critical illness is thought to attenuate stress hypermetabolism and catabolism and is believed to diminish the likelihood of occurrence of colonic bacterial translocation, which can result in sepsis.

Enteral feedings are liquid formula diets that are provided orally directly into either the stomach or the small intestine and are indicated to try and meet the patient's nutritional or metabolic needs. Intermittent bolus feedings infused by gravity are recommended when feedings are instilled into the stomach and are only rarely indicated for critically ill patients. Most critically ill patients receive enteral nutrients via the duodenum or jejunum, either from a nasoduodenal/jejunal tube or via a percutaneous approach (e.g., jejunostomy), using a continuous feeding pump. These sites are preferred because they bypass the stomach, which is often atonic during critical illness; they cause less bowel distention; they cause less fluid and electrolytic imbalance; and they are associated with less aspiration. The type of commercially prepared dietary formula and its strength and rate of infusion are selected based partly on the patient's nutritional and metabolic needs and partly on whether the patient has concomitant illnesses that can be attenuated or accelerated based on the metabolic by-products of the feeding formula chosen.

Preparations

Generally, all products contain carbohydrates, fats, proteins, vitamins, minerals, and water but vary in the amounts and types of each nutrient. Complete (polymeric) formulas require digestion and thus an intact GI tract. Elemental (monomeric or oligomeric) formulas are predigested and can be absorbed in GI tracts with limited digestion. Specially designed products are available in both forms for specific disease states or conditions.

Patients with hepatic encephalopathy may receive Travasorb-Hepatic or Hepatic Aid II because they contain high quantities of branched-chain amino acids. Amin-Aid or Travasorb-Renal may be prescribed for patients in renal failure because these formulas attempt to decrease the urea production. Patients who are burned or septic may be prescribed Stresstein, Criticare, or Traum-Aid, which attempt to stimulate protein synthesis and reduce proteolysis. Patients in respiratory failure having difficulty weaning from the ventilator may be prescribed Pulmocare or formulas with increased fat content, which attempt to reduce CO_2 production, oxygen consumption, and ventilatory requirements. Some formulas contain immunomodulatory agents that may include glutamine or arginine; however, their efficacy in attenuating SIRS or in treating patients with sepsis is controversial.

Most formulas are isotonic and provide about 45 g of protein per liter, although hypertonic formulas are available. High-fiber (Jevity) and low-residue (Resource, Fortison) formulas are available, as are supplements that provide extra calories (Microlipid, ProMode, MCT oil).

Isotonic formulas are usually administered at full strength, and the rate is increased as tolerated. Hypertonic formulas are initially administered either at full strength at a slow rate (25 mL/hr) or half strength at 50 mL/hr. Intolerance of hypertonic formulas may be indicated by severe diarrhea, electrolytic depletion, and dehydration.

Contraindications

There are few contraindications to feeding critically ill patients enterally. It is almost always preferred over the parenteral route for delivering nutrients because it is associated with fewer complications, is less expensive, and is more physiologic. Even patients with diminished peristalsis can still tolerate minimal amounts of feedings, at rates of 15 to 25 mL/hr. Although this minimal infusion rate will not meet nutritional needs, it can preserve the metabolic requirements of the colonic enterocytes, thus preventing the translocation of colonic bacteria and thwarting the onset of sepsis. Enteral feedings are contraindicated only in patients with a high-output fistula, diffuse peritonitis, multiple gut perforations, or a complete mechanical bowel obstruction.

Complications

- Aspiration of feedings
- Diarrhea
- Fluid, electrolyte, or acid-base imbalances

Underfeeding

- Loss of lean body mass
- Difficulty weaning from mechanical ventilation
- Delayed wound healing

Overfeeding

- Hepatic steatosis
- Acute renal failure
- Hyperglycemia

PATIENT CARE MANAGEMENT GUIDELINES

Patient Assessment

1. Assess nutritional status; prealbumin is considered the best indicator of nutritional status. Serum albumin <3.5 g/dL, transferrin <180 mg/dL, and lymphocytes <1500/mL are indications of malnourishment. Skin anergy testing (negative response to antigen) represents malnutrition. A 24-hour urinary urea nitrogen study measures nitrogen balance by subtracting the amount of nitrogen lost from the daily intake in either enteral or parenteral sources. Creatinine-height index measures the amount of creatinine excreted in a 24-hour period proportionately to the height of the patient and reflects muscle wasting. Anthropometric measurements of body size can be taken. Triceps skinfold thickness <3 mm indicates severely depleted fat stores; a midarm circumference <15 cm means muscle wasting. Measure height and weight and compare with desired-weight tables. A decrease of 15% from ideal weight indicates impaired nutrition.

2. Assess GI tolerance: note nausea, vomiting, diarrhea, or cramping and any abdominal distention or absence of bowel sounds; the infusion rate may need to be reduced if these symptoms appear.

3. Monitor flow rates and volumes to ensure that the patient is actually receiving the prescribed amount of calories because continuous feedings are often interrupted.

Patient Management

1. Insufflation of air and aspiration of gastric contents do not confirm placement of nasoenteric tubes. Confirmation with

radiography is necessary before feedings are initiated. Mark feeding tube with indelible marker at exit site once placement is confirmed.

2. With continuous feedings, elevate the HOB 30 degrees at all times (if not otherwise contraindicated) to reduce the risk of aspiration.

3. Small bowel feedings are generally initiated at 50 mL/hr with full-strength isotonic solution. A hypertonic formula can be diluted to quarter strength or half strength. Gradually increase the rate, usually 25 mL every 8 hours, and strength of the formula; evaluate patient tolerance.

4. For intragastric feedings, generally, tube feedings are initiated with an isotonic formula and the nutrient requirements are achieved by increasing the rate over 1 to 2 days.

5. Check residuals at least every 4 hours for patients receiving continuous gastric feedings. If more than 100 to 200 mL (per institutional protocol), hold the feedings and check again for residuals in 2 hours. Metoclopramide (Reglan) or octreotide (Sandostatin) may be ordered to increase gastric motility. Small-bore feeding tubes often collapse when aspirating for residuals. Observe the patient for abdominal distention.

6. Administer using a feeding pump. Change the bag, tubing, and solution every 24 hours to prevent transmission of bacteria or other organisms.

7. Flush the feeding tube with 20 to 50 mL of water once a shift, unless the patient is fluid restricted. Flush the tube if the feeding has been stopped for any reason and after administering medications via the tube.

8. Some medications are available in elixir form and can be administered via tube. Be wary of diarrhea because many elixirs are sorbitol based. Consult with a pharmacist if tablets must be crushed, to ensure that they can be administered efficaciously via this route. Sustained-release and enteric-coated medications may not be crushed. Change to elixirs. Flush the tube before and after medication administration.

9. Provide good oral care because mouth breathing is common in patients who have a nasal tube.

10. When flushing or irrigating small-bore tubing, use the syringe size recommended by the manufacturer. A small syringe can exert greater pressure with minimal effort and may rupture the tube.

11. If the patient develops diarrhea, consider using premixed sterile bags of tube feeding and bulk-forming cathartics.

Critical Observations

Consult physician for the following:

1. Gastric residual >200 mL
2. Uncontrolled diarrhea
3. Increasing abdominal distention, N/V, absent bowel sounds
4. Elevated temperature or signs of infection
5. Possible aspiration or signs of respiratory distress; onset of crackles or cough
6. Elevated serum glucose level
7. Elevated BUN and creatinine; urine output <30 mL/hr or <0.5 mL/kg/hr
8. Electrolyte imbalances
9. Increase in serum liver enzymes and bilirubin
10. Dehydration: dry buccal membranes, nonelastic skin turgor, specific gravity >1.035
11. Tube displacement
12. Mucosal damage from tube

NUTRITION: PARENTERAL

Clinical Brief

In the event the patient does not receive sufficient nutrition with enteral feedings or cannot functionally be fed through the stomach or bowel, parenteral nutrition (PN) containing the required water, nutrients, protein, carbohydrates, fats, electrolytes, vitamins, and minerals may be initiated. PN must be administered via a central line. Parenteral delivery is an option only for patients with limited nutritional and metabolic needs; the higher metabolic requirements of the critically ill can only be met with a highly concentrated solution that must be infused centrally. Dextrose is the primary nutrient source in PN and should comprise approximately 50% to 60% of daily caloric intake. Amino acids, electrolytes, vitamins, and minerals can be tailored to meet additional nutritional needs of the patient. Regular laboratory assessment (nutritional panel) and anthropometric measurements provide information to guard against underfeeding and overfeeding, conditions that can adversely affect pulmonary, renal, and hepatic functioning.

Lipids

Approximately 2% to 4% of nutrients must be given in the form of fats to maintain systemic cellular membrane competency and improve wound healing. This may be accomplished by either giving lipid emulsions (10%, 20%, and 30% solutions) to supplement total parenteral nutrition (TPN) solutions three times weekly or by adding lipids to a total nutrient admixture (TNA) solution that delivers all parenteral nutrients in one solution. Generally, lipids should constitute 15% to 30% of total daily caloric intake.

Complications

- Infection
- Sepsis
- Hyperglycemia

Catheter-related complications (see p. 608)

Underfeeding

- Loss of lean body mass
- Difficulty weaning from mechanical ventilation
- Delayed wound healing

Overfeeding

- Hepatic steatosis
- Acute renal failure
- Hyperglycemia

PATIENT CARE MANAGEMENT GUIDELINES

Patient Assessment

1. Monitor temperature at least once each shift to evaluate the onset of infection. Unexplained fever may be related to central venous catheter (CVC) sepsis.
2. Assess intravenous catheter insertion site for redness, drainage, or tenderness.
3. Check serum glucose level as ordered to identify onset of hyperglycemia. Glucose levels should not exceed 150 mg/dL. Provide glycemic control through administering insulin supplements as needed and as ordered. An acute onset of hyperglycemia may signal sepsis.
4. Review laboratory results for metabolic abnormalities associated with PN therapy: serum glucose, electrolytes, CBC, platelet count, potassium, phosphate, calcium, magnesium, BUN, creatinine, alkaline phosphatase, bilirubin, PT, iron, uric acid, and aspartate aminotransferase (AST) (serum glutamic-oxaloacetic transaminase [SGOT]).
5. Monitor total lymphocyte count and serum albumin and transferrin levels to determine efficacy of PN.
6. Assess fluid volume status: compare daily weights and record I&O. Note signs and symptoms of dehydration or fluid overload.

7. If the patient is mechanically ventilated or has a history of CO_2 retention, assess CO_2 levels.

8. Central line placement must be confirmed via chest radiograph before administration of any solutions through the lines.

Patient Management

1. Do not administer medications, blood products, or any other intravenous solution through the nutrition-dedicated line. If long-term PN is necessary, a long-term central venous access device may be required. See p. 608 for information on central venous access devices.

2. To prevent infection, use aseptic technique when performing dressing or tubing changes. Change dressing and tubing per hospital guidelines or if dressing becomes soiled or nonocclusive. Keep all solutions refrigerated, check expiration dates, and administer within 24 hours of preparation. Do not use the PN if the solution contains particulates or has expired. Each patient's PN solution is formulated specifically for him or her and is not interchangeable with other patients' PN solution. Luer-Lok all tubing connections to prevent inadvertent disconnection and a possible air embolus.

3. Validate correct nutritional components and infuse as ordered. Initial rate is usually 50 to 100 mL/hr and titrated up as tolerated to meet patient's nutritional needs.

4. Do not stop PN abruptly because rebound hypoglycemia can result. If PN is not available, administer $D_{10}W$ at the PN rate until the solution is available. To avoid inconsistent delivery rates that may precipitate rebound hypoglycemia or hyperglycemia reactions, use an infusion pump to administer PN.

5. Insulin added to the PN solution or on a sliding scale is usually required to control hyperglycemia. Check glucose levels every 6 hours.

6. Fat supplements may be prescribed, if the patient is not receiving TNA. Initial therapy requires a slow infusion rate for the first 15 to 30 minutes (1 mL/min for a 10% emulsion, 0.5 mL/min for a 20% emulsion); monitor the patient for respiratory distress associated with hypoxemia and cyanosis. If no adverse effects occur, initiate the prescribed infusion rate. Blood samples to measure serum triglyceride and liver function tests may be obtained to determine the patient's ability to use lipids.

Critical Observations

Consult with physician for the following:

1. Temperature elevation or signs of infection
2. Catheter displacement or thrombosis
3. Fluid overload or dehydration: dry buccal membranes, nonelastic skin turgor, specific gravity >1.035
4. Elevated serum glucose level
5. Electrolyte imbalances
6. Elevated BUN and creatinine; urine output <30 mL/hr or <0.5 mL/kg/hr
7. Increase in serum liver enzymes and bilirubin

GI

PANCREAS TRANSPLANTATION

Clinical Brief

Pancreas transplantation may be considered in patients with type 1 diabetes with end-stage renal disease (or imminent end-stage renal disease) who have had a kidney transplant or plan to have a simultaneous pancreas-kidney (SPK) transplant. If possible, SPK is a preferred procedure to transplanting a donor pancreas at a time after the recipient has already received a donor kidney because rates of rejection are lower with SPK. It is rare that patients are eligible to receive a donor pancreas in the absence of significant renal failure. This may be considered in patients who have recurrent, life-threatening problems associated with being unable to achieve glycemic control.

Contraindications to receiving a donor pancreas include an active neoplasm, positive HIV status, sepsis, severe cardiovascular or pulmonary disease, and a perceived inability to adhere to the immunosuppression regimen.

Complications

- Hyperacute rejection
- Acute rejection
- Infection
- Hemorrhage
- Acute pancreatitis
- Paralytic ileus
- Acute renal failure
- Anastomotic leaks
- Urethritis (in male patients)
- Atelectasis
- Pneumonia

PATIENT CARE MANAGEMENT GUIDELINES

Patient Assessment

1. Assess hemodynamic status: a HR >100 beats/min, SBP <90 mm Hg, CVP <2 mm Hg, and PAWP <4 mm Hg are signs of hypovolemia. Monitor MAP; a MAP <60 mm Hg reflects inadequate tissue perfusion.

2. Assess fluid status: measure I&O hourly, including drainage from all tubes and drains. Urine output should be >30 mL/hr; 50 mL/hr is more desirable. Determine fluid balance every 8 hours. Compare serial weights to evaluate rapid changes (0.5-1 kg/day indicates fluid imbalance). Note skin turgor on inner thigh or forehead, condition of buccal membranes, and development of edema or crackles.

3. Assess tissue perfusion: note level of mentation, skin color and temperature, peripheral pulses, and capillary refill.

4. Continuously monitor ECG for dysrhythmias that may result from electrolyte imbalance, hypoxemia, or hemorrhage.

5. Assess temperature. Monitor for signs of infection. Consider the urinary tract, lungs, and mucous membranes as potential sites of infection, especially because of immunosuppression. Review serial WBC counts and culture reports (if available).

6. Assess respiratory status: note depth, rate, and skin color every 15 minutes postoperatively until stable, then every 1 to 2 hours. Monitor pulse oximetry continuously and ABGs as ordered. Patients with abdominal surgery tend to take shallow breaths secondary to incisional pain.

7. Assess pain using patient's self-report whenever possible. Administer pain medication around the clock to keep pain under control (see Acute Pain in Chapter 2).

8. Assess GI function: palpate graft site for pain, edema, and tenderness, indicating rejection. Be mindful that some patients may not experience pain at the graft site because there is no innervation between the donor organ and the recipient's CNS. Assess for bowel sounds.

9. Monitor for clinical manifestations of acute rejection, which may include fever, headaches, nausea, vomiting, chills, general malaise, increasing weight, and an increasing serum amylase level. Assess glucose level every 30 minutes to 1 hour, urine amylase level every 6 hours, urine pH every 6 hours, and temperature every 4 hours. Glucose is an indicator of

graft perfusion. An upward trend in glucose and temperature and downward trend in urine amylase and urine
pH indicate rejection. A sudden increase in serum glucose
or sudden decrease in urine amylase may indicate thrombosis.

10. Assess acid-base balance. Metabolic acidosis may occur when
urinary diversion is used for exocrine drainage.

11. Assess for signs of anastomotic leaks: lower abdominal pain,
fever, leukocytosis, increased serum amylase and creatinine
levels.

12. Assess for rejection (renal transplant): increased BUN and
creatinine levels, decreased urine output, increased BP,
increased weight, fever, and graft tenderness.

Patient Management

1. Provide supplemental oxygen as ordered (see p. 503 for information on ventilation therapies).

2. Administer intravenous fluids and/or blood products as
ordered to correct intravascular volume and replace blood loss.

3. Monitor serum electrolyte levels and replace as ordered.

4. Use sterile procedure when manipulating GI tubes, surgical
dressings, and indwelling lines. Protect the integrity of the
skin during frequent dressing changes by using skin protectant products. Consult with a wound/skin clinical nurse specialist. Immunosuppressant drugs (e.g., corticosteroids) can
cause delayed wound healing.

5. Maintain patient on bed rest without hip flexion on side of
graft for 48 to 72 hours to prevent thrombosis of graft vessels.

6. Administer corticosteroids, azathioprine, tacrolimus, mycophenolate mofetil, and antilymphocyte globulin (OKT3) as
ordered.

7. Administer anticoagulants as ordered to decrease platelet
aggregation and prevent thrombosis.

8. Administer bladder irrigation as ordered if simultaneous kidney transplant.

9. Maintain patency of the NG tube to prevent undue pressure
on suture line. Do not irrigate or reposition tubes without a
physician's order. Provide good care of the nares and mouth.

10. Administer pain medication and assess level of sedation and
respiratory status. Combine nonopioid analgesics (ketorolac,
ibuprofen) with opioid analgesics (morphine sulfate, hydromorphone, oxycodone) to provide pain relief with lower

doses than would be possible with one drug alone. This approach will produce fewer adverse effects, such as increased sedation and respiratory depression.

11. Administer prophylactic antibiotics, antifungal agents, and antiviral agents as ordered.
12. Administer meticulous skin and mouth care, using nystatin for oral care.

Critical Observations

Consult physician for the following:

1. Signs of fluid imbalance: decreasing SBP >20 mm Hg, increasing HR of >25 beats/min from baseline, decreasing trend in urine output, CVP, and PA pressures
2. Signs of respiratory distress
3. Temperature elevation or signs of infection
4. Upward trend in serum glucose or amylase levels, downward trend in urine amylase level or urine pH
5. Urine output <30mL/hr or <0.5 mL/kg/hr, increasing BUN and creatinine levels
6. Uncontrolled pain
7. Increasing abdominal distention and tenderness

TRANSJUGULAR INTRAHEPATIC PORTOSYSTEMIC SHUNT (TIPS)

Clinical Brief

TIPS is used to treat patients with ascites refractory to pharmacologic intervention or for variceal hemorrhage not controlled by pharmacologic or endoscopic or other nonoperative techniques, to stabilize patients awaiting liver transplant, and to treat patients with cirrhosis in whom surgical decompression of portal hypertension is contraindicated. It is a nonsurgical procedure performed in interventional radiology to create a portosystemic shunt within the vasculature of the liver. An expandable metal stent is inserted via the jugular vein into a tract between the hepatic and portal venous systems to redirect portal blood flow. The result is a decrease in portal venous pressure that decompresses varices and relieves ascites.

Complications

- Stent stenosis, occlusion, or drift
- Acute liver failure (particularly encephalopathy)
- Acute renal failure
- Sepsis

PATIENT CARE MANAGEMENT GUIDELINES

Patient Assessment

1. Assess hemodynamic status: HR >100 beats/min, SBP <90 mm Hg, CVP <2 mm Hg, PAWP <4 mm Hg, and cool, clammy skin may be signs of hemorrhage. The patient is at risk for hemorrhage resulting from damage to blood vessels and liver or inadvertent puncture of hepatic arteries. Recurrent esophageal bleeding may result from a stenotic or occluded stent. Notify physician immediately should you suspect this, and prepare patient for revision of TIPS placement in the interventional radiology suite.

2. Continuously monitor ECG for dysrhythmias.

3. Measure I&O hourly: urine output should be >30mL/hr or >0.5mL/kg/hr. Determine fluid balance every 8 hours; diuresis is desirable. Patient may receive mannitol in the radiology department to aid in excreting contrast media and prevent renal impairment.

4. Monitor respiratory status: depth, rate, and skin color every 15 minutes postprocedure until stable. Continuously monitor oxygen saturation via pulse oximetry.

5. Record temperature and monitor for development of infection.

6. Assess GI function: abdominal pain or abdominal distention, which may indicate hemorrhage, ascites, infection of the stent, or a stenotic or occluded stent. Recurrent esophageal bleeding may signal an occluded or stenotic stent.

7. Assess neurologic status for signs of encephalopathy: personality changes, slurred or slow speech, decreased LOC, asterixis, and increasing serum ammonia levels.

Patient Management

1. Provide supplemental oxygen as ordered.

2. Administer intravenous fluids and/or blood products as ordered.

3. Administer antibiotics as ordered for prophylaxis.

Critical Observations

Consult physician for the following:

1. Signs of hemorrhage

2. Change in LOC and new onset of asterixis

3. Urine output less than 30 mL/hr; increasing BUN and creatinine levels

4. Respiratory depression
5. Elevated temperature and signs of infection
6. Signs of hypovolemia: increasing trend in HR and decreasing trend in urine output, CVP, PA pressures, and BP

ENDOCRINE MODALITIES

INSULIN THERAPY

Clinical Brief

Hyperglycemia and insulin resistance is frequently manifested in critically ill patients even if there is no history of diabetes mellitus (DM). Serum glucose levels greater than 110 mg/dL, in any patient regardless of history, is associated with increased infection, increased incidence of sepsis and systemic inflammation, increased incidence of multiple organ dysfunction syndrome (MODS), increased length of intensive care unit (ICU) and hospital stay, and increased mortality rates.[3]

The cause of the hyperglycemia is unclear. Blood glucose levels increase during the stress response from increased hepatic gluconeogenesis and increased counterregulatory hormones, such as epinephrine, norepinephrine, cortisol, and adrenocorticotropic hormone. Peripheral tissues, such as skeletal muscle, develop insulin resistance, contributing to the hyperglycemia. Glucose is thought to be elevated to provide increased energy for tissues, such as the brain and phagocytes to promote healing, yet there seems to be a relationship between levels of hyperglycemia and mortality rates in critically ill patients.

Tight glycemic control, i.e., a blood sugar between 80 and 110 mg/dL, is associated with as much as a 40% reduction in mortality rates, and a significant reduction in infections, decreased need for renal replacement therapy, decreased need for antibiotics, and reduced time required for mechanical ventilation.[1] Insulin therapy via continuous infusion is used to achieve the targeted blood sugar within the first 24 hours of admission to the ICU.

Complications

• Hypoglycemia

Patient Assessment

1. Determine glucose level via glucometer every hour until glycemic control is achieved. Patients with blood sugars <200

ENDO

rarely have any signs or symptoms. However, if serum glucose falls rapidly, patients may manifest symptoms. It is crucial that bedside glucose be monitored very closely. Traditional blood glucose should be drawn at least once daily to compare values.

2. Assess for adrenergic symptoms: pallor, diaphoresis tachycardia, palpitations, hunger, widened pulse pressure and shakiness. Neuroglycopenic signs include headache, inability to concentrate, confusion, irrational behavior, slurred speech, blurred vision, paresthesias, and somnolence. Obtain serum glucose if symptomatic.

3. ABGs should be monitored to determine acid-base balance in diabetic patients. Ketosis may result in metabolic acidosis.

4. Assess for signs and symptoms of infection; record temperature every 4 hours.

5. Auscultate bowel sounds and assess the abdomen for distention. Hyperglycemia is associated with gastroparesis. Gastroparesis may increase the risk for vomiting and aspiration.

6. Assess hydration status. Hyperglycemia may result in osmotic diuresis and hypovolemia, monitor intake and output every hour initially.

Patient Management

1. Administer insulin infusion as ordered. 50 units of insulin/50 mL 0.9% normal saline (NS) yields 1 unit/mL. Starting dose depends on serum glucose. Typically, an infusion is started at 2 units/kg/hr and is titrated (using a sliding scale) to achieve a serum glucose of 80 to 110 mg/dL. Insulin may be changed to subcutaneously (subQ) when glycemic control is achieved. Follow institution protocol. If blood glucose is less than 80 mg/dL, hold the infusion, notify physician and follow institution protocol (be prepared to administer 50% dextrose IV and recheck blood glucose in 15 minutes).

2. Anticipate dextrose infusions initially for patients who are not diabetic; dextrose is typically added to the IV infusion when blood sugar reaches 250 mg/dL in patients who are diabetic. Monitor patient's response carefully to avoid hypoglycemia.

3. Obtain daily weights. Hypermetabolism and diuresis contribute to weight loss.

4. Consult a nutrition specialist to ensure patient receives only the number of calories required in order to prevent additional hyperglycemia. Enteral feeding is preferred; however, parenteral nutrition may be necessary to prevent malnutrition.

ENDO

5. Insert NG tube as ordered if gastroparesis is present, and elevate the head of the bed 30 to 45 degrees to reduce the risk of aspiration.

Critical Observations

1. Bedside blood glucose <80 mg/dL or >110 mg/dL on insulin drip
2. Signs of hypoglycemia: increasing trend in HR, diaphoresis, tremors, altered LOC
3. Signs of hypovolemia: increasing trend in heart rate, decreasing trend in BP, PA pressures, CVP, urine output
4. Signs of respiratory distress (potential for aspiration)
5. Urine output (U/O) <0.5 mL/kg/hr; increasing BUN and creatinine
6. Gastric residual >200 mL
7. Temperature elevation or signs of infection
8. Abnormal laboratory data

RENAL MODALITIES

RENAL REPLACEMENT THERAPY

Clinical Brief

There are various modes of renal replacement therapy, each having different advantages and disadvantages (Table 7-5). *Hemodialysis* involves pumping the patient's heparinized blood through an extracorporeal filter composed of semipermeable membranes. Blood is removed from and returned to the body through a venous or an arteriovenous (AV) access in the form of femoral lines, a subclavian catheter, AV shunt, AV fistula, or AV graft.

Peritoneal dialysis involves introducing a hypertonic glucose solution (dialysate) into the peritoneal cavity through an abdominal catheter. The dialysate is left to dwell in the abdomen, allowing the exchange of solutes across the peritoneal membrane. The solution is then drained from the abdominal cavity.

Continuous renal replacement therapy (CRRT) is used in the hemodynamically unstable critically ill patient. Ultrafiltration therapies include slow continuous ultrafiltrate (SCUF), continuous arteriovenous hemofiltration (CAVH) (Figure 7-9), and continuous venovenous hemofiltration (CVVH). Dialysis therapies include continuous arteriovenous hemodialysis (CAVHD), continuous arteriovenous

Table 7-5 Comparison of Renal Replacement Therapy Modes

	Peritoneal Dialysis	Hemodialysis	CRRT
Access	Peritoneal catheter	Arteriovenous or venous access	Arteriovenous or venous access
Membrane	Peritoneal	Extracorporeal filter	Extracorporeal filter
Advantages	Continuous, gentle fluid removal	Rapid, efficient fluid and waste removal	Continuous; slow, gentle fluid removal
Disadvantages	Protein loss, poor potassium removal	Hemodynamic instability, heparinization	Heparinization
Contraindications	Abdominal surgery, adhesions, or an undiagnosed acute condition of the abdomen; respiratory insufficiency	Hypotension, bleeding	Bleeding

CRRT, Continuous renal replacement therapy.

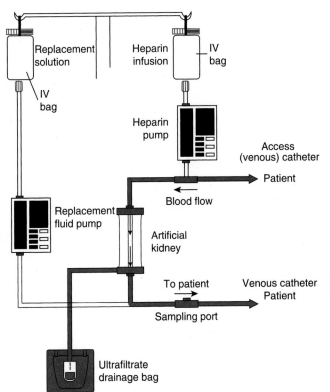

Figure 7-9 Schematic of continuous venovenous hemofiltration system. Various ports are available for fluid replacement, blood drawing, and heparinizing the system. (From Sole ML, Klein DG, Moseley MJ: *Introduction to critical care nursing,* Philadelphia, 2005, Saunders.)

hemodiafiltration (CAVHDF), continuous venovenous hemodialysis (CVVHD), and continuous venovenous hemodiafiltration (CVVHDF).

The modes differ by access, e.g., arterial versus venous cannulation, principles of solute and fluid movement, e.g., diffusion or convection, and whether a special pump is required to propel blood through the circuit.

Complications

All forms of renal replacement therapy
- Hypotension
- Infection
- Dysrhythmias
- Hypoxemia

- Electrolyte imbalances

Hemodialysis
- Disequilibrium syndrome
- Hemolysis
- Air embolus
- Hemorrhage

CRRT
- Hemorrhage
- Blood clotting in the filter

Peritoneal dialysis
- Respiratory insufficiency
- Peritonitis

PATIENT CARE MANAGEMENT GUIDELINES

Hemodialysis

Patient Assessment

1. Perform a head-to-toe assessment.
2. Assess AV shunt, fistula, or graft for bruit and thrill each shift.
3. Assess for signs of infection, including redness, swelling, increased tenderness, and drainage at access site. Obtain temperature every 4 hours.
4. Assess laboratory values.
5. Assess hemodynamic and fluid volume status by monitoring:
   a. Hourly I&O
   b. VS and hemodynamic parameters (if available) every 15 minutes at the onset of treatment until stable, every half hour during treatment once stable, and every 4 hours when not being dialyzed
   c. Breath sounds and heart sounds every 4 hours
   d. Weight daily if no dialysis is done; weight before, during, and after hemodialysis

Patient Management

1. Prevent infection by using good handwashing, initiating good hygiene, separating the patient from other patients with infections, aseptically caring for wounds and all invasive catheters, having the patient turn and C&DB, encouraging early ambulation, and providing good nutrition.
2. Post a sign in the patient's room informing all personnel not to draw blood or check BP in the limb with permanent vascular access device.

RENAL

3. Keep two cannula clamps next to the AV shunt at all times. If the shunt becomes disconnected, apply clamps or direct pressure. Reconnect and assess for blood loss.

4. Aseptically clean insertion sites daily and before initiating dialysis. Change wet, soiled, or loose dressings immediately.

5. Consult with the physician regarding administration of antihypertensive, antiemetic, or opioid agents before hemodialysis because these agents induce hypotension.

6. Adjust schedule for administration of medications based on dialyzability of drug and time of dialysis. Box 7-3 lists common dialyzable medications. Consult physician about administering a postdialysis supplemental dose of any medication that is dialyzed out. Consult physician about obtaining drug levels of dialyzable medications to increase accuracy of dosing.

7. Follow manufacturer's instructions for set-up and operation. Ensure all cannula connections are secure.

8. Assess LOC, presence of chest pain or dysrhythmias, and vital signs.

9. Assess for fluid and electrolyte shifts; monitor serum electrolytes and glucose levels and anticoagulation studies. Administer fluids and medications as ordered to correct imbalances.

10. If the patient becomes hemodynamically unstable, administer normal saline (NS), replacement solution, or vasoactive medications as ordered.

RENAL

Box 7-3 Common Dialyzable Medications

Aminoglycosides: amikacin, gentamicin, kanamycin, neomycin, streptomycin, tobramycin, vancomycin

Cephalosporins: cefazolin, cefuroxime, cefoxitin, ceftazidime, cephalothin, cephaloridine, cephalexin, cephapirin

Penicillins: amoxicillin, ampicillin, carbenicillin, oxacillin, piperacillin, penicillin G, ticarcillin

Other antibiotics: chloramphenicol, sulfonamides, trimethoprim

Cardiovascular agents: procainamide, bretylium, nitroprusside, captopril, enalapril

Immunosuppressives/antineoplastics: azathioprine, methylprednisolone, methotrexate

Miscellaneous: acetaminophen, acetylsalicylic acid, cimetidine, antituberculosis drugs, Librium, theophylline, phenobarbital, phenytoin, ranitidine, lorazepam

These medications often require increased doses during dialysis or supplemental doses after dialysis.

Note: digoxin, propranolol, quinidine, lidocaine, furosemide, heparin, ibuprofen, and morphine sulfate are not removed by hemodialysis.

11. If the patient experiences cramping in the extremities, administer NS or hypertonic saline as ordered and decrease the rate of dialysis.

12. If the patient complains of popping or ringing in ears, dizziness, chest pain, and coughing or if the air is visible entering the patient's vascular return, suspect air embolus. Clamp all blood lines and place the patient in Trendelenburg position and on the left side; administer oxygen.

13. Monitor arterial and venous pressures during treatment for abnormal values, indicating malfunction of dialyzer or access.

14. If the patient develops nausea, vomiting, confusion, headache, hypertension, or seizures, suspect disequilibrium syndrome. Reduce the dialysis rate as ordered and treat the symptoms.

15. If the patient's blood takes on a "cherry pop" appearance and the patient develops chest pain, dyspnea, burning at the access site, and cramping, suspect acute hemolysis. Clamp the blood line, monitor VS, and observe for dysrhythmias. Be prepared to manage a shock state.

RENAL

Critical Observations

Consult physician for the following:

1. Absent bruit or thrill
2. Decrease perfusion to extremities
3. Infected dialysis access site
4. Clotting in circuit
5. Abnormal anticoagulation studies, electrolytes, or hypoxemia
6. Suspected air embolus
7. Disequilibrium syndrome
8. Acute hemolysis
9. Shock
10. Equipment malfunction

Peritoneal Dialysis

Patient Assessment

1. Perform a head-to-toe assessment.
2. Assess for signs of infection, including redness, swelling, increased tenderness, and drainage at peritoneal access site. Obtain temperature every 4 hours.
3. Assess serum electrolytes and glucose during dialysis.
4. Assess fluid volume status by monitoring:
   a. Weight
   b. VS

   c. I&O (including dialysate infused and effluent drained)
      every 4 hours or with each exchange

5. Assess the patient for abdominal pain, rebound tenderness,
   and respiratory compromise, and assess effluent for cloudiness, blood, and/or fibrin clots with each exchange.

Patient Management

1. Prevent infection through good handwashing, initiating good
   hygiene, separating the patient from other patients with
   infections, aseptically caring for wounds and all invasive
   catheters, having the patient turn and C&DB, encouraging
   early ambulation, and providing good nutrition.

2. Until the catheter exit site is healed, use sterile technique to
   clean around the exit site and change the dressing around the
   catheter once per day or when wet. Once the exit site is
   healed, the patient may shower and should clean with povidone-iodine (Betadine) or apply a topical antibiotic ointment around the exit site after the shower.

3. Use strict aseptic technique during exchanges. If the effluent
   is cloudy and peritonitis is suspected, obtain a sample of
   effluent before administering antibiotics.

4. Before an exchange, warm the dialysate solution to body temperature.

5. If ordered, add medications to the dialysate and label the
   dialysate appropriately. (Heparin is often used to prevent
   catheter obstructions by fibrin or blood clots; insulin is
   often used to control glucose in the diabetic patient; antibiotics may be administered in the dialysate to patients with
   peritonitis.)

6. Instill the ordered amount and concentration of dialysate
   with medications via the peritoneal catheter using aseptic
   technique. Allow fluid to dwell in the abdomen for physi-
   cian-ordered time period. When dwell time is over, drain the
   effluent from the abdomen by gravity over 15 to 20 minutes.

7. Patient may experience fullness and shortness of breath during dwell time. Explain that this is normal during this phase.

8. Measure effluent volume by weighing or draining.

9. If difficulty is encountered in draining, check for kinks or
   clamps on tubing, turn the patient from side to side,
   sit the patient up in bed, reposition the drainage bag to
   the lowest possible position, and apply gentle pressure to the
   abdomen.

RENAL

Critical Observations

Consult physician for the following:

1. Symptoms of peritonitis
2. Blood or fibrin clots noted in peritoneal effluent
3. Inability to drain effluent
4. Respiratory distress

Continuous Renal Replacement Therapy (CAVU, CAVH, CAVHD, CVVH, CVVHDF)

Patient Assessment

1. Assess for signs of infection, including redness, swelling, increased tenderness, and drainage at access site. Assess bruit if using AV fistula. Assess circulation distal to limb access site; assess patency of access ports.
2. Assess hemodynamic and fluid volume status by monitoring:
   a. Hourly I&O
   b. VS, CVP, and PA pressures (if available) every 15 minutes at onset of treatment until stable, every half hour during treatment once stable, and every 4 hours after treatment
   c. Breath sounds and heart sounds every 4 hours
   d. Daily weight
   e. Ultrafiltrate rate every 15 minutes until stable and then every hour
   f. Anticoagulation studies
   g. Bleeding at access site and at CCRT circuit

Patient Management

1. Follow manufacturer's instructions to prime filter and blood circuit with heparinized saline. Connect the hemofilter circuit to the patient's access sites, ensuring that all connections are secure.
2. Set blood pump rate and apply air and venous pressure-detecting devices. Monitor venous pressure; an increase in pressure indicates system clotting.
3. If ordered, start dialysate.
4. If ordered, infuse replacement solution. Replacements are based on ultrafiltrate output.
5. If using a gravity drainage bag, keep the bag at least 16 to 20 inches below the filter. The UFR can be increased by lowering the bag or decreased by raising the collection bag (or by increasing the blood pump rate for CVVH).
6. Monitor electrolytes and glucose levels as ordered and administer medications as ordered to correct imbalances.

RENAL

7. Monitor for leaks, disconnections, and clotting in circuit. Keep circuit visible and secure all lines.

8. Monitor anticoagulation studies and assess vascular access for bleeding or clotting.

9. If SBP <90 mm Hg, place the patient flat or in Trendelenburg position. Reduce the ultrafiltrate rate by lowering the bed, raising the collection bag, or decreasing suction (or by decreasing the blood pump rate for CVVH). Administer NS, replacement solution, or vasoactive medications as ordered. If hypotension continues or becomes extreme, clamp ultrafiltrate line.

10. If the amount of ultrafiltrate is reduced, check for kinks in the access site or tubing; check for changes in the blood flow rate (e.g., decreased CO, hypovolemia); raise the bed, lower the collection bag, or increase the suction; and assess for a clotted filter.

11. Hematest ultrafiltrate every 4 hours.

12. If the ultrafiltrate appears pink tinged or the Hematest result is positive, suspect a leak in the filter or a ruptured filter. Treatment should be terminated.

13. If the ultrafiltrate rate decreases and the blood in the circuit is darkened (or venous pressure is increased for CVVH), suspect clotting in the filter. Adjust heparinization; be prepared to replace the circuit.

Critical Observations

Consult physician for the following:

1. Cardiovascular (CV) collapse
2. Blood in ultrafiltrate
3. Clots in filter/clotting in circuit
4. Air embolism
5. Decreased ultrafiltrate
6. Electrolyte imbalances
7. Abnormal glucose levels
8. Abnormal coagulation studies
9. Malfunction of access, dialyzer, or pump

MISC

MISCELLANEOUS THERAPEUTIC MODALITIES

AUTOTRANSFUSION

Clinical Brief

Autotransfusion is a procedure in which the patient's own blood is collected, filtered, and then transfused back to the patient. The advantages of autologous transfusions are that they are readily available, eliminate the risk of transfusion reactions, and eliminate the risk of blood-transmittable diseases. The autotransfuser device is commonly attached to a chest drainage system or wound drain in the case of orthopedic surgery; autotransfused blood should be returned to the patient within 4 hours from collection. The autotransfused blood is usually mixed with an anticoagulant (heparin) to prevent clot formation.

Autotransfusion can be performed preoperatively and saved for future use. In addition, intraoperative and postoperative (e.g., mediastinal chest drainage) blood loss can be replaced by autotransfusion. The trauma patient with massive intrathoracic bleeding can benefit from autotransfusion when banked blood is not yet available.

Contraindications can include blood that is contaminated by bacteria, bile, amniotic fluid, urine, or feces; blood from AIDS, cancer, or sickle cell anemia patients; or blood in patients with wound blood greater than 6 hours old.

Complications

- Coagulopathies
- Infection, e.g., mediastinitis
- Emboli

MISC

PATIENT CARE MANAGEMENT GUIDELINES
Patient Assessment

1. Baseline laboratory data (CBC, platelet count, international normalized ratio [INR], PT, PTT, and electrolyte levels) should be obtained before beginning the autotransfusion.
2. Obtain VS immediately before administering the autotransfusion (T, HR, RR, and BP) and then throughout the procedure as per institutional policy (usually every 30 minutes). Monitor and record urine output and hemodynamics (PAP, PAWP, CVP), hourly or more frequently as patient condition warrants.
3. Monitor the patient for signs and symptoms of excessive bleeding—tachycardia; hypotension; decreased peripheral pulses; cool, clammy skin; decrease in CVP, PA pressures, and PAWP; hematuria; hematemesis; increase in wound drainage; or CT drainage commonly indicate shock or altered hemodynamics.
4. Observe the patient for signs and symptoms of emboli. SOB, change in LOC, and absent or decreased pulses that indicate possible emboli.

5. Observe the patient for signs and symptoms of mediastinitis: increased temperature, purulent wound drainage, wound dehiscence, and/or positive blood cultures. These symptoms can occur from 1 to 6 weeks after autotransfusion.

Patient Management

1. Ensure optimal functioning of the autotransfusion system by following the manufacturer's instructions and institutional policy. (This may include documenting the type and amount of anticoagulant used on the salvaged blood and noting any clot formation.) Maintain aseptic technique during the procedure.
2. Note any foam forming in the blood, which suggests increased hemolysis.
3. Accurately measure and record the amount of collected blood, and infuse as directed.
4. Anticipate administration of blood products (platelets, FFP) if more than 6 L of salvaged blood have been infused.
5. Monitor CBC; platelet count; INR/PT; PTT; and Hgb, Hct, and electrolyte levels during and after the infusion.

Critical Observations

Consult physician for the following:
1. Suspected blood hemolysis or clots in salvaged blood
2. Embolic phenomenon
3. Thrombocytopenia
4. Increasing temperature
5. Unstable BP
6. Excessive bleeding
7. Electrolyte imbalance
8. Decreased SaO_2

BLOOD ADMINISTRATION

Clinical Brief

A variety of blood component products are available for transfusion therapy in the critically ill patient. Adverse reactions with transfusion(s) include infectious and noninfectious complications or bacterial contamination related to product preparation. Despite improved testing in blood collection centers, infectious complications include HIV, hepatitis (viral, low risk), human T-cell lymphotropic virus (HTLV), parvovirus B19 (patients most at risk include pregnant women, those with hemolytic anemia, or those who are immunocompromised), CMV

MISC

(transmitted via blood products that contain WBCs in which the virus is harbored) and new variant Creutzfeldt-Jakob disease (theoretically). Noninfectious complications include hemolytic reactions, transfusion-related "acute lung injury" related to noncardiogenic pulmonary edema, anaphylaxis, allergic reaction, febrile reaction, hypotension, or circulatory overload. Bacterial contamination can occur with platelet collection; storage of platelets longer than 21 days or cell-free products thawing in contaminated water baths. Also, pasteurization does not ensure bacterial decontamination related to albumin.

Transfusion Products

Whole blood: used to replace volume in acute massive hemorrhage. Now most commonly used in acute hemorrhagic shock states of an emergency basis. Rarely used as elective product for transfusion because of allergen factors.

PRBCs: used to increase the oxygen carrying capacity with less risk of fluid overload; increases the patient's Hgb and Hct levels.

Leukocyte-poor (washed) RBCs: contains PRBCs with leukocytes and platelets removed. Used to transfuse patients who have had more than one febrile transfusion reaction, patients who are likely to require multiple transfusions (leukemia), and patients who are immunocompromised and at risk for organisms that can be transmitted via leukocytes.

Platelets: used to restore platelets in patients who have a platelet defect and are bleeding; improve hemostasis in the thrombocytopenic patient who has received a massive transfusion, has undergone cardiac bypass surgery, or has disseminated intravascular coagulation (DIC). Prophylactic platelet transfusion is controversial.

Granulocytes: used to treat patients with decreased WBC count secondary to radiation or chemotherapy. Febrile reactions are common.

FFP: used to treat patients with deficient coagulation factors (e.g., DIC, severe liver disease) and is often administered to patients receiving multiple blood transfusions (PRBCs and/or whole blood) because of massive hemorrhage.

Cryoprecipitate: contains factor VIII, factor XIII, and fibrinogen. Used to treat von Willebrand's disease and hypofibrinogenemia and to correct factor XIII deficiency.

Factor VIII concentrate: contains factor VIII. Used to replace factor VIII in hemophilia A patients.

Factor IX concentrate: contains factor IX. Used to supply factor
   IX in hemophilia B patients.
Albumin: used to expand intravascular volume or replace colloids.
   Available in 5% and 25% solution; 5% is used to correct colloid
   loss, 25% solution is used to correct profound hypoalbuminemia.
Plasma protein fraction (Plasmanate): contains albumin and
   globulins; this product is used to expand intravascular volume
   or correct colloid loss.

Complications

- Hemolytic reaction
- Anaphylactic shock
- Febrile reaction
- Circulatory overload or hypotension
- Allergic reaction
- Transfusion related acute lung injury

PATIENT CARE MANAGEMENT GUIDELINES

Patient Assessment

1. Obtain pretransfusion VS, and assess them again 15 minutes
   after initiating the transfusion. Obtain T, HR, RR, and BP
   every 30 minutes until the transfusion is completed. If trans-
   fusing granulocytes, measure VS every 15 minutes until the
   transfusion is complete.
2. Observe the patient for hemolytic reaction: high fever (102.2° F
   [39° C]); rigors; pain in the chest, loin, neck, or back; hematuria; oliguria; and hypotension.
3. Observe the patient for an anaphylactic reaction: wheezing;
   edema of the tongue, larynx, and pharynx; stridor; hypotension; and cardiopulmonary arrest.
4. Observe the patient for a febrile reaction: fever (100.4° F
   [38.34° C]), chills, flushed skin, headache or backache,
   hypotension, cough, dyspnea, nausea, and vomiting.
5. Observe the patient for fluid overload: SOB, tachycardia,
   hypotension, increased CVP, cough, crackles, distended neck
   veins, and S_3.
6. Observe the patient for an allergic reaction: pruritus,
   urticaria, headache, and edema.
7. Assess the patient's response to therapy; check Hgb and
   Hct levels; PT; platelet count; and sodium, potassium, and
   calcium levels.

MISC

8. Assess the patient for citrate toxicity if the patient is receiving a massive transfusion: tingling of extremities, hypotension, dysrhythmias, and carpopedal spasm.

Patient Management

1. Inspect the blood product for clots, bubbles, and/or discoloration.
2. Only NS can be used to prime or flush the blood administration set or to infuse simultaneously with the blood.
3. Do not administer medications through a blood infusion line.
4. Change blood filters if the infusion rate cannot be maintained and per manufacturer's recommendations; multiunit filters usually are acceptable for 2 to 4 units.
5. Use a blood warmer if large amounts of cold blood products are expected to be given to patients over 4 hours or less, to postoperative hypothermic patients, and to patients with cold agglutinins. Warm blood to body temperature and monitor blood and body temperature throughout the infusion. Do not warm blood >107.6° F (42° C).
6. Verify the patient and blood product according to institution protocol. Generally another licensed professional is required to identify the patient and blood product. Information on the patient's identification (ID) bracelet, transfusion request, and blood product label should match. Do not administer the product if there is not a precise match. Be sure to check the expiration date of the blood product.
7. Ensure patency of the intravenous line. Most blood products can be infused through an 18-gauge catheter.
8. Administer the blood product at a rate of 1 to 2 mL/min during the first 15 minutes and stay with the patient. Anaphylaxis or a hemolytic reaction usually occurs after a small amount of blood has been infused.
9. If no reaction occurs, increase the infusion rate based on the patient's condition and the type of blood product (Table 7-6). Monitor patients with cardiovascular (CV), renal, or liver disease for fluid volume overload.
10. Discontinue the transfusion if the patient manifests any signs and symptoms of a reaction. Save the blood product and tubing for the blood bank, and follow institution protocol.

MISC

Table 7-6 BLOOD COMPONENT ADMINISTRATION GUIDELINES

Blood Component	Infusion Rate	Filter	Volume	Comment
Whole blood	2-4 hr Max: 4 hr	Required	500 mL	Rapid infusion if need is urgent
Packed red blood cells	2-4 hr Max: 4 hr	Required	250 mL	Hgb rises 1 g/dL; Hct rises 3% after 1 unit
Leukocyte-poor red blood cells	2 hr	Required	Variable	
Fresh frozen plasma	1-2 hr, rapidly if bleeding	Use component filter	250 mL	Notify blood bank—takes 20 min to thaw; infuse immediately after thawing
Platelets	Rapidly as patient tolerates	Use component filter	35-50 mL/unit	Usually 6-10 units are ordered. Request that blood bank pool all units
Albumin	1-2 mL/min in normovolemic patients	Special tubing	Varies	Comes in 5% and 25%; can increase intravascular volume quickly; infuse cautiously
Cryoprecipitate	30 min	Use component filter	10 mL/unit	Usually 6-10 units ordered
Granulocytes	2-4 hr	Use component filter	300-400 mL	Request that blood bank pool units VS q15min during infusion

Hct, Hematocrit; *Hgb,* hemoglobin; *VS,* vital signs.

Critical Observations

Consult physician for the following:

1. Allergic reaction
2. Hemolytic reaction
3. Anaphylactic reaction
4. Febrile reaction
5. Volume overload

INTRASPINAL ANALGESIA

Clinical Brief

The term *intraspinal* refers to the spaces or potential spaces surrounding the spinal cord into which medications can be administered. The term is used when referring to the epidural and intrathecal (spinal) routes of administration. Delivery of analgesics by the intraspinal routes can be accomplished by inserting a needle into the subarachnoid space (for intrathecal analgesia) or the epidural space and injecting the analgesic, or by threading a catheter through the needle and taping it in place temporarily for intermittent bolus dosing or continuous administration.

There are three methods for administering intraspinal analgesia: (1) bolus (administered by the clinician), (2) continuous infusion (administered by a pump), and (3) patient-controlled epidural analgesia (administered by the patient using a pump).

Clinician-Administered Bolus Method

Clinicians can provide analgesia by administering a single intrathecal or epidural bolus injection or the catheter can be left in place for intermittent bolus injections (e.g., every 6 hours). The duration of the patient's pain usually determines which bolus method is used.

Continuous Infusion

Continuous pain control with intraspinal analgesia can be accomplished by using an infusion pump to deliver a continuous infusion (also called basal rate) of an analgesic solution. Supplemental bolus doses are prescribed for breakthrough pain and can be administered using the clinician-administered bolus mode available on most infusion pumps.

Patient-Controlled Epidural Analgesia (PCEA)

PCEA permits patients to treat their pain by self-administering doses of epidural analgesics as needed. When PCEA is used, a basal rate usually provides the majority of the patient's analgesic requirement and the PCEA bolus doses are used to manage breakthrough pain. If a basal rate is not provided, it is especially important to remind patients to "stay on top of the pain" to maintain a steady analgesic level. PCEA is appropriate for patients who are alert and oriented enough to manage their pain; for patients who are not, PCEA pumps can be used to administer nurse-managed continuous infusions and rescue doses.

Selected Intraspinal Analgesics

The two main types of drugs administered intraspinally to treat pain are opioids and local anesthetics. These drugs can be administered alone or in combination with each other. The rationale for combining drugs is that they work synergistically to provide better analgesia and fewer side effects at lower doses.

The opioid provides the mainstay analgesia for most patients. The μ-agonist opioids, morphine sulfate and fentanyl, are the most common opioids administered by the epidural route. The primary opioid administered by the intrathecal route is morphine sulfate.

With bolus injection in the opioid-naïve patient, intraspinal morphine sulfate has a slow onset of analgesia (30-60 minutes) and a peak effect of approximately 90 minutes. Additional analgesia usually is required until morphine sulfate takes effect.

Because of its slow onset and rostral (upward) spread that allows binding with opioid receptors in the ventral medulla, large-volume bolus doses (>5 mg) of epidural morphine sulfate have been known to produce late respiratory depression (approximately 2-12 hours after lumbar injection). Earlier respiratory depression at 5 to 10 minutes and before 2 hours also can occur because of vascular uptake of morphine sulfate. Late respiratory depression is uncommon when epidural morphine sulfate is administered in smaller more frequent bolus doses or by continuous infusion.

Fentanyl is used extensively for epidural analgesia, especially for acute pain. Because fentanyl has such a short duration (2-3 hours), administration by continuous infusion or PCEA, rather than intermittent bolus dosing, is preferred for extended pain control. Early-onset respiratory depression is more common than delayed-onset respiratory depression with epidural fentanyl. This reflects vascular uptake of the opioid and occurs most often within an hour of initial injection.

Low (subanesthetic) doses of local anesthetics (usually bupivacaine or ropivacaine) often are combined with epidural opioids for

MISC

the treatment of pain because the drugs work synergistically to provide better analgesia at lower doses than would be possible with the opioid alone. A reduction in doses results in a lower incidence of adverse effects of both opioids and local anesthetics. In addition to improved analgesia and fewer side effects, adding local anesthetics to epidural opioids has been shown to improve GI function and reduce CV, pulmonary, and infectious complications in postoperative patients.

The goal of adding low-dose local anesthetics to epidural opioids for pain management is to provide analgesia, not to produce anesthesia. Patients should be able to ambulate if their condition allows, and epidural analgesia should not hamper this important recovery activity. However, many factors, including location of the epidural catheter, local anesthetic dose, and variability in patient response, can result in patients experiencing motor and sensory deficits and other unwanted local anesthetic effects. Because epidural local anesthetics produce a sympathetic blockade, vasodilation occurs. Orthostatic hypotension and urinary retention are relatively common adverse effects.

Although extremely effective for administering analgesics, intraspinal routes are not without potential for complications. The most serious are intraspinal infection or hematoma. In both cases, the cardinal signs are diffuse back pain or tenderness and pain or paresthesia (abnormal sensations such as numbness and tingling) on intraspinal injection.

MISC

Complications

- Intraspinal infection
- Hematoma at insertion site
- Migration of catheter
- Respiratory depression
- Neurologic sequelae (paresthesia, motor weakness/paralysis)
- Side effects of opioids: nausea/vomiting, urinary retention, pruritus, hypotension
- Allergic reaction to medication used

PATIENT CARE MANAGEMENT GUIDELINES

Patient Assessment

1. Perform systematic initial and ongoing pain assessment (intensity, location, quality, aggravating and relieving factors). See Acute Pain in Chapter 2. Increase and decrease

analgesic based on patient response. Collaborate with anesthesiologist to revise the pain management plan if pain is not adequately controlled.

2. Assess level of sedation (see sedation scale, p. 41) and respiratory status (rate, depth) every 1 to 2 hours during the first 24 hours. Follow institution protocol.

3. Assess for factors that may place the patient at risk for epidural hematoma (e.g., drugs that affect hemostasis, including low-molecular-weight heparin [LMWH]; repeated or difficult spinal punctures; catheter movement).

4. Assess for sensory deficits by asking patient to point to areas of numbness or tingling; assess for motor deficits by asking patient to bend knees and lift buttocks off mattress and press feet against examiner's palm.

5. Assess for urinary retention in patients without a urinary catheter.

6. Obtain temperature every 4 hours.

7. Assess condition of epidural catheter, dressing, and site; reinforce loosened dressing as needed; dressing changes can increase the risk for catheter dislodgment. Contact the anesthesiologist for signs of superficial infection (redness, edema, drainage, soreness) at epidural catheter site or for the need for a dressing change.

8. Have patient dangle at bedside before standing, and assess for postural hypotension.

Patient Management

1. Intraspinal analgesia may be ordered for treatment of pain associated with major thoracic, abdominal, or orthopedic surgery or injuries.

2. Before intraspinal analgesia, evaluate patient for coagulopathies.

3. A multimodality approach (see Acute Pain in Chapter 2) that includes a combination of opioid and local anesthetic intraspinally and parenteral or oral nonopioids, such as ketorolac or ibuprofen, may be used.

4. PCEA should be limited to patients who are able to understand the relationships between pain, pressing a button, and pain relief.

5. Label intraspinal tubing (e.g., epidural catheter) so that it will not be mistaken for other tubings.

6. Use tubing without ports to administer intraspinal analgesia to prevent accidental injection of substances.

MISC

7. Check intraspinal infusion line for loose connections or disconnections. (Cover disconnected catheter end with sterile 4×4 gauze dressing, and notify anesthesiologist.)

8. Use strict aseptic technique when administering epidural boluses or changing drug reservoirs (limit frequent and unnecessary drug reservoir changes); ensure that all solutions administered intraspinally are safe for intraspinal use, sterile, and preservative free (verify correct solution with another nurse before adding).

9. Contact anesthesiologist for unrelieved pain, unresolved adverse effects, signs of infection (including those thought to be unrelated to intraspinal catheterization), patient reports of sore back, or change in sensory or motor function. (Numbness and weakness may be caused by local anesthetic or may be signs of intraspinal infection or hematoma.)

10. Ensure a patent emergency intravenous access; keep naloxone (Narcan) available. If respiratory depression develops, follow institution protocol.

11. Treat adverse effects such as nausea, itching, hypotension, urinary retention, and increased sedation (see sedation scale, p. 41.) with prescribed medications, and consider decreasing analgesic dose by 25% to eliminate the adverse effect rather than repeatedly treating with medications; add or increase dose of nonopioids for additional analgesia.

Catheter Removal

1. Removal of the catheter is done by the anesthesiologist, nurse anesthetist, and in some institutions the critical care nurse. If patient is receiving LMWH, it is recommended that the removal of the catheter be delayed until 10 to 12 hours after a dose of LMWH.

2. After the catheter has been removed, check its tip and note the presence of a colored mark. The colored mark denotes an intact catheter; document your findings. If the patient is to continue on LMWH, it is recommended that LMWH should not be resumed for at least 2 hours after catheter removal.

3. Check the catheter site for signs of infection; apply a sterile dressing to the site.

Critical Observations

Consult anesthesiologist for the following:

1. Inadequate pain control
2. Persistent side effects

3. Presence of back discomfort or pain
4. Presence of paresthesia or motor deficit
5. Hypotension or respiratory depression
6. Signs and symptoms of infection
7. Oversedation

NEUROMUSCULAR BLOCKADE IN THE CRITICALLY ILL

Clinical Brief

Neuromuscular blocking agents (NMBAs) are powerful paralytic agents; NMBAs can be used as a "chemical restraint" when maximal sedation is not effective alone to support patient needs. The most common use of paralysis to fully control the patient's ventilation, and possibly enhance oxygen unloading, is with acute, profound respiratory disease. NMBAs have also been instituted to stabilize cerebral blood flow in patients with elevated intracranial pressure (ICP) and also to manage patients with tetanus and sepsis, in which there is a need to decrease oxygen consumption. NMBAs produce muscle paralysis by blocking the receptor sites at the neuromuscular junction. The goal of neuromuscular blockade is to have less than a 100% block and to use the least amount of drug to achieve the prescribed clinical endpoints (e.g., no movement, no spontaneous ventilation, no ventilator asynchrony). It is imperative to keep in mind that complete muscle paralysis does not alter the patient's LOC; thus NMBAs must be used in combination with other sedation measures to allay patient fear.

There are two main classes of NMBAs. First are the depolarizing NMBAs, which are rarely used outside the OR with the rare exception of assisting in intubating the critically ill patient. The frontrunner or drug standard for this class is succinylcholine, which has a rapid onset of action with a short duration of action. The second type of NMBA is a nondepolarizing agent that has two subclasses. The first subclass is the curare-like agents, such as atracurium (recommended for patients with significant hepatic or renal disease), mivacurium, metocurine, and tubocurarine. The second subclass is steroidal and includes pancuronium (not recommended for patients with coronary artery disease), rocuronium, and vecuronium. It is this second subclass that is more commonly used in the ICU. Side effects to be alert for include tachycardia and hypotension in addition to the loss of intrinsic spontaneous ventilatory ability. With prolonged use, more serious side effects of debilitating muscle tissue weakness and flaccidity can occur.

Objective monitoring of the depth of paralysis is achieved with a peripheral nerve stimulator (PNS). Patients should be comfortably sedated before initiating the NMBA. The PNS electrode is applied to a peripheral nerve; this could be the facial, ulnar, posterior tibial, or peroneal nerve. Before administering the NMBA the patient is sedated. Then a baseline neuromuscular response is assessed, with the delivery of four impulses. A "train-of-four" (TOF) monitoring is used to evaluate the degree of block at the neuromuscular junction. This involves recording the number of twitches in response to four stimuli. If four twitches are observed or palpated, there is less than a 75% block; three twitches correspond to a 75% block; two twitches correspond to an 80% block; and no twitches correspond to a 100% block. A 100% blockade is not desirable because all receptor sites would be occupied and some receptor sites must be available for a reversal agent to be effective should reversal be desired. In addition, if all receptor sites were occupied, continued administration of the drug would cause the drug to be stored. This would lead to prolonged paralysis once the drug therapy was discontinued.

NMBAs do not affect consciousness—patients are able to hear, feel, and think. It is important to keep the patient pain free and anxiety free with analgesics and anxiolytics through the duration of neuromuscular blockade because the inability to move and communicate can be a frightening experience.

Complications

- Immobility, disuse syndrome and/or muscle atrophy
- Side effects of the agent being used, for example, tachycardia
- Weakness after discontinuing the agent, leading to a prolonged recovery
- Acute quadriplegic myopathy syndrome or postparalytic quadriparesis, both from prolonged exposure
- Tachyphylaxis, or tolerance to the drug being administered
- Paralysis
- Inadequate sedation or analgesia
- Inadequate medication for anxiety or pain

PATIENT CARE MANAGEMENT GUIDELINES

Patient Assessment

1. Before NMBA, obtain baseline neuromuscular response with PNS.
2. After drug is initiated, assess depth of paralysis with PNS. Desired blockade is usually one or two twitches in the TOF

mode. With intermittent dosing, check the response before and 15 minutes after the dose. With continuous infusion of the NMBA, check response every 4 hours while the patient's temperature or pH is changing, or if there is a change in concurrent drug therapy.

3. Inspect skin, pressure points, and cornea for dryness and ulceration.

4. Auscultate lungs and assess respiratory effort. Validate ventilator settings and alarms. Assess end-tidal CO_2 if available. Position patient to decrease risk of ventilator-acquired pneumonia.

5. Assess oxygenation status with continuous SpO_2 monitoring and ABG results, and compare results to the prescribed parameters.

6. Assess fluid volume status and hemodynamic parameters: PA pressures (if available), BP, I&O, weight, creatinine and BUN levels, and serial CPK levels for muscle breakdown.

7. Assess VS: T, P, RR, and BP before initiation and hourly thereafter.

8. Assess for pressure ulcer development secondary to immobility.

Patient Management

1. Titrate NMBA to prescribed goal; monitor with PNS after any titration in drug dose. Note that any changes in the patient's temperature, pH, or drug therapy can alter the effects of the NMBA.

2. Ensure that ventilator alarms are on.

3. Prevent complications associated with immobility: reposition patient frequently, maintain patient in proper body alignment, provide ROM exercises, prevent undue pressure on peroneal and ulnar nerves, apply antiembolic hose. Institute DVT prophylaxis.

4. Prevent corneal drying and abrasions: administer an ophthalmic ointment as prescribed; keep eyelids closed with Transpore tape (avoid dressings over the eyes).

5. Provide pulmonary hygiene: suction as necessary and reposition the patient frequently.

6. Administer round-the-clock sedation and analgesics. Administer pain medication before any painful procedure. Consider PCA with baseline delivery dose.

7. Address the patient and family and explain what is going on around them. Reassure the patient and family that the

MISC

paralysis is temporary. Encourage the family to talk to the patient as if the patient were awake.

8. Reorient the patient every time you approach the bed.
9. Consider the use of relaxing music.
10. Place a sign at the head of the bed to communicate to other health care workers that the patient is receiving an NMBA but can still feel pain and hear.
11. Plan uninterrupted periods of rest and promote the sleep-wake cycle.
12. After the NMBA is discontinued, slowly taper sedation and analgesic agents.
13. Have atropine and pharmacologic reversal agents available (e.g., pyridostigmine, neostigmine, edrophonium).

Critical Observations

Consult physician for the following:
1. Inadequate oxygenation or ventilation
2. Hypotension, tachycardia
3. Inadequate neuromuscular blockade
4. Oversedation

SEDATION IN THE CRITICALLY ILL

Clinical Brief

A loss of control, disorientation, and the inability to communicate may potentiate fear and anxiety in the critically ill patient. Agitation increases oxygen consumption, increases the risk for accidental removal of monitoring equipment and invasive catheters, and interferes with diagnostic procedures or therapies that may seem unnatural or are uncomfortable. Balancing oxygen supply and demand is a priority concern to promote physiologic stability and enhance healing for the patient in an ICU. This precarious balance can easily shift askew and lead to tissue ischemia and injury because of patient anxiety, pain, and fear. Sedating a patient in the ICU can promote comfort, improve oxygenation, and protect the patient from injury. The goal of sedation is to keep the patient as calm and comfortable as possible yet not decrease sensorium such that communication becomes difficult. Figure 7-10 shows an algorithm for guiding sedation and analgesia in the mechanically ventilated patient. Monitoring the desired level of sedation can be performed with a sedation scale such as the Riker Sedation-Agitation Scale (SAS), the Motor Activity Assessment Scale (MAAS), or the Ramsay scale or

MISC

modified Ramsay scale (Table 7-7). Sedative agents include anxiolytics, antipsychotics, opioids, and anesthetics. Sedative-hypnotics include the benzodiazepines (e.g., diazepam, lorazepam, and midazolam) and propofol, a nonbarbiturate anesthetic (Table 7-8). Opioids that may be used for sedation in addition to their analgesic properties include morphine sulfate and fentanyl; fentanyl can be given epidurally. Haloperidol, an antipsychotic drug, is used to treat delirium with agitation. See the algorithm for recommended treatment of mechanically ventilated patients regarding sedation and analgesia (Figure 7-10).

Complications

- Oversedation
- Side effects of medications used
- Impaired spontaneous ventilation
- Hypotension
- Risks associated with immobility

PATIENT CARE MANAGEMENT GUIDELINES

Patient Assessment

1. Identify the pathologic cause of agitation (e.g., hypoxia, hypercarbia, inadequate pain control, electrolyte disorder, increased ICP, drug withdrawal, or intoxication with alcohol).
2. Assess for the presence of pain in the sedated patient. Pain should be treated with analgesics; anxiety and agitation should be treated with sedative agents.
3. Be alert for possible paradoxical agitation in older adults.
4. Assess volume status before administering sedatives; changes in HR and BP can be minimized if hypovolemia is corrected.
5. Monitor hemodynamics; be alert for changes in BP and HR and for the development of dysrhythmias, especially in patients receiving haloperidol.
6. Monitor respiratory function; sedatives abolish the hypoxic stimulus. Be alert for hypoventilation and decreased RR.
7. Monitor oxygen saturation with pulse oximetry.
8. Assess airway management in the nonintubated patient.
9. Assess sedation level with the SAS, MAAS or Ramsay scale (p. 602) or other available sedative scale (see p. 41).
10. Monitor triglyceride levels after 2 days with propofol infusions. Include the calories from lipids in the patient's nutritional support.

MISC

MISC

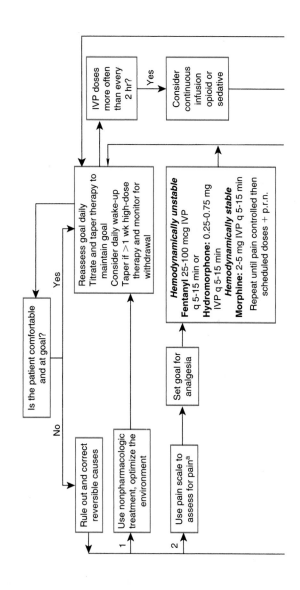

IVP doses more often than every 2 hr? — **Yes** → Consider continuous infusion opioid or sedative

Reassess goal daily
Titrate and taper therapy to maintain goal
Consider daily wake-up
Taper if >1 wk high-dose therapy and monitor for withdrawal

Hemodynamically unstable
Fentanyl 25-100 mcg IVP q 5-15 min or
Hydromorphone: 0.25-0.75 mg IVP q 5-15 min
Hemodynamically stable
Morphine: 2-5 mg IVP q 5-15 min
Repeat until pain controlled then scheduled doses + p.r.n.

Is the patient comfortable and at goal? — **Yes**

No

Rule out and correct reversible causes

1 Use nonpharmacologic treatment, optimize the environment

Set goal for analgesia

2 Use pain scale to assess for pain^a

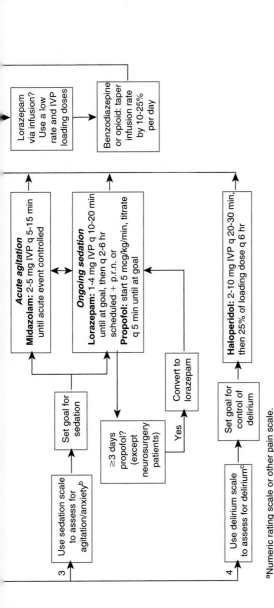

Figure 7-10 This algorithm is a general guideline for the use of analgesics and sedatives. Doses are approximate for a 70-kg adult. IVP = intravenous push. (Modified from Jacobi J et al: Clinical practice guidelines for the sustained use of sedatives and analgesics in the critically ill adult, *Crit Care Med* 30[1]:124, 2002. Used with permission.)

[a]Numeric rating scale or other pain scale.
[b]Riker Sedation-Agitation Scale or other sedation scale (see Table 7-7).
[c]Confusion Assessment Method for the ICU.

MISC

MISC

Table 7-7 SCALES USED TO MEASURE SEDATION AND AGITATION

Score	Description	Definition
RIKER SEDATION-AGITATION SCALE (SAS)		
7	Dangerous agitation	Pulling at endotracheal tube (ETT), trying to remove catheters, climbing over bed rail, striking at staff, thrashing side-to-side
6	Very agitated	Requires physical restraints, biting ETT, does not calm despite frequent verbal reminding of limits
5	Agitated	Anxious or mildly agitated, attempting to sit up, calms down to verbal instruction
4	Calm and cooperative	Calm, awakens easily, follows commands
3	Sedated	Difficult to arouse, awakens to verbal stimulus or gentle shaking but drifts off again, follows simple commands
2	Very sedated	Arouses to physical stimulus but does not communicate or follow commands, may move spontaneously
1	Unarousable	Minimal or no response to noxious stimulus, does not communicate or follow commands
MOTOR ACTIVITY ASSESSMENT SCALE (MAAS)		
6	Dangerously agitated	No external stimulus needed to elicit movement, patient is uncooperative, pulling at tubes and catheters or thrashing side to side, striking at staff, trying to climb out of bed; does not calm down when asked
5	Agitated	No external stimulus needed to elicit movement; attempting to sit up or move limbs out of bed; does not consistently follow commands (e.g., will lie down when asked only to revert back to attempting to sit up or move limbs out of bed)

4	Restless and cooperative	No external stimulus needed to elicit movement; patient is picking at sheets or tubes or uncovering self and follows commands
3	Calm and cooperative	No external stimulus needed to elicit movement; patient is adjusting sheets or clothes purposefully and follows commands
2	Responsive to touch or name	Opens eyes or raises eyebrows or turns head toward stimulus; moves limbs when touched or name is loudly spoken
1	Responsive only to noxious stimulus*	Opens eyes or raises eyebrows or turns head toward stimulus or moves limbs with noxious stimulus
0	Unresponsive	Does not move with noxious stimulus

RAMSAY SCALE

1	Awake	Patient anxious and agitated or restless, or both
2	Awake	Patient cooperative, oriented, and tranquil
3	Awake	Patient responds to commands only
4	Asleep	A brisk response to a light glabellar (space between eyebrows) tap or loud auditory stimulus
5	Asleep	A sluggish response to a light glabellar tap or loud auditory stimulus
6	Asleep	No response to a light glabellar tap or loud auditory stimulus

*Noxious stimulus = suctioning or 5 seconds of vigorous orbital, sternal, or nail bed pressure.
Modified from Jacobi J et al: Clinical practice guidelines for the sustained use of sedatives and analgesics in the critically ill adult. *Crit Care Med* 30(1):125, 2002. Used with permission.

MISC

Table 7-8 COMMONLY USED SEDATIVES FOR CONTINUOUS INTRAVENOUS
ADMINISTRATION

Drug	Dose	Administration Guides
Lorazepam (Ativan)	Bolus: 0.05 mg/kg Infusion: 0.5 mg/hr	Mixture: 10 mg lorazepam in 100 mL D_5W. Increase infusion rate 2-3 mg/hr to achieve desired sedation level. Use lowest rate necessary to maintain level of sedation. Change IV bag after 12 hr.
Midazolam (Versed)	Bolus: 0.1 mg/kg Infusion: 0.05-0.1 mg/kg/hr	Mixture: 100 mg midazolam in 100 mL D_5W
Propofol (Diprivan)	Infusion: 5 mcg/ kg/min	Mixture: propofol comes in a solution of 10% intralipids. Titrate infusion by 5-10 mcg/kg/min increments to desired level of sedation. Use least amount of propofol to maintain the desired level of sedation. Change bottle and tubing every 12 hr. Use strict aseptic technique. Do not administer any other solution or medication in the same line.

MISC

Patient Management

1. Establish at least one other patent intravenous access.
2. Patients receiving continuous intravenous sedation should be mechanically ventilated.
3. Administer continuous infusion of the agent via an intravenous infusion pump, unless the drug is administered by intravenous bolus for short-term use (e.g., an unpleasant procedure may be treated with a dose of benzodiazepine or propofol).
4. Before a painful procedure, patients should be treated with an analgesic agent.
5. Titrate the sedative agent to the prescribed level of sedation, then systematically taper the dose or interrupt continuous dose daily to decrease the prolonged sedative effects.
6. Prevent complications by repositioning the patient, providing meticulous skin care and pulmonary hygiene, and protecting the patient from injury.

7. To prevent withdrawal symptoms in patients receiving sedation longer than 7 days, taper doses systematically.
8. Frequently reorient patient to time and place, optimizing the environment related to lighting and temperature of the room, to establish day and night.

Critical Observations

Consult physician for the following:

1. Hemodynamic instability: bradycardia, hypotension, dysrhythmias
2. Inadequate oxygenation and ventilation
3. Inability to maintain prescribed level of sedation
4. Oversedation

THERMAL REGULATION

Clinical Brief

Cooling and rewarming methods are used to control body temperature. Common thermoregulation disorders treated in the critical care units include hyperpyrexia (fever) and postoperative hypothermia, although heatstroke, malignant hyperthermia, and hypothermia resulting from burns or accidental exposure also are seen in the critical care setting.

External cooling methods can be used alone or in combination with antipyretic therapy. Rewarming methods are generally used in patients who have undergone elective hypothermia (e.g., CV, thoracic, and neurosurgical surgeries).

Cooling methods are used to treat hyperthermia. Hyperthermia refers to a body temperature >99° F (37.2° C) and is classified as (1) *mild*—99° to 102° F (37.2°-38.8° C), (2) *moderate*—102° to 104° F (38.8°-40° C), (3) *critical*—≥105° F (≥40.5° C), and (4) *malignant*—1° F increase every 15 minutes to 109° F (0.5° C increase every 15 minutes to 42.7° C).

Cooling methods are also used to treat brain injury. Mild to moderate therapeutic hypothermia, defined as cooling to 92° F (32°-33° C), can reduce secondary brain injury in those individuals with severe traumatic coma (Glasgow Coma Scale [GCS] <8). Patients receiving therapeutic cooling also receive neuromuscular blockade, sedatives, and analgesics. Generally, cooling occurs for 2 to 5 days after brain injury, and rewarming is controlled so that core temperature is increased 1° per day until a return to 96.8° F (36° C).

Hypothermia induction is recommended for patients who have had an out-of-hospital VF cardiac arrest and are unconscious postresuscitation. Cooling body temperature to 89.6°-93.2° F (32°-34° C) for 12 to 24 hours may improve survial and neurologic outcome.

MISC

Rewarming methods are used to treat hypothermia. Hypothermia refers to a body temperature <98.6° F (37° C) and is classified as (1) *mild*—93.2° to 96.8° F (34°-36° C), (2) *moderate*—86° to 93.2° F (30°-34.5° C), (3) *severe*—<86° F (30° C), and (4) *profound*—<61.7° F (16.5° C).

Complications

External cooling methods
- Vasoconstriction, decreased heat loss
- Frostbite or overshoot—cooling the body temperature too far to hypothermia
- Impaired skin integrity

Rewarming methods
- Shock
- Burns
- Overshoot—rewarming too far to hyperthermia
- Impaired skin integrity

PATIENT CARE MANAGEMENT GUIDELINES

Cooling Methods

Patient Assessment

1. Measure core temperature every 15 to 30 minutes during initial therapy. Anticipate an increase in HR, BP, and RR on initiation of therapy.
2. Assess LOC, presence and quality of peripheral pulses, capillary refill, and skin temperature and condition.
3. Observe for shivering. This will cause an increase in metabolic rate and oxygen consumption. Tensing or clenching of the jaw muscles is an early sign of shivering. An ECG artifact associated with muscle tremor may also be observed.

Patient Management

1. Maintain the environmental temperature at about 70° F (21° C); fans may be required to keep the room cool.
2. Use a wet sheet to cover the patient's torso; tepid baths may be given to lower the patient's temperature. Avoid cold baths because shivering may occur.
3. A cooling blanket may be used:
   a. Precool the blanket if at all possible.
   b. Avoid layers of blankets; a single layer should be used to absorb perspiration.
   c. Turn patient at least every 2 hours and massage skin. Keep blanket in contact with patient during position changes.

MISC

    d. Monitor for drift (T change >1° C in 15 minutes). Avoid overshoot (continual temperature reduction after device is turned off) by stopping the cooling blanket when the core temperature is 102.2° F (39° C).

4. For prolonged moderate hyperthermia (101.8°-104° F [38.8°-40° C]) or critical hyperthermia (≥104.9° F [40.5° C]):
    a. Ice packs can be applied to major artery sites or iced water baths may be given.
    b. Gastric, bladder, and rectal irrigations with iced isotonic solution may be required.
    c. Administer antipyretics as ordered; neuroleptic agents may be required to control shivering.

5. To induce post-resuscitation hypothermia for unresponsive patients after out-of-hospital cardiac arrest, cooling the patient to mild hypothermia (32°–34°C) for 12 to 24 hours may be considered.

Rewarming Methods

Patient Assessment

1. Measure core temperature every 15 to 30 minutes during initial therapy and at least hourly thereafter. Anticipate increase in HR, BP, and RR on initiation of therapy. A drop in BP during rewarming may signal peripheral vasodilation, decreased venous return, and decreased CO (rewarming shock).
2. Continuously monitor ECG for dysrhythmias.
3. Assess LOC (hearing returns at ~93.2° F [34° C]); observe for signs of gastritis or ulceration, excess fluid volume, and thermal injury to skin.

Patient Management

1. Minimize drafts and maintain room temperature; give warm fluids orally if the patient is alert and a gag reflex is present.
2. Apply a bath blanket and cover the head; peripheral vasodilation may occur with use of a hyperthermia blanket.
3. An external hyperthermia blanket may be used; turn the device off when core body temperature is within 1° to 2° of desired temperature. Monitor for drift. (Temperature drift may occur after the device is turned off.)
4. In severe and profound hypothermia (<86° F [30° C]) active rewarming methods may be used: gastric, peritoneal, rectal, or bladder irrigations with heated isotonic solutions or extracorporeal circulation may be required.

MISC

5. If cardiopulmonary arrest occurs, raise the core temperature to 92° F (32°-33° C) to optimize conditions for defibrillation.

6. Monitor the patient for "bolus effect" of pharmacologic agents given during hypothermia; vasodilation occurs with rewarming.

7. Maintain extremities below heart level until vasodilation and hemodynamic stability have been achieved. Cardiac dysrhythmias may result from venous return of acidemic peripheral blood when arms or legs are raised.

8. Do not exceed a rate of 2° C/hr to rewarm the patient.

9. If blood transfusions are required, use a blood warmer.

Critical Observations

Consult physician for the following:

1. Hypothermia or hyperthermia unresponsive to therapy
2. Excessive shivering
3. Hypotension
4. Dysrhythmias
5. Fluid and electrolyte disturbances
6. Hypoxemia and acid-base imbalance
7. Seizures
8. Cardiopulmonary arrest

VENOUS ACCESS DEVICES

Clinical Brief

Selection is based on expected patient need; this considers duration of therapy and type of product(s) to be administered. See Table 7-9 for types and characteristics of commonly used central venous devices.

Complications

- Air emboli, introduced through tubing or connections
- Local or system infection
  —Septic thrombosis, an intravascular infection with high-grade and persistent bacteremia or fungemia
  —Infective nosocomial endocarditis
- Loss of catheter function related to occlusion, dislodgment, migration, or tear

PATIENT CARE MANAGEMENT GUIDELINES

Patient Assessment

1. Review initial and serial chest radiographs to verify central catheter placement.

2. Assess skin integrity at the catheter insertion site or exit site each shift. Note any redness, tenderness, swelling, skin break-down, fluid leakage, or purulent drainage at the site.

3. Monitor VS every 4 hours, noting any increase in temp-erature.

4. Assess for air embolus (increased risk occurs during tubing changes or with procedures requiring exposed catheter hub): chest pain, tachycardia, tachypnea, cyanosis, and hypotension.

5. Monitor for any increase in WBC count or blood glucose levels, which may signal infection.

Patient Management

All Catheters: (Implantable Ports, see p. 612)

Prevent infection:

1. Use strict aseptic technique while manipulating catheters (e.g., dressing changes, accessing ports, changing injection caps). Povidone-iodine can be used as an antiseptic to cleanse the site and injection ports. Consider that a patient may have an allergy to this product.

2. Change dressing per protocol, usually every 24 hours for peripheral catheters and every 72 hours for central lines; change dressings more frequently if the dressing becomes soiled, wet, or loose.

3. Change peripheral access sites every 72 hours maximum.

4. Change injection caps per protocol.

Prevent catheter dislodgment/disconnection:

Secure catheter and extension tubings to prevent catheter dis-lodgment or disconnection. Document catheter position, using markings on the catheter (except totally implanted ports). Have a clamp (without teeth) available. If an air embolus is suspected, clamp the catheter, turn the patient to the left side, and lower the HOB. Administer oxygen.

Catheter malfunction:

1. If unable to aspirate blood from the catheter, raise the patient's arm or have the patient C&DB. Try flushing the catheter gently with NS. Catheter placement may need to be verified by a chest radiograph.

2. If unable to infuse intravenous fluid or medication, try flushing the catheter gently with NS—do not use force. Catheter place-ment may need to be verified by a chest radiograph. If a clot is

MISC

suspected, urokinase may be ordered; follow institution protocol. Generally 1 mL (5000 units/mL) is injected using a tuberculin syringe; wait 5 to 10 minutes and aspirate. The procedure can be repeated twice. If catheter patency has been achieved, withdraw 5 mL of fluid from the catheter and discard. Flush the catheter with NS and resume previous fluid administration. If a medication precipitate is suspected, 0.1 normal hydrochloric acid may be used to clear the catheter of drugs with a low pH; sodium bicarbonate may be used with drugs with a high pH; and 70% ethyl alcohol may be effective if the occlusion is due to fat accumulation from lipid administration.

Obtaining blood samples: peripherally inserted central catheter (PICC) and central venous catheter (CVC)

To obtain blood samples, turn off intravenous solution(s) for 1 minute; attach a syringe to the hub of the catheter; discard three times the volume of the catheter lumen (see Table 7-9); and withdraw the amount of blood needed. Flush the lumen and resume intravenous fluids; if the lumen is not in use, flush with NS; use heparin per institutional policy.

Catheter repair:

Permanent repair for long-term catheters should be done with the manufacturer's repair kit as soon as possible. Short-term multilumen catheters should be changed as soon as possible.

Catheter Removal: Temporary Central Venous Catheter (CVC)

1. If catheter insertion is in a neck vein, place the patient in the Trendelenburg position (to prevent air embolus).
2. Using aseptic technique, remove sutures and steadily pull the catheter back. Apply pressure to the insertion site and apply a sterile occlusive dressing. Check to see if the catheter is intact.

Catheter Removal: PICC

1. Remove dressing.
2. Gently tug on the catheter; if there is resistance, place tension on the catheter, tape it down, and try again in a few minutes.

Single/Multilumen Catheters

Patient Management

1. Tape piggybacked intermittent infusion lines securely to prevent inadvertent disconnection.
2. Flush the catheter lumen with saline every 8 to 12 hours, according to institution protocol when not in use. Flush the

Table 7-9 Characteristics of Central Venous Devices

Device	Use	Volume	Heparinization*	Comment
CENTRALLY PLACED CATHETER				
Single and multilumen	Short-term	0.5-0.6 mL/ lumen	Required	Distal port can be used for CVP monitoring; distal port is 16 gauge; middle and proximal ports are 18 gauge; can be inserted at bedside
PERIPHERALLY INSERTED CENTRAL CATHETER (PICC)				
Single/ multilumen Groshong PICC Per-a-Cath	Moderate- long-term	0.1-0.4 mL/ lumen	Required	Inserted into the basilic or cephalic vein with the tip advanced to the SVC or subclavian veins
IMPLANTABLE PORT				
Porta-Cath Medi-Port	Long-term	2-mL port 2-mL lumen	Required	OR insertion required
Tunneled	Long-term	1.8 mL/lumen	Required	OR insertion required; catheter is tunneled subcutaneously and contains a Dacron mesh cuff to stabilize catheter
Hickman				See Hickman
Broviac	Long-term	1 mL/lumen	Required	
Groshong	Long-term	1.8 mL/lumen	Required	OR insertion required; catheter is tunneled subcutaneously; contains a three-position valve

CVP, Central venous pressure; *OR*, operating room; *SVC*, superior vena cava.
*For catheter lumens not used for continuous infusions.

catheter lumen with 2 mL NS before infusing intermittent medications. After the infusion is complete, flush with NS; use heparin per institutional protocol.

Peripherally Inserted Central Catheter (PICC)

Patient Management

1. Do not take BP in the arm in which the line is inserted.
2. If blood is drawn from the catheter, adequate flushing of the catheter after the specimen has been obtained must occur to prevent clot formation.
3. See the information on single and multilumen catheters.

Groshong

Patient Management

1. Maintain a sterile occlusive dressing to the exit site.
2. Change dressing every 72 hours or more frequently if the dressing becomes soiled, wet, or loose.
3. Change injection caps every 7 days or more frequently (e.g., if blood is in the cap or cap is perforated excessively).
4. Tape piggybacked intermittent infusion lines securely to prevent inadvertent disconnection.
5. Flush catheter vigorously with 5 mL NS after completion of intermittent infusions.
6. Flush the catheter lumen with 10 mL NS after blood infusions or after obtaining blood samples.
7. Inject 20 mL NS before aspirating a blood sample following an infusion of TPN.
8. A Groshong catheter requires no clamping because of its specially designed valve.

Implantable Ports

Patient Management

1. Use aseptic technique when accessing the implanted port. Stabilize the port with the thumb and index finger. If port moves freely, suspect dislodgment.
2. Cannulate the port using a Huber needle and extension tubing that has been flushed with NS. A 90-degree-angled needle is recommended with continuous infusions for patient comfort and ease of dressing applications. Push the Huber needle through the port until it touches the back of the port (to ensure that it is not in the rubber septum).

MISC

3. Aspirate for a blood return and flush the system with NS to confirm patency before initiating the infusion.

4. Flush the catheter with 5 mL NS after a bolus injection; follow with 5 mL heparinized saline if institutional policy so dictates.

5. Flush the catheter with 20 mL NS after a blood sample has been withdrawn or blood has been administered.

6. Maintain a sterile dressing over the needle and port when in use; otherwise no dressing is required.

7. Change Huber needles every 3 to 7 days during continuous infusion.

8. Check the site for irritation or ulceration around the needle; rotate the insertion site PRN; the skin area over the port is approximately 2.5×2.5 cm.

Critical Observations

Consult physician for the following:

1. Febrile state in patient
2. Inability to inject fluid into or withdraw blood from the catheter
3. Onset of chest pain, dyspnea, and cyanosis in the patient
4. Insertion site becomes inflamed and tender or is draining fluid or pus
5. Cracks are noted in the catheter
6. Implantable port is dislodged

MISC

BIBLIOGRAPHY

Neurologic Modalities

Bader MK: *AANN core curriculum for neuroscience nursing,* ed 4, Philadelphia, 2004, Saunders.

Bailes JE: Carotid endarterectomy, *Neurosurgery* 50(6):1290-1295, 2002.

Brain Trauma Foundation. American Association of Neurological Surgeons. Use of barbiturates in the control of intracranial hypertension, *J Neurotrauma* 17(6-7):527-530, 2000.

Censullo JL, Sebastian S: Pentobarbital sodium coma for refractory intracranial hypertension, *J Neurosci Nurs* 35(5):252-262, 2003.

Findlay JM et al: Carotid endarterectomy: a review, *Can J Neurol Sci* 31(1):22-36, 2004.

Greenberg MS: *Handbook of neurosurgery,* ed 5, New York, 2001, Thieme Medical Publishers.

Hickey JV: *The clinical practice of neurological and neurosurgical nursing,* ed 4, Philadelphia, 1977, Lippincott Williams & Wilkins.

Suarez JI: *Critical care neurology and neurosurgery,* Totowa, NJ, 2004, Humana Press.

Pulmonary Modalities

Benditt JO: Surgical therapies for chronic obstructive pulmonary disease, *Respir Care* 49(1):53-61, 2004.

Burns SM: The science of weaning: when and how? *Crit Care Nurs Clin North Am* 16(3):379-386, 2004.

Chapman S, Davies C: Non-invasive positive pressure ventilation in acute respiratory failure, *Care Crit Ill* 19(5):145-149, 2003.

Charnock Y, Evans D: Nursing management of chest drains: a systematic review, *Aust Crit Care* 14(4):156-160, 2001.

Hubble MW, Hubble JP: *Principles of advanced trauma care,* Albany, NY, 2002, Delmar.

Jorgensen K et al: Effects of lung volume reduction surgery on left ventricular diastolic filling and dimensions in patients with severe emphysema, *Chest* 124(5):1863-1870, 2003.

Kruse JA, Fink MP, Carlson RW: *Saunders manual of critical care,* Philadelphia, 2003, Saunders.

Lanuza DM, McCabe MA: Care before and after lung transplant and quality of life research, *AACN Clin Issues* 12(2):186-201, 2001.

Mims BC et al: *Critical care skills: a clinical handbook,* ed 2, Philadelphia, 2004, Saunders.

Stewart CE: *Advanced airway management,* Upper Saddle River, NJ, 2002, Pearson Education, Inc.

Thompson JM et al: *Mosby's clinical nursing,* ed 5, St Louis, 2002, Mosby.

Wilkins RW, Stoller JK, Scanlan CL: *Egan's fundamentals of respiratory care,* ed 8, St Louis, 2003, Mosby, Inc.

Cardiovascular Modalities

American Heart Association Heart Disease and Stroke Statistics—2003 Update. Dallas, Texas, 2003, American Heart Association.

Bosin DM, Flemming M: Electrophysiology testing, *Dimens Crit Care Nurs* 22(1):10-19, 2003.

Braunwald E, Zipes D: *Braunwald's heart disease: a textbook of cardiovascular medicine,* Philadelphia, 2002, Saunders.

Braunwald E et al: ACC/AHA guidelines for the management of patients with unstable angina and non-ST-segment elevation myocardial infarction. A report of the American College of Cardiology/American Heart Association Task Force on Practice Guidelines, *Circulation* 102(10):1193-1209, 2002.

Gragoratos G et al: ACC/AHA/NASPE 2002 guideline update for implantation of cardiac pacemakers and antiarrhythmia devices: a report of the American College of Cardiology/American Heart Association Task Force on Practice Guidelines, *J Cardiovasc Electrophysiol* 13(11):1183-1199, Nov 2002.

Griffin BP, Topol EJ: *Manual of cardiovascular medicine,* ed 2, Philadelphia, 2004, Lippincott Williams & Wilkins.

Gura MT, Forman L: Cardiac resynchronization therapy for heart failure management, *AACN Clin Issues* 15(3):325-339, 2204.

Mancini M et al: The management of immunosuppression, *Crit Care Nurs Q* 27(1):61-64, 2003.

Martgaker MT, Keresztes PA: Evidence-based practice for the use of *N*-acetylcysteine, *Dimens Crit Care Nurs* 23(6):270-273, 2003.

Reiswig TP, Rodeman BJ: Temporary pacemakers in critically ill patients: assessment and management strategies, *AACN Clin Issues* 15(3):305-325, 2004.

Smith AL, Brown CB: New advances and novel treatments in heart failure, *Crit Care Nurse* (Feb Suppl):11-18, 2003.

Stanik-Hutt JA: Drug-coated stents: preventing restenosis in coronary artery disease, *J Cardiovasc Nurse* 19(6):404-408, 2004.

Topol EJ et al: *Textbook of cardiovascular medicine,* Philadelphia, 2002, Lippincott Williams & Wilkins.

Wade CR et al: Postoperative nursing care of cardiac transplant recipient, *Crit Care Nurs Q* 27(1):17-28, 2003.

Gastrointestinal Modalities

Baudouin SV, Evans TW: Nutritional support in critical care, *Clin Chest Med* 24(4):633-644, 2003.

Boyer TD: Transjugular intrahepatic portosystemic shunt: current status, *Gastroenterology* 124(6):1700-1710, 2003.

Burke GW, Ciancio G, Sollinger HW: Advances in pancreas transplantation, *Transplantation* 77(9 Suppl): 62S-67S, 2004.

Elpern E et al: Outcomes associated with enteral tube feedings in a medical intensive care unit, *Am J Crit Care* 13(3):221-227, 2004.

Higgins PD, Fontana RJ: Liver transplantation in acute liver failure, *Panminerva Med* 45(2):85-94, 2003.

Kovacs TO, Jensen DM: Recent advances in the endoscopic diagnosis and therapy of upper gastrointestinal, small intestinal, and colonic bleeding, *Med Clin North Am* 86(6):1319-1356, 2002.

Lenart S, Polissar NL: Comparison of two methods for postpyloric placement of enteral feeding tubes, *Am J Crit Care* 12(4):357-360, 2003.

Mascarenhas R, Mcbarhan S: New support for branched-chain amino acid supplementation in advanced hepatic failure, *Nutr Rev* 62(1):33-38, 2004.

McCashland TM: Current use of transjugular intrahepatic portosystemic shunts, *Curr Gastroenterol Rep* 5(1):31-38, 2003.

NIH: NIH state-of-the-science statement on endoscopic retrograde cholangiopancreatography (ERCP) for diagnosis and therapy, *NIH Consens State Sci Statements* 19(1):1-26, 2002.

Powers J et al: Bedside placement of small-bowel feeding tubes in the intensive care unit, *Crit Care Nurs* 23(1):16-24, 2003.

Roberts SR et al: Nutrition support in the intensive care unit: adequacy, timeliness, and outcomes, *Crit Care Nurs* 23(6):49-57, 2003.

Russo MW et al: Transjugular intrahepatic portosystemic shunt for refractory ascites: an analysis of the literature on efficacy, morbidity, and mortality, *Am J Gastroenterol* 98(11):2521-2527, 2003.

Stechmiller JK, Childress B, Porter T: Arginine immunonutrition in critically ill patients: a clinical dilemma, *Am J Crit Care* 13(1):17-24, 2004.

Weisner RH et al: Recent advances in liver transplantation. *Mayo Clin Proc* 78(2):197-219, 2003.

Willems M et al: Liver transplantation and hepatitis C, *Transpl Int* 15(2-3):61-72, 2002.

Endocrine Modalities

Dickerson LM et al: Glycemic control in medical inpatients with type 2 diabetes mellitus receiving sliding scale insulin regimens versus routine diabetes medications: a multicenter randomized controlled trial, *Ann Fam Med* 1(1):29-35, 2003.

Finney SJ et al: Glucose control and mortality in critically ill patients, *JAMA* 290(15):2041-2047, 2003.

Giddons JF: Nursing management endocrine problems. In Lewis et al, editors: *Medical Surgical Nursing*, ed 6, St Louis, 2004, Mosby.

Graber AL, McDonald T: Newly identified hyperglycemia among hospitalized patients, *South Med J* 93(11):1070-1072, 2001.

Huether S: Alterations of hormone regulation. In Huether SE, McCance KL, editors: *Understanding human pathophysiology*, ed 3, St Louis, 2004, Mosby.

Huether S: Mechanisms of hormone regulation. In Huether SE, McCance KL, editors: *Understanding human pathophysiology*, ed 3, St Louis, 2004, Mosby.

Liolios A: Intensive glucose control in the ICU: an expert interview with James S. Krinsley, MD, *Medscape Gen Med* 6(2):1-4, 2004.

Montori VM, Bistrian BR, McMahon MM: Hyperglycemia in acutely ill patients, *JAMA* 288(17):2167-2169, 2002.

Roberts SR, Hamedani B: Benefits and methods of achieving strict glycemic control in the ICU, *Crit Care Clin North Am* 16(4):537-545, 2004.

Singh, KS et al: Standardization of intravenous insulin therapy improves efficiency and safety of blood glucose control in critically ill adults, *Intensive Care Med* 30(5):804-810, 2004.

Van den Berghe G et al: Intensive insulin therapy in critically ill patients, *N Engl J Med* 345(19):1359-1367, 2001.

Renal Modalities

Al-Khafaj A, Corwin H: Acute renal failure and dialysis in the chronically critically ill patient, *Clin Chest Med* 22(1):165-174, 2001.

Giuliano KK: Continuous renal replacement therapies. In Lynn-McHale DJ, Carlson KK, editors: *AACN procedure manual for critical care*, Philadelphia, 2001, Saunders.

Giuliano KK: Hemodialysis. In Lynn-McHale DJ, Carlson KK, editors: *AACN procedure manual for critical care*, Philadelphia, 2001, Saunders.

Giuliano KK: Peritoneal dialysis. In Lynn-McHale DJ, Carlson KK, editors: *AACN procedure manual for critical care*, Philadelphia, 2001, Saunders.

Kaplow R, Barry R: Continuous renal replacement therapies: a more gentle blood filtering technique allows for fewer complications, *Am J Nurs* 102(11):26-33, 2002.

Paton M: Continuous renal replacement therapy, slow but steady, *Nursing* 33(6):48-50, 2003.

Sole ML, Klein DG, Moseley MJ: *Introduction to critical care nursing*, Philadelphia, 2005, Saunders.

Miscellaneous Modalities

American Heart Association: Highlights of the 2005 American Heart Association guidelines for cardiopulmonary resuscitation and emergency cardiovascular care, *Curr Emerg Cardiovasc Care* 16:4, winter 2005–2006.

Dial S, Nguyen D, Menzies D: Autotransfusion of shed mediastinal blood. A risk factor for mediastinitis after cardiac surgery? Results of a cluster investigation, *Chest* 124(5):1847-1851, 2003.

Evered A: Hypothermia: risk factors and guidelines for nursing care, *Nurs Times* 99(49):40-43, 2003.

Gozzoli V et al: Is it worth treating fever in intensive care unit patients? Preliminary results from a randomized trial of the effect of external cooling, *Arch Intern Med* 161:121-123, 2001.

Jacobi J et al: Clinical practice guidelines for the sustained use of sedatives and analgesics in the critically ill adult, *Crit Care Med* 30(1):119-141, 2002.

Liu S, McDonald S: Current issues in spinal anesthesia, *Anesthesiology* 9:888-906, 2001.

Mermel L et al: Guidelines for the management of intravascular catheter-related infections, *J Intraven Nurs* 24(3):180-205, 2001.

Murray M et al: Clinical practice guidelines for sustained neuromuscular blockade in the adult critically ill patient, *Crit Care Med* 30(1):142-156, 2002.

Park K, Chandhok D: Transfusion-associated complications. *Int Anesthesiol Clin* 42(3):11-26, 2004.

St. Marie B: The complex pain patient: interventional treatment and nursing issues, *Nurs Clin North Am* 38:539-554, 2003.

Taguchi A et al: Effects of a circulating-water garment and forced-air warming on body heat content and core temperature, *Anesthesiology* 100(5):1058-1064, 2004.

Warner C: The use of the orthopaedic perioperative autotransfusion (OrthoPAT) system in total joint replacement surgery, *Orthopaedic Nurs* 20(6):29-32, 2001.

8

Palliative Care in the Critical Care Unit

Inpatient deaths occur more frequently in the critical care unit (CCU) than in any other unit in a hospital. This obliges the CCU nurse to have knowledge, skills, and competencies about end-of-life care. An essential feature of professional nursing practice is to give attention to the range of human experiences and responses to health and illness within the physical and social environments and to alleviate suffering.[1] When health cannot be restored, such as when a person is dying, the focus of nursing care is to assess and manage distressing symptoms.[2]

The most common sources of patient distress when dying in the CCU include pain, dyspnea, and delirium, and nurses have the tools to recognize and treat these phenomena. Withdrawal of mechanical ventilation is a frequent aspect of dying care in the CCU and entails processes that nurses facilitate in collaboration with medical staff and ancillary personnel. Meeting the care needs of the family who is experiencing anticipatory grief, using nursing and other interventions, is a priority when a CCU patient is dying.

SYMPTOM MANAGEMENT: PAIN

Clinical Brief

Pain is a subjective nociceptive phenomenon that is ordinarily measured using a patient's self-report about his or her experience. It is understood to occur when a patient says it does with the intensity that the patient reports.[3] Nociceptive responses activated by pain are expressed cognitively, emotionally, and physiologically. Some patients with pain are unable to provide a self-report due to illness severity, cognitive decline or impairment, or artificial airways (Table 8-1). Pain in CCU patients occurs from trauma, somatic disorders, surgeries, and common CCU procedures and interventions.

Table 8-1 ASSESSING PAIN

Patient Able to Report	Patient Unable to Report	Comments
Numeric rating scale (0-10)	Behaviors: Grimacing Rigidity Wincing Shutting eyes Verbalization Moaning Clenching fists	A combination of measures may be the most valid
Visual analog scale: anchored at "0" = no pain and "10" = worst pain	Physiologic: Tachycardia Tachypnea Increased MAP Diaphoresis	Neuromuscular-blocking agents and sedatives mask signs of pain
Wong FACES scale Verbal descriptors		

Nursing Diagnoses: Acute Pain, Chronic Pain

Outcome Criteria

The patient will report or display signs of pain reduction or elimination.

Interventions

1. Assess for pain frequently.
2. Limit or eliminate painful procedures that are more burdensome than beneficial when the patient is dying, such as turning, suctioning, venipunctures, arterial and central venous lines, nasogastric tubes, and other unpleasant nursing or medical interventions.[4,5]
3. Provide nonsteroidal antiinflammatory drugs for mild to moderate pain or bone pain.[5,6,7]
4. Provide opioids for moderate to severe pain.[5,6,7]
5. Antidepressants and anticonvulsants are useful for reducing neuropathic pain.[6,7]
6. The intravenous route affords the most rapid onset of action.

7. Titrate dosing to patient responses. Opioids have no toxic ceiling and illness severity and tolerance will influence dosing requirements.[5,6,8]

8. See Pain in Chapter 2.

TERMINAL DYSPNEA AND RESPIRATORY DISTRESS

Clinical Brief

Dyspnea is a person's subjective awareness of altered or uncomfortable respiratory functioning. Respiratory distress, an observable corollary to dyspnea, is the physical and/or emotional suffering that results from the experience of dyspnea. It is characterized by behaviors that can be observed and measured.[9] Terminal dyspnea and respiratory distress are highly prevalent in patients dying in the CCU[10,11] (Table 8-2). Many pulmonary, cardiac, and neuromuscular conditions are antecedents to the development of dyspnea.

Nursing Diagnosis: Ineffective Breathing Pattern

Outcome Criteria

The patient will report or display signs of respiratory comfort.

Interventions[9]

1. Assess for dyspnea or respiratory distress frequently in at-risk patients.

Table 8-2 ASSESSING DYSPNEA OR RESPIRATORY DISTRESS

Dyspnea	Respiratory Distress	Comments
Dyspnea numeric rating scale (0-100)	Behaviors: Restlessness Freezing Grunting at end-expiration Fearful facial expression	A combination of measures may be the most valid
Vertical dyspnea visual analog scale: anchored at "0" = no pain, and "100" = worst pain	Physiologic: Tachycardia Tachypnea Accessory muscle use Paradoxical breathing Nasal flaring	
Verbal descriptors		

2. Optimize the patient's position to maximize ventilation and perfusion. The optimal position will vary according to each patient's pathophysiology.

3. Use oxygen if it confers a patient benefit. Nasal cannula is better tolerated than a face mask. Patient signs of distress or respiratory comfort are more valid than SpO_2.

4. Balance rest with activity. Oxygen consumption increases with activity and may worsen hypoxemia, thereby increasing respiratory distress.

5. Administer bronchodilators if indicated.

6. Administer diuretics if respiratory distress is associated with heart failure or volume excess.

7. Administer opioids. Effective doses for treating terminal dyspnea are patient specific but generally lower than those required to treat pain.

8. Administer anxiolytics if fear or anxiety is a component of the patient's dyspnea.

DELIRIUM

Clinical Brief

Delirium is an etiologically, nonspecific cognitive disorder with concurrent disorders in level of consciousness, attention, thinking, perception, memory, emotion, and the sleep-wake cycle.[12] Delirium is produced by organic changes in the brain, metabolic encephalopathies, dehydration, electrolyte imbalances, and medication adverse effects that are all common in the dying CCU patient.[13]

The Confusion Assessment Method for the Intensive Care Unit (CAM-ICU) is a delirium assessment instrument that was designed for use in the CCU with mechanically ventilated patients (see Appendix F). It measures four features of delirium: acute onset or fluctuating course, inattention, disorganized thinking, and altered level of consciousness.[13,14]

Nursing Diagnoses: Disturbed Thought Processes, Acute Confusion, Fear, Impaired Memory, Disturbed Sleep Pattern

Outcome Criteria

The patient's confusion and disturbed thought processes do not produce agitation.

The patient reports less fear.

The patient has periods of sustained, undisturbed sleep.

Interventions

1. Assess for delirium frequently in at-risk patients.
2. Control environmental stimuli to reduce delirium.[15,16]
3. Administer neuroleptics to patients with agitated delirium.[8,17]
4. Nonagitated delirium does not require treatment.
5. Avoid restraints.
6. See Confusion, p. 73 in Chapter 4.

WITHDRAWAL OF MECHANICAL VENTILATION

Clinical Brief

Ventilator withdrawal is a process of liberating a terminally ill patient from mechanical ventilation, recognizing that patient death may follow in minutes to days. Preventing or reducing respiratory distress before, during, and after ventilator withdrawal is a priority. The patient's ability to experience distress predicts the most optimal method for withdrawal. Ventilator withdrawal comprises three processes: premedication, withdrawal method, and extubation (Box 8-1). Discontinuation of neuromuscular blocking agents before

---

Box 8-1 Withdrawal of Mechanical Ventilation

Premedication

- Premedicate patients with signs of respiratory distress before ventilator withdrawal and patients at risk for respiratory distress during or after ventilator withdrawal. Comatose and brain dead patients do not require premedication (Table 8-3).
- Administer morphine as ordered because it has dyspnea-reducing properties. Provide a bolus dose of 5 to 10 mg if patient is opioid naïve. Initiate a continuous infusion at a rate equal to 50% of bolus dose to maintain respiratory comfort.
- Administer lorazepam (2-4 mg) or midazolam (2-5 mg) as ordered if anxiolysis or amnesia is desired. Propofol is useful if complete sedation is indicated.

Method: Incremental reduction in oxygen and ventilatory support

Indication: This method affords the most control and should be employed whenever a patient is at risk for respiratory distress during or after ventilator withdrawal.

NOTE: The process can be stopped at any time during rapid weaning to adjust the patient's medications if signs of distress appear.

Continued

Box 8-1   Withdrawal of Mechanical Ventilation—cont'd

- Provide patient and family with opportunities for privacy and closure. Offer chaplaincy support.
- Premedicate, if indicated.
- Decrease positive end-expiratory pressure (PEEP), FIO_2, and minute volume of ventilation incrementally over 15 to 20 minutes. Observe patient continuously for signs of distress.
- Stop the process to re-bolus and titrate medication if signs of distress are apparent.
- Conclude the rapid wean with placing the patient on a T-piece with humidified room air.

Method: T-piece with humidified room air without weaning

Indication: This method provides a satisfactory withdrawal method when the patient is unlikely to experience respiratory distress because of severely impaired cognition or coma.

- Provide patient and family with opportunities for privacy and closure. Offer chaplaincy support.
- Premedicate, if indicated. Comatose patients may not require premedication.
- Turn off ventilator and place patient on a T-piece with humidified room air.
- Medicate the patient if signs of distress develop after ventilator withdrawal.

Extubation: Patients who will experience distress from a nasotracheal or endotracheal tube should be extubated. Patients may need to retain their tube if there is a large volume of pulmonary secretion; impaired gag/cough reflexes; a large, swollen tongue; inhalation injury; or high risk for postextubation stridor. Balancing burden with benefit will determine when the patient should be extubated. Postextubation stridor or laryngospasm can be reduced with the application of an aerosol mask and administration of nebulized racemic epinephrine.

---

ventilator withdrawal is essential because the paralyzed patient is not able to display signs of distress.[18,19,20]

Dying patients may benefit from transfer from the CCU to a private room on a medical-surgical unit. This affords the patient and family with privacy and quiet. It may also be a benefit to the hospital and the CCU by making a CCU bed available, and reducing the variable costs associated with care in the CCU. Signs of imminent death must be balanced with triage and patient and family needs when deciding about transfer. Signs of imminent death (24 hours) include hypotension, hypoxemia, cool mottled extremities, hypersomnolence, and hypothermia.

Responding to the needs of the attendant family carries the same importance as caring for the dying patient,[21] such as timely and honest

Table 8-3 CONSIDERATIONS FOR WITHDRAWAL OF MECHANICAL VENTILATION ACROSS DIFFERING LEVELS OF PATIENT CONSCIOUSNESS

Brain Death	Coma (Brainstem Function Only)	Impaired Level of Consciousness	Consciousness
PREMEDICATION			
Not indicated	Not indicated	If signs of dyspnea or if dyspnea likely	If patient desires or if dyspnea likely
DRUGS			
None morphine	None	Lorazepam, midazolam, or morphine	Lorazepam, midazolam, or
METHOD			
Turn off ventilator	Rapid wean or T-piece without weaning	Rapid wean then T-piece	Rapid or slow wean then T-piece
EXTUBATION			
Yes	Yes, unless appearance of airway distress can be anticipated	Yes, unless airway compromise and distress can be anticipated	Yes, unless airway compromise and distress can be anticipated

From Kruse JA, Fink MP, Carlson RW: *Saunders manual of critical care*, Philadelphia, 2003, Saunders.

communication; holistic approach to the physical, psychologic, social, and spiritual dimensions of anticipatory grief using multidisciplinary resources; and open visiting.

REFERENCES

1. American Nurses Association: *Nursing's social policy statement,* ed 2, Washington, DC, 2003, American Nurses Association.
2. Center for Ethics & Human Rights Advisory Board: *Pain management and control of distressing symptoms in dying patients,* Washington, DC, 2003, American Nurses Association.
3. McCaffery M, Pasero C: *Pain: a clinical manual,* New York, 1999, Mosby.
4. Campbell ML: Usual care requirements for the patient who is near death. In Campbell ML: *Foregoing life-sustaining therapy: how to care for the patient who is near death,* Aliso Viejo, Calif, 1998, American Association of Critical-Care Nurses.
5. Truog RD et al: Recommendations for end-of-life care in the intensive care unit: the ethics committee of the Society of Critical Care Medicine, *Crit Care Med* 29:2332-2348, 2001.
6. American Pain Society: *Principles of analgesic use in the treatment of acute pain and cancer pain,* ed 5, Glenview, Ill, 2003, American Pain Society.
7. World Health Organization: *Cancer pain relief and palliative care,* Geneva, 1996, World Health Organization.
8. Jacobi J et al: Clinical practice guidelines for the sustained use of sedatives and analgesics in the critically ill adult, *Crit Care Med* 30:119-141, 2002.
9. Campbell ML: Terminal dyspnea and respiratory distress, *Crit Care Clin North Am* 20(3):403-417, 2004.
10. Claessens MT et al: Dying with lung cancer or chronic obstructive pulmonary disease: insights from SUPPORT, *J Am Geriatrics Soc* 48(5 Suppl):S146-S153, 2000.
11. Nelson JE et al: Self-reported symptom experience of critically ill cancer patients receiving intensive care, *Crit Care Med* 2:277-282, 2001.
12. American Psychiatric Association: *Diagnostic statistical manual of mental disorders,* ed 4, Washington, DC, 2000, American Psychiatric Association.
13. Ely EW et al: Evaluation of delirium in critically ill patients: validation of the confusion assessment method for the intensive care unit, *Crit Care Med* 2:1370-1379, 2001.
14. Ely EW, et al: Delirium in mechanically ventilated patients: validity and reliability of the confusion assessment method for the intensive care unit (CAM-ICU), *JAMA* 286:2703-2710, 2001.
15. Breitbart W, Chochinov HM, Passik S: Psychiatric aspects of palliative care. In Doyle D, Hanks GWC, MacDonald D, editors: *Oxford textbook of palliative medicine,* ed 2, London, 1998, Oxford University Press.

16. Harvey MA: Managing agitation in critically ill patients, *Am J Crit Care* 5:7-16, 1996.

17. Breitbart W, Strout D: Delirium in the terminally ill, *Clin Geriatric Med* 16(2):357-372, 2000.

18. Brody H et al: Withdrawing intensive life-sustaining treatment: recommendations for compassionate clinical management, *N Engl J Med* 336:652-657, 1997.

19. Rushton C, Terry PB: Neuromuscular blockade and ventilator withdrawal: ethical controversies, *Am J Crit Care* 4:112-115, 1995.

20. Truog RD, Burns JP: To breathe or not to breathe, *J Clin Ethics* 5(1):39-42, 1994.

21. Kirchhoff KT, Song MK, Kehl K: Caring for the family of the critically ill patient, *Crit Care Clin North Am* 20:453-466, 2004.

BIBLIOGRAPHY

Campbell ML: Do not resuscitate orders. In Kruse JA, Fink MP, Carlson RW editors: *Saunders manual of critical care,* Philadelphia, 2003, Saunders.

Campbell ML, Bizek KS, Thill MC: Patient responses during rapid terminal weaning from mechanical ventilation: a prospective study, *Crit Care Med* 27:73-77, 1999.

Gift A: Validation of a vertical visual analogue scale as a measure of clinical dyspnea, *Rehab Nurs* 14:323-325, 1989.

Kruse JA, Fink MP, Carlson RW: *Saunders manual of critical care,* Philadelphia, 2003, Saunders.

Manz BD et al: Pain assessment in the cognitively impaired and unimpaired elderly, *Pain Manage Nurs* 1(4):106-115, 2000.

Puntillo KA et al: Pain behaviors observed during six common procedures: results from Thunder Project II, *Crit Care Med* 3(2):421-427, 2004.

Puntillo KA, Wilke DJ: Assessment of pain in the critically ill. In Puntillo KA editor: *Pain in the critically ill,* Gaithersburg, Md, 1991, Aspen.

Rubenfeld GD: Principles and practice of withdrawing life-sustaining treatments, *Crit Care Clin* 20(3):435-452, 2004.

Stanik-Hutt JA et al: Pain experiences of traumatically injured patients in a critical care setting, *Am J Crit Care* 10:252-259, 2001.

Tarzian A: Caring for dying patients who have air hunger, *J Nurs Scholar* 32(2):137-143, 2000.

Nursing Care of the Child in the Adult Intensive Care Unit (ICU)

When a child is admitted to an adult ICU, the nurse must be prepared to make necessary modifications in care. Rosenthal[1] proposed the "PEDS framework" to assist the adult intensive care nurse in caring for a child who is admitted to the adult ICU. The PEDS framework includes the following components:

Psychosocial and physical aspects

Environment and equipment

Delivery of fluids, blood components, and medications

Safety issues

PSYCHOSOCIAL AND PHYSICAL ASPECTS

PSYCHOSOCIAL ISSUES

Like most adult patients, the child admitted to the ICU is in the presence of an unfamiliar and threatening ICU environment. For the adult ICU nurse, the care of the critically ill child may also be unfamiliar and threatening. Proactive assessment and planning for the child's and family's psychosocial and developmental needs are prerequisites to therapeutically and effectively communicating with the child and family. Important psychosocial skills for the nurse to incorporate into care include the following:

1. Integrating developmentally sensitive communication skills and behavioral assessment techniques into the nursing care of the child and family

2. Identifying concepts regarding family-centered care and methods of incorporating these concepts into the care of the child and family

COMMUNICATION SKILLS AND BEHAVIORAL ASSESSMENT TECHNIQUES

One of the essential elements of communication is establishing trust with the child and family. Demonstrating developmentally sensitive interaction with the child is important in gaining the family's sense of trust. Information from the admission history, such as cognitive and physical age of the child, and any history of chronic or previous acute illness requiring hospitalization may assist in individualizing care for the child and family.

The young child communicates behaviorally through verbal, nonverbal (body language, behaviors), and abstract (play, drawing, storytelling) cues. Cues such as disinterest in a favorite toy or crying that ceases when a parent approaches the bedside suggest how a child is feeling or perceiving an event or the presence of an individual. The child's normal behavior is more activity oriented and emotional than adult behavior. These qualities of a child's behavior should be viewed as normal in average healthy children and may be used as parameters to contrast the critically ill child (Table 9-1).

Children can be categorized into groups according to physical and cognitive age and common developmental capabilities, tasks, and fears. However, all hospitalized children share common fears despite their cognitive or physical age. These fears include loss of control, threat of separation, painful procedures, and communicated anxiety.[2]

In-depth psychosocial and developmental assessment is beyond the scope of this reference. However, Table 9-2 summarizes specific age-group characteristics with common parental considerations and nursing interventions.

FAMILY-CENTERED CARE

The most essential concept regarding the family is to value, recognize, and support family members in the care of their child. Involving parents in assessing the child's level of comfort or in scheduling daily activities such as bathing, feeding, or physical therapy exercises demonstrates a commitment to the family's involvement in the child's care. An effort should be made to follow the child's home schedule for meals, naps, and playtime as much as possible. The family is the "constant" in the child's life and is ultimately responsible for responding to the child's emotional, social, developmental, physical, and health care needs.[3] Table 9-3 includes some suggested methods of incorporating the family into the care of a critically ill child.

Appropriate support and incorporation of parents in the health care delivery system have the benefit of buffering the threats of the ICU environment on the child. Parents may assist or influence the child's cognitive appraisal or evaluation of the environment,

Table 9-1 Contrasting Affective Nonverbal Behavioral Cues of the Healthy and the Critically Ill Child

Healthy	Critically Ill
POSTURE	
Moves, flexes	May be loose, flaccid
	May prefer fetal position or position of comfort
GESTURES	
Turns to familiar voices	Responds slowly to familiar voices
MOVEMENT	
Moves purposefully	Exhibits minimal movement, lethargy, or unresponsiveness
Moves toward new, pleasurable items	Shows increased movement, irritability (possibly indicating cardiopulmonary or neurologic compromise, pain, or sleep deprivation)
Moves away from threatening items, people	
REACTIONS/COPING STYLE	
Responds to parents coming, leaving	Responds minimally to parent presence, absence
Responds to environment, equipment	Responds minimally to presence, absence of transitional objects
Cries and fights invasive procedures	Displays minimal defensive responses
FACIAL EXPRESSIONS	
Looks at faces, makes eye contact	May not track faces, objects
Changes facial expressions in response to interactions	Avoids eye contact or has minimal response to interactions
Responds negatively to face wash	Minimally changes facial expression during face wash
Blinks in response to stimuli	Has increase, decrease in blinking
Widens eyes with fear	Avoids eye contact
Is fascinated with mouth	Avoids, dislikes mouth stimulation
Holds mouth "ready for action"	Drools, has loose mouth musculature
	Displays intermittent, weak suck on pacifier

Table 9-2 Age-Specific Characteristics, Parental Concerns, and Associated Nursing Interventions

Age-Group Characteristics	Identified Parental Considerations	Nursing Interventions
INFANTS (BIRTH TO 12 MONTHS)		
Develops sense of trust as opposed to mistrust	Needs bonding	Recognize identifiable changes in status
Is not able to provide self-care	Needs encouragement to do passive physiotherapy (range of motion, stroking)	Adhere to handwashing and screen visitors for contagious illnesses
Requires expert respiratory management	Needs encouragement to do parental tasks: feeding, touching, holding, bathing, changing diaper	Converse in a quiet, unhurried manner
Requires strict adherence to infection control		Encourage presence of parents and siblings, and assistance with activities of daily living
Needs stimulation through sight and sound	Needs assistance with interpreting sibling responses to hospitalization of infant	Act as surrogate in absence of parents
Requires active play with toys	Needs information and support for decision regarding continuation of breastfeeding	Provide mobiles to look at and toys to hold
Experiences separation anxiety at approximately 8 months and older		Establish and maintain immediately accessible oxygen and emergency airway equipment
		Anticipate and assist in meeting needs of breastfeeding mother
		Recognize need and establish plan for management of pain and anxiety

TODDLER (1 TO 3 YEARS)

Has prime concern of sense of autonomy and fear of separation	Needs encouragement to provide comfort measures and communication	Encourage parental participation through demonstration
Is a dependent person but has own mind and will	Needs encouragement in holding child at bedside	Offer explanations of thoughts child might feel but cannot express (pain, mommy not here)
Begins speech, albeit limited in use and vocabulary	Needs encouragement to participate in parental tasks: feeding, touching, bathing	Suggest parents avoid participating in painful procedures; instead, offer comfort afterward by holding, stroking
Is concerned about body integrity	Needs assistance with interpreting sibling response to brother's or sister's hospitalization	Use sedation and restraints as necessary for safety
Protects self from environment through avoidance, escape, and denial	Needs education regarding safety measures	Demonstrate procedures and/or illness by dressing up toys and dolls, using puppets (child life worker)
Requires active play		Hold, stroke, spend time with child (especially at bedtime) if parents absent
Requires safe environment for play		Assess level of comfort and establish plan for management of pain and anxiety
Regards parents as most significant people		Offer support to child through simple, short explanations and direction (e.g., "No more," "Mommy's here")
Becomes especially lonely at bedtime		Maintain developmentally appropriate bowel/bladder routines and foster skill development when appropriate

Continued

Table 9-2 AGE-SPECIFIC CHARACTERISTICS, PARENTAL CONCERNS, AND ASSOCIATED NURSING INTERVENTIONS—cont'd

Age-Group Characteristics	Identified Parental Considerations	Nursing Interventions
PRESCHOOL (3 TO 6 YEARS)		
Wants to maintain acquired skills of doing for self; immobility is frightening	Needs encouragement in offering explanations of procedures and events, based on established trust with child	Demonstrate and discuss procedures with parents/family using understandable adult vocabulary
Has vivid imagination and sense of initiative	Needs encouragement to participate in parenting tasks; reading, game playing, activities based on limits of child's illness, holding, stroking, communication	Allow child to participate in acquired tasks
Is acquiring language through limited use of words	Needs assistance with anticipating needs of siblings	Answer questions; understand parent(s) may respond with denial through withdrawal
Imitates adult behavior with potential accompanying sense of guilt		Allow child to demonstrate fears through role playing (e.g., using dressed up toys)
Develops concept of self and nonself by exploring environment and body and by questioning		Facilitate and assist in preparation for sibling visitation when appropriate
Regards family members as significant people		Personalize the room/bedside with familiar toys, pictures, blanket, music
		Assess level of comfort and establish plan for management of pain and anxiety
		Use restraints only as necessary for safety
		Encourage emotional ties with home by encouraging parents to bring in child's favorite toys, games, pictures of pets and siblings, tape recordings

SCHOOL AGE (6 TO 12 YEARS)

Needs recognition of accomplishment; has strong sense of duty	Needs encouragement to promote reading, game playing, activities based on limits of child's illness	Use rewards such as stickers and verbal praise
Experiences inferiority through unattainable achievement, possibly depleting sense of identity	Needs encouragement to provide comfort measures; can act as go-between in communication for explanations and reinforcement	Ascertain child's level of understanding to identify and correct misconceptions and offer explanations at appropriate level
Is capable of verbalizing pain		Permit child participation in progressive self-care
May demand overabundance of love and attention from parent and regress	Needs encouragement to participate in parenting tasks: holding, stroking	Understand and offer comfort for parental separation
Requires that limits be set to foster a sense of security	Needs assistance in reality orientation with news of school and home	Be aware of verbal, nonverbal indications for pain and anxiety
Regards school and related events as main focus of significant people		Use child life worker for play therapy
		Use computer games, videos, etc, as diversional activities
		Offer child choices whenever possible

Continued

Table 9-2 AGE-SPECIFIC CHARACTERISTICS, PARENTAL CONCERNS, AND ASSOCIATED NURSING INTERVENTIONS—CONT'D

Age-Group Characteristics	Identified Parental Considerations	Nursing Interventions
PUBERTY ADOLESCENCE (12 TO 19 YEARS)		
Seeks identity, independence, and clarification of role in society after separation from family	Needs to understand potential for regression	Treat as adult based on level of psychologic adjustment
Is especially vulnerable to depersonalization and regression	Needs encouragement to promote awareness of disease and prognosis	Recognize and foster independence through participation in care
May experience loss of body control, destroying sense of pride in own sexuality	Needs encouragement to treat adolescent as an adult	Set limits but encourage decision making in planning of care
Attempts to identify own sense of belonging, self-esteem	Encourage touching and communication	Encourage personal belongings at bedside
Is concerned with body image change through surgery or illness	Needs assistance with anticipating needs of adolescent	Encourage personal belongings at bedside
Regards peer group as significant people		Include peers in visiting policies, because relationships are moving away from family
		Use music, news of peer group and home events as comfort measures

From Soupios M, Gallagher J, Orlowski JP: Nursing aspects of pediatric intensive care in a general hospital, *Pediatr Clin North Am* 27(3):621-622, 1980.

Table 9-3 SUPPORT OFFERED BY CHILD'S PARENTS, SUGGESTED ACTIVITIES, AND NURSING INTERVENTIONS

Support Offered	Parent Activity	Nurse Intervention
Emotional	Parent presence	Support open visitation Support parent and child while parent takes breaks Assess parents' ability to care for themselves Assess the status of siblings
Tangible	Assist in physical care: bathing, turning, stroking, feeding Assist in diversional activities: playing, reading, music	Assist parent to revise role of a parent of a well child to the role of a parent of a sick child
Informational	Provide facts and knowledge that will assist the child in coping Provide feedback that the child is secure and will recover	Keep parents informed regarding rationale of events and child's progress Support parents in providing appropriate feedback to child

personnel, and events. The child often uses the reactions of the parent as a barometer in interpreting events from the range of threatening to beneficial.

The presence and participation of parents in the care of their critically ill child offer three kinds of support: emotional, tangible, and informational.[4]

Young friends or family members can also offer support by visiting the child hospitalized in the ICU. It is important to remember that the patient's needs and desire to have visitors, as well as the appropriateness of another child visiting the ICU, should be assessed and respected. This need will vary greatly in different age-groups. An infant or young child may only want to see parents, but a teenager may need to see his or her friends because this age-group uses peers as main support figures. The number of visitors may increase when children are hospitalized in the adult ICU, necessitating a structured plan to address epidemiologic issues and educational needs related to the child visitor. A child can be a carrier of organisms that pose a risk to pediatric and adult patients who are immunocompromised or critically ill. Rotavirus and respiratory syncytial virus (RSV) are seen in the adult population as secondary contacts from pediatric cases. Communicable diseases such as chickenpox, measles, or mumps can be hazardous for adult patients and ICU staff who are susceptible to these diseases. Thus in a patient care setting with a mixed population, cross-contamination must be prevented. To decrease this risk, a pediatric health-screening tool can be developed. This tool should ascertain that the child visitor is current with all immunizations, has no communicable diseases such as sore throat, cold, or diarrhea, and has not recently been exposed to such diseases as chickenpox, mumps, or measles. The tool can provide an objective measure to determine if the visitor is eligible to enter the ICU, and it can be easily implemented by ICU staff.

Children who are visitors to the ICU may not know what to expect on entering the ICU or what is expected of them while visiting their friend or relative. Polaroid pictures of the hospitalized child and the ICU environment can provide a visual explanation of what the visiting child can expect to see. The visiting child's response to the pictures can help determine the appropriateness of the visit or any additional preparation needed. It is important to educate the young visitor(s) about policies such as handwashing; identify "safe" places for them to stand or sit; and provide simple explanations of the unusual sights and sounds. Structure the first visit based on the age and needs of both the hospitalized child and the visiting child. For example, the visiting child can count bandages, hold the patient's hand, give kisses, or simply hang a picture that the child has drawn. The visiting child should be accompanied by a supportive adult who is prepared to assist in meeting the needs of that child and can provide explanations and a continuous physical presence throughout the visit.

PHYSICAL ASSESSMENT

Approaching the child in a therapeutic and age-appropriate manner will not only facilitate the assessment process but also lessen the threatening nature of the experience. Always start with the least invasive assessment and move to the more invasive. For example, observe patient's color, work of breathing, respiratory rate, interaction with the environment, and general behavior. Then proceed to the tactile examination, such as feeling for pulses, skin temperature, and listening to breath sounds and abdominal sounds. Finally, do the more invasive part of the examination, such as looking in ears and taking a rectal temperature if required. The reader is encouraged to incorporate the essential psychosocial skills previously discussed into the physical assessment process. Important physical assessment skills include the following:

1. Interpreting vital signs based on age-appropriate norms, as well as the child's present clinical condition
2. Modifying assessment techniques based on the anatomic and physiologic differences and similarities of the child and adult
3. Recognizing the decompensating child using a quick examination approach

INTERPRETING VITAL SIGNS

Although assessment of the child requires a knowledge base of normal physiologic parameters (Table 9-4), it is imperative to understand the importance of observing vital signs before stimulation. Most physiologic parameters such as respiration, heart rate, and blood pressure will vary with the presence of a stranger. Baseline parameters are the most useful and are obtained at rest or sleep if possible. As in the adult, expect that pain, fear, fever, and activity will normally increase the child's vital signs.

It is important to compare the child's vital signs not only to the age-appropriate norms but also to the present clinical condition. Normal vital signs may not be appropriate to the sick child. For example, the child who is ill should compensate by increasing heart

Table 9-4 PEDIATRIC VITAL SIGNS

Age	Heart Rate (beats/min)	Respirations (breaths/min)	Systolic BP (mm Hg)
Newborn	100-160	30-60	50-70
1-6 wk	100-160	30-60	70-95
6 mo	90-120	25-40	80-100
1 yr	90-120	20-30	80-100
3 yr	80-120	20-30	80-110
6 yr	70-110	18-25	80-110
10 yr	60-90	15-20	90-120
14 yr	60-90	15-20	90-130

BP, Blood pressure.
Modified from Seidel JS, Henderson DP: *Prehospital care of pediatric emergencies,* Los Angeles, 1987, American Academy of Pediatrics.

rate, respiratory rate, and temperature in the presence of pneumonia. Because a child's primary means of increasing cardiac output is by increasing heart rate, inability to increase heart rate or a slowing in heart rate may be a sign of decompensation, especially in the face of a worsening clinical picture. Trends in vital signs, rather than single parameters, are usually more reflective of the child's clinical course.

PEDIATRIC ASSESSMENT

An understanding of the anatomic and physiologic differences in children is necessary to make appropriate modifications in assessment techniques and to interpret physical findings. Assessing the pediatric critically ill patient requires flexibility. Assuming the child's physical condition does not require immediate interventions, performing the least invasive assessment techniques first may build trust with the child and family, as well as prevent disruption of the remaining assessment. As with the adult patient, the child's physical and psychologic condition may dictate the priority and sequence in which the data are collected. See Table 9-5 for a guideline for pediatric assessment, including the anatomic differences seen in infants and children versus an adult. The reader is encouraged to review a pediatric textbook for more comprehensive understanding of pediatric issues.

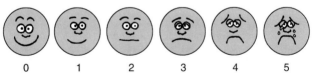

0   1   2   3   4   5

Wong-Baker FACES Pain Rating Scale. Explain to the child that each face is for a person who feels happy because he or she has no pain (hurt) or feels sad because he or she has some or a lot of pain. "Face 0 is very happy because it doesn't hurt at all. Face 1 hurts just a little bit. Face 2 hurts a little more. Face 3 hurts even more. Face 4 hurts a whole lot. Face 5 hurts just as much as you can imagine, although you don't have to be crying to feel this bad." Ask the child to choose the face that best describes how the child is feeling. Rating sale is recommended for children ages 3 and older. **Brief word instructions:** point to each face using the words to describe pain intensity. Ask the child to choose the face that best describes the child's own pain and record the appropriate number. (From Wong DL et al: *Wong's essentials of pediatric nursing,* ed 6, St Louis, 2001, Mosby, p. 1301.)

Table 9-5 PEDIATRIC ASSESSMENT

Differences	Key Points	Interventions
AIRWAY/BREATHING		
Smaller oral cavity with large tongue	More difficult to intubate	Check for appropriate size equipment
Most narrow part of airway is the cricoid ring until about 8 years of age	Secretions, inflammation, edema may obstruct the airway	Suction as needed to keep airway clear
Airway is short (about 5 cm)[5]	It is easy to unintentionally extubate with changes in position	Check artificial airway placement after each position change
Airway is very pliable	An endotracheal tube (ETT) can cause pressure to the trachea	Use an uncuffed ETT until 8 years of age
Large head size (compared to body size), underdeveloped neck muscles, lack of cartilaginous support to the airway	Airway can be compressed and/or obstructed If the child is sitting up and forward to breathe, there is airway compromise	Keep an infant's head in the "sniffing" position A small roll behind the shoulders may be beneficial Avoid overextending or overflexing Keep the child in position of comfort
Infants are obligate nose breathers until 6 months of age	Secretions, nasal cannula, or an NG may obstruct the airway	Keep the nose clear of secretions Replace the NG with an OG Cut the prongs off the nasal cannula

Continued

Table 9-5 PEDIATRIC ASSESSMENT—cont'd

Differences	Key Points	Interventions
Chest wall is thin, muscles poorly developed, and ribs are very flexible	Breath sounds are loud and easy to hear; retractions or unequal chest movement is easy to recognize	Clear description of retractions should be charted Breath sounds must be frequently assessed for presence, absence, or changes
Infants and toddlers use abdominal muscles to assist breathing	May have "see-saw" breathing	
Basal metabolic rate in infants is twice that of an adult, which leads to a higher minute volume	There will be an increased respiratory rate (Table 9-4) and higher oxygen consumption	A slow rate must be monitored closely for respiratory arrest Tachypnea is often the first sign of distress Respiratory rates must be counted for a full minute
Infants have an irregular respiratory rate		
Expiratory grunting is produced when there is an attempt to increase positive end-expiratory pressure (PEEP)	Other breath sounds occur in the same pattern as adults	
CIRCULATORY		
Heart rates are higher in infants and children	Cardiac output changes with rate rather than volume	Heart rates should be counted for a full minute in infants and small children
Tachycardia may reflect pain, fever, shock, hypoxemia, or fear	Hypoxemia may cause bradycardia in infants and tachycardia in older children	Pulses should be documented in each extremity

Bradycardia may reflect a vagal response (tube placement, suctioning, defecation)

Peripheral pulses that are decreased in the legs from the arms can be a sign of cardiac disease

Peripheral pulses can be assessed ... of hypothermia

A child's skin (end-organ perfusion) is thin and will display color changes, temperature, and texture easily and quickly

Normal capillary refill is less than 2 seconds (this has not been scientifically validated)

Cyanosis centrally is abnormal

Blood volume varies with age and weight (80 mL/kg)

A child can compensate for 25% blood loss without a change in systolic blood pressure

Blood pressure (see Table 9-4)

Skin temperature, color, and capillary refill can be altered by environmental factors

Color and skin temperature combined are a good method of assessment for perfusion

Infants may have peripheral cyanosis

Small amounts of blood loss can be significant

Systolic blood pressure may not accurately reflect the situation

May need to use warming devices

Always include environmental factors in the patient assessment

Always note the line of demarcation of skin color and temperature

It is important to trend children's blood pressure

Blood pressures should be documented in each extremity

NEUROLOGIC

At birth infants function at a subcortical level

Continued

Table 9-5 PEDIATRIC ASSESSMENT—cont'd

Differences	Key Points	Interventions
Cortical development is 75% complete by 2 years of age		
Posterior fontanel closes by 3 months of age	Assessment of the fontanels is useful in determining fluid status	The presence or absence of open fontanels should be documented
Anterior fontanel closes at 9 to 18 months of age		Head circumference should be measured daily up until 2 years of age (Table 9-6)
Newborn reflexes include Moro reflex (until 6 months), rooting reflex (until 4 months), grasp reflex (until 3 months), and Babinski's reflex (until 9 to 12 months)		
Meningeal irritation may cause nuchal rigidity, Kernig's sign, Brudzinski's sign, or paradoxical irritability	Soothing interventions may increase irritability More likely to develop "malignant brain edema"[7]	Use a firm rather than a light stroking touch
In the trauma setting children have a lower incidence of mass lesions[6] and increased incidence of intracranial hypertension		
Assessment can be done using the infant Glasgow Coma Scale (see Table 9-1 and Table 9-7)		Use toys and play actions to elicit needed responses

GASTROINTESTINAL

An abdomen will be protuberant until adolescence	Abdomen should always be soft
Stomach will hold:	If there is an abdominal concern, an abdominal girth can be measured just above the umbilicus
90 mL—newborn	
150 mL—1-month-old	The stomach will empty in 2.5-3 hours in a small child, 3-6 hours in an older child	Amount of bolus feeds should not exceed stomach capacity
360 mL—1-year-old		Position for best gastric emptying
2000-3000 mL—adult		
An infant has an immature cardiac sphincter and may have reverse peristalsis	Watch for regurgitation	Position infants side-lying to protect airway if regurgitation occurs
Bowel emptying is involuntary until 14-18 months of age	Children who have become potty trained may regress during times of illness	
Liver margin varies from 3 cm below the costal margin in infants to 1 cm below in a 4- to 5-year-old	Liver enlargement may be a sign of heart failure	
Nutritional needs are high in children because of a high metabolic rate (Table 9-8)	Residuals should be reinserted if possible	Adjust feeds and other needed therapies to maximize the benefit of all treatments
Children should be weighed daily	20%-27% of children in intensive care are undernourished[8]	Weigh at the same time with the same scale without clothes each day

Continued

Table 9-5 PEDIATRIC ASSESSMENT—cont'd

Differences	Key Points	Interventions
RENAL		
Urine output is:	Infants and children have a higher insensible water loss	Intake and output (I&O) must be recorded and monitored carefully
2 mL/kg/hr for infants		
1 mL/kg/hr for children	Specific gravity may run low	
0.5 mL/kg/hr for adolescents		
Infants have less ability to concentrate urine		
Children dehydrate easily	See Table 9-9	Monitor I&O, weight, fontanels, and skin turgor changes
ENDOCRINE		
Glucose production is increased in the neonate and small child	Hypoglycemia is a risk (Box 9-1)	Monitor glucose especially during times of stress
Children have smaller glycogen stores and an increased demand		

IMMUNOLOGIC

Newborns have fewer stored neutrophils and are less able to replenish white blood cells during infectious states

Most immunoglobulin is received from maternal transfer. Physiologic hypogammaglobulinemia occurs at 4-5 months of age

Infants with overwhelming infection may not demonstrate fever or leukocytosis

Children are susceptible to infections during this time, especially *Candida* spp.

Signs of infection may be changes in feeding, glucose levels, or hypothermia

Good handwashing is imperative

PAIN AND AGITATION

Responses to pain are listed in Table 9-10 Children of different ages perceive pain differently

Pain should be assessed using an age-appropriate scale

>4 years old—self report

8-9 years old—numeric scale

3-18 years old—Wong-Baker FACES Pain Rating Scale[9] on p. 640

Suctioning, wound care, and turning were found to be the most painful procedures[10]

The method of pain assessment should be documented with the assessment outcome

Nurses should use vital signs, behavior, and pain assessment scale in determining pain level

DECOMPENSATING CHILD

A child's condition can change very rapidly

See Table 9-11

Extreme vigilance must occur with a sick child

NG, Nasogastric; *OG,* orogastric.

ENVIRONMENT

PSYCHOSOCIAL ENVIRONMENT

The presence of pediatric patients in the adult ICU influences adult patients and their families, as well as fellow health care team members. It is a societal belief that children should not die and parents should not outlive their offspring. Adult patients and staff who are exposed to the sights and sounds of the critically ill child may express a wide variety of emotions such as guilt, anger, and nontherapeutic empathy for the child and family. When another patient expresses concern for a crying child, it may be beneficial to offer a simple update, reassurance, or explanation for the sights and sounds.

Approaching the bedside with confidence goes a long way in reinforcing the child's and family's level of trust in the care that they will receive. Small efforts to decrease anxiety such as sitting down or positioning yourself at the child's eye level when talking to the child can make a difference. A child's uneasy feelings may be in response to the parent's anxiety and the anxiety of the health care team members in the child's immediate environment. Interventions to relieve the anxiety of parents and fellow health team members may include assisting parents and staff in anticipating the child's responses to therapy and illness and guiding parents and staff in therapeutic communication techniques.

All ICU patients, including the young child, may distort reality as a result of sensory overload or sleep deprivation. Interventions to reduce reality distortion in children are similar to interventions for the adult patient (e.g., minimize the instances that the patient may be exposed to procedures or to the procedures experienced by other patients,

Box 9-1 Signs and Symptoms of Hypoglycemia	
Neonate	Infant/child
Pallor	Pallor, sweating
Tremors, jitteriness	Increased heart rate
Tachypnea	Nausea, vomiting
Feeding difficulties	Hunger, abdominal pain
Hypotonia	Irritability
Abnormal cry	Headache, visual disturbances
Apnea, cyanosis	Mental confusion
Convulsions	Convulsions, coma
Coma	

Table 9-6 AVERAGE HEAD CIRCUMFERENCE

Age	Mean (cm)	Standard Deviation (cm)
Birth	35	1.2
1 mo	37.6	1.2
2 mo	39.7	1.2
3 mo	40.4	1.2
6 mo	43.4	1.1
9 mo	45	1.2
12 mo	46.5	1.2
18 mo	48.4	1.2
2 yr	49	1.2
3 yr	50	1.2
4 yr	50.5	1.2
5 yr	50.8	1.4
6 yr	51.2	1.4
7 yr	51.6	1.4
8 yr	52	1.5

Modified from Moran M: Growth and development. In Ashwill JW, Droske SC, editors: *Nursing care of children: principles and practice,* Philadelphia, 1997, WB Saunders.

Table 9-7 ADULT AND INFANT GLASGOW COMA SCALES*

Activity	Adult Best Response	Points	Infant Best Response
Eye opening	Spontaneous	4	Spontaneous
	To verbal stimuli	3	To speech
	To pain	2	To pain
	No response to pain	1	No response to pain
Motor	Follows commands	6	Normal spontaneous movements
	Localizes pain	5	Localizes pain
	Withdrawal in response to pain	4	Withdrawal in response to pain
	Flexion in response to pain	3	Flexion in response to pain
	Extension in response to pain	2	Extension in response to pain
	No response to pain	1	No response to pain
Verbal	Oriented	5	Coos, babbles
	Confused	4	Irritable crying
	Inappropriate words	3	Cries to pain
	Incomprehensible	2	Moans to pain sounds
	No verbal response	1	No verbal response

*Possible points of 3 to 15; score of <8 = coma.

Table 9-8 RECOMMENDED DIETARY ALLOWANCES FOR CALORIES AND PROTEIN BASED ON MEDIAN HEIGHTS AND WEIGHTS

Age	Wt (kg)	Ht (cm)	Kcal/ kg	Kcal/ day	Protein (g/kg)	Protein (g/day)
<6 mo	6	60	108	650	2.2	13
6-12 mo	9	71	98	850	1.6	14
1-3 yr	13	90	102	1300	1.2	16
4-6 yr	20	112	90	1800	1.1	24
7-10 yr	28	132	70	2000	1.0	28
11-14 yr (M)	45	157	55	2500	1.0	45
11-14 yr (F)	46	157	47	2200	0.8	44
15-18 yr (M)	66	176	45	3000	0.9	59
15-18 yr (F)	55	163	40	2200	0.8	44

F, Female; *M,* male.
Modified from *Recommended dietary allowances,* Washington, DC, 1989, National Academy Press.

Table 9-9 SIGNIFICANT WEIGHT GAIN OR LOSS

Weight Gain Related to Fluid Overload	Weight Loss Related to Dehydration
INFANTS	
>50 g/24 hr	Mild: 5% of body weight
	Moderate: 10% of body weight
	Severe: 15% of body weight
CHILDREN	
>200 g/24 hr	Mild: 3% of body weight
	Moderate: 6% of body weight
	Severe: 9% of body weight
ADOLESCENTS	
>500 g/24 hr	Mild: 3% of body weight
	Moderate: 6% of body weight
	Severe: 9% of body weight

Table 9-10 DEVELOPMENTALLY APPROPRIATE RESPONSES
TO PAIN OR AGITATION

Age	Motor Movement	Communication
Newborn (0-3 mo)	Generalized motor movements	Intermittent crying
Young infant (3 mo)	Move/turn slowly	Sustained cry, moan, whimper
Infant (6 mo)	Kick, pull away, wring hands, bite/pinch self	Anticipatory cry, fear cry
9 mo	Push away, elevate, control limb	"Mommy"
12 mo	Resist, tremors, bite towel	"Mommy"
18 mo	Resist, tremors, bite towel	"Ow," "Hurt"

Table 9-11 QUICK EXAMINATION OF A HEALTHY VERSUS
DECOMPENSATING CHILD

Assessment	Healthy Child	Decompensating Child
AIRWAY		
Patency	Requires no interventions; child verbalizes and is able to swallow, cough, gag	Child self-positions; requires interventions such as head positioning, suctioning, adjunct airways
BREATHING		
Respiratory rate	Is within age-appropriate limits	Is tachypneic or brady-pneic compared to age-appropriate limits and condition
Chest movement (presence)	Chest rises and falls equally and simultaneously with abdomen with each breath	Has minimal or no chest movement with respiratory effort
Chest movement (quality)	Has silent and effortless respirations	Shows evidence of labored respirations with retractions

Continued

Table 9-11 QUICK EXAMINATION OF A HEALTHY VERSUS DECOMPENSATING
CHILD—cont'd

Assessment	Healthy Child	Decompensating Child
BREATHING—cont'd		
		Has asynchronous movement (seesaw) between chest and abdomen with respiratory efforts
Air movement (presence)	Air exchange heard bilaterally in all lobes	Despite movement of the chest, minimal or no air exchange is noted on auscultation
Air movement (quality)	Breath sounds normal intensity and duration auscultation location per	Has nasal flaring, grunting, stridor, wheezing, or retractions
CIRCULATION		
Heart rate (presence)	Apical beat present and within age-appropriate limit	Has bradycardia or tachycardia as compared with age-appropriate limits and clinical condition
Heart rate (quality)	Heart rate regular with normal sinus rhythm	Has irregular, slow, or very rapid heart rate; common dysrhythmias include supraventricular tachycardia, brady-dysrhythmias, and asystole
Skin	Has warm, pink extremities with capillary refill ≤2 sec; peripheral pulses present bilaterally with normal intensity	Has pallor, cyanotic or mottled skin color; has cool to cold extremities; capillary refill time is ≥2 sec; peripheral pulses are weak, absent; central pulses are weak
Cerebral perfusion	Is alert to surroundings, recognizes parents or significant others, is responsive to fear and pain, has normal muscle tone	Is irritable, lethargic, obtunded, or comatose; has minimal or no reaction to pain; has loose muscle tone (floppy)
Blood pressure	Has blood pressure within age-appropriate limits	Shows fall in blood pressure from age-appropriate limits (late sign)

manipulate the environment to reduce noise and lights, promote routine nap times, allow family visits, and allow the child's favorite stuffed animal or toy to be at his or her side).

PHYSICAL ENVIRONMENT

Planning a Designated Area

A specific area in the adult ICU should be designated and designed for the care of the child and family. The optimal solution is to physically separate the two populations of patients and to minimize the noise that is inherent in the care of children.

If a permanently designated space in the unit is not possible, modification of an individual bedspace may include the addition of a pediatric supply cart, limitation of extraneous bedside equipment, and placement of the child in a bedspace of the unit that facilitates a balance between low stimulation and adequate observation by nursing staff. Every effort should be made to create a nonthreatening safe place for the child and family that reduces exposure to sights and sounds of an open ICU environment.

Family Support Areas

Family support areas should be in close proximity to the unit. A waiting room, nutritional area, private consultation area, and sleeping accommodations are essential in meeting basic physical needs of families while they support their child through the ICU experience. If the physical environment is not conducive to supporting parents or significant others, it is extremely important that these needs be recognized and addressed daily with a professional resource person.

Pediatric Supply Cart

In the adult-pediatric ICU, it is difficult to predict the number and acuity of the patient census; therefore a mechanism to facilitate bedside equipment access and supply is important. The development of a pediatric supply cart consolidates the required equipment and allows routine intensive care delivery to the infant, child, and adolescent within an adult-oriented unit. Just as the adult equipment is maintained at the bedside ready for use, it is helpful to organize the same supplies in the appropriate sizes for pediatric use in a cart that may be rolled to any bedside if needed. Some suggested items to include on the pediatric supply cart are listed in Box 9-2.

Box 9-2 Pediatric Supply Cart Contents

DRAWER #1: Reference cards and PALS guidelines

Broselow resuscitation tape or guidelines for selection of equipment based on size or
weight

DRAWER #2: Intravenous therapy

20-gauge 1-inch IV catheter

22-gauge 1-inch IV catheter

24-gauge {³⁄₄}-inch IV catheter

21-gauge butterfly needle

23-gauge butterfly needle

25-gauge butterfly needle

Extension set with T-connector

Syringes (1, 3, and 6 mL)

Suture kits

Infant/child soft restraints

Bandages

Infant/child armboards

Tongue blades

$^5/_{16}$ inch and $^1/_2$-inch Penrose drains, rubber bands (infant/child tourniquets)

Safety pins (to secure restraints or armboards)

Cotton balls (to support/pad catheter hub)

IV site protection (commercially made or medicine cup half)

Tape $^1/_2$ inch and 1 inch

Normal saline without preservative

DRAWER #3: Respiratory

Endotracheal tubes

Oxisensors (pediatric, infant)

Oral airways (4, 5, 6, 7 mm)

Nasopharyngeal airways

Tracheostomy tubes (pediatric 00, 0, 1, 2, 3)

Pediatric or small oral suction device

Pediatric chest percussor (small, medium)

Junior or pediatric spirometer

Sterile tracheal suction catheters (5, 8, 10, 12, 14 Fr)

Bulb suction

DRAWER #4: Cardiovascular

Small electrodes

BP cuffs (newborn, child, young adult)

Pediatric stethoscope

Sets of pediatric blood tubes

Sterile mosquito clamps

Box 9-2 Pediatric Supply Cart Contents—cont'd

Sterile needle drivers (small)

Lancets or other device for fingersticks and heelstick

DRAWER #5: GI/GU

Nasogastric tubes (8, 10, 12 Fr)

Feeding tube (5 Fr)

Measuring tape

Bottle

Nipple

Pacifier

Urine bags

Foley catheter (6*, 8, 10, 12 Fr)

DRAWER #6

Pediatric chest drainage collection unit

Trocar catheters (10, 12, 14, 16)

Pediatric tracheostomy tray

Pediatric LP tray

Percutaneous line insertion tray

Central venous catheters (beginning with 4 Fr)

Suture (3-0, 4-0, 5-0 silk)

Intraosseous needles

IV tubing and buretrols, if used

Radiation shield

Baby blanket, medium-sized diapers

---

*May use 5 Fr feeding tube if 6 Fr Foley not available.

BP, Blood pressure; *GI,* gastrointestinal; *GU,* genitourinary; *IV,* intravenous; *LP,* lumbar puncture; *PALS,* pediatric advanced life support.

EQUIPMENT

PHYSICAL ASSESSMENT SUPPLIES

Supplies to perform a physical assessment on a pediatric patient are essentially the same as those for an adult patient. The size of instruments depends on the size of the patient. Basic equipment for physical assessment includes a scale, stethoscope, blood pressure cuff, thermometer, measuring tape, and an otoscope with various size speculums.

Weighing Devices

Because many therapies for the child, such as drug and fluid delivery, are weight specific, obtaining an accurate weight on or soon after admission is vital (see Table 9-9). If a weight cannot be determined, a pediatric resuscitation tape is available to assist in estimation of weight, drug doses, and equipment size selection. Gram scales are also used to measure urine collected in a diaper or blood or body fluid loss on dressings and linen. The total weight of the diaper (g), minus the weight of a dry diaper, indicates the volume of urine (mL).

Stethoscope

Stethoscopes of any size can be used for auscultation; however, the small child may be auscultated more easily using a pediatric stethoscope with the smaller diaphragm and bell.

Blood Pressure Cuffs

The blood pressure cuff should be $^2/_3$ to $^3/_4$ of the upper arm size, and the cuff bladder should completely encircle the child's arm only once. Table 9-12 reviews normal blood pressure cuff sizes in the pediatric patient.

Noninvasive Blood Pressure

Blood pressure values obtained via the indirect method of mercury manometer and auscultation or palpation can be reliable. Research has determined that oscillometric monitors accurately measure blood pressure in the normotensive child. However, in the hemodynamically unstable child, the ability to accurately measure acute pressure changes is questionable.[11] Cuffs that are too small may result in falsely elevated blood pressure readings.[12] It may be necessary to use Doppler to assess blood pressure and peripheral pulses in the hemodynamically compromised child.

Table 9-12   COMMONLY AVAILABLE BLOOD PRESSURE CUFFS

Cuff Name*	Bladder Width (cm)	Bladder Length (cm)
Newborn	2.5-4	5-9
Infant	4-6	11.5-1
Child	7.5-9	17-19
Adult	11.5-13	22-26
Large arm	14-15	30.5-33
Thigh	18-19	36-38

*Cuff name does not guarantee that the cuff will be appropriate size for a child within that age range.
From Report of the Second Task Force on Blood Pressure Control in Children—1987. Task Force on Blood Pressure Control in Children. National Heart, Lung, and Blood Institute, Bethesda, Md, *Pediatrics* 79(1):1-25, 1987.

Temperature Measurement

If using the standard glass thermometer, avoid obtaining the young child's temperature orally. There is a high risk of the child biting and breaking the instrument. In obtaining rectal temperatures, use only rectal-tipped thermometers to minimize the risk of perirectal damage. Rectal temperatures are avoided until a newborn passes the first meconium stool and when a child has diarrhea, rectal irritation, neutropenia, or thrombocytopenia. Tympanic thermometers offer a less invasive option of temperature measurement. The accuracy of the device in children with marked hypothermia and hyperthermia is still being validated. The device is not recommended for infants younger than 3 months of age. Consult the specific product information for age limitations. The accuracy of the tympanic thermometer directly correlates with the skill of the user and compliance with product usage guidelines. Core body temperature may be assessed using a Foley catheter with a bladder thermistor device, or using the thermistor of a pulmonary artery catheter that has been inserted for hemodynamic monitoring.

Measuring Tape

A nonstretch measuring tape that has units in both centimeters and inches should be available to measure head circumferences and abdominal girths. Head circumferences are generally measured in children younger than 2 years.

Otoscope

Because of the high frequency of ear infections in the pediatric population, an otoscope with appropriate-sized speculum covers should be available.

NEEDLES FOR SUBCUTANEOUS OR INTRAMUSCULAR INJECTION

Small, 30-gauge $^1/_2$-inch needles are available for uses such as subcutaneous injection of buffered lidocaine for local anesthesia. Issues regarding intramuscular medication delivery are discussed in the medication delivery section of this chapter.

Intravenous (IV) Catheter Selection

The optimal IV catheter size is one that is the smallest gauge to achieve the intended therapy and not impair blood flow around the catheter. Table 9-13 reviews suggested catheter sizes according to patient age.

Table 9-13 SUGGESTED INTRAVENOUS CATHETER SIZES FOR CHILDREN

Age	Butterfly	Over-the-Needle
Infant	25-27 gauge	24 gauge (range 22-26)
Child	23-25 gauge	22 gauge (range 20-24)
Adolescent	21-23 gauge	20 gauge (range 18-22)

Table 9-14 INTRAVENOUS CATHETER INSERTION AND MAINTENANCE IN CHILDREN

Difference	Result	Interventions
Cooperation	Difficulty is in accessing an uncooperative, moving target	Explanation and preparation of infant is of minimal value, but prepare parent if present Provide comfort and reassurance Preparation of young child should be age appropriate Practice good positioning techniques of child (e.g., mummy wrap) Obtain assistance from another health care team member to hold child if necessary
Security	Once IV is in place, difficulty is securing it because of small size of insertion site and frequent movement of child	Prepare and use an armboard when necessary For infant, make armboards out of padded tongue blades Select an IV site away from a joint or highly mobile area; avoid dominant hand and feet, if ambulatory Use soft restraints on affected extremity to minimize movement and risk of kinking or dislodging the catheter Avoid circumferential taping Use nonadhesive, easily removable, self-adherent wrap to stabilize IV and prevent potential skin breakdown

Continued

Table 9-14 INTRAVENOUS CATHETER INSERTION AND MAINTENANCE IN CHILDREN—cont'd

Difference	Result	Interventions
Technique for venous distention	Because of young child's thin and sensitive skin, warm soaks may burn the patient and large tourniquets may be ineffective	Obtain small latex drains or rubber bands for infants and small children or use a second person's hand to apply circumferential pressure above the insertion site May use disposable diapers with warm water to wrap around extremity to dilate vessels, but keep the bed dry Carefully check the temperature of any moist heat to avoid burning the child's thin skin

IV, Intravenous.

Site Selection

Each site for IV catheterization has its advantages and disadvantages. The clinician should consider the condition of the vessels, the purpose for the IV infusion, and the projected duration of the IV therapy.

Scalp veins are easily found in infants, but they require shaving a portion of the child's head and may be aesthetically unpleasant to the parents. Preferably, upper extremity sites are used and include the dorsum of the hand and cephalic and median basilic veins. When selecting an upper extremity, the clinician should note the child's preference for right-sided or left-sided dominance or an infant's preference of thumbsucking, and use the nondominant hand for the IV therapy. Antecubital veins are infrequently used because they limit the child's mobility and pose a greater risk for dislodgment. In the infant and toddler, veins in the lower extremities such as the saphenous, median marginal, and dorsal arch are used if necessary.

IV access in the infant and young child may be time consuming and difficult. A systematic approach should be in place to ensure efficient IV access in the event a pediatric patient requires resuscitation.

According to pediatric advanced life support (PALS)[13] recommendations, access is attempted in large peripheral veins three times or for a total of 90 seconds, whichever is less. If initial peripheral access is unsuccessful, a percutaneous central venous access or saphenous vein cutdown may be attempted or intraosseous (IO) access should be attempted. There is no age restriction for using intraosseous access in children. Table 9-14 reviews the essential differences in the pediatric patient and the associated, necessary interventions for IV catheter maintenance.

PHLEBOTOMY ISSUES

Blood Volume Requirements for Laboratory Analysis

It is essential to establish minimum blood volumes required for laboratory tests to minimize repeat testing and excessive blood loss. Microtubes and/or pediatric blood tubes should be available along with reference sheets listing the required blood volumes for each test.

Blood Loss

Blood loss associated with the blood drawn for laboratory analysis can be significant. The amount of blood drawn from the patient should be documented in the fluid balance record. Estimating the child's circulatory blood volume (normal is approximately 80 mL/kg) and comparing it with the total amount of blood withdrawn for analysis can assist the clinician in determining the severity of blood loss. When the volume of blood for analysis exceeds 5% to 7% of the circulatory blood volume or if there is a significant decrease in hematocrit levels and accompanying symptomatology, blood replacement should be anticipated.[14]

Blood Sampling

The majority of blood samples in the pediatric population are obtained through IV or intraarterial lines, which increases the chance of sampling error secondary to contamination from IV fluids or flush solutions. An adequate discard volume should be withdrawn to clear the fluid from the sampling port of the catheter without contributing to excessive blood loss. The intravascular access should be flushed with each sampling and the amount of flush solution and discarded volume should be accurately measured and documented. The blood used to clear the line can be reinfused to minimize blood loss.

INTRAOSSEOUS (IO) ACCESS AND INFUSION

Description

Placing an access in the bone marrow cavity offers many advantages because the bone marrow functions as a rigid vein. The marrow sinusoids drain into the venous systems, where fluid or medication can be immediately absorbed into the general circulation. Blood products, fluids, and medications may be administered through the IO route, although it is recommended that hypertonic and alkaline solutions be diluted before infusion.[13,15] Potential complications include tibial fracture, compartment syndrome, skin necrosis, and osteomyelitis. Contraindications include osteogenesis imperfecta, osteoporosis, and a fracture in the extremity to be accessed.

The optimal site for IO placement during a resuscitative effort is the proximal tibia (Figure 9-1), which precludes interference with ventilations and chest compressions. Reusable or disposable bone marrow needles, sizes 15 to 18 gauge, should be available. The needle should stand firmly upward without support, but it should be secured with tape and a sterile dressing. As with any intravascular access, signs of extravasation and patency should be monitored. Heparin-saline flushes may discourage clotting of the access. The IO access is not meant to be permanent; therefore attempts should be made to acquire other IV access and discontinue IO needle as soon as possible.

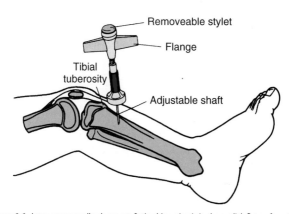

Figure 9-1 Intraosseous needle placement. Optimal insertion is in the medial, flat surface of the anterior tibia approximately 1 to 3 cm below the tibial tuberosity. The needle is directed at a 60- to 90-degree angle away from the growth plate to avoid the epiphyseal plate. (From Fiser DH: Intraosseous infusion, *N Engl J Med* 322[22]:1579-1581, 1990.)

ELECTROCARDIOGRAM (ECG) MONITORING

The optimal pediatric ECG machine must be able to monitor and record rapid heart rates of 250 to 300 beats/min. Because of the infant's irregular respiratory rate and the infant's and young child's propensity toward respiratory rather than cardiac arrest, the machine should also have the capability of monitoring respiratory rate and breathing pattern. Apnea alarm capability is an asset.

Electrodes should be small to allow for sensitivity of the infant's and young child's thinner skin. To decrease the incidence of skin irritation, electrode patches and sites should be rotated regularly. Electrode placement and chest landmarks are the same in the child and in the adult. If using the same system to monitor respiratory function, place the lower electrode on the abdomen to sense respiratory movement.

PULSE OXIMETER

Pulse oximetry is essentially the same technique in the pediatric and adult patient. The child with poor peripheral perfusion is not an optimal candidate for pulse oximetry. In addition, the infant or young child tends to be more active, and movement of the extremity with the probe will lead to inaccurate readings. Site- and size-specific oximetry sensors are used. Alternative sites for the small infant or child include the hand area between the thumb and forefinger or the medial aspect of the infant's foot. Skin under the sensor should be evaluated at least once every 8 hours. Sensor site may be rotated to prevent skin irritation from heat and pressure.

END-TIDAL CO$_2$ MONITORING

The indications and methods for end-tidal CO$_2$ monitoring are the same in the adult and pediatric patient.

PERIPHERAL ARTERY CATHETERIZATION

Indications and Site Selection

The indications and sites for arterial cannulation and monitoring are determined by the stability and size of the artery and the availability of sufficient collateral circulation. Radial artery cannulation is the most commonly used site after verification of collateral ulnar artery circulation using the Allen test. Other optional sites include femoral, pedal, and posterior tibial. Temporal and axillary arterial sites can be used; however, the size and location of the vessels have a higher potential for complications.

Patient Management

The most important issues regarding arterial lines in the child are ensuring patency and security of the line, regulating the amount and pressure of the flush solution, setting appropriate alarm limits, and monitoring for complications. There should be a continuous administration of heparinized intraarterial solution to maintain patency. Consideration of the type of solution and need for heparinization and the amount of fluid that the child receives hourly and daily are important.

For infants and small children, the arterial line should be placed on an infusion pump to regulate the flow and prevent inadvertent administration of unnecessary fluid. Arterial lines should be slowly flushed using a manual rather than the pigtail flush method, regardless of the size of the child. Manual flushing facilitates accurate intake assessment; prevents unnecessary pressures on small, fragile vessels; and limits retrograde embolization into the central circulation. Alarms for all hemodynamic lines should be set for age-appropriate limits and should remain on at all times.

Complications

Children have an increased risk of vasospasm and thrombosis. Infusion of papaverine-containing solutions into arterial catheters has been shown to reduce the risk of catheter failure in pediatric patients.[16] However, its use is not recommended in neonates.

CENTRAL VENOUS CATHETERIZATION

The subclavian vein can be used; however, there is a higher risk of complications associated with this location even by the expert clinician. This is due to the proximity of the subclavian vein to the apex of the lung. A chest radiograph is required to confirm catheter position and evaluate for a potential pneumothorax.

PULMONARY ARTERY CATHETERIZATION

Description

Pulmonary artery catheters are indicated in children who are receiving the most aggressive therapies, such as high ventilator pressures, massive hemodynamic support, and/or barbiturate therapy for increased intracranial pressure.

Insertion

Pediatric pulmonary artery catheters are smaller in diameter than adult catheters, yet they are not much shorter. The femoral vein is a commonly used vessel because it can accommodate the entire length of the catheter and allows for correct placement of catheter ports. Pediatric catheters do not have an additional port for infusion of fluids and medications. The central venous pressure (CVP) port of the 5-French (Fr) catheter is extremely small and clots easily; therefore it is not an optimal port for blood component administration.

Normal Values

The pressures of the cardiac chambers and great vessels are the same in the child older than 2 years as in the adult in the absence of congenital or acquired cardiac disease. Cardiac output varies greatly with size and body; therefore it is prudent to monitor cardiac index in children. The normal cardiac index ranges between 3.5 and 4.5 L/min/m^2.

Patient Management

The amount of solution used for cardiac output injectates is generally 3 or 5 mL rather than 10 mL and should be recorded as a part of the child's hourly intake. When using smaller volumes, iced injectate is recommended. Knowing the dead space or priming volume of catheters is paramount to withdrawing the appropriate amount of discard blood and infusing the minimal amount of flush to clear the catheter.

ASSISTIVE RESPIRATORY DEVICES

Manual Resuscitation Bags

Unlike the adult 1-L manual resuscitation bag, pediatric manual resuscitation bags are available in infant (250 mL) and pediatric (500 mL) sizes. The resuscitation bag should be capable of delivering one and one-half times the child's tidal volume (V_T), or 10 to 15 mL/kg, as well as delivering 100% oxygen. For the pediatric bags to consistently deliver 100% oxygen at rapid respiratory rates, the manual resuscitation bag should have an oxygen reservoir.

Most pediatric resuscitation bags are designed with a pop-off valve to prevent excessive pressure delivery with the average manual breath. Pop-off valves are normally activated with breaths requiring peak inspiratory pressures (PIPs) between 35 and 60 cm H_2O pressure. This reduces the incidence of barotrauma or gastric distention by releasing excessive pressure to the atmosphere rather than to the child. When manual ventilations are essential, the lungs are stiff and require high PIPs. The pop-off valve can be covered with adhesive tape or the clinician's finger during manual breath delivery.

The infant's lung tissue is sensitive to high-pressure ventilation. Pneumothoraces may be induced from manual or mechanical ventilation. A pressure manometer is connected inline to the manual resuscitation bag to minimize excessive PIPs and to provide breaths similar in pressure to the mechanical breaths received from the ventilator. Although a pressure manometer can assist in minimizing pressure and the reservoir can assist in providing 100% oxygen, the only indicator to ensuring adequate V_T delivery is a clinical one. The adequate amount of V_T delivered during a mechanical resuscitation breath is the amount that causes an observable rise and fall of the child's chest.

Resuscitation Masks

Like bags, resuscitation masks come in a variety of sizes, ranging from neonatal to young adult. The ideal mask is one that covers the child's nose and mouth yet prevents pressure on the eyes.

ARTIFICIAL AIRWAYS

All pediatric airways are small compared with the overall body size of the patient. It is important to recognize that the smaller the airway, the more difficult it is to maintain position and patency.

Nasopharyngeal and Oropharyngeal Airways

The correct length for a nasopharyngeal airway in the infant or child is determined by measuring from the tip of the nose to the tragus of the ear. The diameter of the nasopharyngeal airway should be the largest size that easily inserts without causing blanching of the nares. The pediatric patient often has large adenoids and fragile nasal mucosa that can lacerate during the insertion process, causing significant nosebleeds. Nasopharyngeal airways should be maintained as patent as possible because the infant is an obligate nose breather.

An oropharyngeal airway is particularly useful as an assistive device to bag-valve mask ventilations in the unconscious child. The proper size is estimated by placing the airway next to the child's face. The flange should be at the level of the central incisors, and the end should be approximately at the tip of the mandibular angle. Insertion is facilitated by using a tongue depressor to hold the tongue down onto the floor of the child's mouth.

Endotracheal Tube (ETT)

To estimate the correct size of the uncuffed ETT, choose a tube approximately the same size as the child's little finger, or use the following formula:

$$\text{Internal diameter} = \frac{16 + \text{age in yr}}{4}$$

It is important to recognize that both of these methods are estimations of the correct ETT size; tubes one-half size (0.5 mm) larger and one-half size smaller should be available for immediate use. Cuffed ETTs are as safe as uncuffed tubes and may be indicated in the patient with stiff, noncompliant lungs. Use the following formula to determine the size of a cuffed ETT:

$$(\text{Age in yr} \div 4) + 3$$

Keep cuff pressure <20 cm H_2O. ETT position should be confirmed with colorimetric detector or capnography in children with perfusion rhythms.

Pediatric Intubation

Every effort should be made to intubate the child under controlled conditions, using appropriately sized equipment (Table 9-15). Awake intubations should be considered only for resuscitation situations or when there is considerable question about whether the child can be ventilated by bag and mask when sedated and pharmacologically paralyzed. Rapid-sequence sedation and paralysis with IV medications provide the clinician satisfactory visualization of the larynx in most cases. Cricoid pressure should be considered in all pediatric intubations to minimize aspiration.

Tracheostomy Tubes

Tracheostomy tubes are available in neonatal and pediatric internal diameters. The difference between the neonatal and pediatric sizes is in length of the airway. Pediatric-size tracheostomy tubes are not available with cuffs unless the tube is custom ordered.

Patient Management

Humidification

Respiratory distress can drastically increase the child's insensible water loss. Humidity will minimize insensible water loss, excessive

Table 9-15 Recommended Resuscitation Equipment for the Child

Age	0-6 mo	6-12 mo	1 yr	18 mo	3 yr	5 yr	6 yr	8 yr	10 yr	12 yr	14 yr
Weight (kg)	3-5	7	10	12	15	20	20	25	30	40	50
Resus mask	0-1	1	1-2	2	3	3	3	3	3	4	4-5
Laryngoscope	0	1	1	1	2	2	2	2	2	2	3
ETT	3	3.5	3.5	4	4.5	5	5.5	6	6	6.5	7
Suction (ETT/trach)	6	6	8	8	10	10	10	10	10	14	14
Suction (OP/NP)	10	10	10	10	14	14	14	16	16	16	16
Chest tube	10-12	10-12	16-20	16-20	16-20	20-28	20-28	20-28	28-32	28-32	32-42
NG/OG	8	8	8	8	10	10	10	10	12	12	14
Foley	6*	6*	8	8	10	10	10	10	12	12	14
Trach (pediatric)	00,0	1	1	1-2	2-3	3	3	4	4	5	6

Modified from Widner-Kolberg MR: Baltimore, 1989, Maryland Institutes for Emergency Medical Services Systems.

ETT, Endotracheal tube; *NG*, nasogastric; *NP*, nasopharyngeal; *OG*, orogastric; *OP*, oropharyngeal; *resus*, resuscitation; *trach*, tracheostomy.

*May use 5 Fr feeding tube.

Box 9-3   Formula for Determination of Suction Catheter Size

ETT size (mm) $\times$ 2 = suction catheter size (Fr)*

Example: 4.5 mm $\times$ 2 = 9 or

            = 8 Fr suction catheter

---

*Round to next lowest size.

drying of respiratory secretions, and the risk of occluding the artificial airway with mucus plugs. Humidity also prevents excessive drying and irritation of the airways.

Suctioning

Suctioning the child is the most common method used to determine patency of the artificial airway and to clear accumulated secretions.[17] Despite the frequency of this nursing intervention, care must be taken in the actual performance of the procedure to minimize complications (Box 9-3).

Each pass of the suction catheter should not exceed 10 seconds. During suctioning, the wall suction pressure gauge should not exceed 100 mm Hg. Another intervention to prevent mucosal damage that is practiced in some pediatric facilities includes measuring the suction catheter so that the catheter extends only beyond the end of the tracheostomy or ETT *during* the procedure. Once this measurement is determined, an example of the marked suction catheter should be posted at the child's bedside.

MECHANICAL VENTILATION OF THE CHILD

The Optimal Ventilator

A ventilator must be able to deliver small but accurate V_T ($\leq$100 mL) against high airway resistance and low lung compliance because the young child has a higher basal metabolic rate, larger body surface area (BSA), and smaller airway diameter with higher airway resistance. Pediatric ventilators must be able to generate low and high inspiratory flow rates. A flow rate that is too high may result in the premature delivery of volume, the generation of unnecessary high pressures, and inadequate inspiratory/expiratory (I:E) ratios. A flow rate that is too low may not deliver the total V_T in the short inspiratory time available. Pediatric ventilators must have rapid response times or there will be poor coordination of the ventilator with the child's own breathing, thus increasing the child's work of breathing and the risk of not reversing the respiratory failure.

MODES OF MECHANICAL VENTILATION

A pediatric patient may be ventilated using a variety of modes: volume cycled, pressure cycled, and time cycled. Pressure-cycled ventilation is commonly used in the newborn or infant population because of the low V_T needed and because a continuous-flow system requires no extra energy to initiate a breath.

Pressure-controlled ventilation (using Siemens Servo C) is often used with pediatric patients. This mode of ventilation permits airflow to reach a preset inspiratory pressure quickly in the inspiratory phase as opposed to near the end of the inspiratory phase (as occurs in pressure cycled). In pressure-controlled ventilation, the ventilator delivers breaths with a constant preset pressure at a preset rate. The pressure is maintained during the inspiratory effort. This mode may be advantageous because it encourages partially collapsed alveoli to open with sustained inspiratory pressure. This mode of ventilation may decrease the mean airway pressure in some patients.

Volume-cycled ventilation may be used to ventilate even small children if proper consideration is given to the compliance factor of the ventilator circuit. It is also important to assess whether the ventilator has a backup ventilation mode with parameters programmed that may be deleterious to the infant or child. For example, a machine with a backup ventilation mode that has a V_T of 500 mL could cause barotrauma in a child weighing 15 kg.

The choice of ventilator control may be critical to its success with a volume-cycled ventilator. Because small or weak children may have trouble opening the demand valve in the intermittent mandatory ventilation (IMV) circuit, hypoventilation is a real concern. Most current volume-cycled ventilators that are used in children have the options of assist control, IMV, synchronized intermittent mandatory ventilation (SIMV), and pressure support. The use of SIMV with pressure support generally overcomes the problem of opening the demand valve and still allows the child the opportunity to breathe independently between ventilator breaths.

Time-cycled ventilation provides a continuous flow of gas in the respiratory circuit, which can decrease the work of breathing for the ill infant. In this situation the infant does not have to open a demand valve to access the next breath. The disadvantage of time-cycled ventilation is that the machine may have too low inspiratory flow capabilities and may not provide adequate flows for children who weigh more than 15 kg. Inspiration and expiration timing may be adjusted in an attempt to provide optimal ventilation. Sedation and paralysis may be required in order for the child to tolerate these adjustments.

INDICATIONS FOR MECHANICAL VENTILATION

In addition to the broad, generic reasons for mechanical ventilation such as respiratory failure, pediatric patients commonly require mechanical ventilation to decrease the work and the oxygen cost of breathing.

Some key points for ventilator management are following:
1. Rate should be age appropriate and relate to condition of the patient.
2. Minute ventilation (V_E) should be maintained within normal range.
3. V_T can be affected by air leaks around the ETT or in the ventilator circuit.
4. Normal V_T is 7 to 10 mL/kg. A higher ventilator rate will keep V_T at 7 mL/kg and a lower rate will keep the V_T at 10 L/kg.
5. PEEP assists the young child in preventing alveoli collapse, which has a tendency to occur; 2 to 3 cm H_2O PEEP is recommended.

A common complication of ventilation devices is barotrauma with air leaks. The infant may experience spontaneous pneumothorax. Thin chest walls may lead to referred breath sounds over collapsed lung fields, and the ability of pediatric patients to maintain their blood pressures for prolonged periods despite a tension pneumothorax may mask the classic signs of pneumothorax. See Table 9-16 for other complications.

RESUSCITATION EQUIPMENT AND SUPPLIES

Table 9-15 provides a list of essential resuscitation equipment based on the age and weight of the child. The items are suggested as additions to other equipment listed in the chapter and are not inclusive. Additional recommended supplies include:
1. Infant and pediatric internal and external defibrillator paddles
2. External pacemaker machine with appropriately sized pacer electrodes
3. Chest drainage systems. A critical bleed following postoperative cardiac surgery is defined as 3 mL/kg of body weight for more than 2 hours and requires surgical intervention.[18]
4. Gastrointestinal (GI) drainage devices, which should not exceed 100 mm Hg wall suction. There is a greater incidence of aspiration and impedance to ventilatory efforts with abdominal distention (see Table 9-16).

Table 9-16 COMPLICATIONS OF MECHANICAL VENTILATION

Complication	Developmental/Situational Risks	Interventions
Extubation (inadvertent)	Infant/child is cognitively too immature to understand rationale for tube placement and security	Use soft restraints or elbow restraints
	Infant/child is more activity oriented	Keep soft restraints for all extremities at the bedside
	Infant/child is usually intubated with uncuffed tube	Provide adequate sedation and analgesia
	Although cuffed tube does not ensure security, it does assist in stability	Increase use of paralytic agents
		Assess and document security of tube and markers at teeth/gums every hour
		Consider nasotracheal intubation for long-term ventilation to increase stability and comfort
		If using adhesive tape to secure ETT, use benzoin under tape to enhance adhesiveness
Aspiration, gastric distention	Infant/child has delayed gastric emptying	Place NG tube early
	Use of uncuffed ETTs is increased	Facilitate gastric emptying with enteral medication delivery or feedings by placing patient on right side
	Infant/child is prone to vomiting when extremely upset	Check residuals frequently
	Weak cardiac sphincter and large manual ventilation breaths increase the risk of introducing air into the stomach	Assess stomach contents before upsetting procedures, chest physiotherapy, Trendelenburg position
	Infant/child swallows air when upset and crying	Manually ventilate only with as much air that raises and lowers the child's chest

ETT, Endotracheal tube; *NG*, nasogastric.

5. Urinary drainage devices. Urine output is an indicator of end-organ perfusion in the infant and young child and should be accurately measured every hour. In the newborn or small infant, a 5 Fr feeding tube may be used as a urinary catheter and connected to a volu-feeder or baby bottle for collection and measurement. Urinary drainage bags or stoma bags may be used to collect urine. To test the specific gravity or pH of urine collected in a child's diaper, follow these steps:
   a. Remove the top dry liner of the inside of the diaper to obtain urine-saturated fibers.
   b. Place fibers into the barrel of a syringe.
   c. Replace the plunger of the syringe and push the plunger, squeezing the urine from the syringe into a medicine cup.

6. Over-the-bed radiant warmers. Infants and young children are at risk for hypothermia. Infants cannot shiver to keep warm, and hypothermia shifts the oxyhemoglobin dissociation curve to the left, preventing the release of oxygen to the tissue and increasing oxygen consumption and glucose utilization. It is recommended that the child remain uncovered, the skin temperature probe attached, and that the warmer be used to regulate the child's temperature. Clinicians and parents should avoid using oil-based solutions on the child while the child is under the warmer because this may lead to thermal burns similar to sunburn.

7. Hypothermia/hyperthermia devices. Hyperthermia blankets are rarely used in the infant and young child because over-the-bed radiant warmers are so efficient. Cooling blankets are often helpful in controlling body temperature. Cover the blanket with liners to prevent thermal tissue damage.

8. Blood warmers. It may be necessary to add an IV pump or to manually draw the warmed blood into a 60-mL syringe and deliver it directly.

DELIVERY OF FLUIDS, MEDICATIONS, AND BLOOD

FLUID MANAGEMENT

Fluid Requirements by Weight

Each child is individually assessed for the amount and type of prescribed IV fluid. The average child's maintenance fluid requirements may be determined by body weight (Table 9-17).

Table 9-17 Calculation of Daily Maintenance Fluid Requirements

Weight	Fluid Requirement	Example
0-10 kg (>72 hr old)	100 mL/kg	Patient weight = 5 kg Patient weight (kg) × fluid requirement: 5 × 100 = 500 mL/day Hourly rate = 500 ÷ 24 = 21 mL/hr
11-20 kg	100 mL/kg for the first 10 kg or 1000 mL/day plus 50 mL/kg for each kg 11 through 20	Patient weight = 13 kg For the first 10 kg: 10 kg × 100 = 1000 mL For kg >10 and ≤20 (total of 3): 3 kg × 50 = 150 mL 1000 mL +150 mL TOTAL 1150 mL/day Hourly rate = 1150 ÷ 24 = 48 mL/hr
21-30 kg	100 mL/kg for the first 10 kg or 1000 mL/day plus 50 mL/kg for each kg 11 through 20 plus 25 mL/kg for each kg 21 through 30	Patient weight = 26 kg For the first 10 kg: 10 kg × 100 = 1000 mL For kg >10 and ≤20 (total of 10): 10 kg × 50 = 500 mL For kg >20 and ≤30 (total of 6): 6 kg × 25 = 150 mL 1000 mL 500 mL +150 mL TOTAL 1650 mL/day Hourly rate = 1650 ÷ 24 = 69 mL/hr

Continued

Table 9-17 Calculation of Daily Maintenance Fluid Requirements—cont'd

Weight	Fluid Requirement	Example
31-40 kg	100 mL/kg for the first 10 kg or 1000 mL/day	Patient weight = 32 kg
	plus 50 mL/kg for each kg 11 through 20	For the first 10 kg; 10 kg × 100 = 1000 mL
	plus 25 mL/kg for each kg 21 through 30	For kg >10 and ≤20 (total of 10): 10 kg × 50 = 500 mL
	plus 10 mL/kg for each kg 31 through 40	For kg >20 and ≤30 (total of 10): 10 kg × 25 = 250 mL
		For kg >30 and ≤40 (total of 2): 2 kg × 10 = 20 mL
		1000 mL
		500 mL
		250 mL
		+20 mL
		TOTAL 1770 mL/day
		Hourly rate = 1770 ÷ 24 = 74 mL/hr

Fluid Requirements by Body Surface Area (BSA)

The child's maintenance fluid requirements may also be calculated according to BSA. (To determine BSA, see nomogram in Appendix C.) Maintenance fluid requirements are 1500 mL/m^2/day. For example, a child weighing 8 kg who is 35 cm long and has a BSA of 0.43 m^2 requires 645 mL/day (1500 mL × 0.43 m^2 = 645 mL) at an hourly rate of 27 mL (645 ÷ 24 hr = 27 mL/hr).

Alteration in Maintenance Fluid Requirements

Maintenance fluid requirements may be altered based on the child's disease state. Often a child recovering from postoperative cardiac surgery, a neurologic disorder, or a renal disorder is placed on restricted maintenance fluid requirements such as two-thirds maintenance fluid or replacement of insensible fluid loss only.

Accurate Monitoring and Delivery of Fluid

It is imperative that fluid be administered accurately and safely. Even the volume of fluid used to mix and deliver medications should be added into the I&O totals. IV fluids are administered most commonly via an infusion device.

ADMINISTRATION OF FLUID BOLUSES

Fluid boluses include the intermittent delivery of either colloid or crystalloid fluid in an attempt to restore intravascular volume. For bolus fluid resuscitation therapy, PALS standards recommend 20 mL/kg of isotonic crystalloid solution delivered as rapidly as possible (over approximately 20 minutes).

Important considerations regarding pediatric fluid boluses include (1) determination of the accurate amount and type of fluid, (2) rapid administration of fluid (given over 20 to 30 minutes), and (3) reevaluation of the patient for the need of another fluid bolus. Fluid boluses are often drawn up in a 60-mL syringe and manually pushed. Dextrose-containing solutions are contraindicated for fluid resuscitation because of the risk for hyperglycemia and cerebral edema.

BLOOD COMPONENT ADMINISTRATION

The fundamental principles in blood component administration are the same in the adult and pediatric patient. The primary difference is the prescribed dose, which is determined by the child's weight. Table 9-18 reviews blood component therapy, suggested dose, and rates of administration.

Table 9-18 BLOOD COMPONENT ADMINISTRATION IN CHILDREN

Blood Component	Usual Dose	Rate of Infusion	Comments
Whole blood	20 mL/kg initially	As rapidly as necessary to restore volume and stabilize the child	Administration is usually reserved for massive hemorrhage
Packed RBCs	10-15 mL/kg	5 mL/kg/hr or 2 mL/kg/hr if heart failure develops	1 mL/kg will increase Hct approximately 1%. Infuse within 4 hr. If necessary, divide the unit into smaller volumes for infusion.
Platelets	0.1 unit/kg	Each unit over 5-10 min via syringe or pump	The usual dose will increase platelet count by 50,000/mm³
Fresh frozen plasma	Hemorrhage: 15-30 mL/kg Clotting deficiency: 10-15 mL/kg	Hemorrhage: rapidly to stabilize the child Clotting deficiency: over 2-3 hr	Monitor for fluid overload
Granulocytes	Dependent on WBC counts and clinical condition, 10 mL/kg/day initially	Slowly over 2-4 hr because of fever and chills, side effects commonly associated with infusion	Granulocytes have a short life span. Transfuse as soon after collection as possible.
Albumin 5%	1 g/kg or 20 mL/kg	1-2 mL/min or 60-120 mL/hr	Monitor for fluid overload. Type and cross match are not required.
Albumin 25%	1 g/kg or 4 mL/kg	0.2-0.4 mL/min or 12-24 mL/hr	Monitor for fluid overload. Type and cross-match are not required.

Hct, Hematocrit; *RBC,* red blood cell; *WBC,* white blood cell.

MEDICATION ADMINISTRATION

Dose Determination

Medications are prescribed on a microgram, milligram, or milliequivalent per kilogram of body weight. This same weight should be used during the child's entire hospitalization unless the child substantially loses or gains lean muscle mass.

Oral Medications

For administration of oral medications to the young child, it is important to account for the child's developmental capabilities. The developmental level will determine the method of administering the oral medication (spoon, cup, nipple, or single-dose system with needleless syringe). Generally a child younger than 8 years is unable to swallow a pill. Many forms of medication cannot be crushed (e.g., sustained-released products); therefore it may be necessary to order the liquid dose form.

Intramuscular (IM) Medications

Table 9-19 and Table 9-20 identify the proper needle size and injection sites for intramuscular medications.

Continuous Vasoactive Infusions

See Table 9-21 for select vasoactive drugs and usual dosage range.

Pain Management

The bedside nurse must often act as an advocate for pain management in a young child. The child may be subject to painful procedures and/or postoperative pain. Before initiating any procedure, an age-appropriate explanation of the procedure, as well as the amount

Table 9-19 Intramuscular Injections According to Age Group

Age Group	Needle Length (in)	Needle Gauge	Maximum Volume (mL)
Infant	$5/8$	25-27	1
Toddler	1	22-23	1
Preschooler	1	22-23	$1-1^{1}/_{2}$
School age	$1-1^{1}/_{2}$	22-23	2
Adolescent	$1-1^{1}/_{2}$	22-23	2

Table 9-20 SITES FOR INTRAMUSCULAR INJECTIONS

Site	Landmarks	Interventions
VASTUS LATERALIS: preferred in children <3 yr (rectus femoris muscle also possibly used)	Greater trochanter and knee	Give injection in middle third of anterolateral aspect of thigh

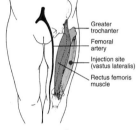

| DORSOGLUTEAL: preferred in children >3 yr and who have been walking more than 1 yr | Posterosuperior iliac crest and greater trochanter | Give injection superior and lateral to imaginary line connecting landmarks |

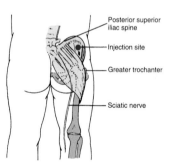

| VENTROGLUTEAL: use in children >3 yr and who have been walking more than 1 yr | Greater trochanter, anterior iliac spine, and posterior edge of iliac crest | Give injection at center of *V* that is formed when the index finger is placed on anterior iliac crest, middle finger on posterior iliac crest while palm of the hand is resting on greater trochanter
Use right hand to find landmarks when injecting into left ventrogluteal site; use left hand to find landmarks when injecting into right ventrogluteal site |

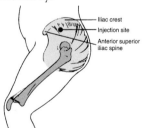

Table 9-21 CONTINUOUS INFUSIONS DOSAGE RANGE

Drug	Dosage Range
Alprostadil (PGE$_1$)	0.1-0.4 mcg/kg/min
Dobutamine	2-20 mcg/kg/min
Dopamine	2-20 mcg/kg/min
Epinephrine	0.1-1 mcg/kg/min
Isoproterenol	0.1-1 mcg/kg/min
Lidocaine	20-50 mcg/kg/min
Nitroglycerin	1-25 mcg/kg/min
Nitroprusside	1-8 mcg/kg/min
Norepinephrine	0.1-1 mcg/kg/min

and duration of discomfort, should be communicated to the child. Before a painful procedure, an analgesic and/or local anesthetic should be administered as well as an anxiolytic or sedative to reduce anxiety (anxiolytics and sedatives do not relieve pain).

Postoperative pain may be managed with opioid and nonopioid analgesics. Around-the-clock or continuous infusion is recommended. Patient-controlled analgesia can be used in the pediatric population. IM injections are painful and frightening and should be used only under exceptional circumstances; the oral route is recommended as soon as the child can tolerate oral intake.

The primary difference between adult and pediatric management is the dosing. Table 9-22 is a table of usual dosages for analgesics and sedatives. An important consideration for medication dosing in children is whether they are experiencing a growth spurt. A child undergoing a growth spurt may metabolize medications very quickly and may need more frequent dosing to relieve pain.

Physiologic dependence (withdrawal) may develop with opioid and benzodiazepine administration. A child may demonstrate increased irritability, wakefulness, tremors, tachypnea, refusal to eat,

Table 9-22 Usual Dosages for Children (Older Than 6 Months and Weighing Less Than 50

Drug	Oral Dosage (mg/kg)	Parenteral Dosage
Acetaminophen	10-15 q4h	—
Aspirin	10-15 q4h	—
Ibuprofen	10 q6-8h	—
Codeine	1 q3-4h	—
Fentanyl	—	0.5-1.5 mcg/kg/hr
Hydromorphone	0.06 q3-4h	0.015 mg/kg q3-4h
Levorphanol	0.04 q6-8h	0.02 mg/kg q6-8h
Midazolam	—	0.05-0.1 mg/kg q1-2h
		0.05-0.2 mg/kg/hr
Nalbuphine	—	0.1-0.2 mg/kg q1-2h
		0.1-0.4 mg/kg/hr

or diarrhea after 3 to 5 days of dosing. Steadily decreasing doses by a predetermined percentage, as opposed to abruptly stopping a medication, may prevent withdrawal syndrome.

Precalculated Drug Sheets

Pediatric doses may be unfamiliar to the adult clinician; therefore a precalculated emergency drug sheet is very helpful. All emergency medication doses are based on the child's weight (in kilograms). The emergency drug sheet should include the recommended resuscitation medication doses, medication concentration, and final medication dose and volume that the individual child is to receive. A listing of select pediatric drugs and doses can be found in Table 9-23.

Medication Pitfalls

1. Several medications are available in multiple concentrations. Table 9-24 includes commonly used medications available in adult and pediatric concentrations.
2. Dose calculations. It is imperative that calculations be double-checked with a second registered nurse or a pharmacist. A calculator should be used to determine pediatric dose calculations.
3. Single-dose system. A pediatric patient may require doses that are substantially smaller and thus more difficult to estimate from a multiple-dose syringe. Therefore a single-dose system is recommended for pediatric patients.

Table 9-23 PEDIATRIC DRUGS AND DOSES*

Drug	Usual IV Dose	Comments
Adenosine	0.1 mg/kg	Rapid IV push; maximum dose
Amiodarone	5 mg/kg	= 6 mg (child), 12 mg (adolescent)
Atropine	0.02 mg/kg	Maximum single dose: 0.5 mg (child); 1 mg (adolescent)
	Minimum dose 0.1 mg	May repeat dose after 5 min; maximum total 1 mg child; 2 mg adolescent
Bretylium	Initial: 5 mg/kg Repeat: 10 mg/kg	
Calcium chloride 10%	20 mg/kg (0.2 mL/kg)	Give slowly
Dextrose 50%	0.5-1 g/kg	Requires 1:1 dilution with NS (peripheral IV)
Diazepam	0.1 mg/kg	
Epinephrine	0.01 mg/kg (1:10,000)	
Ketamine	1-2 mg/kg (normovolemia) 0.5 mg/kg (hypovolemia)	
Lidocaine	1 mg/kg	
Naloxone	0.1 mg/kg	Children >5 yr may be given 2 mg. Give slowly and titrate to desired effect
Phenobarbital	20 mg/kg	
Phenytoin	15 mg/kg	Use with NS. Do not exceed 50 mg/min
Procainamide	5 mg/kg	Do not exceed 50 mg/min
Propranolol	0.1 mg/kg	Give slow IVP
Sodium bicarbonate	1 mEq/kg or 0.3 × kg × base deficit	If child <1 yr, dilute one to one with D_5W; infuse only after adequate ventilation is achieved
Verapamil	0.1 mg/kg	Do not use if child <1 yr

IV, Intravenous; *IVP,* intravenous push; *NS,* normal saline.
*Use central line if available; flush line after medication administration.

Table 9-24 RECOMMENDATIONS FOR THE USE OF MEDICATIONS WITH
MULTIPLE DRUG CONCENTRATIONS IN CHILDREN

Drug Name	Neonate/Child (<20 kg)	Child (>20 kg)
Naloxone	Neonatal 0.02 mg/mL	Adult 0.4 mg/mL
Digitalis	Neonatal 0.1 mg/mL	Adult 0.25 mg/mL
Ketamine	Pediatric 10 mg/mL	Adult 100 mg/mL
Sodium bicarbonate	4.2% (0.5 mEq/mL)	8.4% (1 mEq/mL)

4. Preparation of the first-line resuscitative medications. Preparing and labeling syringes containing the child's first-line resuscitative drugs such as epinephrine and atropine ahead of time can save time in the event of an emergency. These prepared syringes must be replaced every 24 hours. Medications that can be delivered via an ETT create the acronym ALIEN (Box 9-4). However, the IV or IO route is preferred to ETT drug administration.

5. Sodium chloride flushes. Manual flushing rather than gravity or pump-assisted flushing is preferred in the pediatric patient. The recommended volume for a flush should not exceed 3 mL for an infant and 5 mL for a child.[13] Flushes should be considered as intake and calculated in fluid intake totals.

SAFETY

ENVIRONMENTAL SAFETY

When working with small children, additional safety issues must be considered. Choking hazards exist because young children tend to put everything into their mouths. The fascinating knobs and

---

Box 9-4 Emergency Medications That May Be Delivered Via ETT*

Atropine
Lidocaine
Isuprel
Epinephrine[†]
Naloxone

*Dilute medications for administration; follow with 1 to 2 mL normal saline (NS) and several ventilations.
†Requires higher dose (0.1 mg/kg).

switches found on IV pumps and ventilators must be kept out of reach or turned away from the child.

SOFT RESTRAINTS

In the pediatric critical care setting the availability and use of soft restraints is generally considered an important safety measure. In an effort to provide optimal safety without awkward positioning, the ties may be secured to the infant's or small child's diaper. A confirmatory medical order for restraint(s) is required.

PREPARING THE CRITICALLY ILL CHILD FOR TRANSPORT

If a critically ill child must be transported to or from any critical care area within a hospital or to another health care facility, a safe transport must be planned. Guidelines and interventions[19] that can be used for transporting the critically ill child include the following:

1. Knowledge of the destination: to determine the length of time the patient will be at the alternate setting and what is needed, call ahead.

2. Evaluation of patient stability: determine the risk/benefit of transport. Assess the level of intervention the patient has needed in the past 2 to 4 hours.

3. Maintenance of the airway: anticipate potential emergencies and associated equipment needs. Secure ETT with tape that is well anchored around the tube and face. Assign someone to manually hold the ETT while bagging and moving the patient. Disconnect the ETT from Ambu bag when moving the patient to and from the stretcher.

   Suction the ETT just before leaving the unit. Take extra pediatric suction catheters.

   Take a self-inflatable bag and correct size mask for all patients who have an ETT.

   Take an extra ETT, tape, and pediatric intubation equipment if the patient is going to an area that is not familiar with pediatric patients. Take an extra tracheostomy (trach) tube, ties, and scissors for all patients who have a tracheostomy tube. Full E-cylinder oxygen tanks should be used. Check the gauge on the tank, and take oxygen masks for delivery of supplemental oxygen.

4. Continuous monitoring: check battery on all portable ECG, respiratory, and pressure waveform monitors. Take vital signs every 5 to 30 minutes, including a check of neurologic func-

tion. Monitor arterial pressure, intracranial pressure, or pulmonary artery pressure if applicable. Always take a blood pressure cuff and monitor pulse oximetry.

5. Maintenance of IV access: check for a blood return and check the skin around IV catheter site. Make sure IV is anchored to the skin and protected from dislodgment.

 Have extra vascular volume expanders (normal saline [NS], lactated Ringer's [LR], blood) for those patients who require frequent fluid boluses. IVs should be regulated by a pump if the patient is fluid restricted or has vasoactive medications (attach more than one IV pump to one IV pole).

6. Immobilization: immobilize combative or active patients to protect them from injury.

 For infants, use stockinette restraints for arms and legs. These can be safely pinned to the bedding, but detach them when transferring the infant out of the bed. For children, use arm and leg restraints (even on those patients who are recovering from anesthesia).

 Maintain cervical spine (C-spine) precautions for all children with a suspected head or neck injury. Cervical collars that fit all ages, infant to adult, are commercially available. If an appropriate-size collar is not available for a small child, rolled towels, pillowcases, or baby blankets can be used. Rolled towels should be placed on either side of the infant or toddler's head, with tape applied across the forehead to each towel and the backboard beneath for stabilization. Sandbags or liter bags of fluid should never be used because they can put pressure on the head when the infant or child is logrolled. For older children, maintain neck collar placement.

 Use as many trained health care team members as needed to help move the patient. Secure drainage bags to the bed or stretcher. Avoid securing items to the side rail.

7. Temperature regulation: cover the child sufficiently with blankets. For infants, swaddle them in blankets and use head covering (stockinette caps). Have warming lights, blankets, and radiant warmers ready on return from the transport. Use battery-powered warmed Isolette for neonates.

8. Medications: emergency IV push medications include atropine, epinephrine 1:10,000, sodium bicarbonate, and 25% dextrose (50% dextrose is too caustic on small vessels and should be diluted). Have a pediatric emergency drug card with drug doses calculated for the patient's weight; and have analgesics, sedatives, or anticonvulsants available.

REFERENCES

1. Rosenthal CH: Immunosuppression in pediatric critical care patients, *Crit Care Nurs Clin North Am* 1:775-785, 1989.

2. Wong D: *Nursing care of infants and children,* St Louis, 2003, Mosby.

3. Hazinski MF: Psychosocial aspects of pediatric critical care. In Hazinski, MF, *Manual of pediatric critical care,* St Louis, 1999, Mosby.

4. Macnab A, Macrae D, Henning R: *Care of the critically ill child,* London, 1999, Churchill Livingstone.

5. Krantz BE, editor: *Advanced trauma life support for doctors: student course manual,* Chicago, 1997, American College of Surgeons.

6. Vernon-Levett P: Traumatic brain injury in children. In Moloney-Harmon P, editor: *Nursing care of the pediatric trauma patient,* St Louis, 2003, Saunders.

7. McQuillan K et al: *Trauma nursing from resuscitation through rehabilitation,* Philadelphia, 2002, WB Saunders.

8. Torres A, Wiggins P: Nutrition in the pediatric intensive care unit patient. In Tobias JD, editor: *Pediatric critical care: the essentials,* Armonk, N.Y., 1999, Futura.

9. Wong DL et al: *Wong's essentials of pediatric nursing,* ed 6, St Louis, 2001, Mosby, p. 1301.

10. Puntillo KA et al: Patient's perceptions and responses to procedural pain: results from Thunder Project II, *Am J Crit Care* 10(4):238-251, 2001.

11. Craig J, Smith JB, Fineman LD: Tissue perfusion. In Curley MAQ, Moloney-Harmon PA, editors: *Critical care nursing of infants and children,* ed 2, Philadelphia, 2001, WB Saunders.

12. Fuhrman B, Zimmerman J: *Pediatric critical care,* St Louis, 1998, Mosby.

13. Hazinski MF, editor: *PALS provider manual,* Dallas, 2002, American Heart Association.

14. Hazinski MF: Critical care of the pediatric cardiovascular patient, *Nurs Clin North Am* 16:671-697, 1981.

15. Fiser DH: Intraosseous infusion, *N Engl J Med* 322:1579-1581, 1990.

16. Heulitt M et al: Double-blind, randomized, controlled trial of papaverine-containing infusions to prevent failure of arterial catheters in pediatric patients, *Crit Care Med* 21:825-838, 1993.

17. Burg F et al, editors: *Gellis and Kagan's current pediatric therapy,* Philadelphia, 1999, WB Saunders.

18. Hazinski MF: Hemodynamic monitoring in children. In Daily EK, Schroeder JS, editors: *Techniques in bedside hemodynamic monitoring,* ed 5, St Louis, 2000, Mosby.

19. Bowen SL: Transporting the critically ill child. In Moloney-Harmon PA, Czerwinski SJ, editors: *Nursing care of the pediatric trauma patient,* St Louis, 2003, Saunders.

BIBLIOGRAPHY

American Heart Association: Highlights of the 2005 American Heart Association guidelines for cardiopulmonary resuscitation and emerging cardiovascular care, *Curr Emerg Cardiovasc Care* 16:4, winter 2005-2006.

American Red Cross, Council of Community Blood Centers, American Association of Blood Banks: *Circular of information: for the use of human blood and blood components*, August, 2000. Available online at www.aabb.org/all_about_blood/coi/aabb_coi.htm.

Anand KJ: Effects of perinatal pain and stress, *Prog Brain Res* 122:117-129, 2000.

Behrman RE, Vaughan VC, Nelson WE: *Nelson textbook of pediatrics*, ed 17, Philadelphia, 2004, WB Saunders.

Bernardy KS: The child with a gastrointestinal alteration. In James SR, Ashwill JW, Droske SC, editors: *Nursing care of children: principles & practice*, Philadelphia, 2002, WB Saunders.

Bowden V: Alterations in neurologic status. In *Children and their families: the continuum of care*, Philadelphia, 1998, WB Saunders.

Brem A: An overview of renal structure and function. In Fuhrman B, Zimmerman J, editors: *Pediatric critical care*, St Louis, 1998, Mosby.

Curley MAQ, Moloney-Harmom PA, editors: *Critical care nursing of infants and children*, ed 2, Philadelphia, 2001, WB Saunders.

Guyton AC: *Textbook of medical physiology*, ed 10, Philadelphia, 2000, WB Saunders.

Haines C, Walstenholme M: Family support in paediatric intensive care. In Williams L, Asquith J, editors: *Paediatric intensive care nursing*, Edinburgh, 2000, Churchill Livingstone.

Hata JS: Acute respiratory distress syndrome in children. In Tobias JD, editor: *Pediatric critical care: the essentials*, Armonk, N.Y., 1999, Futura.

Hazinski MF: *Manual of pediatric critical care*, St Louis, 1999, Mosby.

Hazinski MF: *Nursing care of the critically ill child*, ed 2, St Louis, 1992, Mosby.

Hazinski MF: Psychosocial aspects of pediatric critical care. In Hazinski MF, *Manual of pediatric critical care*, St Louis, 1999, Mosby.

Kidder C: Reestablishing health factors influencing the child's recovery in pediatric intensive care, *J Pediatr Nurs* 4(2):96-103, 1989.

Kirsch CSB: Pharmacotherapeutics for the neonate and the pediatric patient. In Kuhn MM, editor: *Pharmacotherapeutics: a nursing process approach*, ed 4, Philadelphia, 1998, FA Davis.

Krantz BE, editor: *Advanced trauma life support for doctors: student course manual*, Chicago, 1997, American College of Surgeons.

Landier WC, Barrell ML, Styffe EJ: How to administer blood components to children, *Am J Matern Child Nurs* 12(3):178-184, 1987.

Lansdown R: *Children in the hospital: a guide for family and careers*, Oxford, 1994, Oxford University Press.

LeMoine MAS: The child with a genitourinary alteration. In James SR, Ashwill JW, Droske SC, editors: *Nursing care of children: principles & practice,* Philadelphia, 2002, WB Saunders.

Liebman MA: Initial resuscitation of the pediatric trauma victim. In Moloney-Harmon P, editor: *Nursing care of the pediatric trauma patient,* St Louis, 2003, Saunders.

McCaffery M, Pasero C: *Pain: clinical manual,* ed 2, St Louis, 1999, Mosby.

Moloney-Harmon PA, Adams P: Trauma. In Curley M, Moloney-Harmon PA, editors: *Critical care nursing of infants and children,* ed 2, Philadelphia, 2001, WB Saunders.

Moran M: Growth and development. In Ashwill JW, Droske SC, editors: *Nursing care of children: principles and practice,* Philadelphia, 1997, WB Saunders.

Morrison H: Pain in the critically ill child. In Puntillo K, editor: *Pain in the critically ill: assessment and management,* Gaithersburg, Md, 1999, Aspen.

Muir R, Town DA: Spinal cord injury. In Moloney-Harmon P, editor: *Nursing care of the pediatric trauma patient,* St Louis, 2003, Saunders.

Pain Management Guideline Panel, Agency for Health Care Policy and Research, US Health and Human Services: Clinician's quick reference guide to acute pain management in infants, children, and adolescents: operative and medical procedures, *J Pain Symptom Manage* 7(4):229-242, 1992.

Report of the Second Task Force on Blood Pressure Control in Children—1987. Task Force on Blood Pressure Control in Children. National Heart, Lung, and Blood Institute, Bethesda, Md, *Pediatrics* 79(1):1-25, 1987.

Rosenthal CH: *Pediatric critical care nursing in the adult ICU: essentials of practice, national conference on pediatric critical care nursing,* New York, 1990, Contemporary Forums.

Schechter NL, Zeltzer LK: Pediatric pain: new directions from a developmental perspective, *J Dev Behav Pediatr* 20(4):209-210, 1999.

Seidel JS, Henderson DP: *Prehospital care of pediatric emergencies,* Los Angeles, 1987, American Academy of Pediatrics.

Soupios M, Gallagher J, Orlowski JP: Nursing aspects of pediatric intensive care in a general hospital, *Pediatr Clin North Am* 27(3):621-622, 1980.

Susla GM, Dionne RE: Pharmacokinetics-pharmacodynamics: drug delivery and therapeutic drug monitoring. In Holbrook P, editor: *Textbook of pediatric critical care,* Philadelphia, 1993, WB Saunders.

Tobias JD, editor: *Pediatric critical care: the essentials,* Armonk, N.Y., 1999, Futura.

Tobias JD, Wilson, Jr. WR: Postoperative cardiac care. In Tobias JD, editor: *Pediatric critical care: the essentials,* Armonk, N.Y., 1999, Futura.

Widner-Kolberg MR: Maryland Institutes for Emergency Medical Services Systems, Baltimore, 1989.

Wong DL: *Whaley & Wong's nursing care of infants and children,* ed 7, St Louis, 2003, Mosby.

Zaloga G, Grenvik A: Endocrinology, metabolism, nutrition, and pharmacology. In Shoemaker W et al, editors: *Textbook of critical care,* ed 4, Philadelphia, 2000, WB Saunders.

10

Pharmacology in the Critically Ill Patient

Clinical Brief

The goal of drug therapy in the critically ill is the same for any individual: to achieve the desired effect while minimizing adverse effects. Various factors can alter pharmacodynamics and pharmacokinetics, which ultimately can affect the efficacy of drug therapy.

PHARMACODYNAMICS

A drug that combines with a receptor and enhances a physiologic response is referred to as an *agonist*.

A drug that combines with a receptor and prevents the stimulation of the receptor is an *antagonist*.

Receptor responsiveness can be decreased with repeated doses of drugs. This is known as down-regulation. Up-regulation results in exaggerated drug responses and is associated with an increase in the number of receptors.

Drug-drug interactions can be additive, synergistic, or antagonistic.

Therapeutic index refers to the drug concentration needed to produce a therapeutic response. The index is a ratio; if close to 1, there is a greater possibility that the drug will produce toxic effects.

Drug responses can be predictable (e.g., side effects, toxic effects) and unpredictable (e.g., allergic reaction, idiosyncratic reaction) adverse effects.

The mechanism of action of a drug, or how the drug works in the body, is the interaction between the drug and the receptor. The patient's response to the drug is the drug's effect. The drug effects can be related to the dose and time that the drug is administered. Ideally, the drug should elicit a therapeutic response. The therapeutic range is a drug concentration at the site of action between the minimum effective concentration and the maximum effective concentration.

Drug concentrations outside of range will produce either toxic manifestations or no therapeutic response. Predictable adverse effects are dose related. A drug with a narrow therapeutic index requires close monitoring for adverse effects. A drug can cause toxicity to body structures, such as the liver, kidney, eyes, ears, and hematologic and sexual organ systems. Combination of drugs can be administered to treat various conditions. The effects of multiple drugs can be additive, synergistic, or antagonistic. Multiple-drug therapy is often used in the severely ill patient, thus close monitoring of the patient for drug-drug interactions is critical.

PHARMACOKINETICS

Absorption

Most drugs are absorbed in the small intestine because of the large surface area created by mucosal villi.

For the oral or nasogastric tube route, the dose form (e.g., tablet, elixir), gastrointestinal (GI) tract pH and motility, blood flow to stomach or intestine, food, antacids, and other concurrent drug therapy affect the rate and completeness of drug absorption.

Intramuscular (IM) and subcutaneous routes may produce erratic absorption rates secondary to changes in blood flow to the injection site and to a decrease in muscle mass and subcutaneous tissue.

Topical agents can be affected by skin conditions and changes in blood flow to the area.

Because bioavailability of the drug may be decreased secondary to diminished or erratic absorption in the critically ill patient, the intravenous (IV) route is commonly used. A number of conditions, such as shock, diarrhea, and paralytic ileus, experienced by the critically ill patient can adversely affect the absorption of pharmacologic agents. The IV route allows for direct introduction of the drug into the circulation to produce an immediate drug concentration to achieve the therapeutic effect.

Distribution

Distribution is dependent on blood flow.

The area to which a drug is distributed is referred to as the volume of distribution.

Once a drug enters the circulation, it can be distributed to various body fluids and tissues (e.g., fatty tissue).

Once a drug enters the circulation, it can bind to plasma proteins (particularly albumin), making it unavailable to interact at the receptor sites. Only free or unbound drug is pharmacologically active.

An abnormal accumulation of fluid (e.g., edema, ascites, pleural effusion) can increase the volume of distribution and may affect the plasma concentration of a drug.

Distribution is affected by body size, properties of the drug, tissue and protein binding, and blood flow. Drugs can be hydrophilic (water soluble) or lipophilic (lipid soluble). These drug properties allow for the drug to move across tissue membranes. Drugs that are not lipophilic do not distribute well to fatty tissues. Thus obese individuals may experience adverse effects if the dose of the non-lipophilic drug is based on actual body weight of the individuals. Some drugs have a high affinity for protein. Protein binding may be affected by malnutrition or renal failure. In addition, low serum protein may be present in patients with burns, heart failure, liver disease, sepsis, and inflammatory diseases. Patients with hypoalbuminemia may experience adverse effects of the drug because more unbound drug is available to exert its effect. Dose reduction may be needed in these individuals. Disease states that affect cardiac output (CO) (e.g., cardiac failure, shock) in the critically ill patient may alter drug distribution. In addition, an edematous patient or patient with fluid volume overload can have a large volume of distribution and require increased drug doses. When the fluid volume overload is corrected, a reduced drug dose may be required. Patients with fluid volume deficits may also require reduced drug doses.

Biotransformation

The major organ responsible for changing the drug molecule either into an active or inactive compound is the liver.

First-pass metabolism affects the bioavailability of the drug.

Biotransformation prepares the drug for elimination from the body.

Enzyme activity can be induced by certain drugs (e.g., phenobarbital, phenytoin), cigarette smoking, cruciferous vegetables, and char-broiled meats.

Reduced enzyme activity results in drug accumulation.

The half-life of a drug can be markedly increased or decreased depending on enzyme activity.

Because the major organ of biotransformation is the liver, any reduction in blood flow to the liver can affect the functioning of this organ. Liver disease can decrease enzyme activity that in turn causes drugs to accumulate in the body. Drugs can also cause hepatotoxicity, diminishing the liver's ability to transform drugs. Patients in critical care units may experience shock, have reduced CO, or receive hepato-toxic drugs that can affect liver function. Thus critically ill patients may be at risk for toxic effects and may require a reduction in drug dose. In addition, some critically ill patients may be receiving drugs that cause enzyme induction. In these cases, higher drug doses may be required.

Elimination

The kidneys are the major organs for drug elimination; however, drugs can also be excreted via other routes (e.g., lungs, intestines, sweat, saliva).

Reduction in renal blood flow reduces the clearance of drugs.

A decrease in glomerular filtration rate reduces renal elimination of drugs.

Only free drug is filtered at the glomerulus; protein-bound drugs do not cross the glomerular membrane.

The renal tubules are responsible for eliminating some drugs.

Lipid-soluble drugs are reabsorbed in the renal tubules.

The pH of urine affects tubular reabsorption.

A decrease in tubular function reduces renal elimination of drugs.

The half-life of renally cleared drugs is affected by renal function.

Critically ill patients who have renal failure will have reduced drug clearance. Drugs can accumulate in the blood, resulting in drug toxicity. Changes in the acid-base balance of urine can either enhance or inhibit drug excretion from the body. Patients experiencing conditions that reduce CO and consequently renal blood flow will be at risk for drug accumulation and adverse drug effects. Critically ill patients with renal disease or reduced renal function may require reduced drug doses, otherwise drugs will not be eliminated from the body and toxic effects will result.

PATIENT CARE MANAGEMENT

Drug administration in the critically ill patient requires knowledge of the drug and knowledge of the patient. The critical care nurse's knowledge base of the drug should include: the indication, dose, pharmacodynamics, contraindications and precautions, and pharmacokinetics (absorption, distribution, biotransformation, elimination). The critical care nurse's knowledge of the patient should include history of the present illness, health history including drug allergies, history of over-the-counter medications and herbal medicines, developmental and psychosocial history, physical findings, and results of laboratory and diagnostic testing.

DOSE FORM

In addition, understanding the dose form and its impact on absorption is important. Not all drug forms can be crushed. For example, enteric-coated tablets are designed to be absorbed in the intestine. Crushing these tablets may cause gastric irritation and/or adverse effects if absorbed in the stomach. Likewise, sustained-release capsules should be swallowed whole. Swallowing the contents of an opened capsule or administering the contents down a nasogastric tube could result in an overdose of the medication. Changing dose forms may require changes in the dose of the drug. For example, a liquid form of a drug may be absorbed more rapidly and more completely than a tablet, requiring an adjusted dose.

ASSESSMENT

Assess for changes in the patient's condition that may alter absorption, distribution, biotransformation, and elimination. Be alert to changes in CO, changes in renal and liver function, and any changes in nutrition. Monitor renal and hepatic laboratory results closely. Be aware of a drug's therapeutic index. Patients may experience toxic effects from small changes in drug dosing, biotransformation, or elimination if a drug has a narrow margin of safety. Equally important is obtaining accurate weights and fluid balances so that accurate dosing can be prescribed.

EVALUATION

Evaluate the patient's response to therapy. Are the drugs effective? Does the patient manifest adverse effects? Because multiple-drug therapy is common in the critically ill patient, could there be drug-drug interactions? (Consider over-the-counter medications and herbal remedies that the patient may have taken before admission.) Is the drug in the therapeutic range? A steady state takes approximately five half-lives.

DRUG LEVELS

Drug-level monitoring is sometimes performed, particularly if the drug has a narrow margin of safety or the patient is at risk for developing adverse effects. Some drugs require specific timing to obtain the blood sample for drug-level measurements. For example, a digoxin level should be drawn at least 6 hours after the dose, whereas a lithium level should be drawn just before the next dose.

Peak and trough drug levels are also obtained through blood samples taken at specific times. Peak drug concentration is measured 30 minutes after a 30-minute infusion of the drug; the trough is measured immediately before a dose.

AGING

Although young adults are admitted to critical care units, older adults may be more at risk for developing adverse effects from drug therapy. Physiologic changes that occur with aging can affect pharmacokinetics of drug therapy. For example, lean body mass decreases, yet adipose tissue increases. Lipid-soluble drugs will be stored in fatty tissue and be slowly released into the bloodstream, resulting in a longer half-life of the drugs. Protein levels can be lower than normal in older adults, thus drugs that are highly protein bound will have a reduced bound fraction. This results in more unbound drug, which is pharmacologically active. Glomerular filtration rate decreases with aging, reducing renal elimination of drugs. With the decrease in lean body mass, creatinine production decreases. Thus the serum creatinine level is less useful in estimating glomerular filtration rate. However, creatinine clearance can be used to estimate glomerular filtration rate in older adults. Hepatic blood flow is reduced with aging, compromising hepatic biotransformation. Drugs that are administered orally undergo first-pass metabolism. Older adults experience a decreased first-pass effect, which can result in increased drug bioavailability. With decreased function of the renal and hepatic systems, an illness may further impair the function of these organs in older adults.

In addition, older adults may experience exaggerated or diminished responses to drug therapy. The older adult may have a reduction in the number or function of receptors. Homeostasis mechanisms may be altered, and there may be reduced compensatory responses. Older patients may have exaggerated responses to blood pressure (BP) medication. They may also have more intense or prolonged effects of neuromuscular blocking agents. Therefore critical assessment of older adults and the effects of drug therapy is essential to determine if the desired goal is met and adverse effects are minimized.

CLINICAL BRIEFS OF EMERGENCY DRUGS IN THE ADULT PATIENT

NOTE: Check product information for dosing and administration before administering any medication.

ABCIXIMAB (REOPRO)

Classification

Glycoprotein (GP) IIb/IIIa inhibitor, platelet aggregation inhibitor, antithrombotic, monoclonal antibody

Effects

Inhibits platelet aggregation

Indications

Non–Q-wave myocardial infarction (MI) or unstable angina with planned percutaneous coronary intervention (PCI)

Contraindications

Active internal bleeding, severe uncontrolled hypertension, history of intracranial hemorrhage, history of cerebrovascular accident (CVA) within 2 years, major surgery or trauma within 1 month, thrombocytopenia, aneurysm, arteriovenous malformation (AVM), bleeding disorders within 30 days, use of IV dextran before or during PCI, concomitant use of another GP IIb/IIIa inhibitor

Administration

Dose

For acute coronary syndrome (ACS) with planned PCI within 24 hours: 10 to 60 minutes before procedures give 0.25 mg/kg IV bolus, then 0.125 mcg/kg/min IV infusion. For PCI only: 0.25 mg/kg IV bolus followed by 10 mcg/min IV infusion.

Precautions

Abciximab binds irreversibly with platelets. Hypersensitivity may develop with repeated administration; 48 hours is required for platelet recovery.

Patient Management

1. Administer through inline, nonpyrogenic, low-protein-binding filter (if not used during drug preparation).
2. Institute bleeding precautions (e.g., avoid IM injections, handle the patient with care, avoid sharp objects).
3. Assess for bleeding: femoral sheath access site, current and prior IV sites; note bleeding gums, ecchymosis, petechiae, hematuria, melena, epistaxis, hemoptysis, change in neurologic signs (intracranial bleed), and retroperitoneal bleeding (back pain, leg weakness).

4. Monitor lab results (e.g., complete blood cell count [CBC], platelets and coagulation studies).
5. Keep the patient on bed rest with extremity immobile.
6. Check pulses of affected extremity, including after sheath removal.
7. Follow institutional protocol.
8. Discontinue abciximab infusion if (1) unable to control bleeding with application of pressure, (2) patient experiences hypersensitivity reaction, (3) PCI failed, and (4) decrease in platelet count (<1,000, 000/mm³ or decrease of 25% of pretreatment value).
9. Observe for adverse effects: major bleeding, intracranial hemorrhage, bleeding at femoral artery and other access sites, thrombocytopenia, abdominal pain, back pain, chest pain, dysrhythmias, hypotension, limb embolism, pericardial effusion, and pulmonary edema.

ADENOSINE (ADENOCARD)

Classification

Antidysrhythmic

Effects

Adenosine restores normal sinus rhythm (NSR) by slowing conduction time through the atrioventricular (AV) node

Indications

Narrow-complex paroxysmal supraventricular tachycardia (PSVT), including PSVT associated with Wolff-Parkinson-White (WPW) syndrome. Does not convert atrial fibrillation, atrial flutter, or ventricular tachycardia (VT)

Contraindications

Hypersensitivity to adenosine, second- or third-degree AV heart block, sick sinus syndrome (unless functioning artificial pacemaker is present), and asthma; not recommended in the treatment of atrial fibrillation, atrial flutter, and VT

Administration

Dose

Administer 6-mg (undiluted) IV bolus over 1 to 2 seconds; follow with a rapid 20-mL saline flush to ensure that the drug reaches the circulation. Give 12-mg rapid IV bolus if the first dose fails to eliminate the PSVT within 1 to 2 minutes. Repeat the 12-mg dose if needed. Do not give second dose if high-level block occurs with first dose.

Precautions

A short-lasting first-, second-, or third-degree heart block may result. Patients developing high-level block after one dose of adenosine should not be given additional doses. New dysrhythmias may develop during conversion (e.g., premature ventricular contractions [PVCs], premature atrial contractions [PACs], sinus bradycardia, sinus tachycardia, and AV blocks), but are generally self-limiting because the half-life of adenosine is less than 10 seconds. Higher degrees of heart block may result in patients taking carbamazepine. Dipyridamole potentiates effects of adenosine. Larger doses may be required in patients taking theophylline or other methylxanthine products because the effects of adenosine are antagonized by methylxanthines.

Patient Management

1. Check patency of IV and rapidly flush IV after adenosine administration to ensure that the drug reaches the circulation.
2. Evaluate heart rate (HR) and rhythm 1 to 2 minutes after administering adenosine and monitor for dysrhythmias during conversion; BP is not adversely affected with the usual dose of adenosine, but larger doses may result in hypotension.
3. Measure PR interval for development of AV block.
4. Observe for adverse effects: nonmyocardial chest discomfort, hypotension, and dyspnea. Patients may report facial flushing, sweating, headache, lightheadedness, tingling in the arms, blurred vision, heaviness in arms, burning sensation, neck and back pain, numbness, metallic taste, tightness in throat, and pressure in groin. These are usually short lived. However, notify physician if effects last longer than a minute.
5. Individualize treatment for prolonged adverse effects (e.g., external pacemaker for prolonged third-degree block). Aminophylline is an antagonist.

ALTEPLASE (ACTIVASE)

Classification

Thrombolytic, fibrinolytic

Effect

Lyses clots

Indications

Acute myocardial infarction (AMI), acute ischemic stroke

Contraindications

Hypersensitivity; active internal bleeding within 21 days (except menses); major surgery or trauma within 14 days; history of cardio-vascular, intracranial, or intraspinal event within 2 months (stroke, AVM, neoplasm, aneurysm, recent trauma, or recent surgery); aortic dissection; severe uncontrolled hypertension; and bleeding disorders. Prolonged cardiopulmonary resuscitation (CPR) with evidence of thoracic trauma, lumbar puncture within 7 days, recent arterial puncture at noncompressible site.

Administration

Dose

AMI: If weight is ≥67 kg: 15-mg IV bolus over 2 minutes, followed by 50 mg IV infusion over the next 30 minutes, followed by 35 mg over the next 60 minutes. If weight is <67 kg: 15 mg IV bolus over 2 minutes, then 0.75 mg/kg (do not exceed 50 mg) infusion over 30 minutes, followed by 60-minute infusion of 0.5 mg/kg (do not exceed 35 mg)

Three-hour infusion: if weight is ≥65 kg, administer 6 to 10 mg over 2 minutes; follow with an infusion of 50 to 54 mg (total 60 mg) over 1 hour. Then follow with 20 mg/hr for 2 additional hours.

Three-hour infusion: if weight is <65 kg: total dose to be given is 1.25 mg/kg. Administer 3/5 of the dose divided as above into a bolus and first-hour dose. Follow with 1/5 of the total calculated dose/hour for 2 hours.

Acute ischemic attack: infuse 0.9 mg/kg (maximum 90 mg) over 60 minutes; give 10% of the total dose as an initial bolus over 1 minute; give remainder of alteplase over the next 60 minutes.

Follow infusion with at least 30 mL normal saline (NS) or D_5W to ensure administration of total dose.

Patient Management

1. Initiate two peripheral IV lines with one dedicated for fibri-nolytic agent only. Aspirin and heparin will be administered concurrently for AMI.
2. Assess for bleeding: bleeding gums, petechiae, ecchymosis, hematuria, melena, epistaxis, and hemoptysis; assess neuro-logic signs carefully (intracranial hemorrhage).

3. Initiate bleeding precautions, e.g., minimize bleeding: avoid IM injections and use of noncompressible pressure sites during fibrinolytic therapy; avoid invasive procedures; handle the patient carefully, maintain strict bed rest.

4. Monitor continuous electrocardiogram (ECG) for dysrhythmia development in the treatment of AMI. Follow institutional protocol. Monitor neurologic status frequently for intracranial hemorrhage. Discontinue alteplase if suspected. Notify physician.

5. Observe adverse effects: cerebral hemorrhage, spontaneous bleeding, dysrhythmias, cardiac arrest, cardiogenic shock, and cardiac decompensation and notify physician.

AMIODARONE (CORDARONE)

Classification

Antidysrhythmic

Effects

Prolongs duration of action potential, depresses conduction velocity, slows conduction at AV node. Decreases cardiac workload and myocardial oxygen consumption through its vasodilatory effects.

Indications

Atrial and ventricular tachydysrhythmias

Contraindications

Severe sinus bradycardia, second- or third-degree AV block (unless pacemaker is functioning), cardiogenic shock

Administration

Dose

In cardiac arrest, give 300 mg IV push; repeat with 150 mg intravenously in 3 to 5 minutes (maximum dose is 2.2 g in 24 hours) for recurrent bouts of ventricular tachycardia/ventricular fibrillation. If spontaneous circulation is restored, administer 360 mg at 1 mg/min over 6 hours, followed with a maintenance infusion of 0.5 mg/min over 18 hours. May continue maintenance infusion until ventricular dysrhythmias are stabilized.

In supraventricular dysrhythmias: give 150 mg intravenously over 10 minutes; follow with a loading infusion of 360 mg at 1 mg/min over 6 hours; then with a maintenance infusion of 0.5 mg/min.

Precautions

Hypokalemia and hypomagnesemia should be corrected before amiodarone is administered. Amiodarone is prodysrhythmic; existing dysrhythmias may worsen or new dysrhythmias may develop. QT interval may increase. Hypotension and negative inotropic effects may occur. Pulmonary toxicity may occur with long-term use.

Patient Management

1. Monitor HR, rhythm, and BP continuously during infusion.
2. Be alert for QT interval prolongation.
3. Assess for visual impairment (may progress to permanent blindness) and report onset to physician.
4. Observe for adverse effects: hypotension, dysrhythmias including bradydysrhythmias and heart block, hepatotoxicity, visual impairment, and cardiac arrest. Notify physician of adverse effects.
5. Monitor patient response to drug interactions even after amiodarone has been discontinued because the half-life of amiodarone is long (40 days).

ANISTREPLASE (EMINASE)

Classification

Thrombolytic, fibrinolytic

Effect

Lyses clots

Indication

AMI

Contraindications

Hypersensitivity; active internal bleeding within 21 days (except menses); major surgery or trauma within 14 days; history of cardiovascular, intracranial, or intraspinal event within 3 months (stroke, AVM, neoplasm, aneurysm, recent trauma, or recent surgery); aortic dissection; severe uncontrolled hypertension; and bleeding disorders. Prolonged CPR with evidence of thoracic trauma; lumbar puncture within 7 days; recent arterial puncture at noncompressible site

Administration

Dose

30 international units IV over 2 to 5 minutes

Precautions

Renal and hepatic disease, subacute bacterial endocarditis

Patient Management

1. Initiate two peripheral IV lines with one dedicated for fibrinolytic agent only. Aspirin and heparin will be administered concurrently for AMI.
2. Draw blood for coagulation studies and type and crossmatch.
3. Assess for bleeding: bleeding gums, petechiae, ecchymosis, hematuria, melena, epistaxis, and hemoptysis; assess neurologic signs carefully (intracranial hemorrhage); assess for retroperitoneal bleeding (back pain, leg weakness, diminished pulses). If bleeding is evident, stop infusion and notify physician.
4. Minimize bleeding: avoid IM injections and use of noncompressible pressure sites during fibrinolytic therapy; avoid invasive procedures; handle the patient carefully.
5. Monitor continuous ECG for dysrhythmia development in the treatment of AMI.
6. Observe adverse effects: cerebral hemorrhage, spontaneous bleeding, dysrhythmias, cardiac arrest, cardiogenic shock, and cardiac decompensation.

ATENOLOL (TENORMIN)

Classification

β-Adrenergic blocking agent

Effects

Reduces HR, CO, BP, and myocardial oxygen consumption. Promotes redistribution of blood flow from adequately supplied areas of the heart to ischemic areas. Reduces incidence of recurrent MI, size of the infarct, and incidence of fatal dysrhythmias. Converts supraventricular tachydysrhythmias to NSR.

Indications

AMI, supraventricular tachycardia (SVT)

Contraindications

Sinus bradycardia, second- and third-degree heart block, cardiogenic shock, overt heart failure

Administration

Dose

Administer 5 mg IV over 5 minutes; wait 10 minutes; repeat 5-mg dose slowly IV. If tolerated, may give 50 mg by mouth (PO) 10 minutes after the last IV bolus. Maintenance: 50 mg PO bid.

Precautions

Use cautiously in patients with heart failure, lung disease or bronchospasm, and severe abnormalities in cardiac conduction. Abrupt withdrawal in patients with thyroid disease may precipitate thyroid storm. May mask tachycardia associated with hyperthyroidism or hypoglycemia.

Patient Management

1. Monitor cardiac rhythm, HR, and BP; notify physician if bradycardia (<60 beats/min) or hypotension (systolic blood pressure [SBP] <100 mm Hg) develops.
2. Assess CO and signs of myocardial ischemia (e.g., angina, dysrhythmias, ST segment, T-wave changes).
3. Assess the patient for development of heart failure.
4. Monitor blood glucose levels, especially in patients with diabetes.
5. Observe for adverse effects: breathing difficulties, bradycardia, heart block, ventricular dysrhythmias, hypotension, and cardiac failure.

ATROPINE

Classification

Anticholinergic, muscarinic antagonist

Effects

Atropine increases conduction through the AV node and increases the HR.

Indications

Symptomatic sinus bradycardia, asystole, or bradycardic pulseless electrical activity

Contraindications

Adhesions between the iris and lens, advanced renal and hepatic impairment, asthma, narrow-angle glaucoma, obstructive disease of the GI and urinary tracts, myasthenia gravis, and paralytic ileus

Administration

Dose

For bradycardia, administer 0.5 mg IV bolus every 3 to 5 minutes until adequate response or a total dose of 3 mg is given. Doses of less than 0.5 mg can cause further bradycardia. For asystole, or pulseless electrical activity, administer 1 mg intravenously; repeat every 3 to 5 minutes if needed up to 3 doses.

Atropine can be given intraosseously (IO) if IV is not available in emergency situations. Atropine may also be given via the endotracheal tube, however, intraosseous (IO) or IV route is preferred.

Precautions

In the presence of an acute myocardial infarction, atropine can increase cardiac irritability. Avoid in hypothermic bradycardia.

Patient Management

1. Monitor HR for response to therapy (>60 beats/min is desirable); be alert for development of ventricular fibrillation (VF) or VT.
2. Excessive doses can result in tachycardia, flushed hot skin, delirium, coma, or death.

CALCIUM CHLORIDE

Classification

Electrolyte replenisher, cardiotonic

Effects

Calcium chloride replaces and maintains calcium in body fluids.

Indications

Hypocalcemia, hyperkalemia, and calcium channel blocker overdose

Contraindications

VF, hypercalcemia, renal calculi, and digitalis toxicity

Administration

Dose

For hyperkalemia and calcium channel blocker overdose, give 8 to 16 mg/kg IV. Repeat if needed. One gram of calcium chloride in a 10% solution is equivalent to 13.6 mEq of calcium.

Precautions

The dose of calcium may need to be adjusted in patients with renal or cardiac disease. Cardiac dysrhythmias may be evidenced when calcium is administered to patients who are receiving digitalis glycosides or who have been digitalized. Severe necrosis and sloughing of tissues will occur with infiltration. Calcium chloride is three times more potent than calcium gluconate

Patient Management

1. Administer calcium through a central line.
2. Assess patency of IV; note any precipitate.
3. Monitor BP because peripheral vasodilatation will occur.
4. Monitor serial serum calcium levels.
5. Continuously monitor ECG for onset of dysrhythmias.
6. Monitor for electrolyte imbalances.
7. Observe for adverse effects: bradycardia, cardiac arrest, constipation, fatigue, venous irritation, depression, loss of appetite, and tingling.

DALTEPARIN

Classification

Anticoagulant, low-molecular-weight heparin

Effects

Inhibits thrombin generation by factor Xa inhibition and indirectly by forming a complex with antithrombin III

Indications

ACS, non–Q-wave MI, unstable angina

Contraindications

Platelet count <100,000/mm^3, hypersensitivity

Administration

Dose

1 mg/kg subcutaneous bid for 2 to 8 days

Precautions

Blood dyscrasias, peptic ulcer disease, recent lumbar puncture, hepatic disease, pericarditis, and other conditions at risk for bleeding

Patient Management

1. Assess for bleeding: bleeding gums, petechiae, ecchymosis, epistaxis, hematuria, melena, and change in neurologic signs (intracranial hemorrhage).
2. Assess IV sites and previous puncture sites.
3. Assess for covert bleeding, e.g., retroperitoneal or epidural hematoma (patients with current or recent intraspinal catheters or lumbar punctures).
4. Monitor hematocrit (Hct) level, complete blood cell count (CBC), and platelet counts.
5. Minimize bleeding: avoid IM injections, use electric razors.
6. Observe for adverse effects: thrombocytopenia, bleeding.

DIGOXIN (LANOXIN)

Classification

Cardiac glycoside, inotropic, antidysrhythmic

Effects

Digoxin increases myocardial contractility, decreases HR, and enhances CO, which improves renal blood flow and increases urinary output.

Indications

Patients with heart failure, cardiogenic shock, and atrial dysrhythmias such as atrial fibrillation, atrial flutter, and PSVT

Contraindications

Patients who demonstrate signs and symptoms of digitalis toxicity, VF, VT, carotid sinus syndrome, and second- or third-degree heart block

Administration

Dose

Doses must be individualized. Usual loading dose is 10 to 15 mcg/kg (lean body weight). Maintenance dose is usually 0.125 to 0.5 mg per day.

Precautions

Use cautiously in older adults and in patients with acute myocardial infarction or renal impairment. Administer IV digoxin with caution in the hypertensive patient because a transient increase in BP may occur. Patients with partial AV block may develop complete heart block. Patients with WPW may experience fatal ventricular dysrhythmias. Avoid electrical cardioversion in patients on digoxin unless life-threatening condition exists.

Patient Management

1. Check potassium and magnesium levels before administration because hypokalemia and hypomagnesemia are associated with increased risk of digitalis toxicity.
2. Check calcium level because hypercalcemia can increase the risk of digitalis toxicity and hypocalcemia can nullify the effects of digoxin.
3. Take apical pulse before administration; if <60 beats/min, consult with physician.
4. Measure serial PR intervals for development of heart block.
5. Evaluate the patient for controlled dysrhythmia (decreased ventricular response to atrial fibrillation or atrial flutter).
6. Evaluate the patient for resolution of heart failure.
7. Be prepared to treat overdose with IV magnesium sulfate or digoxin immune Fab (Digibind) if the patient has severe, life-threatening refractory dysrhythmias (Box 10-1).
8. Observe for digitalis toxicity: nausea and vomiting, anorexia, epigastric pain, unusual fatigue, diarrhea, dysrhythmias, excessive slowing of HR, blurred or yellow vision, irritability or confusion, ST segment sagging or prolonged PR interval.

DILTIAZEM (CARDIZEM)

Classification

Calcium channel blocker, antidysrhythmic

Effects

Depresses impulse formation and conduction velocity. Dilates coronary arteries and arterioles.

Indications

Control of rapid ventricular response in atrial fibrillation and flutter; conversion of PSVT

Contraindications

Wide QRS tachycardias of uncertain origin, atrial fibrillation, or flutter when associated with an accessory bypass tract (WPW, short PR syndrome), second- or third-degree heart block, severe hypotension,

Box 10-1 Digibind, DigiFab

The dose of Digibind/DigiFab varies according to the amount of digoxin to be neutralized. Each vial will bind with 0.6 mg of digoxin. Usual initial dose of 20 vials has been administered. If amount of ingested digoxin is unknown, 10 vials can be considered. Digibind must be given through a 0.22-micron membrane filter over 15 to 30 minutes; DigiFab can be administered as an infusion over 30 minutes. If the toxicity has not been reversed after several hours, repeating a single dose may be required. Monitor patient for acute anaphylaxis, life-threatening hypokalemia, and heart rate because the withdrawal of digoxin effects in patients with atrial fibrillation or atrial flutter may cause a return of rapid ventricular rate. Heart failure may worsen secondary to withdrawal of the inotropic effects of digitalis.

cardiogenic shock, heart failure, and sick sinus syndrome unless functioning pacemaker in place

Administration

Dose

Initially, administer 0.25 mg/kg intravenously over 2 minutes; in 15 minutes give 0.35 mg/kg if needed. If an infusion is required, rate is 5 mg/hr; maximum dose is 15 mg/hr. Infusion is not recommended greater than 24 hours.

Precautions

Life-threatening tachycardia with severe hypotension in atrial fibrillation or flutter in patients with an accessory bypass tract can occur; periods of asystole can occur in patients with sick sinus syndrome. Use cautiously in patients with preexisting impaired ventricular function; condition may exacerbate. May cause AV block. Severe hypotension in patients receiving IV β-blocking agents, do not give concomitantly.

Patient Management

1. Evaluate dysrhythmia control.
2. Monitor HR, rhythm, and BP. Notify physician if hypotension or bradycardia develops.
3. Measure PR interval for onset of AV block.
4. Monitor CO and assess for signs of heart failure.
5. Observe for adverse effects: dysrhythmias, hypotension, flushing, heart block, chest pain, heart failure, dyspnea, and edema.

DOBUTAMINE (DOBUTREX)

Classification

Inotrope, β_1-agonist

Effects

Dobutamine increases myocardial contractility and increases CO without significant change in BP. It increases coronary blood flow and myocardial oxygen consumption.

Indications

Heart failure, cardiac decompensation

Contraindications

Idiopathic hypertrophic subaortic stenosis, shock without adequate fluid replacement; sulfite sensitivity

Administration

Dose

IV infusion is 2 to 20 mcg/kg/min titrated to desired patient response. A concentration of 250 mg/250 mL D$_5$W yields 1 mg/mL. Concentration of solution should not exceed 5 mg/mL of dobutamine (Table 10-1). Avoid if systolic blood pressure (SBP) <100 mm Hg and signs of shock are evident.

Table 10-1 DOBUTAMINE DOSAGE CHART (DOBUTAMINE: 250 MG/250 ML*; CONCENTRATION: 1000 MCG/ML)

mcg/kg/min	Weight (kg)											
	45	50	55	60	65	70	75	80	85	90	95	100
	Flow Rate (mL/hr)											
5	14	15	17	18	20	21	23	24	26	27	29	30
7.5	20	23	25	27	29	32	34	36	38	41	43	45
10	27	30	33	36	39	42	45	48	51	54	57	60
12.5	34	38	41	45	49	53	56	60	64	68	71	75
15	41	45	50	54	59	63	68	72	77	81	86	90
17.5	47	53	58	63	68	74	79	84	89	95	100	105
20	54	60	66	72	78	84	90	96	102	108	114	120

*Dobutamine—advanced cardiac life support (ACLS): patient weight in kg × 15 determines the amount of dobutamine (mg) to be added to 250 mL of IV fluid. The rate set on the infusion pump = mcg/kg/min.

Precautions

Hemodynamic monitoring is recommended for optimal benefit when dobutamine is administered. Fluid deficits should be corrected before infusion of dobutamine. At doses greater than 20 mcg/kg/min, an increase in HR may occur. Dobutamine facilitates conduction through the AV node and can cause a rapid ventricular response in patients with inadequately treated atrial fibrillation. CV effects are intensified by monoamine oxidase (MAO) inhibitors and tricyclic antidepressants. Concurrent use with general anesthetics may increase the potential for ventricular dysrhythmias.

Patient Management

1. Use large veins for administration; an infusion pump should be used to regulate flow rate.
2. Correct hypovolemia before starting.
3. Titrate so HR does not exceed >10% of baseline.
4. Check BP and HR every 2 to 5 minutes during initial administration and during titration of the drug.
5. Monitor CI, PAWP, and urine output continuously during administration.
6. Observe for adverse effects: tachycardia, hypertension, chest pain, shortness of breath, and cardiac dysrhythmias.

DOPAMINE (INTROPIN)

Classification

Sympathomimetic, vasopressor, inotropic

Effects

Dopamine in low doses (1-2 mcg/kg/min) increases blood flow to the kidneys, thereby increasing glomerular filtration rate, urine flow, and sodium (Na) excretion. In low to moderate doses (2-10 mcg/kg/min), it increases myocardial contractility and CO. In high doses (10-20 mcg/kg/min), it increases peripheral resistance and renal vasoconstriction.

Indications

Shock state, symptomatic bradycardia

Contraindications

Uncorrected tachydysrhythmias, pheochromocytoma, VF

Administration

Dose

Initially, 2 to 10 mcg/kg. Increase infusion by 5 to 10 mcg/kg/min every 1 to 30 min until desired effect. A concentration of 400 mg/500 mL D_5W yields 800 mcg/mL (Table 10-2).

Precautions

Concurrent use with β-blockers may antagonize the effect of dopamine. CV effects are intensified by MAO inhibitors and tricyclic antidepressants. Some general anesthetics can increase risk of dysrhythmias. Use cautiously in patients with occlusive vascular disease, arterial embolism, and diabetic endarteritis. Correct hypovolemic states before administering dopamine. Extravasation may cause necrosis and sloughing of surrounding tissue.

Patient Management

1. Use large vein; check vein frequently for blanching or pallor, which may indicate extravasation.
2. Notify physician if extravasation occurs. Treat with phentolamine (5-10 mg in 10-15 mL NS) via local infiltration as soon as possible.

Table 10-2 DOPAMINE DOSAGE CHART (DOPAMINE: 400 MG/500 ML*; CONCENTRATION: 800 MCG/ML)

	Weight (kg)											
	45	50	55	60	65	70	75	80	85	90	95	100
mcg/kg/min	Flow Rate (mL/hr)											
1	3	4	4	5	5	6	6	6	6	7	7	8
2	7	8	8	9	10	11	11	12	13	14	14	15
3	10	11	12	14	15	16	17	18	19	20	21	23
5	17	19	21	23	24	26	28	30	32	34	36	38
7	24	26	29	32	34	37	39	42	45	47	50	53
10	34	38	41	45	49	53	56	60	64	68	71	75
13	44	49	54	59	63	68	73	78	83	88	93	98
15	51	56	62	68	73	79	84	90	96	101	107	113
20	68	75	83	90	98	105	113	120	128	135	143	150
25	84	94	103	113	122	131	141	150	159	167	178	188
30	101	113	124	135	146	158	169	180	191	203	214	225

*Dopamine—advanced cardiac life support (ACLS): patient weight in kg ×15 determines the amount of dopamine (mg) to be added to 250 mL of IV fluid. The rate set on the infusion pump = mcg/kg/min.

3. Do not use the proximal port of a pulmonary artery (PA) catheter to infuse the drug if CO readings are being obtained.
4. Monitor BP and HR every 2 to 5 minutes initially and during titration of the drug.
5. Measure urine output hourly to evaluate renal function. Doses greater than 20 mcg/kg/min decrease renal perfusion.
6. Determine pulse pressure because a decrease indicates excessive vasoconstriction.
7. Taper infusion gradually to prevent sudden hypotension.
8. Observe for adverse effects: tachycardia, headache, dysrhythmias, nausea and vomiting, hypotension, chest pain, shortness of breath, and vasoconstriction (numbness, tingling, pallor, cold skin, decreased pulses, decreased cerebral perfusion, and decreased urine output).
9. Report the drug's inability to maintain a desired response despite increased dose.

ENALAPRILAT

Classification

Angiotensin-converting enzyme (ACE) inhibitor, antihypertensive, vasodilator

Effects

Reduces peripheral arterial resistance, reduces preload and afterload in patients with heart failure, improves CO, helps prevent adverse left ventricular (LV) remodeling in post-MI patients, delays heart failure post MI, and decreases sudden death and recurrent MI

Indications

Heart failure, hypertension, MI with LV failure

Contraindications

Hypersensitivity, pregnancy, angioedema

Administration

Dose

Enalaprilat: 1.25 mg intravenously over 5 minutes, followed by 1.25 to 5 mg intravenously every 6 hours. Usual oral dose is 2.5 mg and titrated to 20 mg bid.

Enalapril is the oral form, Enalaprilat is the parenteral form. May cause precipitous drop in BP after initial dose and in patients who are volume depleted. Hyperkalemia may occur. Use caution in renal disease.

Patient Management

1. Monitor HR and BP.
2. Evaluate patient response to treatment (e.g., edema, dyspnea, crackles resolved, BP controlled).
3. Monitor electrolyte levels and renal function.
4. Observe for adverse effects: hypotension, chest pain, dysrhythmias, agranulocytosis, neutropenia, renal failure, and hyperkalemia.

ENOXAPARIN (LOVENOX)

Classification

Anticoagulant, low-molecular-weight heparin

Effects

Inhibits thrombin generation by factor Xa inhibition and indirectly by forming a complex with antithrombin III

Indications

ACS, non–Q-wave MI, unstable angina

Contraindications

Platelet count <100,000/mm^3; hypersensitivity

Administration

Dose

1 mg/kg subcutaneous bid for 2 to 8 days

Precautions

Blood dyscrasias, peptic ulcer disease, recent lumbar puncture, current or recent spinal or epidural puncture, hepatic disease, pericarditis, and other conditions at risk for bleeding

Patient Management

1. Assess for bleeding: bleeding gums, petechiae, ecchymosis, epistaxis, hematuria, melena, and change in neurologic signs (intracranial hemorrhage).

2. Assess IV sites and previous puncture sites.
3. Assess for covert bleeding, e.g., retroperitoneal or epidural hematoma (patients with current or recent intraspinal catheters or lumbar punctures); patients who need neuraxial anesthesia or spinal puncture may be at risk for developing epidural or spinal hematoma. Monitor neurologic function.
4. Monitor Hct level, CBC, and platelet counts.
5. Minimize bleeding: avoid IM injections, use electric razors.
6. Observe for adverse effects: thrombocytopenia, bleeding, neurologic injury when used with spinal or epidural puncture.

EPINEPHRINE (ADRENALIN)

Classification

Bronchodilator, vasopressor, cardiac stimulant

Effects

Epinephrine increases myocardial contractility, HR, SBP, and CO. It also relaxes bronchial smooth muscle.

Indications

Cardiac arrest, hypersensitivity reactions, anaphylaxis, acute asthma attacks, symptomatic bradycardia, severe hypotension

Contraindications

Acute narrow-angle glaucoma and coronary insufficiency

Administration

Dose

For patients in cardiac arrest, give 1 mg intravenously or intraosseously if no IV is available, every 3 to 5 minutes. Follow with five forceful inhalations. As a vasopressor, administer as an IV infusion at 2 to 10 mcg/min and titrate to desired response; 1 mg/250 mL D_5W yields 4 mcg/mL (Table 10-3).

For bronchospasm or anaphylaxis, give 0.1 to 0.5 mg (0.1-0.5 mL of 1:1000 solution) subcutaneously and repeat every 10 to 20 minutes. If using an IV route, give 0.1 to 0.25 mg (1-2.5 mL of 1:10,000 solution). Note: Epinephrine 1:1000 solution contains 1 mg/mL; epinephrine 1:10,000 solution contains 0.1 mg/mL.

Precautions

Use cautiously in older patients and patients with angina, hypothyroidism, hypertension, psychoneurosis, and diabetes. Epinephrine

Table 10-3 Isoproterenol and Epinephrine Doses (Isoproterenol and Epinephrine: 1 mg/250 mL; Concentration: 4 mcg/mL)

Dose (mcg/min)	Rate (mL/hr)
1	15
2	30
3	45
4	60

should be administered cautiously in patients with long-standing bronchial asthma and emphysema who have developed degenerative heart disease. Do not administer concurrently with isoproterenol—death may result. Epinephrine increases myocardial oxygen demand and may cause angina and myocardial ischemia. MAO inhibitors and tricyclic antidepressants can prolong and intensify the effects of epinephrine. Repeated local injections or extravasation of epinephrine can cause tissue necrosis.

Patient Management

1. Monitor continuous ECG.
2. Monitor BP and HR every 2 to 5 minutes during the initial infusion and during drug titration.
3. Use an infusion device; validate correct drug and infusion rate. Use central venous access.
4. Do not use the proximal port of a PA catheter for infusing epinephrine if CO readings are being obtained.
5. Evaluate patient's response; monitor CI.
6. Observe for adverse effects: chest pain, dysrhythmias, headache, restlessness, dizziness, nausea and vomiting, weakness, hypertensive crisis, and decreased perfusion to fingers/toes.
7. Report the drug's inability to maintain a desired effect despite increased doses.

EPTIFIBITIDE

Classification

GP IIb/IIIa inhibitor, platelet aggregation inhibitor, antithrombotic, monoclonal antibody

Effects

Inhibits platelet aggregation

Indication

Non–Q-wave MI or unstable angina managed medically or undergoing percutaneous coronary intervention (PCI)

Contraindications

Active internal bleeding, severe uncontrolled hypertension, history of intracranial hemorrhage, major surgery or trauma within 1 month, thrombocytopenia, aneurysm, AVM, bleeding disorders within 30 days, concomitant use of another GP IIb/IIIa inhibitor

Administration

Dose

ACS: IV bolus of 180 mcg/kg; followed by IV infusion of 2 mcg/kg/min

PCI: IV bolus 180 mcg/kg; followed by IV infusion of 2 mcg/kg/min. Repeat bolus of 180 mg/kg 10 minutes after initial bolus

Precautions

Platelet function recovers within 4 to 8 hours after eptifibitide is discontinued

Patient Management

1. Administer through inline nonpyrogenic low-protein-binding filter (if not used during drug preparation).
2. Assess for bleeding: femoral sheath access site, current and prior IV sites; note bleeding gums, ecchymosis, petechiae, hematuria, melena, epistaxis, hemoptysis, change in neurologic signs (intracranial bleed), and retroperitoneal bleeding (back pain, leg weakness).
3. Monitor lab results (e.g., CBC, platelets, and coagulation studies).
4. Keep the patient on bed rest with extremity immobile.
5. Check pulses of affected extremity, including after sheath removal.
6. Follow institutional protocol.
7. Institute measures to minimize bleeding (e.g., avoid IM injections, handle the patient with care, avoid sharp objects, avoid automatic BP cuffs).

8. Observe for adverse effects: major bleeding, intracranial hemorrhage, bleeding at femoral artery and other access sites, thrombocytopenia, abdominal pain, back pain, chest pain, dysrhythmias, hypotension, limb embolism, pericardial effusion, and pulmonary edema.

ESMOLOL (BREVIBLOC)

Classification

β-Adrenergic blocking agent

Effects

Esmolol decreases HR, BP, contractility, and myocardial oxygen consumption.

Indications

ACS, SVT

Contraindications

Sinus bradycardia, heart block greater than first degree, cardiogenic shock, and overt heart failure. Do not use concurrent with epinephrine

Administration

Dose

Administer 0.5 mg/kg over 1 minute; follow by an infusion 0.05 mg/kg/min. Titrate to desired effect, not to exceed 0.3 mg/kg/min. A concentration of 5 g/500 mL D_5W yields 10 mg/mL.

Precautions

Use cautiously in patients with impaired renal function, diabetes, bronchospasm, or hypotension.

Patient Management

1. Monitor BP every 2 minutes during titration. Hypotension can be reversed by decreasing the dose or by discontinuing the infusion. Half-life of esmolol is 2 to 9 minutes.
2. Evaluate dysrhythmia control.
3. Monitor ECG for bradycardia or heart block.
4. Evaluate the patient for heart failure.
5. Monitor blood glucose levels, especially in patients with diabetes.

6. Observe for adverse effects: hypotension, pallor, lightheadedness, paresthesias, urinary retention, nausea and vomiting, wheezing, and inflammation at the infusion site.

7. Report signs of overdose: tachycardia or bradycardia, dizziness or fainting, difficulty in breathing, bluish palmar surface of hands, seizures, cold hands, fever, sore throat, or unusual bleeding.

FUROSEMIDE (LASIX)

Classification

Diuretic, antihypertensive

Effects

Furosemide promotes the excretion of fluid and electrolytes and reduces plasma volume.

Indications

Edematous states: heart failure, pulmonary edema, hepatic and renal disease, and hypertension

Contraindications

Sensitivity to furosemide or sulfonamides

Administration

Dose

IV dose is 0.5 to 1 mg/kg over 1 to 2 minutes; if no response can give 2 mg/kg over 1 to 2 minutes.

Precautions

Profound electrolyte and water depletion can occur.

Patient Management

1. Check potassium level before administering furosemide; hypokalemia should be corrected before administering the drug.
2. Evaluate hearing and assess for ototoxicity.
3. Assess lungs to evaluate patient response to therapy.
4. Monitor urine output to evaluate drug effectiveness.
5. Monitor serial blood urea nitrogen (BUN) and creatinine levels to assess renal function.

6. Assess the patient for volume depletion and electrolyte imbalance.
7. Monitor BP and intake and output (I&O) and assess serial weights (1 kg is equal to approximately 1000 mL fluid) to evaluate fluid loss.
8. Monitor the patient receiving digitalis for digitalis toxicity secondary to diuretic-induced hypokalemia.
9. Advise the patient to report ringing in ears, severe abdominal pain, or sore throat and fever. These symptoms may indicate furosemide toxicity.
10. Observe for adverse effects: volume depletion, orthostatic hypotension, electrolyte imbalance, transient deafness, glucose intolerance, and hepatic dysfunction.

HEPARIN

Classification

Anticoagulant, antithrombotic

Effects

Inhibits antithrombin III, prevents conversion of fibrinogen to fibrin and prothrombin to thrombin

Indications

Treatment of thrombosis and emboli; adjuvant therapy in AMI

Contraindications

Hypersensitivity, active bleeding (except disseminated intravascular coagulation [DIC]); hemophilia; recent intracranial, intraspinal, or eye surgery; severe thrombocytopenia; severe hypertension; or bleeding disorders

Administration

Dose

Adjuvant treatment in AMI: bolus with 60 international units/kg (maximum 4000 international units) follow with infusion 12 international units/kg/hr (maximum 1000 international units/hr for patients >70 kg); adjust infusion to activated partial thromboplastin time (aPTT) (1.5-2 times control for 48 hours or until angiography)

Precautions

Any condition or procedures in which there is a risk of hemorrhage; heparin is available in many strengths. Read label carefully.

Patient Management

1. Assess for bleeding: bleeding gums, petechiae, ecchymosis, hematuria, epistaxis, hemoptysis, and melena; check all catheter sites and prior puncture sites; assess neurologic signs (intracranial bleeding); assess for retroperitoneal bleeding (back pain, leg weakness).
2. Monitor aPTT results. Follow institutional heparin protocol.
3. Monitor Hct and hemoglobin (Hgb) levels and platelet count.
4. Monitor HR and BP.
5. Minimize bleeding: avoid IM injections and other invasive therapies; handle patient gently.
6. Observe for adverse effects: bleeding, thrombocytopenia.

IBUTILIDE (CORVERT)

Classification

Antidysrhythmic

Effect

Prolongs duration of action potential and the effective refractory period

Indications

Atrial fibrillation, atrial flutter

Contraindications

Hypersensitivity

Administration

Dose

For patients ≥60 kg, 1 mg intravenously over 10 minutes. A second dose may be administered 10 minutes later. For patients <60 kg, 0.01 mg/kg intravenously over 10 minutes

Precautions

Second- or third-degree AV block, sinus node dysfunction; ventricular dysrhythmias can develop. May cause torsades de pointes.

Patient Management

1. Monitor ECG continuously for development of dysrhythmias during the infusion and for 4 to 6 hours after the infusion is completed. Prolonged QT interval can occur.
2. Monitor BP and HR closely.
3. Observe for adverse effects: sinus arrest, bradycardia, dysrhythmias, hypotension, and congestive heart failure.

INAMRINONE (INOCOR)

Classification

Inotrope, vasodilator

Effects

Inamrinone increases myocardial contractility and CO. It decreases afterload and preload.

Indication

Heart failure refractory to traditional therapies

Contraindications

Hypersensitivity to amrinone or bisulfites; severe aortic or pulmonic valvular disease

Administration

Dose

IV loading dose is 0.75 mg/kg over 10 to 15 minutes. The drug can be given undiluted. As an infusion, administer at 5 to 15 mcg/kg/min. Do not mix with dextrose; protect from light.

Precautions

Avoid administration with disopyramide; can cause excessive hypotension. Use cautiously in patients who have hepatic or renal disease. Outflow tract obstruction may worsen in patients with hypertrophic subaortic stenosis.

Patient Management

1. Monitor BP, pulmonary artery wedge pressure (PAWP), mean arterial pressure (MAP), systemic vascular resistance index (SVRI), pulmonary vascular resistance index (PVRI), cardiac index (CI), and HR during infusion. Decrease rate of infusion or stop infusion for excessive hypotension.

   2. Monitor intake and output, electrolytes, and renal function.
   3. Observe for adverse effects: thrombocytopenia, hypotension, dizziness, dysrhythmias, chest pain, hypokalemia, nausea and vomiting, abdominal pain, anorexia, hepatic toxicity, and fever.

ISOPROTERENOL (ISUPREL)

Classification

Sympathomimetic, β-adrenergic agonist

Effects

Isoproterenol increases CO, coronary blood flow, and stroke volume and relaxes bronchial smooth muscle.

Indications

Bronchial asthma, obstructive pulmonary disease, bronchospasm, heart block, refractory torsades de pointes, and shock states

Contraindications

Digitalis-induced tachycardia, heart block, angina, or patients receiving β-blockers

Administration

Dose

In torsades de pointes, titrate infusion to increase HR until VT is suppressed. A concentration of 1 mg/250 mL D_5W yields 4 mcg/mL (see Table 10-3).

Precautions

Volume deficit should be corrected before initiating isoproterenol. Administer cautiously in patients with hypertension, coronary artery disease, hyperthyroidism, and diabetes. The drug is not indicated in cardiac arrest. Do not use concurrently with epinephrine; VF and VT may develop. Myocardial oxygen demand increases; which may increase myocardial ischemia. Isoproterenol's effects are enhanced by MAO inhibitors and tricyclic antidepressants.

Patient Management

   1. If the HR exceeds 110 beats/min, the dose may need to be decreased. If the HR exceeds 130 beats/min, ventricular dysrhythmias may be induced.

2. Monitor BP, MAP, central venous pressure (CVP), urinary output, and peripheral blood flow; evaluate for therapeutic response.
3. An infusion pump should be used to control infusion rate.
4. Observe for adverse effects: headache, tachycardia, anginal pain, palpitations, dysrhythmias, flushing of the face, nervousness, sweating, hypotension, and pulmonary edema.

LABETALOL (NORMODYNE, TRANDATE)

Classification

α/β-Adrenergic blocking agent, antihypertensive, antianginal

Effects

Labetalol decreases BP and renin secretion and can decrease HR and CO.

Indications

Acute coronary syndrome, hypertension

Contraindications

Bronchial asthma, cardiac failure, heart block, cardiogenic shock, and bradycardia

Administration

Dose

ACS: 10 mg intravenously over 1 to 2 minutes; may repeat or double dose every 10 minutes to a maximum of 150 mg; or 10 mg intravenously followed by an infusion 2 to 8 mg/min. A concentration of 200 mg/160 mL D_5W yields 1 mg/mL.

Precautions

Use cautiously in patients with heart failure, hepatic impairment, chronic bronchitis, emphysema, and preexisting peripheral vascular disease.

Patient Management

1. Check HR and BP before administering labetalol.
2. Monitor BP every 2 to 5 minutes during titration of infusion; avoid rapid BP drop because cerebral infarction or angina can occur.

3. Have the patient remain supine immediately following injection.
4. Assess the patient for heart failure development.
5. Monitor blood glucose levels especially in patients with diabetes.
6. Observe for adverse effects: dizziness, orthostatic hypotension, fatigue, nasal stuffiness, edema, paresthesias, dysrhythmias, AV block, agranulocytosis, thrombocytopenia, and wheezing.

LIDOCAINE

Classification

Antidysrhythmic

Effect

Lidocaine suppresses the automaticity of ectopic foci.

Indications

Cardiac arrest from VF and VT; stable VT, and wide complex tachycardias of uncertain type. Prophylactic use in AMI is not recommended.

Contraindications

Patients with Adams-Stokes syndrome and severe heart block without a pacemaker; WPW syndrome

Administration

Dose

The loading dose is 1 to 1.5 mg/kg IV push; repeat with 0.5 to 0.75 mg/kg every 5 to 10 minutes. Maximum is 3 mg/kg. Maintenance infusion is 1 to 4 mg/min. A concentration of 2 g/500 mL D_5W yields 4 mg/mL (Table 10-4).

Table 10-4 LIDOCAINE, BRETYLIUM, AND PROCAINAMIDE DOSES (LIDOCAINE, BRETYLIUM, PROCAINAMIDE: 2 G/500 ML; CONCENTRATION: 4 MG/ML)

Dose (mg/min)	Rate (mL/hr)
1	15
2	30
3	45
4	60

Precautions

Concurrent use with phenytoin can produce excessive cardiac depression. Use with β-blockers or cimetidine may slow hepatic metabolism of lidocaine. Older patients are more susceptible to adverse effects. Do not use lidocaine solutions containing epinephrine.

Patient Management

1. Monitor continuous ECG and evaluate dysrhythmia control.
2. Measure serial PR intervals.
3. Evaluate CO/CI.
4. Assess for central nervous system (CNS) effects such as twitching and tremors, which may precede seizures.
5. Use infusion pump, do not exceed 4 mg/min.
6. Observe for adverse effects: dizziness, restlessness, confusion, twitching, paresthesias, dysarthria, convulsions, drowsiness, bradycardia, itching, rash, anxiety, respiratory depression, blurred vision, tinnitus, vomiting, and malignant hyperthermia.

LISINOPRIL

Classification

ACE inhibitor, antihypertensive, vasodilator

Effects

Reduces peripheral arterial resistance, reduces preload and afterload in patients with heart failure, improves CO, helps prevent adverse LV remodeling in post-MI patients, delays heart failure post MI, and decreases sudden death and recurrent MI

Indications

Heart failure, hypertension, AMI

Contraindications

Hypersensitivity, pregnancy

Administration

Dose

In AMI, 5 mg PO within 24 hours of onset of symptoms followed by 5 mg after 24 hours, then 10 mg after 48 hours, then 10 mg daily for 6 weeks; for hypertension, 10 to 40 mg daily

Precautions

Renal disease, hyperkalemia, and renal artery stenosis

Patient Management

1. Monitor HR and BP.
2. Evaluate patient response to treatment (e.g., edema, dyspnea, crackles resolved, BP controlled).
3. Monitor electrolyte levels and renal function.
4. Observe for adverse effects: hypotension, agranulocytosis, renal failure, hyperkalemia, and angioedema.

MAGNESIUM SULFATE

Classification

Electrolyte replenisher, antidysrhythmic, anticonvulsant

Effects

Magnesium sulfate replaces and maintains magnesium levels in body fluids. It depresses the CNS, producing anticonvulsant effects; decreases incidence of dysrhythmias.

Indications

Seizures associated with eclampsia and preeclampsia, hypomagnesemia, torsades de pointes, life-threatening ventricular dysrhythmias secondary to digitalis toxicity

Contraindications

Heart block, myocardial damage, and renal failure; also contraindicated for the pregnant patient within 2 hours of expected delivery

Administration

Dose

For cardiac arrest if torsades or hypomagnesemia is suspected: 1 to 2 g diluted in 10 mL D_5W IV push. For torsades de pointes: infusion: 1 to 2 g in 50 to 100 mL D_5W over 5 to 60 minutes; followed with 0.5 to 1 g/hr to control torsades. For AMI: infusion: 1 to 2 g in 50 to 100 mL D_5W over 5 to 60 minutes; followed with 0.5 to 1 g/hr for 24 hours. For seizures, give 1 to 4 g as a 10% solution. Administer 1.5 mL of a 10% solution intravenously over 1 minute. As an infusion of 4 g/250 mL D_5W, do not exceed a rate of 4 mL/min.

For hypomagnesemia, give an infusion of 5 g/1000 mL D_5W over 3 hours (rate not to exceed 3 mL/min).

Precautions

Use cautiously in patients with renal disease and in the presence of heart failure or myocardial damage. CNS effects are potentiated when the drug is administered with other CNS depressants. If magnesium toxicity occurs in a patient receiving digitalis who requires calcium to treat the toxicity, heart block may occur. Hypotension may occur with rapid administration. Magnesium sulfate crosses the placenta and can produce adverse effects on the baby.

Patient Management

1. Monitor continuous ECG for suppression of torsades de pointes.
2. Monitor HR and BP every 2 to 5 minutes during drug titration.

For eclampsia/preeclampsia:

1. Evaluate presence of patellar reflexes before each dose. If they are absent, magnesium should not be given until they return.
2. Monitor respirations: respirations must be at least 16 breaths/min before a dose can be given to reduce the risk for respiratory arrest.
3. Monitor renal status: urine output should be at least 25 mL/hr.
4. Monitor for signs of heart block and hypotension.
5. Have emergency equipment available in case of respiratory or cardiac arrest.
6. Calcium 5 to 10 mEq can be given to reverse respiratory depression and heart block.
7. Observe for adverse effects: absent patellar reflex; flushing; hypotension; sweating; flaccid paralysis; prolonged PR, QRS, and QT intervals; respiratory depression; and cardiac arrest.

MANNITOL

Classification

Osmotic diuretic

Effects

Increases osmotic pressure of fluid in renal tubules and decreases reabsorption of water and electrolytes; increases urine output and Na and chloride (Cl) excretion

Indication

Increased intracranial pressure (ICP)

Contraindications

Active intracranial bleeding, anuria, severe pulmonary congestion, severe heart failure, fluid and electrolyte depletion, and renal dysfunction

Administration

Dose

IV infusion of 0.5 to 1 g/kg over 5 to 10 minutes; additional doses of 0.25 to 2 g/kg every 4 to 6 hours as needed

Precautions

Dehydration, renal dysfunction, cardiac disease

Patient Management

1. Monitor HR, BP, and ICP (if available); CVP and PAP (if available).
2. Assess hydration status and monitor urine output every hour.
3. Monitor serum electrolyte, BUN, and creatinine levels and arterial blood gases (ABGs).
4. Monitor serum osmolality. Serum levels should not exceed 310 mOsm/kg.
5. Observe for adverse effects: seizures, rebound increased ICP, pulmonary congestion, acidosis, hypotension, fluid and electrolyte imbalance, and fluid overload.

METOPROLOL (LOPRESSOR)

Classification

β-Adrenergic blocking agent, antidysrhythmic

Effects

Reduces incidence of recurrent MI, size of the infarct, and incidence of fatal dysrhythmias

Indications

ACS, PSVT, hypertensive crisis

Contraindications

Bradycardia (<45 beats/min), second- and third-degree heart block, cardiac failure, hypotension (SBP <100 mm Hg), first-degree heart block (PR >0.24)

Administration

Dose

Administer 5 mg slowly intravenously at 5-minute intervals to a total of 15 mg. Oral metoprolol can be initiated 15 minutes after the last IV bolus. Usually 50 mg PO every 6 hours for 48 hours, then 100 mg PO bid. However, dose and frequency are based on patient tolerance.

Precautions

Use cautiously in patients in heart failure, lung disease, or bronchospasm. May mask tachycardia associated with hyperthyroidism or hypoglycemia. Concurrent therapy with calcium channel blocking agents may cause severe hypotension. May cause severe bradycardia in patients with WPW syndrome

Patient Management

1. Monitor cardiac rhythm, HR, and BP. Notify physician if hypotension (SBP <100 mm Hg), bradycardia (HR <45 beats/min), or heart block greater than first degree develops.
2. Evaluate the patient for development of heart failure.
3. Monitor blood glucose levels, especially in patients with diabetes.
4. Observe for adverse effects: breathing difficulties, bradycardias, heart block, hypotension, and cardiac failure.

MILRINONE (PRIMACOR)

Classification

Inotrope, vasodilator, antidysrhythmic

Effects

Arterial vasodilation and increase in myocardial contractility

Indication

Treatment of heart failure

Contraindication

Hypersensitivity to milrinone; severe aortic or pulmonic valvular disease

Administration

Dose

Loading dose is 50 mcg/kg intravenously slowly over 10 minutes. Titrate (0.375-0.75 mcg/kg/min) to patient hemodynamic response.

Precautions

Outflow tract obstruction may worsen in patients with obstructive aortic or pulmonic valve disease or hypertrophic subaortic stenosis. Ventricular dysrhythmias may develop. Increase in ventricular response in atrial fibrillation/atrial flutter may occur. Infusion rates should be reduced in patients with renal function impairment.

Patient Management

1. Monitor HR and rhythm every 2 to 5 minutes during titration of infusion; evaluate MAP, SVRI, PVRI, CI, and PAWP.
2. Monitor I&O, daily weights and creatinine, BUN, and serum electrolyte levels.
3. Titrate infusion to maximum hemodynamic effect.
4. Reduce infusion rate if hypotension occurs.
5. Observe for adverse effects: dysrhythmias, hypotension, angina, hypokalemia, and thrombocytopenia.

MORPHINE SULFATE

Classification

Opiate analgesic

Effects

Decreases pain impulse transmission; decreases myocardial oxygen requirements; relieves pulmonary congestion

Indications

Chest pain with ACS unresponsive to nitrates, cardiogenic pulmonary edema

Contraindications

Hypersensitivity, respiratory rate <12 breaths/min

Administration

Dose

2 to 4 mg intravenously over 1 to 5 minutes every 5 to 30 minutes

Precautions

Compromised respiratory state, hypovolemia. May increase ventricular response in presence of PSVT

Patient Management

1. Dose is individualized based on patient response; administer slowly via IV route.
2. Assess pain using the patient's self-report whenever possible.
3. Monitor respiratory rate.
4. Monitor HR and BP and level of sedation.
5. Observe for adverse effects: bradycardia, orthostatic hypotension, respiratory depression, and apnea.

NALMEFENE (REVEX)

Classification

Opioid antagonist

Effect

Nalmefene competes for opioid receptor sites in the CNS. It has no pharmacologic activity of its own.

Indications

Patients with known or suspected opioid-induced respiratory depression

Contraindications

Hypersensitivity

Administration

Dose

IV: 0.5 mg/70 kg; follow with 1 mg/70 kg in 2 to 5 minutes. Additional doses are not recommended.

Precautions

Use cautiously in patients with cardiac irritability and opioid addiction.

Patient Management

1. Monitor respiratory depth and rate continuously; duration of opioid may exceed that of naloxone, and the patient may lapse into respiratory depression.
2. Provide O_2 and artificial ventilation as necessary.
3. Observe for adverse effects: side effects are dose related and may be caused by abrupt reversal of the effects of opioid: hypertension, nausea and vomiting, tachycardia, pulmonary edema.

NALOXONE (NARCAN)

Classification

Opioid antagonist

Effect

Naloxone competes for opioid receptor sites in the CNS. It has no pharmacologic activity of its own.

Indications

Patients with known or suspected opioid-induced respiratory depression

Contraindications

Hypersensitivity

Administration

Dose

Administer 0.4 to 2 mg intravenously over 15 seconds; dose may be repeated every 2 to 3 minutes.

Precautions

Use cautiously in patients with cardiac irritability and opioid addiction. Drug is not effective in respiratory depression caused by anesthetics, barbiturates, or other nonopioid agents.

Patient Management

1. Monitor respiratory depth and rate continuously; duration of opioid may exceed that of naloxone, and the patient may lapse into respiratory depression.
2. Provide O_2 and artificial ventilation as necessary.
3. Observe for adverse effects: nausea and vomiting, sweating, tachycardia, hypertension, pulmonary edema, VT, and VF.

NESIRITIDE (NATRECOR)

Classification

Cardiotonic, vasodilator

Effect

Dilates arteries and veins; decreases PAWP and SBP

Indications

Congestive heart failure

Contraindications

Not recommended as the primary treatment for cardiogenic shock; patients with SBP <90 mm Hg, restricted or obstructive cardiomyopathy, pericarditis, pericardial tamponade, or patients with low filling pressures.

Administration

Dose

Administer 2 mcg/kg IV bolus over 1 minute; follow with an infusion 0.01 mcg/kg/min.

Precautions

Nesiritide is a recombinant protein—use caution in patients with allergies.

Patient Management

1. Monitor BP frequently. Stop infusion for excessive drop in blood pressure.
2. Monitor HR and rhythm, CI and PAWP, renal function, urine output, and fluid/electrolytes.
3. Observe for adverse effects: lightheadedness, dizziness, dysrhythmias, hypotension, dyspnea, angina, abdominal pain, impaired vision, hemoptysis, paresthesias, and allergic reactions.

NITROGLYCERIN (TRIDIL, NITROL)

Classification

Vasodilator, antianginal, antihypertensive

Effects

Nitroglycerin decreases venous return, preload, myocardial oxygen demand, BP, MAP, CVP, PAWP, PVRI, and SVRI. It improves coronary artery blood flow and oxygen delivery.

Indications

Angina, hypertension, and heart failure in AMI

Contraindications

Patients with hypersensitivity to nitrites; patients with head trauma, cerebral hemorrhage, severe anemia, pericardial tamponade, constrictive pericarditis, or RV infarction; those with hypertrophic cardiomyopathy who are experiencing chest pain. Patients who are severely bradycardic or tachycardic and patients who have taken sildenafil (Viagra) within 24 hours.

Administration

Dose

Initial IV infusion is 5 mcg/min; increase by 5 mcg every 3 to 5 minutes and titrate to desired response. In patients with unstable angina and congestive heart failure (CHF) associated with MI, 12.5 to 25 mcg followed with an infusion of 10 to 20 mcg/min may be given. A concentration of 50 mg/500 mL D_5W yields 100 mcg/mL. No fixed maximum dose has been established (Table 10-5).

Precautions

Use with tricyclic antidepressants may result in additive hypotension. Orthostatic hypotension may be potentiated with antihypertensives or vasodilators. Correct volume deficit to prevent profound hypotension. Tolerance may develop within 12 to 24 hours of nitroglycerin use.

Table 10-5 NITROGLYCERIN DOSES (NITROGLYCERIN: 50 MG/500 ML; CONCENTRATION: 100 MCG/ML

Dose (mcg/min)	Rate (mL/hr)
5	3
10	6
15	9
20	12
25	15
30	18
35	21
40	24
45	27
50	30

Patient Management

1. Monitor HR; a 10 beat/min increase suggests adequate vasodilation.
2. Monitor BP every 2 to 5 minutes while titrating.
3. Stop infusion and lift the patient's lower extremities if SBP <90 mm Hg or if the patient complains of dizziness or light-headedness.
4. Calculate coronary perfusion pressure (CPP); monitor PAWP, SVRI, and PVRI; and evaluate CI.
5. Observe for adverse effects: headache, dizziness, dry mouth, blurred vision, orthostatic hypotension, tachycardia, angina, flushing, palpitations, nausea, and restlessness. Discontinue if blurred vision or dry mouth occurs.
6. Report unrelieved angina, side effects and cyanotic lips and palmar surface of hands, extreme dizziness, pressure in head, dyspnea, fever, muscle twitching, seizure, and weak or fast HR.

NITROPRUSSIDE (NIPRIDE)

Classification

Vasodilator, antihypertensive

Effects

Nitroprusside decreases BP and peripheral resistance and usually increases CO.

Indications

Hypertension, acute heart failure

Contraindication

Coarctation of aorta

Administration

Dose

IV infusion is 0.1 to 5 mcg/kg/min. Maximum is 10 mcg/kg/min. Titrate in small increments every 3 to 5 minutes to desired effect. Do not exceed 10 mcg/kg/min. A concentration of 50 mg/250 mL D_5W yields 200 mcg/mL (Table 10-6).

Precautions

Use cautiously in patients with hypothyroidism, increased intracranial pressure, or hepatic or renal disease and in those receiving

Table 10-6 NITROPRUSSIDE DOSAGE CHART (NITROPRUSSIDE: 50 MG/
250 ML; CONCENTRATION: 200 MCG/ML)

	Weight (kg)											
	45	50	55	60	65	70	75	80	85	90	95	100
mcg/kg/min	Flow Rate (mL/hr)											
1	14	15	16	18	20	21	23	24	26	27	29	30
2	27	30	33	36	39	42	45	48	51	54	57	60
4	54	60	66	72	78	84	90	96	102	108	114	120
6	81	90	99	108	117	126	135	144	153	162	171	180
8	108	120	132	144	156	168	180	192	204	216	228	240

antihypertensive agents. Infusion rates greater than 2 mcg/kg/min are associated with increased risk of cyanide toxicity.

Patient Management

1. Monitor BP continuously; if hypotension develops, discontinue IV nitroprusside. BP should return to pretreatment level within 1 to 10 minutes.
2. Use an IV infusion device; validate concentration and dosage.
3. Protect solution from light; it normally is brownish.
4. Assess the patient for chest pain, dysrhythmias, and fluid retention.
5. Observe for adverse effects: headache, dizziness, excessive sweating, nervousness, restlessness, ataxia, delirium, loss of consciousness, ringing in the ears, abdominal pain, retrosternal discomfort, bradycardia, tachycardia, and increased ICP.
6. Tolerance to nitroprusside may indicate toxicity. Monitor thiocyanate levels. Thiocyanate levels of greater than 100 mcg/mL indicate toxicity.
7. Assess for signs of toxicity: profound hypotension, air hunger, confusion, metabolic acidosis, dyspnea, headache, loss of consciousness, vomiting, and bright red venous blood. Have available cyanide antidote kit.

NOREPINEPHRINE (LEVOPHED)

Classification

Sympathomimetic, vasopressor

Effects

Norepinephrine produces vasoconstriction, increases myocardial contractility, and dilates coronary arteries.

Indications

Hypotensive states

Contraindications

Mesenteric or peripheral vascular thrombosis or use with cyclopropane or halothane anesthesia

Administration

Dose

IV infusion is 0.5 to 1 mcg/min; titrate every 3 to 5 minutes, up to 30 mcg/min, to desired BP. A concentration of 4 mg/250 mL D_5W yields 16 mcg/mL (Tables 10-7 and 10-8).

Precautions

Concurrent administration with MAO inhibitors increases the risk of hypertensive crisis. When the drug is administered with tricyclic antidepressants, severe hypertension may result. Use cautiously in patients with history of hypertension, hyperthyroidism, and severe cardiac disease. Correct fluid volume deficit before administering norepinephrine.

Table 10-7 NOREPINEPHRINE DOSAGE CHART (NOREPINEPHRINE: 4 MG/ 250 ML; CONCENTRATION: 16 MCG/ML)

mcg/kg/ min	Weight (kg)											
	45	50	55	60	65	70	75	80	85	90	95	100
	Flow Rate (mL/hr)											
0.1	17	19	21	23	24	26	28	30	32	34	36	38
0.2	34	38	41	45	49	53	56	60	64	68	71	75
0.3	51	56	62	68	73	79	84	90	96	101	107	113
0.4	68	75	82	90	98	105	112	120	128	135	142	150
0.5	85	94	103	113	122	132	141	150	160	169	178	188
0.6	101	113	124	135	146	158	168	180	191	203	214	225
0.7	118	132	144	158	171	184	197	210	223	237	249	263
0.8	135	150	165	180	195	210	225	240	255	270	285	300
0.9	152	169	185	203	220	237	253	270	287	304	320	338
1.0	169	188	206	225	244	263	281	300	319	338	356	375

Table 10-8 NOREPINEPHRINE DOSES* (NOREPINEPHRINE: 4 MG/250 ML; CONCENTRATION: 16 MCG/ML)

Dose (mcg/min)	Rate (mL/hr)
1	4
2	8
3	11
4	15
5	19

*Dose is closest to mcg/min due to rounding of rate in mL/hr to nearest whole number.

Patient Management

1. Monitor BP continuously until stabilized at desired level, then check BP every 5 minutes. Avoid hypertension.
2. Monitor continuous ECG and evaluate CO/CI.
3. Assess patency of IV site (avoid peripheral veins in hands, legs; use large veins) and observe for extravasation; blanching may indicate extravasation. If extravasation occurs, stop the infusion and call physician. Be prepared to infiltrate the area with phentolamine 5 to 10 mg in 10 to 15 mL NS.
4. Use an infusion pump to regulate flow.
5. Assess for signs and symptoms of excessive vasoconstriction: cold skin, pallor, decreased pulses, decreased cerebral perfusion, and decreased pulse pressure.
6. Report decreased urinary output.
7. Taper medication gradually and monitor vital signs.
8. Observe for adverse effects: headache, VT, bradycardia, VF, angina, dyspnea, decreased urinary output, metabolic acidosis, restlessness, and hypertensive state.

PROCAINAMIDE (PRONESTYL)

Classification

Antidysrhythmic

Effects

Procainamide depresses cardiac automaticity, excitability, and conductivity.

Indications

Premature ventricular complexes, VT, and atrial dysrhythmias

Contraindications

Second- or third-degree heart block, hypersensitivity to procaine, myasthenia gravis, torsades de pointes, and lupus erythematosus

Administration

Dose

Administer 20 mg/min intravenously until the dysrhythmia is abolished, hypotension occurs, QRS widens by 50%, or a total of 17 mg/kg has been given. IV infusion is 1 to 4 mg/min; a dose of 2 g/500 mL D_5W yields 4 mg/mL (see drug dosage chart, Table 10-4). When starting oral maintenance dose, wait at least 4 hours after last IV dose.

Precautions

Concurrent administration with cimetidine, β-blockers, ranitidine, or amiodarone may result in increased procainamide blood levels. Use cautiously in patients with conduction delays, hepatic or renal insufficiency, and heart failure. Patients with atrial fibrillation and atrial flutter may develop increased ventricular rate. Use caution with other drugs that prolong QT interval.

Patient Management

1. Monitor BP and ECG continuously during IV titration.
2. Measure PR, QT, and QRS intervals. If QRS widens >50% and QT interval is prolonged, notify physician.
3. Assess for heart failure development.
4. Evaluate CI.
5. Monitor procainamide and NAPA serum levels.
6. Observe for adverse effects: prolonged PR, QRS and QT intervals; hypotension, agranulocytosis, neutropenia, joint pain, fever, chills, bradycardia, VT, VF, nausea and vomiting, anorexia, diarrhea, bitter taste, maculopapular rash, and lupus erythematosus–like syndrome.

PROPRANOLOL (INDERAL)

Classification

β-Adrenergic blocking agent, antidysrhythmic

Effects

Propranolol decreases cardiac oxygen demand, HR, BP, and myocardial contractility.

Indications

ACS, cardiac dysrhythmias, hypertension

Contraindications

Asthma, chronic obstructive pulmonary disease (COPD), allergic rhinitis, sinus bradycardia, heart block greater than first degree, cardiogenic shock, and right ventricular failure secondary to pulmonary hypertension

Administration

Dose

IV dose is 0.1 mg/kg divided into three equal-dose intervals. Administer slowly over 2 to 3 minutes. Do not exceed 1 mg/min. Wait 2 minutes and repeat if needed. Subsequent doses may not be given for at least 4 hours, regardless of route to be administered.

Precautions

Additive effects may result when the drug is administered with diltiazem or verapamil. Use with digoxin may result in excessive bradycardia, with potential for heart block. Concurrent use with epinephrine may result in significant hypertension and excessive bradycardia. Propranolol may mask certain symptoms of developing hypoglycemia. Use cautiously in patients with heart failure or respiratory disease and in patients taking other antihypertensive drugs. The dose should be adjusted in older patients.

Patient Management

1. Continuously monitor ECG with IV administration; report rhythm change to physician; if bradycardia develops, do not administer propranolol and notify physician.
2. Monitor BP and other hemodynamic parameters (e.g., CVP, PAWP) frequently during IV administration; if SBP <90 mm Hg, notify physician.
3. Assess the patient for development of heart failure.
4. Monitor blood glucose levels, especially in patients with diabetes.
5. Do not abruptly withdraw medication.
6. Observe for adverse effects: bradycardia, hypotension, heart failure, intensification of AV block, nausea and vomiting, abdominal cramps, hypoglycemia, and difficulty in breathing.

RAMIPRIL (ALTACE)

Classification

ACE inhibitor, antihypertensive, vasodilator

Effects

Reduces peripheral arterial resistance, reduces preload and afterload in patients with heart failure, improves CO, helps prevent adverse LV remodeling in post-MI patients, delays heart failure post MI, and decreases sudden death and recurrent MI

Indications

Heart failure, hypertension, AMI

Contraindications

Hypersensitivity, pregnancy

Administration

Dose

Oral dose of 2.5 mg titrated to 5 mg bid

Precautions

Hypovolemia, impaired liver or renal function, blood dyscrasias, COPD, renal artery stenosis

Patient Management

1. Monitor HR and BP.
2. Evaluate patient response to treatment (e.g., edema, dyspnea, crackles resolved, BP controlled).
3. Monitor electrolyte levels and renal function.
4. Observe for adverse effects: hypotension, chest pain, dysrhythmias, eosinophilia, leukopenia, renal failure, hyperkalemia, and angioedema.

RETEPLASE (RETAVase)

Classification

Thrombolytic, fibrinolytic

Effect

Lyses clots

Indication

AMI

Contraindications

Hypersensitivity; active internal bleeding within 21 days (except menses); major surgery or trauma within 14 days; history of cardiovascular, intracranial, or intraspinal event within 3 months (stroke, AVM, neoplasm, aneurysm, recent trauma, or recent surgery); aortic dissection; severe uncontrolled hypertension; and bleeding disorders. Prolonged CPR with evidence of thoracic trauma; lumbar puncture within 7 days; recent arterial puncture at noncompressible site.

Administration

Dose

10 units IV bolus over 2 minutes; followed by a second 10 units IV bolus 30 minutes later

Patient Management

1. Initiate two peripheral IV lines, with one dedicated for fibrinolytic agent only. Aspirin and heparin will be administered concurrently for AMI.
2. Assess for bleeding: bleeding gums, petechiae, ecchymosis, hematuria, melena, epistaxis, and hemoptysis; assess neurologic signs carefully (intracranial hemorrhage).
3. Minimize bleeding: avoid IM injections and use of noncompressible pressure sites during fibrinolytic therapy; avoid invasive procedures; handle the patient carefully.
4. Monitor continuous ECG for dysrhythmia development in the treatment of AMI.
5. Observe adverse effects: cerebral hemorrhage, spontaneous bleeding, dysrhythmias, cardiac arrest, cardiogenic shock, and cardiac decompensation.

SODIUM BICARBONATE

Classification

Alkalinizer, antacid, electrolyte replenisher

Effects

Sodium bicarbonate increases the plasma bicarbonate, buffers excess hydrogen ion concentration, and increases blood pH.

Indications

Metabolic acidosis, hyperkalemia, and need to alkalinize the urine

Contraindications

Metabolic or respiratory acidosis, hypocalcemia, hypertension, hypochloremia, impaired renal function; not recommended for routine use in cardiac arrest unless other interventions have been instituted and specific clinical circumstances exist (e.g., preexisting metabolic acidosis)

Administration

Dose

IV dose is 1 mEq/kg initially, then 0.5 mEq/kg every 10 minutes if indicated by arterial pH and P_{CO_2}. IV infusion is 2 to 5 mEq/kg; drug may be administered over 4 to 8 hours in less acute acidosis.

Precautions

Rapid administration of sodium bicarbonate may result in severe alkalosis. Tetany or hyperirritability may occur with increased alkalosis.

Patient Management

1. Assess patency of IV; extravasation may cause necrosis or sloughing of tissue.
2. Obtain arterial blood pH, P_{O_2}, and P_{CO_2} results before administering sodium bicarbonate.
3. Flush line before and after administration of sodium bicarbonate.
4. Observe for adverse effects: restlessness, tetany, hypokalemia, alkalosis, and hypernatremia.

STREPTOKINASE (STREPTASE)

Classification

Thrombolytic, fibrinolytic

Effect

Lyses clots

Indication

AMI

Contraindications

Hypersensitivity; active internal bleeding within 21 days (except menses); major surgery or trauma within 14 days; history of cardio-vascular, intracranial, or intraspinal event within 3 months (stroke, AVM, neoplasm, aneurysm, recent trauma, or recent surgery); aortic dissection; severe uncontrolled hypertension; and bleeding disorders. Prolonged CPR with evidence of thoracic trauma; lumbar puncture within 7 days; and recent arterial puncture at noncompressible site.

Administration

Dose

1.5 million international units IV infusion over 1 hour

Patient Management

1. Initiate two peripheral IV lines with one dedicated for fibri-nolytic agent only. Aspirin and heparin will be administered concurrently for AMI.
2. Assess for bleeding: bleeding gums, petechiae, ecchymosis, hematuria, melena, epistaxis, and hemoptysis; assess neuro-logic signs carefully (intracranial hemorrhage). Assess for retroperitoneal bleeding (back pain, leg weakness, dimin-ished pulses). If bleeding is evident, stop infusion and notify physician.
3. Institute bleeding precautions: keep patient on bed rest, avoid IM injections and use of noncompressible pressure sites dur-ing fibrinolytic therapy; avoid invasive procedures; handle the patient carefully.
4. Monitor coagulation studies.
5. Monitor VS frequently, and monitor continuous ECG for changes in ST segment and dysrhythmia development in the treatment of AMI.
6. Observe adverse effects: allergic reaction, cerebral hemor-rhage, spontaneous bleeding, dysrhythmias, cardiac arrest, cardiogenic shock, and cardiac decompensation.

TENECTEPLASE (TNKase)

Classification

Thrombolytic, fibrinolytic

Effect

Lyses clots

Indication

AMI

Contraindications

Hypersensitivity; active internal bleeding within 21 days (except menses); major surgery/trauma within 14 days; history of cardiovascular, intracranial, or intraspinal event within 3 months (stroke, AVM, neoplasm, aneurysm, recent trauma, or recent surgery); aortic dissection; severe uncontrolled hypertension; and bleeding disorders. Prolonged CPR with evidence of thoracic trauma; lumbar puncture within 7 days; and recent arterial puncture at noncompressible site.

Administration

Dose

30 to 50 mg IV bolus, depending on body weight: <60 kg, 30 mg; 60 to 69.9 kg, 35 mg; 70 to 79.9 kg, 40 mg; 80 to 89.9 kg, 45 mg; >90 kg, 50 mg

Precautions

Renal and hepatic disease, subacute bacterial endocarditis

Patient Management

1. Initiate two peripheral IV lines with one dedicated for fibrinolytic agent only. Aspirin and heparin will be administered concurrently for AMI.
2. Draw blood for coagulation studies and type and crossmatch.
3. Assess for bleeding: bleeding gums, petechiae, ecchymosis, hematuria, melena, epistaxis, and hemoptysis; assess neurologic signs carefully (intracranial hemorrhage); assess for retroperitoneal bleeding (back pain, leg weakness, diminished pulses). If bleeding evident, stop infusion and notify physician.
4. Institute bleeding precautions. Minimize bleeding: avoid IM injections and use of noncompressible pressure sites during fibrinolytic therapy; avoid invasive procedures; handle the patient carefully; maintain patient on bed rest.
5. Monitor continuous ECG for dysrhythmia development in the treatment of AMI.
6. Observe adverse effects: cerebral hemorrhage, spontaneous bleeding, dysrhythmias, cardiac arrest, cardiogenic shock, and cardiac decompensation.

TIROFIBAN (AGGRASTAT)

Classification

GP IIb/IIIa inhibitor, platelet aggregation inhibitor, antithrombotic, monoclonal antibody

Effect

Inhibits platelet aggregation

Indication

Non–Q-wave MI or unstable angina with planned PCI

Contraindications

Active internal bleeding, severe uncontrolled hypertension, history of intracranial hemorrhage, major surgery or trauma within 1 month, thrombocytopenia, aneurysm, AVM, bleeding disorders within 30 days, liver disease, acute pericarditis, and concomitant use of another GP IIb/IIIa inhibitor

Administration

Dose

0.4 mcg/kg/min intravenously over 30 minutes; followed by 0.1 mcg/kg/min infusion

Precautions

Patients with platelet count <150,000/mm^3. Platelet function recovery occurs within 4 to 8 hours after tirofiban is discontinued.

Patient Management

1. Administer through inline, nonpyrogenic, low-protein-binding filter (if not used during drug preparation). Monitor VS frequently.
2. Assess for bleeding: femoral sheath access site, current and prior IV sites; note bleeding gums, ecchymosis, petechiae, hematuria, melena, epistaxis, hemoptysis, change in neurologic signs (intracranial bleed), and retroperitoneal bleeding (back pain, leg weakness).
3. Monitor lab results (e.g., CBC, platelets, and coagulation studies).
4. Keep the patient on bed rest with extremity immobile.
5. Check pulses of affected extremity, including after sheath removal.

6. Follow institutional protocol.
7. Institute bleeding precautions: e.g., avoid IM injections, handle the patient with care, avoid sharp objects.
8. Observe for adverse effects: major bleeding, intracranial hemorrhage, bleeding at femoral artery and other access sites, thrombocytopenia, abdominal pain, back pain, chest pain, dysrhythmias, hypotension, limb embolism, pericardial effusion, hemoptysis, and pulmonary edema.

VASOPRESSIN (PITRESSIN)

Classification

Vasopressor, antidiuretic hormone

Effect

Causes vasoconstriction of the vascular bed.

Indications

Shock-refractory ventricular fibrillation

Contraindications

Hypersensitivity

Administration

Dose

One dose only: 40 units intravenously. May be administered intraosseously if IV not available.

Precautions

May cause cardiac ischemia, myocardial infarction. May produce water intoxication

Patient Management

1. Vasopressin can be used in emergency cardiac care. Follow advanced cardiac life support (ACLS).
2. Continuously monitor ECG; obtain BP frequently and assess fluid/electrolyte balance.
3. Maintain airway, breathing, and circulation.

CALCULATIONS

The critical care environment requires that nurses be able to calculate infusion drips to determine the amount of drug being administered.

Medications are often administered as continuous IV infusions and titrated to achieve the desired response.

DRUG CONCENTRATION IN MG/ML OR MCG/ML

$$1 \text{ mg} = 1000 \text{ mcg}$$
$$1 \text{ g} = 1000 \text{ mg}$$

To determine the amount of drug in one milliliter, divide the amount of drug in solution by the amount of solution (mL).

Example: 200 mg of drug in 500 mL

Determine mg/mL:

$$\frac{200 \text{ mg}}{500 \text{ mL}} = 0.4 \text{ mg/mL}$$

Determine mcg/mL:

First change mg to mcg:

$$200 \text{ mg} \times 1000 \text{ mcg/mg} = 200,000 \text{ mcg}$$

Then divide mcg by mL of solution:

$$\frac{200,000 \text{ mcg}}{500} = 400 \text{ mcg/mL}$$

CALCULATING MCG/KG/MIN

Drug dosages are often expressed in mcg/kg/min. Three parameters must be known to determine the amount of medication the patient is receiving:

1. Patient weight in kg (1 kg = 2.2 lb)
2. Infusion rate (mL/hr)
3. Drug concentration

The drug concentration is multiplied by the infusion rate and divided by the patient weight × 60 min/hr:

$$\text{mcg/kg/min} = \frac{\text{mcg/mL} \times \text{mL/hr}}{\text{kg} \times 60 \text{ min/hr}}$$

Example: A patient weighing 75 kg is receiving dobutamine at 20 mL/hr. There is 250 mg of dobutamine in 250 mL D_5W.

1. The patient weight is 75 kg.
2. The infusion rate is 20 mL/hr.
3. The drug concentration must be determined in mcg/mL:

First change mg to mcg:

$$250 \text{ mg} = 250,000 \text{ mcg}$$

Next, divide the dose by the amount of solution:

$$\frac{250,000 \text{ mcg}}{250 \text{ mL}} = 1000 \text{ mcg/mL}$$

Because all three parameters are known, now determine mcg/kg/min:

$$\text{mcg/kg/min} = \frac{\text{mcg/mL} \times \text{mL/hr}}{\text{kg} \times 60 \text{ min/hr}}$$

$$= \frac{1000 \times 20}{75 \times 60}$$

$$= \frac{20,000}{4500}$$

$$= 4.44 \text{ mcg/kg/min}$$

CALCULATING THE AMOUNT OF FLUID TO INFUSE (ML/HR)

Three parameters must be known to determine the infusion rate for the IV pump:

1. The patient weight in kg (1 kg = 2.2 lb)
2. The dose ordered by the physician in mcg/kg/min
3. The drug concentration in mcg/min

Multiply the dose ordered by the patient weight × 60 minutes and divide by the drug concentration:

$$\text{mL/hr} = \frac{\text{mcg/kg/min ordered} \times \text{kg} \times 60 \text{ min}}{\text{mcg/mL}}$$

Example: A patient weighing 70 kg is to receive dopamine at 6 mcg/kg/min. There is 400 mg of dopamine in 250 mL D_5W.

1. The patient weight is 70 kg.
2. The dose ordered is 6 mcg/kg/min.
3. The drug concentration must be determined in mcg/mL:

First change mg to mcg:

$$400 \text{ mg} \times 1000 \text{ mcg/mg} = 400,000 \text{ mcg}$$

Next, divide the dose by the amount of solution:

$$\frac{400,000 \text{ mcg}}{250 \text{ mL}} = 1600 \text{ mcg/mL}$$

Because all three parameters are known, determine mL/hr:

$$mL/hr = \frac{mcg/kg/\min ordered \times kg \times 60 \min}{mcg/mL}$$

$$= \frac{6 \times 70 \times 60}{1600}$$

$$= \frac{25,200}{1600}$$

$$= 16 \; mL/hr$$

BIBLIOGRAPHY

Brundage RC, Mann HJ: General principles of pharmacokinetics and pharmaco-dynamics. In Fink MP et al, editors: *Textbook of critical care,* Philadelphia, 2005, WB Saunders.

Devlin JW, Zarowitz BJ: Alterations in drug disposition in the elderly. In Grenvik A et al, editor: *Textbook of critical care,* Philadelphia, 2000, WB Saunders.

Gahart BL, Nazareno AR: *Intravenous medications,* St Louis, 2005, Mosby.

Gutierrez K: Older adult pharmacotherapeutics. In Gutierrez K, Queener SF editors: *Pharmacology for nursing practice,* St Louis, 2003, Mosby.

Hazinski MF, Cummins RO, Field JM: *Handbook of emergency cardiovascular care for the healthcare providers,* Dallas, 2000, American Heart Association.

Lehne RA: *Pharmacology for nursing care,* St Louis, 2004, Saunders.

Mosby's drug consult, St Louis, 2004, Mosby.

Turkoski BB, Lance BR, Bonfiglio MF: *Drug information handbook for nursing,* Hudson, Ohio, 2004, Lexi-Comp.

11

Complementary Therapies

Clinical Brief

Alternative and complementary therapies continue to increase in popularity. Some are used as adjuncts to reduce pain and anxiety, and many are valuable in all patient age groups. Many can be taught to patients and their families, as well as to other nurses and health care providers. Critical care nurses who have an understanding of the therapies and know that patients may be incorporating these into their health care practices can be a resource for patients and families and support their self-healing.

Alternative is the term used for therapies that serve as substitutes for conventional treatments or medications.

Complementary is the term used for therapies that serve as adjuncts or additions to conventional care.

Integrative health care means a synthesis or blend of alternative, complementary, and conventional therapies, treatments, and medications. Interventions from all healing systems are options for care.

Holistic health care integrates the body, mind, and spirit. People are more than the sum of their parts.

POTENTIAL HARMFUL EFFECTS

1. Some therapies have serious side effects.
2. Interactions with other treatments and medications or foods can occur, especially with some herbal products or nutritional supplements.
3. Some products do not contain the ingredients on the label or may contain less or more than stated. Products may also contain herbicides, pesticides, or other substances that can cause serious reactions.

4. Few therapies have been studied for their use in children, so effectiveness, safety, dosage, or length of intervention is unknown.

HEALING SYSTEMS AND HEALING THERAPIES

A healing system is a body of knowledge and skills with its own perspective and methods of assessing, diagnosing, and treating conditions or symptoms. Examples of healing systems are homeopathy, osteopathy, and traditional Chinese medicine (TCM).

Healing therapies are interventions that may or may not have evolved from a particular healing system. Examples of therapies that have evolved from a healing system include acupuncture and homeopathic remedies. Examples of therapies that have not evolved from a specific healing system include music, reflexology, and therapeutic touch.

ACUPRESSURE

Acupressure is the application of pressure using the fingers on the same points at which needles are used in acupuncture. A single point, or a combination of points, is pressed for 1 to 2 minutes for symptom relief.

Clinical Examples

One commonly used acupressure treatment can be effective in helping headache. The point, called large intestine 4, can be found by using the thumb and index finger of one hand to squeeze the fleshy portion (the part between the thumb and index finger) of the opposite hand for 1 to 2 minutes. This point should not be used during pregnancy.

Another commonly used pressure point, called pericardium 6, can help people with nausea and is used also for relief of angina. On the center of the inner wrist, two fingers down from where the wrist creases, place the thumb very firmly for 1 to 2 minutes; repeat on the other arm and as often as needed.

Spleen 6, located four fingerwidths above the inside anklebone and just behind the tibia, is also used for relief of angina. This point should not be used during pregnancy.

Clinical Cautions

Several acupressure points should not be used during pregnancy because of their potential for stimulating labor. Large intestine 4 (described previously for headache) and spleen 6 (described previously for relief of angina) are two such points.

Although there are continuing education courses on acupressure, no specific preparation is needed to practice the techniques. Many books give easy-to-follow detailed instructions.

ACUPUNCTURE

Acupuncture uses needles, heat, and electrical stimulation to manipulate the body's network of energy pathways (called *meridians*) to activate the body's energy, called *qi* (pronounced chee). Small feather-like needles are inserted at specific points for about 15 to 20 minutes. An herbal substance called *moxa* is burned or low-level electrical stimulation is used to increase stimulation of the acupuncture points.

Clinical Examples

Acupuncture can be used for a variety of conditions including many types of pain and discomfort. For example, postoperative and chemotherapy nausea and vomiting, nausea associated with pregnancy, and postoperative dental pain have been treated effectively with needle acupuncture.

Patients with other conditions such as headache, lower back pain, and fibromyalgia may also benefit. Many patients respond to acupuncture for back pain when other treatment has not been effective.

Clinical Cautions

Patients may need to sign a separate informed consent for acupuncture.

Only disposable needles should be used to reduce the risk of blood-borne pathogen transmission.

Regulations for the education or training and experience of acupuncturists vary by state.

The American Academy of Medical Acupuncture certifies most physicians who practice acupuncture. Applicants take a proficiency examination and meet training and experience requirements.

The National Commission for the Certification of Acupuncturists can certify other providers; applicants take a national examination.

AROMATHERAPY

Aromatherapy is the use of essential oils to promote relief of a particular symptom or condition. Oils can be used directly on the skin, diluted with water or alcohol, or released into the air and inhaled.

Clinical Examples

Lavender is an essential oil commonly used to relieve nasal congestion and lower anxiety. Lavender oil has been used as well to promote sleep in critical care patients.

Eucalyptus and peppermint are other natural decongestants.

Clinical Cautions

Some people have allergies to some of the natural oils that have flowers as their source. Although not reported in studies, aromatherapy should be used with caution in those with reactive airway disease.

HERBAL PREPARATIONS

Herbal preparations are plants that are used for medicinal purposes. They are most commonly available in their dried form as tablets or capsules, tinctures, teas, and poultices.

Clinical Examples

Nonprescription herbal products are used to prevent or treat specific illnesses.

Valerian *(Valeriana officinalis)* is a nonaddicting herb that can be used to reduce anxiety and insomnia. Melatonin is thought by some to increase sleep in critically ill patients as well.

St. John's wort *(Hypericum perforatum)* can be used for mild to moderate depression.

Hawthorn *(Crataegus laevigata)* is often used for mild to moderate congestive heart failure (CHF) and angina. It inhibits vasoconstriction and dilates blood vessels.

Black cohosh *(Cimicifuga racemosa)* is commonly used by women during menopause.

Saw palmetto *(Serenoa repens)* is often used by men who have benign prostatic hypertrophy.

Chamomile can have a calming effect on gastritis.

Clinical Cautions

Herbal preparations are not regulated, so consumers need to obtain them from a reputable source. One of the best indicators is that a company uses an independent laboratory to conduct random audits of its products.

Herbs sold as standardized extracts are more likely to contain the accurate amount of the active component of the herb as stated on the label and less likely to contain inactive plant parts or pesticides.

Some herbal products have actions and effects that work in a manner similar to prescription medications. For example, patients should not be taking hawthorn and digitalis at the same time because hawthorn may potentiate the action of cardiac glycosides. Patients should not be using a selective serotonin reuptake inhibitor (SSRI) antidepressant and St. John's wort at the same time.

Some herbs (e.g., black cohosh) have effects similar to estrogen and should not be taken by women who are pregnant.

HOMEOPATHY

Homeopathy is a healing system based on the "law of similars"; that is, a much diluted preparation of a substance that can cause symptoms in a healthy person can cure those same symptoms in a sick person. Homeopathic medicines, called *remedies,* are made from naturally occurring plant, animal, and mineral substances. Homeopathic preparations are so dilute that most remedies have no detectable amount of the original substance. The more dilute the preparation, the more potent that remedy is thought to be.

Clinical Examples

Homeopathic remedies commonly used for different types of pain include belladonna or bryonia for headache, arnica for traumatic or surgical pain, and Traumeel cream for sprains and injuries.

Many people use the homeopathic remedy oscillococcinum for flu symptoms or homeopathic lozenges or nasal gel of zinc gluconate to reduce the duration and severity of cold symptoms.

Clinical Cautions

The U.S. Food and Drug Administration (FDA) regulates the manufacture of homeopathic preparations so these remedies are safe to purchase over-the-counter.

Because these remedies contain no active ingredients, they are considered safe for use by children and older adults.

There is no standard training program for those who practice homeopathy. The American Institute of Homeopathy can certify physicians; the allopathic board and the board of homeopathic examiners must license those in Arizona, Connecticut, and Nevada.

IMAGERY

Imagery is the use of all the senses to encourage changes in attitudes, behavior, or physiologic reactions. Visualization is a specific form of imagery that allows a person to see something with the mind's eye. Patients can be encouraged to use any technique that helps them to relax and then to use any image that helps them to reduce anxiety during painful procedures or stressful situations. Some practitioners can also use a specific form of imagery called *interactive guided imagery*, allowing a person to communicate with a symptom to help identify ways of relieving distress.

Clinical Examples

Imagery can also help people to understand the connections between stressful circumstances and physical symptoms and ways of releasing unconscious blocks to improvement. Sample scripts are available in many imagery articles and books to address specific symptoms or concerns, as well as strategies for developing a guided imagery program in critical care. Also, using imagery tapes requires little instruction or time on the nurse's part.

It can be helpful to help patients to "time travel" (i.e., to imagine a time when their pain is relieved or surgery is completed successfully).

Patients who had coronary artery bypass graft (CABG) surgery and who used self-hypnosis were more relaxed postoperatively and used less pain medication. A replication study with the same type of patients showed reduced pain, fatigue, anxiety, narcotic use, length of stay, and increased patient satisfaction.

Patients having colorectal surgery who listened to guided imagery tapes for 3 days preoperatively, during induction, and for 6 days postoperatively had less anxiety and pain and used 50% less narcotics postoperatively.

Clinical Cautions

Care is needed to help patients select scripts, rather than nurses selecting for patients. There is always the possibility that an image that is upsetting, rather than calming, can be selected.

There is no standard training program in imagery, but there are several that are reputable. One of the best known and respected is that conducted by the Academy of Guided Imagery (Mill Valley, Calif).

MASSAGE

Massage is the systematic manual manipulation of body soft tissues, most commonly using gliding strokes with the palms of the hands in a slow, rhythmic fashion, using firm, steady pressure. Massage has been a component of nursing practice for many years.

Clinical Examples

Massage as brief as 5 to 10 minutes can promote sleep and sleep quality. This can be especially helpful for patients who cannot or should not take any additional medications. Massage has been shown to reduce anxiety, heart rate, respiratory rate, muscle tension, and oxygen consumption.

A 5-minute foot massage has been shown to decrease heart rate, mean arterial blood pressure, and respirations, while increasing relaxation. Patients do not have to be in a particular position and the time involved in a full massage is not needed.

Six-minute massages one or two times a day on developmentally and medically stable premature infants 1360 g and over led to an increased weight gain. Many other benefits have been shown in previous work; these include improved digestion, sleep-wake cycles, bonding, and pain tolerance. Guidelines for infant massage are easily found in published articles.

Clinical Cautions

Years ago massage was thought to be contraindicated in patients with myocardial infarction because of sympathetic nervous system stimulation, but recent studies have shown no evidence of that. Massage should not be performed over a fracture or incisional site, within 48 hours after immunization at the site, or in people who have contagious or painful disorders or bleeding disturbances.

MUSIC THERAPY

Music therapy is the use of sound to promote relaxation and reduce stress and pain. Music is an inexpensive therapy and one that seems very familiar to people and can be less threatening when exploring alternative therapies. Music therapists focus on pitch (highness or lowness), rhythm (organized flow of pitches), harmony (sound combinations), and tempo (beat).

Clinical Examples

Inexpensive audiocassettes of compact discs can be used; music seems to work better if people select which type of music they prefer. Headphones can help if rooms are not private.

Music found to be most relaxing does not have lyrics, and has slow, flowing rhythms with 60 to 80 beats per minute.

The beat of music can be used to synchronize heart rate and breathing.

Patients receiving music intraoperatively (conscious sedation) required significantly less sedation and analgesia.

A single 30-minute music therapy intervention was found safe and effective in decreasing anxiety, heart rate, and respiratory rate in patients receiving mechanical ventilation.[1]

One study of patients who listened to self-selected music during chest tube removal found no significant difference in pain, psychologic responses, and narcotic requirements. Most patients though reported liking listening to the music even though there were no differences in pain.[2]

Patients may have differing music preferences depending on their culture, experiences, and taste. Music that is relaxing for one person may be stressful for another.

Lullabies increased the development of nonnutritive sucking of premature infants.

Music can be used to reduce pain, decrease feelings of isolation, buffer noise, decrease myocardial oxygen demand, increase a sense of control and separation from environmental stressors, and improve mood. Chlan and Tracy[3] developed guidelines for using music therapy in critical care, and a music therapy assessment and intervention tool for use in patient care.

Many organizations employ musicians or music therapists in patient care settings. For example, there are several hospices with therapists who play live harp or guitar. Music needs to be private, based on a report of a comatose patient who thought he had died and was in heaven because he heard harp music playing.

Clinical Cautions

There is no standardized program in music for conventional practitioners. Names of music therapists can be obtained through the National Association of Music Therapists.

NUTRITION AND NUTRITIONAL SUPPLEMENTS

Nutrition and nutritional supplements include the use of foods, vitamins, and other dietary supplements to promote health and treat some health problems.

Clinical Examples

Supplements commonly used for osteoarthritic pain include glucosamine sulfate (with or without chondroitin) and capsaicin.

Garlic is a natural antibiotic and has antihypertensive and cholesterol-lowering effects.

Ginger and gugulipid can lower serum cholesterol, as well as improve the ratio of high-density lipoproteins (HDL) to low-density lipoproteins (LDL).

Ginger can help reduce nausea.

Coenzyme Q10 is used to decrease symptoms in those with mild to moderate CHF. Some studies show that it improves ejection fraction, stroke volume, cardiac output, cardiac index, and end-diastolic volume. It is also used to reduce cardiotoxicity associated with some chemotherapeutic drugs.

L-Carnitine increases myocardial oxygen use and lowers triglycerides and total cholesterol while increasing HDL.

Some people with coronary atherosclerosis follow a program with a 10% fat, vegetarian diet as its foundation. The program, developed by Ornish and colleagues,[4] includes other components such as moderate exercise, support groups, and yoga. Reversal of atherosclerosis has been documented in several research studies.

Substituting soy protein (at least 25 g) for high-fat animal protein diets lowers serum total cholesterol and LDL levels. Psyllium fiber seems to have a similar effect when added to the diet.

Clinical Cautions

Garlic and ginger can increase bleeding time, especially in those taking aspirin or warfarin.

Many conventional practitioners do not have an extensive background or current knowledge in this area. Practitioners of other healing systems, such as naturopathy, TCM, and Ayurveda, have strong content in nutrition in their educational programs.

REFLEXOLOGY

Reflexology is a form of massage to the foot or hand based on the premise that any discomfort or pain in a specific area of the foot or hand corresponds to a body part or to a disorder. Pressure on a specific area on the foot or hand is thought to release the blockage in that area and to allow energy to flow freely through that part of the body. Color-coded charts are available that show the locations of corresponding foot or hand sites. People can use these charts to locate the appropriate point on the foot to massage to relieve pain.

Clinical Examples

Massage of specific points, most especially on the feet, can be effective in relieving common symptoms such as headache, constipation, diarrhea, and anxiety.

Clinical Cautions

Although there are continuing education courses on reflexology, no specific preparation is needed to practice the techniques. Many books give easy-to-follow detailed instructions. The International Institute of Reflexology sponsors respected certification programs.

SPIRITUALITY AND PRAYER

Spirituality and prayer are used to assist people in their inward sense of something greater than the individual self or the meaning one perceives that transcends the immediate circumstances. Spirituality is a sense of meaning and purpose in life or belief in a higher power or source of energy without any limits. It involves the person's core and the need to reach out beyond oneself. Prayer can be the outward, concrete expression of those feelings, although not all people meet their spiritual needs through prayer or religion. Spirituality can be seen in relationships with ourselves, others, nature, and a divine being or life force.

Clinical Examples

Nurses' use of spiritual interventions can be very helpful when patients are faced with a life-threatening illness or condition.

If patients and/or their families are interested, prayer can help provide a source of strength during a critical care experience and the accompanying crisis.

More studies show an association between religion or spirituality and health outcomes such as hypertension, surgical recovery, coping with illness, and the will to live.

Respecting patients' spiritual and religious beliefs includes asking them which ones they would like included in their care. Those with serious illness or who are dying often look toward spirituality for helping them understand why they are critically ill or dying. Also, religious beliefs can affect care decisions such as feeding, ventilator support, and blood transfusions. People may feel abandoned by a supreme being and be in spiritual distress or crisis.

A nursing research study showed that even patients who report never or rarely attending religious services still can view religion as very important in their lives.

Nursing interventions can include practicing compassionate presence, conducting a spiritual assessment, and integrating spiritual or religious practices when appropriate. Often patients will share with nurses what gives them meaning and purpose in life.

Clinical Cautions

Some patients are not religious and nurses need to approach prayer with care. Chaplains can be a good resource for help in meeting the spiritual needs of patients and families.

THERAPEUTIC TOUCH (TT)

TT is used to facilitate healing using the palms of one's hands. While holding the palms 2 to 3 inches away from another person's body, TT practitioners can pick up any unevenness or imbalance in the energy of that person. Then, TT practitioners can change those imbalances and help the energy flow smoothly throughout the body, fostering a sense of well-being and relaxation.

Clinical Examples

TT has demonstrated positive effects on reducing pain and anxiety, promoting wound healing, and improving quality of life. TT has been found to promote sleep and relaxation in critically ill patients, while they remain hemodynamically stable. One study showed that TT reduced anxiety in those with burns.

Clinical Cautions

TT must be used carefully and for shorter durations with older adults, infants, or those who are severely debilitated.

TT practiced by qualified practitioners rarely has side effects, so it can be used to help critically ill patients and their family members to relieve stress and many symptoms.

TT practitioners and teachers are recognized by the national organization of TT, Nurse Healers—Professional Associates International.

REFERENCES

1. Chlan L: Effectiveness of a music therapy intervention on relaxation and anxiety for patients receiving ventilatory assistance, *Heart Lung* 27:169-176, 1998.
2. Broscious SK: Music: an intervention of pain during chest tube removal after open heart surgery, *Am J Crit Care* 8:410-415, 1999.
3. Chlan L, Tracy MF: Music therapy in critical care: indications and guidelines for intervention, *Crit Care Nurse* 19:35-41, 1999.
4. Ornish D et al: Intensive lifestyle changes for reversal of coronary artery disease, *JAMA* 280 (23):2001-2007, 1998.

BIBLIOGRAPHY

Ashton C et al: Self-hypnosis reduces anxiety following coronary artery bypass surgery, *J Cardiovasc Surg* 38:69-75, 1997.

Beachy JM: Premature infant massage in the NICU, *Neonatal Network*, 22:39-45, 2003.

Beck SL: The therapeutic use of music for cancer-related pain, *Oncol Nurs Forum* 18:1327-1337, 1991.

Braeckman J: The extract of *Serenoa repens* in the treatment of BPH: a multicenter open study, *Curr Ther Res* 55:776-785, 1994.

Buckle J: *Clinical aromatherapy: essential oils in practice,* San Diego, 2003, Singular.

Clark, A et al: The effect of therapeutic touch on pain and anxiety in burn patients, *J Adv Nurs* 28:10-20, 1998.

Cox C, Hayes J: Physiologic and psychodynamic responses to the administration of therapeutic touch in critical care, *Intens Crit Care Nurs* 15:363-368, 1999.

Crane B: *Reflexology: the definitive practitioner's manual,* Rockport, Me, 1997, Element.

Cummings S, Ullman D: *Everybody's guide to homeopathic medicines,* New York, 1991, Putnam.

Deisch P et al: Guided imagery: replication study using coronary artery bypass graft patients, *Nurs Clin N Am,* 35:417-425, 2000.

Denison B: Touch the pain away: new research on therapeutic touch and persons with fibromyalgia syndrome, *Holist Nurs Pract* 18:142-151, 2004.

Dossey BM et al: *Holistic nursing: a handbook for practice,* ed 3, Gaithersburg, Md, 1999, Aspen.

Faymonville ME et al: Psychological approaches during conscious sedation: hypnosis versus stress-reducing strategies; a prospective randomized study, *Pain* 73:361-367, 1997.

Gach MR: *Acupressure's potent points: a guide to self-care for common ailments,* New York, 1990, Bantam.

Good M et al: Cultural differences in music chosen for pain relief, *J Holistic Nurs* 18:245-260, 2000.

Guzzetta CE: Critical care research: weaving a body-mind-spirit tapestry, *Am J Crit Care* 13:320-327, 2004.

Hays J, Cox C: Immediate effects of a five-minute foot massage on patients in critical care, *Intens Crit Care Nurs* 15:77-82, 1999.

Helms J: An overview of medical acupuncture, *Altern Ther Health Med* 4(3):35-45, 1998.

Holt-Ashley M: Nurses pray: use of prayer and spirituality as a complementary therapy in the intensive care setting, *AACN Clin Issues* 11:60-67, 2000.

Jacobs J et al: Treatment of acute childhood diarrhea with homeopathic medicine: a randomized clinical trial in Nicaragua, *Pediatrics* 5:719-725, 1994.

Krieger D: *Accepting your power to heal: the personal practice of therapeutic touch,* Santa Fe, NM, 1993, Bear.

Kub JE et al: Religious importance and practices of patients with a life-threatening illness: implications for screening protocols, *Appl Nurs Res* 16:196-200, 2003.

Loman DG: The use of complementary and alternative health care practices among children, *J Ped Health Care* 17:2, 2003.

Milton D: Escaping the "Prozac syndrome," *Adv Nurse* 3(6):25-26, 2001.

Milton D: Alternative and complementary therapies in emergency nursing, *J Emerg Nurs* 24:500-508, 1998.

Milton D: Integrating alternative and complementary therapies into cancer care, *J Occ Health Nurs* 46:454-461, 1998.

Morelli V et al: Alternative therapies, part II. Congestive heart failure and hypercholesterolemia, *Am Fam Physician* 62:1325-1330, 2000.

Mossad SB et al: Zinc gluconate lozenges for treating the common cold: a randomized double-blind placebo controlled study, *Ann Intern Med* 125:81-88, 1996.

Murray M: *The healing power of herbs,* ed 2, Rocklin, Calif, 1995, Prima.

Murray M: *Encyclopedia of nutritional supplements,* Green Bay, Wis, 1996, Impakt Communications.

National Institutes of Health: *Consensus statement: acupuncture,* 15:1-34, 1997.

Norman L: *Feet first: a guide to foot reflexology,* New York, 1988, Simon & Schuster.

Nussbaum GB: Spirituality in critical care: patient comfort and satisfaction, *Crit Care Nurs Q* 26:214-220, 2003.

Puchalski C: Spirituality in health: the role of spirituality in critical care, *Crit Care Clin* 20:487-504, 2004.

Richards KC, Gibson R, Overton-McCoy AL: Effects of massage in acute and critical care, *AACN Clin Issues* 11:77-96, 2000.

Rossman M: *Guided imagery for self-healing,* ed 2, Tiburon, Calif, 2000, Kramer Press.

Seskevich JE et al: Beneficial effects of noetic therapies on mood before percutaneous intervention for unstable coronary syndromes, *Nurs Res* 53:116-121, 2004.

Standley JM: The effect of contingent music to increase non-nutritive sucking of premature infants, *Pediatr Nurs* 26:493-499, 2000.

Tracy MF, Lindquist R: Nursing's role in complementary and alternative therapy use in critical care, *Crit Care Nurs Clin N Am* 15:289-294, 2003.

Tussek DL, Cwynar R: Strategies for implementing a guided imagery program to enhance patient experience, *AACN Clin Issues* 11:68-76, 2000.

White J: State of the science of music interventions: critical care and perioperative practice, *Crit Care Nurs Clin N Am* 12:219-225, 2000.

Wirth DP et al: Non-contact therapeutic touch intervention and full-thickness cutaneous wounds: a replication, *Complementary Ther Med* 2(4):237-240, 1996.

Scoring Tools

TRAUMA SCORE

Assessment Parameter		Trauma Score
Glasgow Coma Scale score	14-15	5
	11-13	4
	8-10	3
	5-7	2
	3-4	1
Respiratory rate	10-24	4
	25-35	3
	>35	2
	1-9	1
	0	0
Respiratory expansion	Normal	1
	Shallow	0
	Retractive	0
Systolic blood pressure	>90	4
	70-90	3
	50-69	2
	1-49	1
No carotid pulse	0	0
Capillary refill	Normal	2
	Delayed	1
	None	0

From Champion HR, Gainer PS, Yackee E: A progress report on the trauma score in predicting a fatal outcome, *J Trauma* 26:927-931, 1988; and Champion HR et al: Trauma score, *Crit Care Med* 9(9):672-676, 1981.

Continued

Trauma Score: Projected Estimate of Survival

Trauma Score	Percentage Survival
16	99
15	98
14	96
13	93
12	87
11	76
10	60
9	42
8	26
7	15
6	8
5	4
4	2
3	1
2	0
1	0

THERAPEUTIC INTERVENTION SCORING SYSTEM (TISS)

4 Points	2 Points
a. Cardiac arrest and/or counourtershock within past 48 hr*	a. CVP (central venous pressure)
b. Controlled ventilation with or without positive end-expiratory pressure (PEEP)*	b. Two peripheral IV catheters
c. Controlled ventilation with intermittent or continuous muscle relaxants*	c. Hemodialysis—stable patient
d. Balloon tamponade of varices*	d. Fresh tracheostomy (<48 hr)
e. Continuous arterial infusion*	e. Spontaneous respiration via endotracheal tube or tracheostomy (T-piece or tracheostomy mask)
f. Pulmonary artery catheter	f. Gastrointestinal (GI) feedings
g. Atrial and/or ventricular pacing*	g. Replacement of excess fluid loss*
h. Hemodialysis in unstable patient*	h. Parenteral chemotherapy
i. Peritoneal dialysis	i. Hourly neurologic vital signs
j. Induced hypothermia*	j. Multiple dressing changes
k. Pressure-activated blood infusion*	k. Pitressin infusion IV
l. G-suit	
m. Intracranial pressure monitoring	
n. Platelet transfusion	
o. IABA (intraaortic balloon assist)	
p. Emergency operative procedures (within past 24 hr)*	
q. Lavage of acute GI bleeding	
r. Emergency endoscopy or bronchoscopy	
s. Vasoactive drug infusion (>1 drug)	

THERAPEUTIC INTERVENTION SCORING SYSTEM (TISS)—CONT'D

3 Points	1 Point
a. Central intravenous (IV) hyperalimentation (includes renal, cardiac, hepatic failure fluid)	a. Electrocardiogram (ECG) monitoring
b. Pacemaker on standby	b. Hourly vital signs
c. Chest tubes	c. One peripheral IV catheter
d. Intermittent mandatory ventilation (IMV) or assisted ventilation*	d. Chronic anticoagulation
e. Continuous positive airway pressure (CPAP)	e. Standard intake and output (I&O) (q24h)
f. Concentrated K⁺ infusion via central catheter	f. STAT blood tests
g. Nasotracheal or orotracheal intubation*	g. Intermittent scheduled IV medications
h. Blind intratracheal suctioning	h. Routine dressing changes
i. Complex metabolic balance (frequent I&O)*	i. Standard orthopedic traction
j. Multiple arterial blood gases (ABGs), bleeding, STAT studies (>4/shift)	j. Tracheostomy care
k. Frequent infusions of blood products (>5 units/24 hr)	k. Decubitus ulcer*
l. Bolus IV medication (nonscheduled)	l. Urinary catheter
m. Vasoactive drug infusion (one drug)	m. Supplemental oxygen (nasal or mask)
n. Continuous antiarrhythmia infusions	n. Antibiotics IV (two or fewer)
o. Cardioversion for arrhythmia (not defibrillation)	o. Chest physiotherapy
p. Hypothermia blanket	p. Extensive irrigations, packings, or debridement of wound, fistula, or colostomy
q. Arterial line	q. GI decompression
r. Acute digitalization—within 48 hr	r. Peripheral hyperalimentation/ intralipid therapy
s. Measurement of cardiac output by any method	
t. Active diuresis for fluid overload or cerebral edema	

THERAPEUTIC INTERVENTION SCORING SYSTEM (TISS)—CONT'D

3 Points	1 Point
u. Active Rx for metabolic alkalosis	
v. Active Rx for metabolic acidosis	
w. Emergency thoracentesis, paracentesis, pericardiocentesis	
x. Active anticoagulation (initial 48 hr)*	
y. Phlebotomy for volume overload	
z. Coverage with more than 2 IV antibiotics	
aa. Rx of seizures, metabolic encephalopathy (48 hr of onset)	
bb. Complicated orthopedic traction*	

From Keene AR, Cullen DG: Therapeutic intervention scoring system: update 1983, *Crit Care Med* 11(1):2, 1983.

Therapeutic Intervention Scoring System explanation code:

4-Point Interventions: (a) Point score for 2 days after most recent cardiac arrest. (b) Does not mean intermittent mandatory ventilation (3-point intervention). Means that regardless of the internal plumbing of ventilator, the full ventilatory needs are being supplied by the machine. Whether the patient is ineffectively breathing around the ventilator is irrelevant as long as it is providing the needed minute ventilation. (c) For example, D-tubocurarine chloride, pancuronium (Pavulon), metocurine (Metubine). (d) Use Sengstaken-Blakemore or Linton tube for esophageal or gastric bleeding. (e) Pitressin infusion via inferior mesenteric artery (IMA), superior mesenteric artery (SMA), gastric artery catheters for control of gastrointestinal bleeding, or other intraarterial infusion. Does not include standard 3 mL/hr heparin flush to maintain catheter patency. (g) Active pacing even if a chronic pacemaker. (h) Include first two runs of an acute dialysis. Include chronic dialysis when medical situation renders dialysis unstable. (j) Continuous or intermittent cooling to achieve temperature 91.4° F (33° C). (k) Use of a blood pump or manual pumping in those requiring rapid blood replacement. (p) May be the initial emergency procedure—precludes diagnostic tests.
3-Point Interventions: (d) The patient is supplying some ventilatory needs. (g) Not a daily point score. Patient must have been intubated in the intensive care unit (ICU) (elective or emergency) within previous 24 hr. (i) Measurement of I&O above normal 24-hr routine. Frequent adjustment of intake according to total output. (x) Includes Rheomacrodex. (bb) For example, Stryker frame, CircOlectric.
2-Point Interventions: (g) Replacement of clear fluids over and above the ordered maintenance level.
1-Point Intervention: (k) Must have a decubitus ulcer. Does not include preventive therapy.

APACHE III SCORING

An APACHE III score consists of points assigned to the following components: age, presence of chronic health problems, physiology/laboratory data, and neurologic function.

Age

Age (years)	Points
≤44	0
45-59	5
60-64	11
65-69	13
70-74	16
75-84	17
≥85	24

Chronic Health Problems

Condition	Points
Cirrhosis	4
Immunosuppression	10
Leukemia/multiple myeloma	10
Metastatic cancer	11
Lymphoma	13
Hepatic failure	16
AIDS	23

Acid-Base Points

pH	$Paco_2$	Points
<7.2	<50	12
<7.2	≥50	4
7.2-<7.35	<30	9
7.2-<7.3	30-<40	6
7.2-<7.3	40-<50	3
7.2-<7.3	≥50	2
7.35-<7.5	<30	5
7.3-<7.45	30-<45	0

APACHE III SCORING—CONT'D

Acid-Base Points—Cont'd

pH	Paco$_2$	Points
7.3-<7.45	≥45	1
7.45-<7.5	30-<35	0
7.45-<7.5	35-<45	2
7.45-<7.5	>45	12
7.5-≥7.65	≥40	12
7.5-<7.6	<40	3
≥7.6	<25	0
≥7.6	25-<40	3

Neurologic Scoring[*]

	Oriented, Converses	Confused Speech	Inappropriate Words and Incoherent Sounds	No Response
Obeys verbal command	0	3	10	15 16[†]
Localizes pain	3	8	13	15 16[†]
Flexion withdrawal/ decorticate rigidity	3	13	24 24[†]	24 33[†]
Decerebrate rigidity/no response	3	13	29 29[†]	29 48[†]

[*]Points assigned if eyes open spontaneously or to painful/verbal stimulation.
[†]Points assigned if eyes do not open spontaneously or to painful/verbal stimulation.

APACHE III PHYSIOLOGIC SCORING FOR VITAL SIGNS AND LABORATORY TESTS

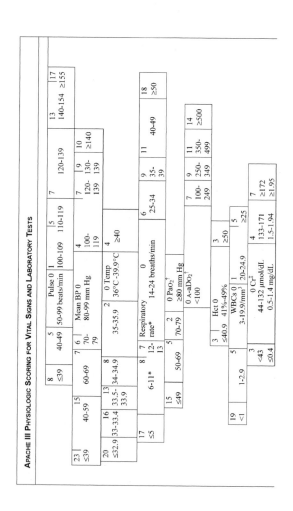

Creatinine (Cr§)

Points	0	10
	0-132 µmol/dL	≥133
	0-1.4 mg/dL	≥1.5

u/o

Points	1	0	4	5	7	8	15
mL/day	≥4000	2000-3999	1500-1999	900-1499	600-899	400-599	≤399

BUN

Points	0	2	7	11	12
mmol/L	≤6.1	6.2-7.1	7.2-14.3	14.4-28.5	≥28.6
mg/dL	≤16.9	17-19	20-39	40-79	≥80

Na

Points	0	2	3	4
mmol/L	135-154	120-134	≤119	≥155
mEq/L	135-154	120-134	≤119	≥155

Albumin

Points	0	4	6	11
g/L	25-44	≥45	20-24	≤19
g/dL	2.5-4.4	≥4.5	2.0-2.4	≤1.9

Bilirubin

Points	0	5	6	8	16
µmol/L	≤34	35-51	52-85	86-135	≥136
mg/dL	≤1.9	2-2.9	3-4.9	5-7.9	≥8.0

Glucose

Points	0	3	5	8‖	9‖
mmol/dL	3.4-11.1	11.2-19.3	≥19.4	≤2.1	2.2-3.3
mg/dL	60-199	200-349	≥350	≤39	40-59

Modified from Knaus WA et al: The APACHE III prognostic system, *Chest* 100:1619-1636, 1991.

A-aDO2, Alveolar-arterial oxygen gradient; *BP*, blood pressure; *BUN*, blood urea nitrogen; *Cr*, creatinine; *Hct*, hematocrit; *Na*, sodium; *PaO2*, arterial oxygen tension or partial pressure; *Temp*, temperature; *u/o*, urine output; *WBCs*, white blood cells (count).

*For patients on mechanical ventilation, no points are given for respiratory rates 6-12.

†Only use A-aDO2 for intubated patients with FIO_2 ≥0.5. Do not use PaO_2 weights for these patients.

‡Creatinine without acute renal failure (ARF). ARF is defined as creatinine ≥1.5 dL/day and urine output <410 mL/day and no chronic dialysis.

§Creatinine with ARF.

‖Glucose ≤39 mg/dL is lower weight than 40-59.

Organ and Tissue Donation

Organs, including the kidneys, heart, pancreas, and liver, can be donated for transplantation. A heart-beating, brain-dead cadaver is mandatory, and blood type is required.

Tissues including skin, bone, eye, ear, heart valves, and soft tissues can also be transplanted. Tissue donation does not require a heart-beating cadaver because the tissues are avascular when transplanted. Organs and tissues may also be donated for medical research.

POTENTIAL DONOR IDENTIFICATION

1. Brain-dead patients (see p. 11 for brain-death criteria)
2. No active infection
3. No history of transmissible disease
4. No previous disease of the organ or tissue (e.g., renal disease, type 1 diabetes mellitus [insulin-dependent], rheumatoid arthritis, malignancy [except brain tumor], bone disease)
5. Any age (physiologic age is considered)
6. Anyone, regardless of medical history or age, is eligible for eye donation and donation of organs and tissues for biomedical research.

GENERAL GUIDELINES: CARE OF THE DONOR*

Respiratory Function

Outcome Criteria

pH 7.35 to 7.45
Pao$_2$ 70 to 100 mm Hg

---

*Organ-specific protocols are used—contact your local organ-procurement agency.

Pa_{CO_2} >16 and <60 mm Hg to maintain pH

O_2 sat ≥95%

Absence of peripheral cyanosis

Absence of adventitious lung sounds

Interventions

Regulate ventilator settings as needed.

Draw arterial blood gases (ABGs) q4h or as needed (PRN)

Monitor peak inspiratory pressure (<40 cm H_2O) and plateau airway pressures (<35 cm H_2O)

Avoid positive end-expiratory pressure (PEEP) levels >5 cm H_2O and high FI_{O_2} levels

Maintain nasogastric (NG) tube patency (if present)

Suction PRN.

Assess nail beds.

Auscultate lung fields.

Turn patient frequently, if appropriate.

Assess chest wall excursion.

Prevent or aggressively treat pneumothorax.

Cardiovascular Function

Outcome Criteria

Systolic blood pressure (SBP) 100 to 170 mm Hg

Heart rate 60 to 130

Central venous pressure (CVP) 12 to 15 mm Hg

Interventions

Administer crystalloids/colloids to mean arterial pressure (MAP) 65 to 70 mm Hg.

If hypertensive, labetalol or nicardipine may be ordered

If hypotensive, norepinephrine or phenylephrine may be ordered to maintain MAP

Anticipate packed red blood cells (PRBCs), if hematocrit (Hct) <30%.

Monitor fluid losses.

Monitor for fluid overload (central venous pressure [CVP], pulmonary artery pressure [PAP]).

Monitor cardiac output/cardiac index (CO/CI), systemic vascular resistance index (SVRI), and left ventricular stroke work index (LVSWI)

If LVSWI is <35 g-m/m^2, anticipate dopamine or dobutamine

Monitor coagulation studies

Maintain sequential compression devices

Renal Function

Outcome Criteria

Urine output 75 to 150 mL/hr
CVP 12 to 15 mm Hg
Serum glucose 8 to 120 mg/dL
Sodium (Na) 135 to 145 mEq/L
Potassium (K^+) 3.5 to 4.5 mEq/L
Blood urea nitrogen (BUN) 10 to 20 mg/dL
Creatinine (Cr) 0.6 to 1.2 mg/dL

Interventions

Administer fluids such as Ringer's lactate, hetastarch in sodium chloride (Hespan), or plasma protein fraction (Plasmanate) as ordered to maintain CVP.
Administer electrolyte supplements as ordered, e.g., potassium, calcium, phosphorus, magnesium.
Anticipate diuretics (mannitol, furosemide) to increase urine output if patient is hydrated and blood pressure (BP) is stable.
Monitor BP, CVP, and urine output every hour.
Monitor kidney function (blood urea nitrogen [BUN], Cr) and electrolyte levels.
If diabetes insipidus occurs:
· Administer aqueous vasopressin (Pitressin) as an infusion and titrate to keep urine output between 150 and 300 mL/hr.
· Replace urine output milliliter for milliliter.
· Administer additional fluids as necessary.
· Monitor serum glucose q4h and fingerstick q2h.
· Anticipate insulin subQ or IV infusion for hyperglycemia; check blood sugars q30min.

Thermal Regulatory Function

Outcome Criterion

Temperature (T) 96.8° to 99.5° F (36°-37.5° C)

Interventions

Monitor core temperature every hour.
Use warming blanket or heat shields.
Avoid unnecessary exposure of patient.
Warm blood products and intravenous (IV) fluids if T <95° F (35° C).
Warm inspired gas from ventilator to 101.3° F (38.5° C)

Administer acetaminophen (Tylenol) suppository as ordered for
T >100.94° F (38.3° C).
Use cooling blanket to decrease temperature.

GUIDELINES FOR AVASCULAR TISSUES

Cornea

Apply ophthalmic saline solution to eyes; tape eyes closed.
Apply cold compresses to eyes.
Elevate head of bed (HOB) 30 to 40 degrees.

Skin

Turn patient frequently.
Assess for skin breakdown and infection.

BIBLIOGRAPHY

McCoy J, Argue PC: The role of critical care nurses in organ donation: a case
study, *Crit Care Nurse* 19:48-52, 1999.
Powner DJ, Darby JM, Kellum JA: Proposed treatment guidelines for donor
care, *Prog Transplant* 14(1):16-26, 2004.

Appendix C

Body Surface Area (BSA) Nomogram

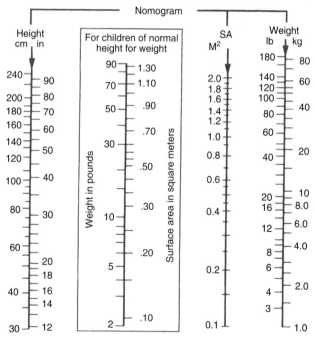

(From Behrman RE, Vaughn VC, editors: *Nelson's textbook of pediatrics*, ed 12, Philadelphia, 1983, Saunders.)

Nomogram for calculation of body surface area. Place a straight edge from the patient's height in the left column to the weight in the right column. The point of intersection on the body surface area column indicates the body surface area.

Formulas

CARDIOPULMONARY PARAMETERS

CORONARY PERFUSION PRESSURE (CPP)

CPP is the driving pressure influencing coronary blood flow. Coronary blood flow ceases when CPP reaches 40 mm Hg.

Equation: CPP = DBP − PAWP (LVEDP)
Normal: 60-80 mm Hg

DBP = diastolic blood pressure
PAWP = pulmonary artery wedge pressure
LVEDP = left ventricular end-diastolic pressure

PULSE PRESSURE (PP)

PP reflects stroke volume (SV) and arterial compliance. Widened PP is associated with a decrease in peripheral resistance and/or increase in SV. Narrowed PP is associated with an increase in peripheral resistance and/or decrease in SV.

Equation: PP = SBP − DBP
Normal: 30-40 mm Hg

SBP = systolic blood pressure

RATE PRESSURE PRODUCT (RPP)

RPP is also known as double product (DP); it is an indirect measurement of myocardial oxygen demand. Activities performed at lower heart rates (HRs) and SBPs are better tolerated by individuals with coronary artery disease.

Equation: RPP = HR × SBP
Normal: <12,000

MEAN ARTERIAL PRESSURE (MAP)

MAP is a measure of the average arterial perfusion pressure, which determines blood flow to the tissues.

$$\text{Equation: } MAP = 1/3\,PP + DBP \text{ or } \frac{2(DBP) + SBP}{3}$$

Normal: 70-105 mm Hg

CARDIAC OUTPUT (CO)

CO is the measurement of the amount of blood ejected by the ventricles each minute. It reflects pump efficiency and is a determinant of tissue perfusion.

$$\text{Equation: } CO = HR \times SV$$

Normal: 4-8 L/min

CARDIAC INDEX (CI)

CI is a measurement of the CO adjusted for body size. It is a more precise measurement of pump efficiency than CO.

$$\text{Equation: } CI = \frac{CO}{BSA}$$

Normal: 2.5-4.0 L/min/m^2

BSA = body surface area

STROKE VOLUME (SV)

SV represents the volume of blood ejected from the ventricle with each cardiac contraction. It is influenced by preload, afterload, and contractility.

$$\text{Equation: } SV = \frac{CO(mL/min)}{HR}$$

Normal: 60-120 mL/beat

STROKE INDEX (SI)

SI is a measurement of SV adjusted for body size.

$$\text{Equation: } SI = \frac{SV}{BSA} \text{ or } \frac{CI(mL/min)}{HR}$$

Normal: 30-65 ml/beat/m^2

SYSTEMIC VASCULAR RESISTANCE (SVR)

SVR is a measurement of left ventricular afterload. A diseased aortic valve and resistance in the systemic arterial circulation increase left ventricular afterload.

$$\text{Equation: } SVRI = \frac{MAP - CVP}{CO} \times 80$$

Normal: 900-1400 dynes/sec/cm^{-5}

SYSTEMIC VASCULAR RESISTANCE INDEX (SVRI)

SVRI is a measurement of left ventricular afterload, adjusted for body size.

$$\text{Equation: } SVRI = \frac{MAP - CVP}{CI} \times 80$$

Normal: 1700-2600 dynes/sec/cm^{-5}/m^2

PULMONARY VASCULAR RESISTANCE (PVR)

PVR is a measurement of right ventricular afterload. A diseased pulmonic valve and resistance in pulmonary arterial circulation increase right ventricular afterload.

$$\text{Equation: } PVR = \frac{PAMP - PAWP}{CO} \times 80$$

Normal: 100-250 dynes/sec/cm^{-5}

PAMP = pulmonary artery mean pressure

PULMONARY VASCULAR RESISTANCE INDEX (PVRI)

PVRI is a measurement of right ventricular afterload, adjusted for body size.

$$\text{Equation: } PVRI = \frac{PAMP - PAWP}{CI} \times 80$$

Normal: 200-450 dynes/sec/cm^{-5}/m^2

LEFT VENTRICULAR STROKE WORK INDEX (LVSWI)

LVSWI is a measurement of amount of work the left ventricle does per cardiac contraction, adjusted for body size. It is an indirect method of measuring myocardial contractility.

Equation: $LVSWI = SI \times (MAP - PAWP) \times 0.0136$

Normal: 45-60 g-m/m^2

RIGHT VENTRICULAR STROKE WORK INDEX (RVSWI)

RVSWI is a measurement of amount of work the right ventricle does per cardiac contraction, adjusted for body size. It is an indirect method of measuring myocardial contractility.

Equation: $RVSWI = SI \times (PAMP - CVP) \times 0.0136$

Normal: 7-12 g-m/m^2

EJECTION FRACTION (EF)

EF is a measurement of the ratio of the amount of blood ejected from the ventricle to the amount of blood remaining in the ventricle at end diastole. It is an indirect measurement of contractility.

Equation: $EF = \dfrac{SV}{EDV} \times 100$

Normal: *60% or greater*

EDV = end-diastolic volume

ALVEOLAR AIR EQUATION (P_{AO_2})

P_{AO_2} is a measurement of alveolar partial pressure of oxygen.

Equation: $P_{AO_2} = F_{IO_2}(Pb - PH_2O) - \dfrac{Paco_2}{0.8}$

Normal: 100 mm Hg

Pb = barometric pressure
PH$_2$O = water vapor pressure
Pb − PH$_2$O = 713

EXPECTED Pao$_2$ (Pao$_2$)

Pao$_2$ is a measurement of lung function when the expected Pao$_2$ is compared with the actual Pao$_2$. For people older than 60 years, subtract 1 mm Hg for each year older than 60.

Equation: $Pao_2 = F_{IO_2} \times 5$

ALVEOLAR-ARTERIAL OXYGEN GRADIENT (P[A-a]O$_2$) OR A-a GRADIENT

P(A-a)O$_2$ is a measurement of the difference between partial pressure of oxygen in the alveoli and arterial blood and an indication of oxygen transfer in the lung. However, supplemental oxygen and age can affect the gradient in individuals who do not have an acute condition of the lung.

Equation: $P(A\text{-}a)O_2 = PAO_2 - PaO_2$

Normal: <15 mm Hg (room air); 10-65 mm Hg (100% O$_2$)

ARTERIAL-ALVEOLAR OXYGEN TENSION RATIO (P[a/A]O$_2$ RATIO)

P(a/A)O$_2$ ratio is a measurement of the efficiency of gas exchange in the lung. Supplemental oxygen does not affect the ratio. A value less than 0.75 can indicate ventilation-perfusion ($\dot{V}/\dot{Q}$) inequalities, shunt abnormalities, or diffusion problems.

Equation: $\dfrac{PaO_2}{PAO_2}$

Normal: 0.75-0.90

ARTERIAL OXYGEN CONTENT (CaO$_2$)

CaO$_2$ is a measurement of oxygen content in arterial blood, including oxygen bound to hemoglobin (Hgb) and oxygen dissolved in blood. A decreased value may indicate a low PaO$_2$, SaO$_2$, and/or Hgb.

Equation: $CaO_2 = (SaO_2 \times Hgb \times 1.34) + (PaO_2 \times 0.003)$

Normal: 18-20 mL/100 mL

VENOUS OXYGEN CONTENT (CvO$_2$)

CvO$_2$ is a measurement of oxygen content in venous blood. It takes into account SvO$_2$, PvO$_2$, and Hgb; thus any change in these indices affects the CvO$_2$.

Equation: $CvO_2 = (SvO_2 \times Hgb \times 1.34) + (PvO_2 \times 0.003)$

Normal: 15.5 mL/100 mL

ARTERIOVENOUS OXYGEN CONTENT DIFFERENCE (C[a-v]o$_2$)

C(a-v)o$_2$ is a measurement that reflects oxygen uptake at the tissue level. An increased value indicates inadequate cardiovascular functioning. A decrease in CO results in more O$_2$ extracted, thus reducing the O$_2$ content of venous blood. A decreased value indicates poor tissue utilization of oxygen.

$$\text{Equation: } C(a\text{-}v)o_2 = Cao_2 - Cvo_2$$

Normal: 4-6 mL/100 mL

ARTERIAL OXYGEN DELIVERY ($\dot{D}o_2$) OR OXYGEN TRANSPORT

$\dot{D}o_2$ is a measurement of volume of O$_2$ delivered to tissues every minute. A decrease in $\dot{D}o_2$ may be due to a decrease in oxygen content (Pao$_2$, Sao$_2$, Hgb) or decrease in CO.

$$\text{Equation: } \dot{D}o_2 = CO \times 10 \times Cao_2$$

Normal: 900-1200 mL/min

ARTERIAL OXYGEN DELIVERY INDEX ($\dot{D}o_2I$)

$\dot{D}o_2I$ is a measurement of $\dot{D}o_2$ adjusted for body size.

$$\text{Equation: } \dot{D}o_2I = CI \times 10 \times Cao_2$$

Normal: 500-600 mL/min/m^2

OXYGEN CONSUMPTION ($\dot{V}o_2$)

$\dot{V}o_2$ is a measurement of volume of oxygen used by tissues every minute, and determines the amount of oxygen delivered to the cells. A decreased value may indicate that metabolic needs of tissues are not being met, usually as a result of inadequate O$_2$ transport.

$$\text{Equation: } \dot{V}o_2 = CO \times 10 \times C(a\text{-}v)o_2$$

Normal: 200-250 mL/min

OXYGEN CONSUMPTION INDEX ($\dot{V}o_2I$)

$\dot{V}o_2I$ is a measurement of $\dot{V}o_2$ adjusted for body size.

$$\text{Equation: } \dot{V}o_2I = CI \times 10 \times C(a\text{-}v)o_2$$

Normal: 115-165 mL/min/m^2

OXYGEN UTILIZATION COEFFICIENT OR OXYGEN EXTRACTION RATIO (ERo$_2$)

ERo_2 is a measurement that indicates the balance between oxygen supply and demand. It is the fraction of available O_2 that is used by the tissues. Values greater than 25% indicate that cellular oxygenation is threatened.

$$\text{Equation: } ER_{O_2} = \frac{C(a-v)o_2}{Cao_2} \text{ or } \frac{\dot{V}o_2}{\dot{D}o_2}$$

Normal: 25%

PHYSIOLOGIC SHUNT (Qs/Qt)

Qs/Qt is a measurement of the efficiency of the oxygenation system. It reflects the portion of venous blood that is not involved in gas exchange. High values are indicative of lung dysfunction (e.g., atelectasis or pulmonary edema).

$$\text{Equation: } Qs/Qt = \frac{Cco_2 - Cao_2}{Cco_2 - Cvo_2}$$

Normal: 0%-8%

$Cco_2 = O_2$ content in capillary blood
$Cco_2 = (Hgb \times 1.34) + (Pao_2 \times 0.003)$

Qs/Qt APPROXIMATION

$$\text{Equation: } \frac{Pao_2}{Fio_2}$$

Values: 500 = 10%
        300 = 15%
        200 = 20%

DYNAMIC COMPLIANCE

Dynamic compliance is a measure of maximum airway pressure required to deliver a given tidal volume. It reflects lung elasticity and airway resistance during the breathing cycle. A low value reflects a reduced compliance (bronchospasm, secretions in airway).

$$\text{Equation: } \frac{V_T}{PIP - PEEP}$$

Normal: 33-55 mL/cm H_2O

V_T = Tidal volume; PIP = peak inspiratory pressure;
PEEP = positive end-expiratory pressure

STATIC COMPLIANCE

Static compliance is a measurement of airway pressure required to hold the lungs at end-inspiration (after a tidal volume has been delivered and no airflow is present). It reflects only lung elasticity not affected by gas flow. A low value reflects lung stiffness.

$$\text{Equation: } \frac{V_T}{\text{Plateau pressure - PEEP}}$$

Normal: 50-100 mL/cm H_2O

NEUROLOGIC PARAMETERS

CEREBRAL PERFUSION PRESSURE (CPP)

CPP is a measurement of the pressure necessary to provide adequate cerebral blood flow. A value <60 mm Hg is associated with cerebral ischemia.

$$\text{Equation: CPP = MAP} - \text{ICP}$$

Normal: 60-100 mm Hg

ICP = intracranial pressure

METABOLIC PARAMETERS

ANION GAP (GAP) OR DELTA

GAP is a measurement of excess unmeasurable anions used to differentiate the mechanisms of metabolic acidosis. GAP will remain normal in metabolic acidosis resulting from bicarbonate loss.

$$\text{Equation: GAP = Na} - (HCO_3 + Cl)$$

Normal: 8-16 mEq/L

BASAL ENERGY EXPENDITURE (BEE) OR HARRIS-BENEDICT EQUATION

BEE is a measurement of basal energy expenditure required to support vital life functions.

$$\text{Equation: Men: } = (66.47 + 13.7W + 5H) - (6.76A)$$

$$\text{Women: } = (655.1 + 9.56W + 1.8H) - (4.68A)$$

$$W = \text{wt (kg); } H = \text{ht (cm); } A = \text{age}$$

$$\text{Total energy expenditure (TEE)} = \text{BEE} \times \text{AF} \times \text{IF}$$

AF = activity factor (bed rest = 1.2; ambulatory = 1.3)

IF = injury factor (surgery = 1.2; trauma = 1.35; sepsis = 1.6; burn = 2.1)

RESPIRATORY QUOTIENT (RQ)

RQ is a measurement of the state of nutrition. The relationship of oxygen consumption and carbon dioxide production reflects the oxidative state of the cell and energy consumption.

$$\text{Equation: RQ} = \frac{CO_2 \text{ production}}{O_2 \text{ consumption}}$$

Normal: 0.8-1

0.7 = lipolysis or starvation

0.8 = protein is primary source of energy

0.85 = carbohydrates, protein, and fat are energy sources

1 = carbohydrate is primary source of energy

>1 = lipogenesis; state of being overfed

RENAL PARAMETERS

GLOMERULAR FILTRATION RATE (GFR)

GFR is a measurement of amount of blood filtered by glomeruli each minute. GFR is affected by blood pressure and glomerular capillary membrane permeability. A decreased value may indicate renal disease or decreased perfusion to the kidneys.

$$\text{Equation: Male}: \frac{(140 - \text{age}) \times \text{wt(kg)}}{75 \times \text{serum Cr}}$$

$$\text{Female}: \frac{(140 - \text{age}) \times \text{wt(kg)}}{85 \times \text{serum Cr}}$$

Normal: 80-120 mL/min

Cr = creatinine

OSMOLALITY

Osmolality is a measurement of solute concentration per volume of solution. An increased value is associated with dehydration, a decreased value with overhydration. Renal concentrating ability can be assessed with simultaneous urine and serum osmolality measurements.

$$\text{Equation: } (2Na) + K + \frac{BUN}{3} + \frac{Glucose}{18}$$

Normal: 275-295 mOsm (serum)

Appendix E

Confusion Assessment Method

Confusion Assessment Method

	Absent	Present
1. Acute Onset or Fluctuating Course		
A. Is there evidence of an acute change in mental status from baseline? **OR**		
B. Did the (abnormal) behavior fluctuate during the past 24 hours, that is, tend to come and go or increase and decrease in severity, as evidenced by fluctuation on a sedation scale (e.g., Richmond Agitation-Sedation Scale), Glasgow Coma Scale, or previous delirium assessment?		
2. Inattention	Absent	Present
Did the patient have difficulty focusing attention, as evidenced by a score of less than 8 on either the auditory or visual component of the Attention Screening Examination?		
3. Disorganized Thinking	Absent	Present
Is there evidence of disorganized or incoherent thinking, as evidenced by incorrect answers to 2 or more of the 4 questions or the inability to follow commands?		

Questions (use either set A or set B):

Set A	Set B
1. Will a stone float on water?	1. Will a leaf float on water?
2. Are there fish in the sea?	2. Are there elephants in the sea?
3. Does 1 pound weigh more than 2 pounds?	3. Do 2 pounds weigh more than 1 pound?
4. Can you use a hammer	4. Can you use a hammer to cut

Other:

1. Are you having any unclear thinking?
2. Hold up this many fingers (examiner holds two fingers in front of patient).
3. Now do the same thing with the other hand (do not repeat the number of fingers).

	Absent	Present
4. Altered Level of Consciousness		
Is the patient's level of consciousness anything other than alert, such as vigilant, lethargic, or stuporous (i.e., Richmond score other than 0 at time of assessment)?		
Alert: spontaneously fully aware of environment and interacts appropriately		
Vigilant: hyperalert		
Lethargic: drowsy but easily aroused; unaware of some elements in the environment or not spontaneously interacting appropriately with the interviewer; becomes fully aware and appropriately interactive when prodded minimally		
Stuporous: becomes incompletely aware when prodded strongly; can be aroused only by vigorous and repeated stimuli, and as soon as the stimulus ceases, lapses back into the unresponsive state		

	Yes	No
Overall Assessment: Presence of Features 1 and 2 and Either Feature 3 or Feature 4:		

From Fink MP et al, *Textbook of critical care*, ed 5, Philadelphia, 2005, Saunders.

STEP ONE: SEDATION ASSESSMENT

The Richmond Agitation and Sedation Scale (RASS)

+4	Combative	Combative, violent, immediate danger to staff
+3	Very agitated	Pulls or removes tube(s) or catheter(s); aggressive
+2	Agitated	Frequent nonpurposeful movement, fights ventilator
+1	Restless	Anxious, apprehensive but movements not aggressive or vigorous
0	Alert and calm	
−1	Drowsy	Not fully alert but has sustained awakening to voice (eye opening and contact >10 sec)
−2	Light sedation	Briefly awakens to voice (eye opening and contact <10 sec)
−3	Moderate sedation	Movement or eye opening to voice (but no eye contact)
−4	Deep sedation	No response to voice but movement or eye opening to physical stimulation
−5	Unarousable	No response to voice or physical stimulation

If RASS is −4 or −5, the **Stop** and **Reassess** patient at a later time.
If RASS is above −4 (−3 through +4) then **Proceed to Step 2.**

STEP TWO: DELIRIUM ASSESSMENT

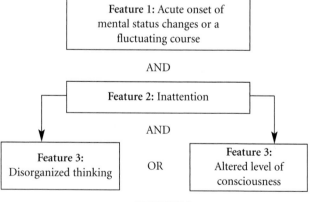

= **DELIRIUM**

Modified from Sessler CN et al: The Richmond Agitation-Sedation Scale: Validity and reliability in adult intensive care unit patients. Am J Respir Crit Care Med 2002;166:1338-1344; and Ely EW, Truman B, Shintani A, et al: Monitoring and sedation status over time in ICU patients: Reliability and validity of the Richmond Agitation-Sedation Scale (RASS), JAMA 2003;289:2983-2991.

Glossary

acute coronary syndromes
Term that refers to unstable angina, non–ST segment elevation myocardial infarction, and ST segment elevation myocardial infarction

afterload
The force the ventricles must overcome to eject blood

alternative therapy
Term used for therapies that serve as substitutes for conventional treatments or medications

angioedema
Giant wheal; reaction of the subcutaneous or submucosal tissue resulting in localized edema

antrectomy
The surgical excision of the pyloric part of the stomach

anuria
Absence of urine formation, usually <75 mL/day

areflexia
Absence of reflexes

asterixis
Flapping tremor, usually a sign of neurologic irritation

atelectasis
Collapse of alveoli that results in a loss of surface area available for gas exchange

autoregulation
The body's ability to control blood flow despite changes in arterial blood pressure

azotemia
Presence of nitrogen compounds in the blood (elevated blood urea nitrogen [BUN] level)

balanced analgesia
An approach to pain management that combines analgesics from the three analgesic groups (nonopioids, opioids, and adjuvant analgesics)

brain attack
A term that refers to stroke or cerebrovascular accident (CVA)

Brudzinski's sign
Flexion of the knee and hip in response to bending the patient's head toward the chest; a sign of meningeal irritation

cardiovert
Application of electrical current synchronized to the QRS complex to terminate a tachydysrhythmia

carpopedal
The wrist (carpal) and foot (pedal)

Chvostek's sign
Spasm of facial muscles elicited on tapping the area over the facial nerve; sign of tetany

circumoral
Around the mouth; circumoral pallor or cyanosis refers to paleness or bluish color around the mouth

colloid
Solutions that cannot pass through semipermeable membranes (e.g., dextran, albumin); usually retained in the intravascular space and used to restore volume

complementary therapy
Term used for therapies that serve as adjuncts or additions to conventional care

contractility
Ability of the cell to shorten and lengthen its muscle fiber

contralateral
Pertaining to the opposite side

crystalloid
Solutions that can pass through semipermeable membranes (e.g., D_5W, normal saline [NS])

decerebrate
Bilateral extension, internal rotation, and wrist flexion of upper extremities; bilateral extension, internal rotation, and plantar flexion of lower extremities

decorticate
Bilateral adduction of shoulders; extension, internal rotation, and plantar flexion of lower extremities; pronation and flexion of elbows and wrists

defibrillate
Application of nonsynchronized electrical current to the myocardium to terminate a life-threatening dysrhythmia

dehiscence
Separation or splitting open of a surgical wound

dermatome
Area of skin supplied by nerve fibers

distal
Farthest from the point of origin

dysesthesia
Impaired sensation (out of proportion to the stimulus)

dysphasia
Impairment of speech (e.g., inability to arrange words in the proper order)

dysrhythmia
Any disorder of rate, rhythm, electrical impulse origin, or conduction within the heart

ecchymosis
Nonraised, purplish hemorrhagic spot larger than a petechia

ectopy
Arising from an abnormal site (e.g., ectopic beats are impulses arising outside the normal electrical conduction system of the heart)

empyema
Pus accumulation in a body cavity

encephalopathy
Degeneration of the brain caused by several conditions or diseases

endocardium
Layer of cells that line the cavity of the heart

escharotomy
Surgical incision of the burned body part to reduce pressure on tissues and restore blood flow

eupnea
Normal respiration

flaccid
Weak muscles

gastroduodenostomy
Surgical connection of the duodenum and stomach (Billroth I procedure)

gastroenterostomy
Surgical connection of the stomach and intestine

gastrojejunostomy
Surgical connection of the stomach and jejunum (Billroth II procedure)

gastroparesis
Paralysis of the stomach

gavage
Feeding through a tube

hemianopsia
Blindness in half of the visual field

hemoptysis
Blood in sputum; coughing up of blood

hypercapnea
Elevated carbon dioxide in the blood

hypercarbia
Elevated carbon dioxide in the blood

hyperpyrexia
Elevated temperature, fever, hyperthermia

hypertonic
An osmolality greater than fluid a solution is being compared with (i.e., hypertonic IV fluids such as D_5NS and $D_{10}W$ refer to an osmolality >300 and, if infused, can cause cells to shrink and cause circulatory overload)

hypokinesia
Decreased movement or motion (e.g., a hypokinetic ventricle refers to decreased contraction [motion] of the ventricle)

hypotonic
An osmolality less than fluid a solution is being compared with (i.e., hypotonic IV fluids such as 0.45NS refer to an osmolality <300 and, if infused, can cause swelling of cells, hypotension, and fluid depletion)

hypoxemia
Deficient oxygenation in the blood

hypoxia
Reduced oxygen availability to the tissues

inotropic
Pertaining to the force or strength of muscular contraction

ipsilateral
Pertaining to the same side

isotonic
The same osmolality of fluid a solution is being compared to (i.e., isotonic IV fluids such as 0.9NS and lactated Ringer's refer to solutions that do not affect flow of water across the cell membranes)

Kernig's sign
Inability to completely extend the leg when the thigh is flexed on the abdomen

Kussmaul's sign
A rise, instead of a fall, in the venous pressure during inspiration

lateralizing
Pertaining to one side

lavage
Irrigation of a cavity or organ such as the stomach

leukocytosis
Increase in number of leukocytes (e.g., basophils, eosinophils, neutrophils, monocytes, lymphocytes)

leukopenia
Decrease in number of leukocytes (usually <5000/mL)

myoglobinuria
Presence of myoglobin (globulin from muscle) in the urine

nuchal rigidity
Stiff neck

oliguria
Urine volume <400 mL/day

otorrhea
Discharge from the ear

papilledema
Edema of the optic disk

paraplegia
Paralysis of the lower extremities

parenchyma
The essential elements of an organ

petechiae
Nonraised, round, purplish spots caused by intradermal or submucous hemorrhages

pharmacodynamics
The action and effects of drugs in the body

pharmacokinetics
How the body works on the drug (e.g., absorption, distribution, biotransformation, and excretion)

pheochromocytoma
A tumor of the adrenal medulla that secretes epinephrine and norepinephrine, resulting in severe hypertension, increased metabolism, and hyperglycemia

photophobia
Intolerance to light

polydipsia
Excessive thirst

polyuria
Excessive urination

postictal
Following a seizure

preload
Volume of blood in the ventricles at the end of diastole

proprioception
Pertaining to the position of the body; involves balance, coordination, and posture

proximal
Closest or nearest to the point of origin

pyloroplasty
Surgery involving the pylorus, usually to enlarge the communication between the stomach and duodenum

quadriplegia
Paralysis of all four extremities

rhabdomyolysis
Skeletal muscle injury that results in release of substances, such as myoglobin, that are potentially toxic to the kidney

rhinorrhea
Discharge from the nose

stomatitis
Inflammation of the oral mucosa

tetraplegia
Paralysis of all four extremities

thrombocytopenia
Reduction in the number of platelets

tonic-clonic
Involuntary muscular contraction and relaxation in rapid succession

Trendelenburg position
The patient is supine and the head is down

Trousseau's sign
Carpal spasm on compression of the upper arm; sign of tetany

urticaria
Hives; vascular reaction that results in wheals and itching (pruritus)

vagotomy
The surgical interruption of the vagus nerve, usually performed to reduce gastric secretions in the treatment of ulcers

ventilation
Movement of air between the lungs and environment

Index

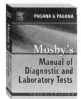

Cardiopulmonary Parameter Values

Abbreviation	Parameter name	Normal
PAS (mm Hg)	Pulmonary artery systolic	15-30
PAD (mm Hg)	Pulmonary artery diastolic	5-15
PAM (mm Hg)	Pulmonary artery mean	10-20
PAWP (mm Hg)	Pulmonary artery wedge pressure	4-12
CVP (mm Hg)	Central venous pressure	2-6
MAP (mm Hg)	Mean arterial pressure	70-105
PP (mm Hg)	Pulse pressure	30-40
CO (L/min)	Cardiac output	4-8
CI (L/min/m^2)	Cardiac index	2.5-4.0
SV (mL/beat)	Stroke volume	60-120
SI (mL/beat/m^2)	Stroke index	30-65
LVSWI (g-m/m^2)	Stroke work index, left ventricular	45-60
RVSWI (g-m/m^2)	Stroke work index, right ventricular	7-12
PVR (dynes/sec/cm^{-5})	Pulmonary vascular resistance	100-250
PVRI (dynes/sec/cm^{-5}/m^2)	Pulmonary vascular resistance index	200-450
SVR (dynes/sec/cm^{-5})	Systemic vascular resistance	900-1400
SVRI (dynes/sec/cm^{-5}/m^2)	Systemic vascular resistance index	1700-2600
Cao_2 (mL/100 mL)	Oxygen content, arterial	18-20
Cvo_2 (mL/100 mL)	Oxygen content, venous	15.5
$C(a-v)o_2$ (mL/100 mL)	Oxygen content, arteriovenous difference	4-6
$\dot{V}o_2$ (mL/min)	Oxygen consumption	200-250
$\dot{V}o_2I$ (mL/min/m^2)	Oxygen consumption index	115-165
$\dot{D}o_2o_2$ (mL/min)	Oxygen delivery, arterial	900-1200
$\dot{D}o_2I$ (mL/min/m^2)	Oxygen delivery index, arterial	500-600
ERo_2	Oxygen extraction ratio	25%